HurstReviews

Medical-Surgical
Nursing Review

NOTICE

Medicine is an ever-changing science. As new research and clinical experience broaden our knowledge, changes in treatment and drug therapy are required. The authors and the publisher of this work have checked with sources believed to be reliable in their efforts to provide information that is complete and generally in accord with the standards accepted at the time of publication. However, in view of the possibility of human error or changes in medical sciences, neither the authors nor the publisher nor any other party who has been involved in the preparation or publication of this work warrants that the information contained herein is in every respect accurate or complete, and they disclaim all responsibility for any errors or omissions or for the results obtained from use of the information contained in this work. Readers are encouraged to confirm the information contained herein with other sources. For example and in particular, readers are advised to check the product information sheet included in the package of each drug they plan to administer to be certain that the information contained in this work is accurate and that changes have not been made in the recommended dose or in the contraindications for administration. This recommendation is of particular importance in connection with new or infrequently used drugs.

HurstReviews

Medical-Surgical Nursing Review

**Marlene Hurst,
RN, MSN, FNP-R, CCRN-R**

President
Hurst Review Services
Brookhaven, Mississippi

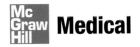 **Medical**

New York   Chicago   San Francisco   Lisbon   London   Madrid   Mexico City
Milan   New Delhi   San Juan   Seoul   Singapore   Sydney   Toronto

1 2 3 4 5 6 7 8 9 0   CTP/CTP   14 13 12 11

Set ISBN 978-0-07-159752-4
Set MHID 0-07-159752-2
Book ISBN 978-0-07-159753-1
Book MHID 0-07-159753-0
CD-ROM ISBN 978-0-07-159754-8
CD-ROM MHID 0-07-159754-9

This book was set in Minion by Glyph International.
The editors were Joseph Morita and Robert Pancotti.
The production supervisor was Catherine H. Saggese.
The illustration manager was Armen Ovsepyan.
Project management was provided by Madhu Bhardwaj, Glyph International.
The text designer was Alan Barnett; the cover designer was David Dell'Accio.
China Translation & Printing Services, Ltd. was printer and binder.

Library of Congress Cataloging-in-Publication Data

Hurst, Marlene, author.
     Medical-surgical nursing review / Marlene Hurst
          p. ; cm. — (Hurst reviews)
     Includes bibliographical references and index.
     ISBN-13: 978-0-07-159753-1 (paperback : alkaline paper)
     ISBN-10: 0-07-159753-0 (paperback : alkaline paper)
     ISBN-13: 978-0-07-159752-4 (set)
     ISBN-10: 0-07-159752-2 (set)
        [etc.]
     1. Operating room nursing—Examinations, questions, etc.   I. Title.   II. Series: Hurst reviews.
[DNLM: 1. Perioperative Nursing—Examination Questions.   WY 18.2]
RD32.3.H86 2011
617'.917—dc22

                                                                2010044506

CONTENTS

CONTRIBUTORS AND REVIEWERS

Pamela Black, BSN, MSN
Instructor
Southeastern Louisiana University
Hammond, Louisiana

Tanya Boyd, RN, MSN
Instructor
Southwest Mississippi Community College
Summit, Mississippi

Cathy Bridge, RN, BSN, MEd, CIC, CPHQ
Compliance Officer
King's Daughters Medical Center
Brookhaven, Mississippi

Rebecca Brumfield, BS, MS
Faculty
Hurst Review Services
Brookhaven, Mississippi

Danny Dunaway, RN
Staff Nurse
Select Specialty Hospital
Jackson, Mississippi

Charles Dykes, BSN, MSN
Instructor
Southeastern Louisiana University
Hammond, Louisiana

Stephanie Greer, RN, MSN
Instructor
Southwest Mississippi Community College
Summit, Mississippi

Teresa Harvey, RN, CPHRM
Nursing Support Coordinator
Hurst Review Services
Brookhaven, Mississippi

Mary F. King, RN, MS
Faculty
Hurst Review Services
Brookhaven, Mississippi

Carol Owens, BSN, MSN
Instructor
Louisiana Tech University
Ruston, Louisiana

Lisa Samuel, BS, MA
Regional Director
Hurst Review Services
Brookhaven, Mississippi

Jena Smith, RN, MSN, NP-C
Faculty
Hurst Review Services
Brookhaven, Mississippi

Debra Strong, BS, MS
Curriculum Coordinator
Hurst Review Services
Brookhaven, Mississippi

Medical-surgical nursing (also known as med-surg) is considered by many to be the foundation of all nursing practice. When I completed nursing school in 1986, it was a common requirement to work on a med-surg unit before entering another specialty area such as labor and delivery or critical care. In my opinion, medical-surgical nursing is one of the most challenging and demanding areas of nursing practice. Why? Because the med-surg nurse has to be ready for anything and everything! Medical-surgical nursing is no longer considered to be just an entry-level position, but a complex, adult health specialty.

Typically, when we think of medical-surgical nursing, we think first of a hospital setting. However, medical-surgical nurses may work in clinics, home health care, urgent care centers, surgery centers, the military, or long-term care facilities. The patients in this area exhibit a wide variety of clinical conditions.

Some patients may be recovering from surgery; other patients may be in the final stages of a chronic disease.

In some hospitals, medical-surgical nursing is separated into medical nursing and surgical nursing. Medical nursing units may be divided further into units such as oncology, orthopedics, or pulmonary nursing. Surgical nursing units may be divided further into units such as neurosurgical nursing or cardiovascular surgical nursing. The bigger the hospital, the more likely it is that each area will be divided into more specialty areas.

The term med-surg encompasses many different diseases, conditions, procedures, and patient ages. When working in a med-surg unit, you may have two patients going for surgery, one who is returning from a heart catheterization, one who is a newly diagnosed diabetic, and another who was just transferred from the intensive care unit post-coronary artery bypass! In addition, many of these patients are unstable and have rapidly changing conditions. Like the emergency department nurse, the med-surg nurse must be ready for anything including emergencies! To work in this area of nursing, you must have a comprehensive knowledge base, excellent prioritization skills, judgment, and intuition. Just because someone is on a med-surg floor does not mean they aren't critical and very unstable.

In this Preface, you will see examples of the features that I use throughout this text, with some things to keep in mind as you progress through the book and into your career.

Many "sneaky" emergencies can occur on the medical-surgical unit. A simple sinus surgery can suddenly develop into shock. A reaction to a common antibiotic can quickly result in renal failure. Only quick

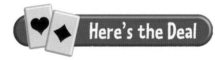

Here's the Deal

The med-surg nurse loves a *challenge* and new experiences and looks forward to what the day may bring although they never know exactly what that may be!

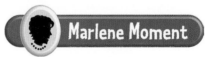

Marlene Moment

The Academy of Medical-Surgical Nurses states that Medical-Surgical Nurses are the backbone of every adult-care clinical agency. All adult patients are eventually cared for by medical-surgical nurses. Medical-Surgical nurses can and will "DO IT ALL!" (For more information, please see the website for the Academy of Medical-Surgical Nurses: www.amsn.org)

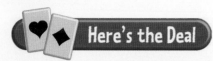

The medical-surgical unit is a con-glomeration of all kinds of non-pregnant adults who have all sorts of health problems. Therefore, nurses assigned to such a unit must be versatile and on their toes at all times!

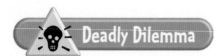

The most "stable looking" patient can deteriorate into an emergency situation in a moment's notice.

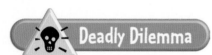

Do not depend on the report that you receive from the outgoing shift of staff members to tell you what is going on with your patient. Take time to read the chart, perform your OWN thorough physical assessments, and really get to know your patient.

recognition of these emergencies followed with immediate action by **YOU**, the nurse, may save your patient's life.

Subtle changes in the patient can signal the onset of dangerous, life-threatening conditions. Scary, isn't it? Yes, but close patient assessments and thorough knowledge of each patient's signs and symptoms can make all the difference in the world. Medical-surgical nurses must be prepared for the *worst* to occur at any time. Medical-surgical patients may have multiple health problems, all of which may flare up at the same time.

CASE IN POINT When caring for patients, don't just focus on the admitting diagnosis. Most med-surg patients have multiple health problems. For example, a patient's primary admitting diagnosis may be congestive heart failure. However, the physical assessment that you perform may show that the problem that needs immediate attention is a deep vein thrombosis.

CASE IN POINT You may have a bedridden patient with a diagnosis of pneumonia. During your assessment, however, you note that the patient has ankle edema. Just because someone has pneumonia doesn't mean they usually have ankle edema too.

Something else, besides pneumonia, is going on. You had better be looking for something else because pneumonia won't make a patient's feet swell, and a bedridden patient probably isn't dangling his legs off the side of the bed, so this can't be dependent edema either.

All hospitalized patients are acutely ill or they would not have been admitted to the hospital. Do not allow a routine admission diagnosis such as dehydration to make you think that the patient is completely stable. Always look for the worst possible thing that could go wrong and assume that the worst is going to happen. Always be suspicious! Assume the worst. Be a pessimist! It's OK! This attitude could prevent a fatal complication. After all of this stress and worrying, there will be times when *absolutely nothing* is going wrong and you may feel as if you over-reacted. Whatever! It's better to feel as if you have overreacted than to overlook a potentially life-threatening problem. Assuming the worst helps assure safe, effective care for your patients.

In closing, let me assure you that it is normal to get an "overwhelmed" feeling when studying all of the different diseases. I'm sure you have already had that feeling since you started nursing school!

When you first begin learning about medical-surgical nursing, you have to learn about many diseases in great detail. However, over time, you will see that many diseases are dealt with in similar ways and that you can apply what you have learned about one problem to several other problems. It just takes time and experience. Take this journey into nursing practice one day at a time. Learn and understand all you can every day for the rest of your career. Know that you will never know it all (no one ever does). Understand that you will have questions every day and that it is *okay* to have questions and *not* to know it all. Be aggressive in seeking out answers. Every patient is a puzzle and it is up to us to solve the puzzle as soon as possible before a problem occurs. The time you spend with each patient may be the only opportunity that your patient has to have problems identified and solved. When the patient is discharged, he or she may not have someone as observant, caring, and diligent as you looking after them. Help the patient all you can while you can! This may be their only chance for help and you may be the only person who cares enough to take the time to do so.

1 Introduction to Medical-Surgical Nursing

OBJECTIVES

In this chapter you will review:

- The function and purpose of the medical-surgical unit.
- The scope and role of the medical-surgical nurse.
- The impact of culture on the provision of care in the medical-surgical setting.
- Patient safety in the medical-surgical setting.
- Utilization of the nursing process in the medical-surgical setting.
- Documentation of care in the medical-surgical setting.

THE MEDICAL-SURGICAL UNIT

Hospitals organize patients in order to create the optimal healing environment. The medical-surgical unit has often been described as a "catch-all" for different types of patients. This is not to be confused with patients who are uncomplicated or do not require specialized care. Patients who are hospitalized in today's health care environment are most likely experiencing a serious acute illness or the exacerbation of a chronic illness. This patient mix includes surgical patients, cardiac patients, cancer patients, renal patients, and everything else that doesn't fit into one of the specialized categories.

The medical-surgical unit is a conglomeration of all kinds of nonpregnant adults having all sorts of health problems; therefore, nurses on such a unit must be versatile and on their toes at all times! Emergency Department nurses (who expect emergencies) are well equipped to deal with emergency situations because they deal with life-and-death emergencies on a daily basis, and they are always looking for complications secondary to trauma. Nurses on a medical-surgical unit must be careful not to develop a "ho-hum" attitude toward routine nursing care, as their patients can experience rapid changes in condition and quickly become unstable even though they were admitted for the predictable kinds of conditions commonly seen on a medical-surgical unit.

The largest percentage of medical-surgical nurses are employed by acute care facilities; however, there are opportunities for provision of care by medical-surgical nurses in other settings. These settings include but are not limited to clinics, outpatient surgery centers, physician offices, long-term care facilities. In other words, patients require medical-surgical care across a wide expanse of the health care spectrum.

✚ The nursing process

The nursing process is how we do what we do! The nurse has a scientific knowledge base from all nursing research and other disciplines (anatomy and physiology, psychology, nutrition, chemistry, etc.), and uses the nursing process to provide evidence-based nursing care. A sound understanding of the nursing process is mandatory for all nurses in any practice area.

The nursing process is the organizing framework for all nursing care. The phases of the nursing process are:

- Assessment
- Diagnosis
- Planning
- Implementation
- Evaluation

Assessment

Nursing assessment is the initial and most important phase of the nursing process. If you miss something, how can the best nursing diagnosis

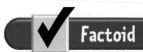

Here's the Deal

Hospital admissions are necessary when a sick person needs a nurse around the clock.

Factoid

Specialized units (pediatrics, intensive care, obstetrics) have sick patients with more predictable needs, but the nurse on a medical-surgical unit must be prepared to take care of adult patients across the life span who have all kinds of acute and chronic health issues, many of which can deteriorate into emergency situations.

be assigned? It can't! The RN always has to complete the admission assessment, because this is the time when the patient is assessed from head to toe, just to make sure that something important is not being missed.

CASE IN POINT   What if the patient is admitted with an ingrown toenail and all that we focused on was the toe? If I missed night sweats, remittent fever, and a chronic cough, then I could possibly spread TB all over the surgical unit! The admission nursing assessment and history is too important to delegate to non-nurses! Does this mean that the CNA cannot get your admission vital signs and weigh my patient? Certified nurse aides are supposed to be able to correctly perform these tasks; however, since drug dosing is based on weight and comparisons of vital signs refer back to baseline, the RN obtains these initial data. Does this mean that the RN has to go through every pill bottle in a 10-pound grocery sack of medications to write down every dosage and schedule, plus when it was taken last? No, it does not. The LPN is a licensed staff member who is perfectly capable of filling out the medication reconciliation record! But the RN is required to sign the admission form verifying all data. And the RN oversees all aspects of care; but we will discuss this more with principles of management and delegation.

Subjective Versus Objective Data

Some aspects of physical assessment can be seen by the nurse, and other aspects of physical assessment must be based on what the patient tells you.

Nursing diagnosis

The second phase of the nursing process requires what your nursing instructors call "critical thinking."

- First, you assess your patient and differentiate normal versus abnormal findings.
- Then, determine what is normal for your patient depending on the history and disease process.
- Next, analyze data from your complete nursing assessment, and interpret what the data mean.
- Once you determine the patient's problem, you're ready to go to the list of patient problems that NANDA (North American Nursing Diagnosis Association) put together for us, and pick out the appropriate nursing diagnosis! Now we are ready to roll!

Planning

If you miss the boat on the nursing diagnosis, your planning isn't worth a "toot!" That's why your data (objective and subjective) needs to be

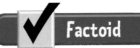

The admission physical assessment and nursing history are only performed by the registered nurse!

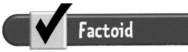

Objective data=can be observed
The big "O"= Observed
Anything that can be observed (seen by the nurse, such as moist rales in a lung, lesions on the body, vital signs, or lab tests) are always objective data.

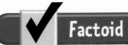

Anything that the nurse cannot detect independently is subjective data, because the patient will have to tell you about the complaint. The nurse can see the patient grimacing and limping with each step (objective data because the nurse can see this), but the nurse must share these observations with the patient and ask if pain is present (subjective feeling experienced by the patient).

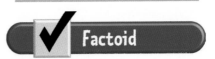

Subjective = Has to be stated (said) by the patient
The big "S" = Stated (by the patient)

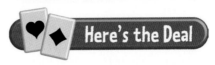

When performing patient assessments, the first step is to compare everything you see with normal physical assessment findings. Then, based on patient history, consider what is normal for that particular patient.

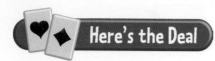

Here's the Deal

Now you see why "thinking" is critical! All those notes you have written down, the patient lab work and X-rays, plus the subjective data obtained from the patient are all pieces of the puzzle that you put together with the processes of analysis and interpretation to come to a conclusion about the patient's problem.

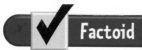

Factoid

Sometimes you will find that you need additional data in order to come to a conclusion about your patient's problem. That's when you go back to the drawing board!

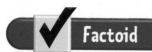

Factoid

The ABC method is always good to use when setting priorities, but don't pick airway as the priority if your patient does not have an airway problem!

- A = airway
- B = breathing
- C = circulation

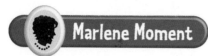

Marlene Moment

If your diabetic patient has an airway problem, but you decide to do foot care first, nobody except the mortician will see what a good job you did because they don't usually open the lower half of the casket for viewing.

complete and verified with the patient. Planning always starts with deciding which patient problems need attention first!

In addition to setting priorities, the planning phase of the nursing process is also a time for setting realistic, attainable patient goals that provide the direction for selecting interventions to accomplish the desired patient outcomes.

Implementation

Now we are ready to carry out the planned actions (nursing interventions) during this caregiving phase of the nursing process.

- These interventions can be independent, interdependent, or dependent actions.
- A large portion of nursing interventions come from the nursing domain: things that nurses have been taught to do that are based on scientific, outcome-based, nursing knowledge.

As nurses we cannot do everything independently, so we collaborate with other members of the health care team to carry out interdependent nursing interventions. For example, you know (independently) your patient who has an endotracheal (ET) tube needs mouth care and a lemon-glycerin swab will not suffice. Here's what to do:

- Collaborate with the physician for a peroxide-based oral solution.
- Wait for the respiratory therapist (RT) to change the mouth piece/bite block and the Velcro strap holding the ET tube.
- Enlist assistance of the RT to secure and stabilize the endotracheal tube.
- Clean, suction, and rinse the patient's mouth during a time when everything is out of the mouth and you can see what you are doing!
- We all work together (interdependently); because none of us want the patient to develop a lung infection from a yucky, bacteria-filled mouth!

We aren't finished with the implementation phase until we do the paperwork! We have to document the patient response (during and after the intervention) and share this information with other health care team members.

Charting (documentation) may be done using pen-and-paper; nurse's notes or flow sheets, or may be computerized charting, done at the bedside. Regardless of how you chart, institutional guidelines for use of accepted abbreviations must be followed to the letter! Because so many errors are preventable, abbreviations are changing to protect the patient.

Evaluation

During the evaluation phase of the nursing process, you have to determine whether or not the plan is working. You ask yourself:

- Have goals been met?
- Are the short-term goals being met with progress toward long-term goals?

- Is this plan of care working to accomplish the patient's highest possible level of wellness?

The nurse has to reassess whether the plan of care is accomplishing the expected outcomes! Notice that we have to assess again!

- We are always assessing and reassessing the patient's response to everything!
- And we are always evaluating and re-evaluating everything too!

The evaluation phase is never ending.

- Some patient issues resolve and are no longer priority.
- Other problems change or new problems present themselves!

That's why nursing is so FUN! Nothing is ever the same (static)! Patient needs and related nursing care are constantly changing (dynamic) from minute to minute and day to day.

SBAR form of communicating the patient status in terms of recovery, risk reduction, or rehab concerns. This format originated with commanders in the armed forces, and was used when one commander "handed-off" to another:

S = Situation: Describe the current problem.

B = Background: Give the doctor a rundown on the patient (admission diagnosis and vital signs, treatments, previous lab results, or whatever is relevant).

A = Assessment: Share conclusions (based on assessment) about the patient's problem.

R = Recommendation: Offer a statement of what you believe would be helpful to remedy the patient's problem.

+ Therapeutic communication

Therapeutic communication is sending, receiving, and interpreting information necessary for all interactions with patients, families, and health care personnel. Communication is verbal, which includes the written and spoken word, as well as nonverbal, which includes tone, gestures, body language, and physical presence when silence is used. All therapeutic communication is "for good" and is goal oriented rather than just "shooting the breeze" (talking to be talking) about trivia, or making social conversation.

- Beginning with the birth cry, communication is a basic human need: the ability to make needs known, to understand, and respond.
- Therapeutic communication is powered by the need to know, understand, and validate.
- Therapeutic communication facilitates acceptance of health care offered.
- Information must be elicited from patients and family members in order to understand and prioritize needs for planning care.
- Continuation of care demands effective goal-directed communication.

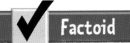

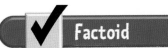

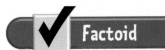

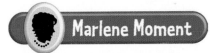

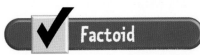

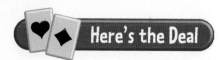

With experienced nurses reaching retirement age, and existing nurses leaving the profession sooner, the nursing workforce is experiencing change.[1] What factors will impact the future of nursing and the quality of medical-surgical nursing the most? New nurses meet the challenge with these essential attributes:

- Nursing knowledge
- Nursing skills
- Clinical judgment
- The ability to analyze assessment findings
- The ability interpret clues from the patient.[1]

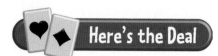

The introduction sets the tone, whether you are a new graduate meeting with a nurse recruiter, or you are meeting your patient for the first time.

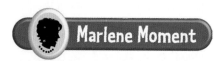

Always select the proper PLACE. Never correct a coworker in front of another health care worker, in the hallway or in the patient's presence. And always shut the door and wait until the patient is alone before discussing personal stuff!

- Information must be communicated to other members of the health care team for integrated and uninterrupted patient care.

Therapeutic communication is for the purpose of enabling health care providers to:
- collect data necessary for creating a diagnosis.
- formulate the patient treatment plan.
- enhance understanding and acceptance of the plan of care.
- obtain feedback that the patient understands his or her role in the plan.

You must use communication skills while conducting the admission interview, completing the patient history, and performing the admission assessment. This may be challenging because you are talking with a sick patient who may be:

- frightened of a "bad diagnosis."
- anxious about health care costs and missing work.
- intimidated by white coats.
- feeling vulnerable in a peek-a-boo gown!

The "Four Ps" is a good place to start:

- Always be POLITE and show respect for the individual.
- Always select the PROPER time. Don't ask about personal information in the presence of visitors.

In addition to communicating with your patient, you will be required to communicate with everyone else too: family members, visitors, physicians, and other members of the health care team. You cannot conduct a patient interview or perform any management or delegation function without using therapeutic communication. Here are some other basic principles:

- Always be nonjudgmental.
- Use active listening: Don't be thinking about what YOU are going to say next, or what else you have to do. Focus on the patient and what he or she is saying!
- Keep all patient communication and patient data confidential. If it is not relevant to the nursing care needs, you don't share this communication with others. Even computer screens and assignment boards in hospitals are not available for public viewing.
- If the patient is in pain or distress or distracted by other issues, don't attempt any interview, patient teaching, or long conversations requiring patient attention or input.
- Don't use big words to let people know how smart you are! If they can't understand what you are saying, then your message will not be received. And don't use slang terms, either! You want to make sure that your message is clear, so avoid any terms that can be misunderstood.

Be sure to use all of the above basic principles of therapeutic communication and refer to Table 1-1 for specific communication techniques.

Table 1-1 Techniques of therapeutic communication

Communication technique	Description and examples of how used
Silence	Keep your mouth shut! But make sure the patient knows that you are actively listening to every word and constantly engaged. Face the patient and use nonverbal communication (relaxed, open body language, with facial expressions) to demonstrate interest in what the patient is saying or NOT saying. Sometimes patients need more time to process information and respond. Silence gives the patient time to formulate his or her thoughts. Don't let yourself feel uncomfortable or hurried: stay focused on the goal of therapeutic communication! Sometimes just being with a patient is what he or she needs. Maybe the surgeon has just returned a bad verdict on a biopsy and the patient is alone with this "ton of bricks." Ask for permission if it seems appropriate. For example, "May I just sit with you?" Or show that you value the patient by saying, "I'd like to be here with you (during this time, or until family member or clergy arrives)."
Sharing observations	Make a note of patient behaviors, and share observations. For example, "You seem angry ... or ... you seem tense today." Make note of congruence between verbal and nonverbal communication (ie, do they match). For example, the patient may tell you that the biopsy showed invasive cancer, and yet he or she is laughing. Share the observation this way: "Sometimes when people are really nervous, or don't know how to respond, they laugh at really bad news." Then ask for validation (see technique below).
Broad opening statements	This technique lets the patient lead the conversation and select topics of personal concern. For example, "How are you doing with your hospitalization today?" opens the door for just about anything from health concerns, to family or job issues secondary to hospitalization.
General leads	This technique keeps the patient on track by directing the patient to an area that the nurse wishes to explore. For example, "I would like to hear more about.... (whatever)."
Open-ended questions	This technique allows the nurse to gather more information while keeping the patient focused. For example, "And then you...."? Or, "And then he responded by...."
Validating	This technique allows the nurse to gain feedback from the patient to make sure that both parties (sender and receiver) are interpreting the message the same way. For example, the nurse might say, "I hear you saying that you are unhappy with your treatment plan."
Restating	Repeat what the person said (in his or her own words), allowing the patient to hear what he or she said for the purpose of seeking clarification and/or keeping the patient focused on the topic. You may feel like "Polly Parrot," but this technique really works! Just don't overuse this technique or you may find yourself on the roost with other pigeons!

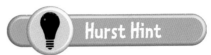

Hurst Hint

Silence. If you're one of those kinesthetic (hyped-up) people who always have to be moving, twisting your hair, or thumping a pencil, this will help you to be able to sit still and quiet: With your mouth SHUT, rub the tip of your tongue back and forth across your teeth (front, bottom works well and your need to move doesn't bother anybody).

(Continued)

Table 1-1   Techniques of therapeutic communication (*Continued*)

Communication technique	Description and examples of how used
Giving information	Providing factual information to replace myths and "old wives' tales" or misconceptions. The nursing diagnosis "Fear of the unknown related to knowledge deficit" can be effectively dispelled with factual information presented in language that the patient can understand.
Direct questioning	This technique is commonly used when filling out the admission history. (Check all that apply.) For example, "Are you a diabetic, or do you have any diabetes in your family?" Direct questioning is mandatory when you must get straight to the point and elicit an immediate answer, such as is necessary when your patient expresses suicidal ideation. For example, you MUST say, "Are you thinking of killing yourself"? Yes, you have to be just that abrupt; otherwise, you may not get another chance to ask.
Summarizing	This wraps up a conversation/interview by stating briefly what has been discussed. For example, "During the past few minutes we've talked about...blah, blah, blah."[2]

*This table uses concepts from *Hurst Reviews: NCLEX-RN Review,* 2008.

✚ Cultural considerations

The concept of culture is derived from anthropology, the study of human beings and how they live, customs, practices, and patterns of behavior. All patients have beliefs handed down by families that influence their behavior and health-seeking practices.

Culture is a population's specific set of values, beliefs, traditions, social norms, and patterns of behavior that are passed down over generations from one family to the next.

Growing up in a particular family, in a particular neighborhood, and locale exposes the individual to different patterns of behavior, speech, and belief systems. Your patients have different cultures and respond to illness and hospitalization in ways that vary because:

- Patients come from many different cultural backgrounds.

- Depending on cultural orientation, health and illness have different meanings.

- Persons from different cultures may experience communication based on the impact a specific culture has on communication.

- Many patients experience culture shock, and demonstrate anxiety and confusion when facing the many stressors of hospitalization.

- Communication styles, appropriateness of eye contact, touch, and particular health care belief systems are specific factors that demand cultural competence to prevent a negative impact on communication and the nurse–patient relationship.

Table 1-2 contrasts communication styles, the dos and don'ts of touch and eye contact, and some cultural beliefs about health, health care, and health care providers. Please note that the term "Black" refers to a highly diverse group of Americans coming to the United States from all over the world (rather than solely from Africa). Therefore, this cultural term is used in Table 1-2 rather than African American.[3] Refer to Table 1-2 for specific guidelines.

Table 1-2   Cultural barriers to communication

Culture	Communication patterns/methods	Eye contact and touch	Orientation to values and beliefs
Black Americans: from Caribbean, Haiti, Dominican Republic, and Africa	Have a need for solidarity and seek refuge in family, church, and community especially in times of illness. Bonds of kinship are strong. Self-identity is tied to the group and from an early age they are socialized to be in control and independent. Condescending attitudes will NOT be tolerated! Personal questions may feel like an invasion of privacy. Blacks tend to be highly expressive, and emotion is expressed freely and naturally. Communication may be expressed in "Black" English even though they are competent and articulate in the formal English language.	Some cultures maintain eye contact while speaking to a person, but look away while listening to that same person. Most African Americans born in America are comfortable with eye contact, viewing it as a sign of respect. African immigrants view eye contact as rude behavior. Touch is acceptable with family members and close personal friends.	Some use prayer for healing, and lying on of hands for anointing power. Some hold on to ancestral beliefs of illness as a state of disharmony with nature and use folk remedies and supernatural healing rituals. Some have a fatalistic view of illness and pain. Folk healers are "Grannies," Voodoo Priests, or Root Doctors depending on the country of origin. Self-treatment with use of over-the-counter medications is usually a first-line health care practice.
Asian Americans: from China, India, Japan, Philippines, Korea, Laos, Cambodia, Vietnam, Thailand, and Pacific Islands	Family hierarchy must be respected, and health care providers can do so by recognizing and addressing the oldest male in the family or group first, before addressing or greeting the patient. When an elderly parent is the patient, children have a moral obligation to protect them and care for them, which means that the nurse must recognize this and involve grown children in all planning and implementations of nursing care. Problems are kept within the family and confidentiality is critical.	Do not like to be touched by members of the opposite sex. Touch is avoided during conversations, and touching the head is particularly disrespectful because the head is considered sacred.	Respect elders and those in authority such as health care providers. Hold to the belief system that life is a cycle of suffering and rebirth, so suffering is natural and to be endured. Many delay seeking health care and believe that healing is spiritual as well as scientific. Karma as well as biology causes illness. Chinese medicine integrates body, mind, and spirit, and a balance of yin and yang (hot and cold) is essential to achieve health. Herbalists and shamans are healers. Ayurveda (means knowledge of life) is the traditional approach to healing for Asians. India's holistic approach calls for balance in body and mind through yoga, meditation, and herbal medicine.

(Continued)

Table 1-2   Cultural barriers to communication (*Continued*)

Culture	Communication patterns/methods	Eye contact and touch	Orientation to values and beliefs
European American: A conglomeration from all over Europe! Whites and Caucasians!	Silence can show respect or disrespect for someone, depending on the situation. Consumers of health care expect explanations in language they can understand, and they ask questions freely, expecting answers.	Direct eye contact is an indicator of trustworthiness, honesty, and attentiveness. Touch is acceptable with permission and respect for privacy. Handshakes are customary as formal greetings.	Increasingly health conscious and seeking alternative medicine. Desire to be active participant in health care and informed decision maker. Depending on subculture, many use preventive health care practices. The uninsured and underinsured delay health care because of financial hardship. Most respect health care professionals, but some degree of bias is present in mainstream society.
Hispanic American (H) from Caribbean, Mexico, Puerto Rico, and Central and South America; and Italian American from Italy! (I)	Both cultures are very gregarious and sociable. Behavior is demonstrative, with dramatic nonverbal communication, gestures/facial expressions, and verbal expressiveness, especially when pain or pleasure is experienced. An audience of family members and friends are welcomed and expected during times of illness. (H) Hispanics respect health care professionals and will verbally express disagreement or doubt, so nurses must ask questions and seek validation.	(H) Averting the eyes to avoid a direct gaze is common and is a sign of respect and attentiveness. If the patient is older than the nurse, the gaze should be directed below eye level. (I) Eye contact is appropriate and expected. Both cultures are very tactile and are comfortable with close physical contact and touch. Hugs and handshakes are welcome and socially appropriate among friends and family members. (I) Kissing on the cheek among men and women is appropriate when the relationship is close.	(H) Older women who serve as health practitioners are called curanderos, and they provide health care information. Recovery from illness is a result of the skill of the doctor and God's power and will. Some Hispanics believe that illness results from witchcraft, the "evil eye," or is punishment for sins. Some Hispanic cultures may not value preventive health care, and miss appointments, showing up an hour or a day late, still expecting to see the doctor. (I) See European Americans.
Native American: from North America, not immigrants (they were here first!)	Speaking in a quiet tone shows respect. Loud talk is considered rude, so keep the tone down! Wait and be patient, as members from different tribes may require extra time to mull over explanations. Silence is a communication technique that works well.	Direct eye contact is rude and may be considered confrontational. Touch may be considered unacceptable unless the persons know each other very well. Light touch in greeting is acceptable by some tribes. Health care professionals should ask permission before any touch just to be sure! Touching the dead is prohibited.	Believe that wellness and health occur when a person is in harmony with nature and natural laws of the universe. Illness is thought to occur when the person is in a state of disharmony or dis-equilibrium. Evil spirits, fear, and jealousy of other nations as well as failure to live according to the native code of life promote disharmony and can also cause illness. Shamans are sought out as holistic healers, and folk medicine and rituals are used. Hospitalization is a last resort when other approaches fail. Tribal practices to induce healing may include: • Prayer • Chanting • Smudging (brushing smoke from herbs or incense over the patient) • Herbalism • Laying on of hands[3]

Source: Young C, Koopsen C. *Spirituality, Health and Healing.* Mississauga, Ontario: Jones & Bartlett Learning; 2006.

The nurse who is culturally insensitive may cause the patient to refuse needed health care. Other adverse outcomes include:

- Lack of respect for health care providers.
- Misunderstanding of concepts necessary for promotion of wellness.
- Low self-esteem and feelings of rejection because a belief system and way of behavior is not valued or respected.
- Impaired communication between the patient and health care providers.

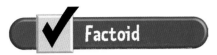

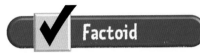

Culturally competent care opens the door to effective cross-cultural communication.

The only way to "diagnose" potential cultural problems is to include "those" questions on the admission form:

- "Do you have any religious beliefs or needs that we can assist you with during this hospitalization?"
- "Do you have any cultural beliefs that we should discuss so we can provide appropriate care during this hospitalization?"
- "Do you have any cultural needs that we need to incorporate into your plan of care?"

All patients need to feel valued, regardless of race, creed, and cultural and religious preferences. My patient needs to have access to the shaman, curanderos, or voodoo priest as desired, and healers are to be respected and welcomed. If practices require a special setting (such as smudging, in which smoke from fire is used), the nurse can assist in making arrangements for a satisfactory room within the hospital.

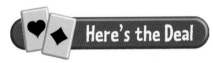

Talk is NOT cheap! Communication is basic to everything that we do!

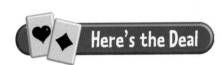

First and foremost: Respect for religious practices and acceptance of cultural beliefs are priority for establishing the nurse–patient relationship. Patient's cultural beliefs must be identified to provide direction for nursing care planning.

PATIENT TEACHING

You will be required to teach patients about all aspects of their unique health care needs from the disease process, to medications, treatments, risk reduction, and self-care monitoring associated with discharge teaching. In doing so, you will use principles of therapeutic communications with cultural considerations:

- To determine the patient's learning needs and preferred learning style.
- To conduct teaching sessions with the patient and/or family member(s).
- To deal with conflict when teaching is contrary to what "grannie" believes.
- To show respect for grannie (never belittling) and find culturally acceptable ways to accomplish identified teaching goals.

When creating your plan for any patient teaching, please refer to the Hurst 5 Rights for patient teaching:

- Right time: Pick a time when the patient is pain free and not experiencing distress or distraction.
- Right setting: If the patient does not have a private room, it might be best to accompany the patient to a classroom, depending on the nature of the material to be taught.

It would be totally inappropriate to give the patient written instructions about home care if he or she is illiterate!

- Right method: Depending on the material to be taught and your assessment of the patient's preferred method for learning, select from videos, brochures, one-to-one question-and-answer, or group teaching. Psychomotor (hands-on) techniques (example, an orange and an insulin syringe) would be appropriate for teaching skills.
- Right material: The content must match what the patient needs to learn about his or her medical condition, self-care and monitoring, risk reduction, and recovery. Keep it simple and in terms that the patient can understand.
- Right evaluation: Just because you taught something, it doesn't necessarily mean that the patient has learned. You must get feedback from the patient to make sure that learning has occurred. If teaching nutrition, it might be appropriate to allow the patient to select items from a menu that are to be included or avoided in a prescribed diet.

Standards for care have been established for cultural competence, and agencies that accredit hospitals look for evidence that patients are receiving this consideration. Mandatory in-service education requires that health care providers fulfill the agency objectives for periodically reviewing guidelines for culturally competent care.

A recent study using community lay educators and patient navigators to deliver culturally tailored health information showed positive outcomes in terms of increased knowledge about self-care and decreasing barriers to health care, and had the added benefit of improving the cultural knowledge base of the health care providers![4]

THE MEDICAL-SURGICAL NURSE TODAY

The medical-surgical nurse was once considered an entry-level or "starter" position. In the past a new nurse had to "pay his or her dues" on the medical-surgical unit before moving on to a specialty unit. Today, however, medical-surgical nursing is considered an adult health specialty.

The Academy of Medical-Surgical Nurses refers to this group as "the backbone of every adult-care clinical agency," which is an accurate description. The organization also goes on to outline the scope of this increasingly specialized group of caregivers (Table 1-3).

Table 1-3   Academy of Medical-Surgical Nurses: description of the medical-surgical nurse today

Skill set	• Knowledge related to all aspects of adult health; • Excellent assessment, clinical, organization, and prioritization skills; and • Educator for patients, families, peers, and other health professionals.
Patient advocate	• Participates in the measurement and improvement of the quality of care delivered; • Is dedicated to making patient safety a top priority; and • Supports patients in identifying and meeting their interests and needs.

(Continued)

Table 1-3   Academy of Medical-Surgical Nurses: description of the medical-surgical nurse today (*Continued*)

Diversity	• Provides care for patients of all ages; • Manages the care of patients with multiple medical, surgical, and/or psychiatric diagnoses as well as diagnoses across all medical specialties; • Embraces opportunities to learn new skills; and • Can practice across a wide array of health care settings, both inpatient and outpatient.
Making a difference	• Provides comfort and care to people who, at that moment, need someone genuinely interested in their lives and well-being; • Heals patients physically and emotionally through intuitive experiences that rely on observation and touch; • Assists patients in reaching the goal of returning to their highest level of functioning; and • Provides dignity and respect in end-of-life decision making and care.

Data from Academy of Medical-Surgical Nurses web site: http://www.amsn.org

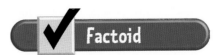

Factoid

Nurses on a medical-surgical unit must be able to provide a wide variety of specialized care and be ready for emergencies too!

PRACTICE QUESTIONS

1. A medical-surgical nursing unit suddenly becomes short staffed when a nurse scheduled to work 7 a.m. to 7 p.m. does not report to work. Which option by the nurse manager offers the LEAST effective solution for providing safe effective care for the existing patients?

   A. Employ a PRN agency nurse whose salary is double that of the regular staff nurse.

   B. Request that the nursing supervisor pull a float nurse from another area of the hospital.

   C. Take the patient assignments that would have been given to the absent nurse.

   D. Call the nursing administrator to temporarily suspend any additional admissions to this nursing unit.

2. A Spanish-speaking patient who can speak, read, and understand very little English has just signed a permit for surgery after receiving preoperative information in English. Which priority action by the nurse best exemplifies the role of the nurse as a patient advocate?

   A. Refuse to sign the operative permit as a witness to the signature.

   B. Notify the hospital ethics committee of this breach in standards for informed consent.

   C. Delay surgery until arrival of a Spanish interpreter who can translate all previous preoperative information.

   D. Report the physician/surgeon to the Peer Review Organization (PRO) for illegal/unethical action.

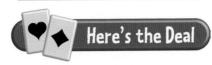

Here's the Deal

On a "routine" day, the nurse may have a patient with gastroenteritis (diarrhea, diarrhea, diarrhea) in one room and another with pneumonia in the other room. It is easy to get lulled into complacency when everything is so "routine," isn't it? People don't just come in and DIE with routine stuff! Better think again! Unexpected occurrences can and do occur on all patient care units.

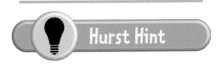

Hurst Hint

When things change on a medical-surgical unit, they usually change fast!

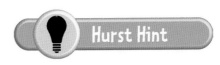

Hurst Hint

Always assume the worst!

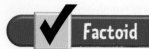

Factoid

Your patient should never be worse off AFTER a procedure than he or she was before! Something is wrong!

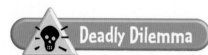

Deadly Dilemma

Because of the effect of illness on diabetes, your patient in room 210 who appears sound asleep is now breathing rapidly and is very lethargic! Metabolic acidosis (ketoacidosis, we call it because he is a diabetic)! This is a medical emergency! The medical-surgical nurse has to be continuously observant for these types of patient care emergencies.

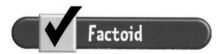

Factoid

Illness + diabetes = diabetic ketoacidosis

3. Upon completion of a nursing history when the patient is scheduled for excision and biopsy of a breast nodule, which of the following is of greatest and most immediate concern to the nurse?

A. An aunt and two cousins have had cancer of the breast.

B. An uncle had a febrile response during surgery and "almost died."

C. A previous surgery was complicated by postoperative nausea and vomiting.

D. A latex allergy was discovered during a previous hospitalization.

4. After an above-the-knee amputation on a diabetic patient, which postoperative intervention is the priority?

A. Keep a tourniquet clearly visible at the head of the bed.

B. Medicate the patient as needed for phantom pain with PRN analgesia.

C. Administer prescribed antibiotics IVPB (intravenous piggy back) as ordered.

D. Allow ample time for the patient to discuss concerns about body image change related to the amputated limb.

5. An elderly adult develops watery foul-smelling diarrhea after bowel surgery. After notifying the physician, which next nursing implementation is the priority?

A. Administer prescribed antidiarrheal agents.

B. Monitor cardiac output and blood pressure.

C. Caution the patient not to strain with stools.

D. Place the patient in protective (reverse) isolation.

6. Which of the following items is most important to keep at the bedside following an above-the-knee (AK) amputation when the patient is an African American pastor in the rural south?

A. A Bible.

B. A tourniquet.

C. A bedside commode.

D. A blood pressure cuff.

7. On the third postoperative day after a vaginal hysterectomy, a middle-aged woman verbalizes all of the following subjective complaints. Which one would be of most concern to the nurse?

A. Numbness and tingling from left knee to ankle.

B. An uncomfortable feeling of lower pelvic fullness.

C. Pain in the calf when ambulating to the restroom.

D. Nausea occurring 30 minutes after a codeine-based oral analgesia.

8. A nurse is reviewing the admission history of an elderly woman who has adult onset diabetes (Type II) and is NPO for a radiologic procedure using iodine-based dye for contrast. Which lab results are the most critical to report to the physician?

   A. BUN 26 mg/dL

   B. Serum creatinine 2.8 mg/dL

   C. Urine specific gravity 1.027

   D. Blood sugar 2-hour postprandial 120 mg/dL

9. Which of the following lab tests would assist the med-surg nurse to evaluate both the preoperative patient's nutritional readiness for surgery and unexplained ankle edema on a medical patient who has been on prolonged bed rest?

   A. Serum glucose

   B. Serum sodium

   C. Serum albumin

   D. Serum magnesium

10. A patient is receiving a nitroglycerin drip, and the primary nurse is titrating the IV flowrate to maintain blood pressure. To which, if any, licensed or unlicensed assistive personnel could the task of monitoring blood pressure readings be delegated?

   A. Another RN (registered nurse).

   B. The UAP (unlicensed assistive personnel).

   C. The LPN/LVN (licensed practical or vocational nurse).

   D. The primary RN may not delegate blood pressure monitoring.

References

1. Plauntz LM. Preoperative assessment of the surgical patient. *Nurs Clin N Am.* 42:361–377, 2007.

2. Hurst M. Everything you ever wanted to know about therapeutic communication. In: Hurst M. *Hurst Reviews: NCLEX-RN Review.* New York: McGraw-Hill; 2008.

3. Young C, Koopsen C. *Spirituality, Health and Healing.* Mississauga, Ontario: Jones & Bartlett Learning; 2006.

4. Fisher TL, Bumet DL, Huang ES, Chin MH, Cagney KA. Cultural leverage: Interventions using culture to narrow racial disparities in health. *Med Care Res Rev.* 64:243S–282S, 2007.

5. Pagana KD, Pagana TJ. *Mosby's Diagnostic and Laboratory Test Reference.* St Louis: Mosby; 2007.

2 Fluids and Electrolytes

OBJECTIVES

In this chapter you will review:

- Differences and similarities in the effect of excess and deficits of fluids and electrolytes (cations and anions).
- Medical-surgical and clinical conditions that contribute to fluid loss, fluid gain, and electrolyte imbalance.
- The body's compensatory response to rapid fluid loss or gain.
- The effects of altered fluid and electrolyte balance related to priority needs of oxygenation, circulation, and physical safety.
- Priorities for care when the patient is experiencing fluid/electrolyte imbalance.
- Treatment modalities and nursing care to promote restoration of fluid and electrolyte balance.
- Nursing measures to create and maintain a safe, effective care environment for the patient experiencing fluid and/or electrolyte imbalance.
- Components of a teaching plan to enhance self-care monitoring for the patient recovering from a fluid/electrolyte imbalance.

Let's get the normal stuff straight first!

Fluid and electrolyte imbalances are seen in every area of nursing practice. These imbalances are usually secondary to some other problem, such as cardiac, renal, adrenal, parathyroid, pituitary dysfunction; and can even be related to medications. In other words, when there is a fluid and/or electrolyte imbalance, it's usually the **result** (or a symptom) of **another** problem rather than being the **primary** problem itself. As a general rule, something else causes the imbalance to start with. For example, if the kidneys aren't functioning properly, the patient may retain potassium and become hyperkalemic. If the adrenal glands aren't functioning properly, aldosterone may be overproduced, causing sodium and water retention (fluid volume excess). If there is a pituitary problem resulting in decreased production of ADH (antidiuretic hormone), the patient will begin to lose significant amounts of water, leading to fluid volume deficit and hypernatremia. Relax if you haven't learned these concepts yet! The point is, you HAVE to understand fluids and electrolytes and the relationship to disease processes because you will encounter it on a regular basis (especially in med-surg). If you do not have a **solid** foundation on the basics of fluids and electrolytes, we highly encourage you to refer to Hurst Review's **Pathophysiology Review** book. You will be so glad you did! In fact, my pathophysiology book will help you throughout medical-surgical nursing.

FLUID IMBALANCES

. . . .

✚ Fluid volume excess

What is it?

Fluid volume excess (or FVE, also called hypervolemia) is too much fluid in the vascular space. The term *vascular space* refers to veins, arteries, capillaries, arterioles, and the chambers of the heart. In fluid volume excess, sodium and water are being retained which will expand the vascular space. (Fig. 2-1).

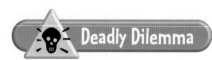

Deadly Dilemma

The patient may not have a fluid and electrolyte imbalance on admission; however, they may develop one during their hospital stay. Being familiar with key signs and symptoms of fluid and electrolyte imbalances may help you pick up on a life-threatening problem before it's too late.

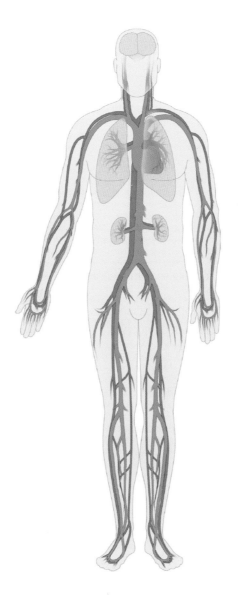

◄ Figure 2-1. Vascular Space. The vascular space where fluid volume excess and deficit occur.

Causes and why?

The following table demonstrates the causes of FVE and why it occurs.

Causes	Why
Renal failure	The kidneys are normally responsible for the majority of fluid elimination. In renal failure or renal insufficiency, the kidneys lose their ability to efficiently excrete fluid (in the form of urine); therefore, fluid builds up in the vascular space.
CHF	Decreased cardiac output from a weak heart leads to decreased kidney perfusion, causing renal insufficiency. Renal insufficiency leads to decreased urine output causing excessive fluid retention.

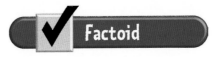

Factoid

Even a small decrease in renal function can lead to the kidney's inability to properly excrete fluid (and electrolytes) in the form of urine.

(Continued)

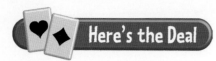

Here's the Deal

Aldosterone is a steroid (specifically a mineralocorticoid) produced by the adrenal cortex. The normal action of aldosterone is to conserve sodium and water when the body has lost too much.

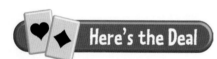

Here's the Deal

Medications can cause fluid retention in the vascular space OR the interstitial space (tissue).

Causes	Why
Steroid excess	Cushing's syndrome—retention of sodium and water because of excessive aldosterone production. Hyperaldosteronism—overproduction of steroids (mineralocorticoids) by the adrenal cortex. Hyperaldosteronism—too much aldosterone regardless of the cause. For example, if aldosterone excess is caused by an adrenal tumor, it is referred to as Conn's syndrome. Another cause of excessive aldosterone is adrenal hyperplasia (enlarged adrenal cortex).
Excessive sodium (various sources): • IV normal saline • Lactated ringers • Foods	Excessive sodium intake (from any source) causes fluid retention in the vascular space.
Blood product administration	Blood products are infused directly into the vascular space leading to increased fluid volume.
Increased ADH (antidiuretic hormone)	The normal action of ADH is to retain water when needed. The syndrome of inappropriate antidiuretic hormone (SIADH) is a disease in which the body produces too much ADH. This causes excessive water to be retained in the vascular space leading to fluid volume excess (FVE).
Medications	Steroids, anti-inflammatories, Alka-Seltzer, oral contraceptives, oral hypoglycemics (diabetes medications), and fleet enemas all lead to fluid retention.
Liver disease	Excess production of aldosterone, which causes sodium and water retention.
Burn treatment	In a major burn, the vessels are severely damaged leading to fluid leakage from the vascular space. To combat the excessive fluid leakage, IV fluids will be rapidly infused to prevent fluid volume deficit (FVD) or "shock." 24 hours post-burn, the damaged vessels begin to repair, leading to less fluid leakage. This is a critical time because continued rapid IV infusions for FVD could now lead to fluid volume excess.
Albumin infusion	Albumin is a large protein. The protein exerts a fluid "pull" from the interstitial space back into the vascular space possibly leading to fluid retention.

Source: Created by the author from Reference 1.

Signs and symptoms and why?

The following table shows the signs and symptoms associated with FVE and why these occur.

Signs and symptoms	Why
Jugular vein distention (JVD) and/or peripheral vein distention	As the vascular space expands to a volume in which the heart can no longer compensate for, the pressure in the right ventricle and atrium rises, leading to JVD.
Bounding pulse and tachycardia	Heart pumps hard and fast to keep the fluid moving forward.
Increased central venous pressure (CVP)	More vascular volume leads to increased central venous pressure.
Increased BP	More vascular volume leads to increased blood pressure.
Dyspnea and tachypnea	Excess fluid in the lungs impairs respiratory efforts.
Abnormal breath sounds	Excess fluid collects in the lungs; lungs sound wet.
Productive cough	Fluid collects in the lungs, causing a productive cough; the body is trying to rid of the excess fluid through mucous.
Edema	Vascular spaces leak fluid into the tissues.
Polyuria	Kidneys excrete the excess fluid.
Decreased urine specific gravity	Excess urine leads to dilute urine.
Third spacing can develop in FVE. The most common places are the abdomen and around the lungs in the pleural space.	The vascular space can no longer compensate for the excessive volume; therefore, the fluid shifts from the vascular space to alternative spaces.
Weight gain	Fluid retention causes weight gain.

Source: Created by the author from Reference 1.

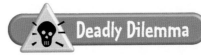

FVE can lead to pulmonary edema, a life-threatening complication.

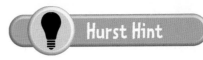

If the patient is on bedrest, he or she may have sacral edema rather than peripheral edema.

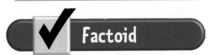

Third spacing occurs when fluid has moved to places it shouldn't be.

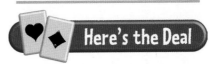

Some doctors prefer for ALL lab work to be immediately reported (depending on how critical the patient's condition is). You will learn their preferences with time. BUT, critical lab values should ALWAYS be reported to the physician immediately. Know your hospital's policy related to reporting of critical lab values!!

Testing, testing, testing

The lab work ordered (and the results) will vary depending on the *cause* of the problem. For example, in fluid volume excess related to increased aldosterone (sodium *and* water are retained equally…or *isotonic overhydration*), the sodium level will be **normal** in conjunction with FVE. However, in SIADH, in which the patient is retaining a large volume of fluid, the sodium level will be abnormally low secondary to dilution. This is also known as *water intoxication.*

Test	Clinical significance	Nursing care
BUN (blood urea nitrogen)—the liver converts ammonia to urea, which is excreted by the kidneys. BUN tells us how the liver and the kidneys are functioning. Renal disease results in inadequate urea excretion, but it can also be elevated in a high protein diet or GI bleeding. It can also be a marker for hydration status—up in dehydration and down in FVE. BUN is also interpreted along with creatinine in determining renal function. This is called renal function studies. Normal BUN: Adult—10–20 mg/dL. Critical value—↑100 mg/dL—significant renal function impairment.	Decreased blood urea nitrogen resulting from plasma dilution.	Make sure the lab work is ordered properly. Make sure the lab comes and draws the blood. Report critical values to the physician.
Electrolytes Normal adult sodium—136–145 mEq/L. Critical value is <120 or >160 Normal adult potassium—3.5–5.0 mEq/L. Critical value is <2.5 or >6.5 mEq/L.	When there is too much aldosterone secretion (primary hyperaldosteronism), sodium and water are retained and potassium is excreted. The patient will be hypernatremic (elevated serum sodium) and hypokalemic (decreased serum potassium).	Make sure the lab work is ordered properly. Make sure the lab comes and draws the blood. Monitor for cardiac arrhythmias and other s/s of hypokalemia (see chart). Assessment for signs of fluid and electrolyte imbalance. Monitor blood pressure. Patients with primary aldosteronism have high blood pressure, high serum sodium levels, low serum potassium, and headache. Monitor for complications after surgery such as s/s infection, fluid and electrolyte imbalance, hypertension, hypokalemia, or hyperkalemia because the patient will probably be treated with potassium-sparing diuretics to rid the body of excess fluid. The patient could also be started on a potassium supplement to compensate for hypokalemia. Report critical values to the physician.

Aldosterone level can be measured in the blood or the urine. Blood (supine)—3–10 ng/dL (female). Blood (upright)—5–30 ng/dL (female). Blood (upright)—6–22 ng/dL (male). Urine—2–26 mcg/24 hour.	When there is too much aldosterone secretion (hyperaldosteronism or Cushing's disease), sodium and water are retained and potassium is excreted. The patient will be hypernatremic (elevated serum sodium) and hypokalemic (decreased serum potassium). Aldosterone will be increased in primary aldosteronism, which is usually either a tumor of the adrenal cortex (Conn's syndrome) or hyperplasia of the adrenal glands.	Report critical values to the physician.
CT or MRI to detect tumor	If a tumor is suspected (primary hyperaldosteronism), CT or MRI will confirm. Surgery may be required.	Make sure patient has no jewelry or other items that could interfere with X-ray.
Urinary output—normal urinary output is 1 mL/kg/hour.	In CHF, the heart is weak with decreased cardiac output. This leads to decreased kidney perfusion and the urinary output will go down. In renal failure, the kidneys aren't functioning properly and the urinary output will go down.	Assess the urinary output and call the doctor if less than 30 mL/hour Report critical values to the physician. Monitor for s/s of FVE when the urine output is low. Always think "heart" problems first and watch for s/s of congestive heart failure.
Decreased Hematocrit Normal value: Adult male—42%–52%. Adult female—37%–47%. Critical value—↓15% or ↑60%.	Decreased hematocrit is caused by plasma dilution.	Make sure the lab work is ordered properly. Make sure the lab comes and draws the blood. Report critical values to the physician.

(Continued)

Test	Clinical significance	Nursing care
Chest X-ray The chest X-ray may reveal the presence of fluid if any.	Detects presence of pulmonary edema (fluid in the lungs), pleural effusion (in the pleural space), or pericardial effusion (in the pericardial space).	There should be no metal (jewelry). Patient should take a deep breath and hold it in order to expand the lungs. After the picture is taken, remind the patient to breathe!
Urine and serum osmolality may be measured simultaneously in FVE if SIADH is suspected.	SIADH (syndrome of inappropriate antidiuretic hormone)—too much ADH resulting in fluid retention, serum hypoosmolality, dilutional hyponatremia, hypochloremia, and concentrated urine.	See causes of SIADH for nursing care related to FVE and SIADH. Be alert for decreased urinary output with high specific gravity along with dilute serum (low specific gravity). Remember...concentrated makes numbers go up. Dilute makes numbers go down. The patient may be on seizure precautions related to hyponatremia. In hyponatremia, the patient may be given IV hypertonic saline solution. It should be infused slowly and with an infusion pump to prevent the sodium from rising too quickly. Fluids may be restricted to 800–1000 mL per day. In severe hyponatremia, the fluid may be restricted to 500 mL per day. Ice chips and/or chewing gum may help with thirst.
CVP (central venous pressure) is the measurement of the pressure in the right atrium (also right ventricular preload) using a central venous catheter via the internal jugular or subclavian vein. The catheter tip is placed inside the superior vena cava close to but not inside the right atrium.	Increased CVP indicates FVE (volume overload). Decreased CVP indicates hypovolemia (fluid volume deficit). This is also known as *hemodynamic monitoring or invasive pressure monitoring* and takes place inside the intensive care unit. Used to assist with management of patients with cardiac, pulmonary, or vascular volume problems by giving an indication of the pressure in the right side of the heart.	The critical care nurse monitors trends in hemodynamic readings *simultaneously* with nursing observation of pertinent s/s.

Interventions and why?

The primary goal of treatment for FVE is to decrease the amount of fluid to relieve symptoms without causing further fluid and electrolyte imbalances. In addition, it is imperative that the underlying cause be identified and treated.

The patient needs volume reduction, which will be accomplished through prescribed diuresis and a low-sodium diet. Fluid intake may be limited according to the patient's condition (i.e., heart or renal failure).

- Physical assessment: To determine severity of signs and symptoms and degree of illness.

- Monitor lab values daily or more often as ordered by the physician: Be alert for a low hematocrit, low BUN (caused by plasma dilution), as well as abnormal potassium and sodium levels (caused by electrolyte imbalances).

- Daily weights: Same time, same scales, same clothes, and void first! Abrupt weight gain indicates worsening of FVE.

- Anterior and posterior chest auscultation at regular intervals: Early detection, documentation, and reporting of wet crackles/rales. The increased volume may overload the heart, causing fluid to back up into the lungs.

- 24-Hour I&O: Keep accurate records of everything going in, such as IV fluids, oral intake with meals and medications; and everything going out, including urine, excreta, and gastric fluid by suction or vomitus. I&O is an essential part of assessing fluid and electrolyte balance.

- Bed rest: Bed rest induces diuresis by increasing kidney perfusion as well as decreasing the workload on the heart for patients with an underlying heart condition as the cause of their FVE.

- Diuretics as ordered (Tables 2-1). These medications induce diuresis.

- Monitor for the presence of peripheral edema, which indicates worsening of FVE.

Table 2-1   Diuretics in a nutshell

Name of diuretic generic/trade	How the drug works	What to teach my patient
HCTZ/HydroDIURIL (hydrochlorothiazide) furosemide (Lasix)	Acts on the proximal, distal, or loop of Henle in the renal tubules to promote excretion of sodium and water.	- Take medication early in the morning, so you won't be up all night going to the bathroom! - Monitor BP. Hold medicine and call your doctor if systolic <90 mm Hg.

(Continued)

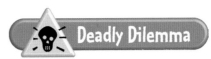

Deadly Dilemma

Never start a potassium supplement and a potassium *sparing* diuretic at the same time. This can result in hyperkalemia.

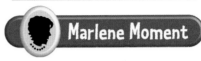

Marlene Moment

Sit the patient up if possible and be sure to listen to those posterior lung bases first, we want to catch "wet lungs" early; if you wait till you hear "wet lung" sounds anteriorly right below the clavicle your patient is DROWNING!

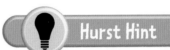

Hurst Hint

Don't forget to include excess perspiration and drainage from wounds in output. You will have to estimate these!

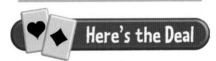

Here's the Deal

If fluids are limited, give oral medications with fluids served at mealtime, reserving some water for later in the day (or night) to quench thirst.

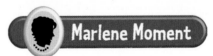

Marlene Moment

Don't just look at Maw-maw's feet when you assess your patient for peripheral edema, especially if she has been on bed rest. Edema will form in the most dependent areas first, so check the sacrum and back if her feet haven't touched the ground lately. Another thing to be alert for is skin breakdown. (Edematous skin is just waiting to breakdown!)

Table 2-1   Diuretics in a nutshell (*Continued*)

Name of diuretic generic/trade	How the drug works	What to teach my patient
bumetanide (Bumex) torsemide(Demadex) Metolazone (Zaroxolyn)		• Weigh daily. • Hold medicine and call doctor for loss of 2–3 lb overnight. • Eat foods high in potassium, such as fresh produce. • Stand slowly to prevent a drop in BP (orthostatic hypotension). • Hold medicine and call your doctor for ringing or roaring in your ears.
Spironolactone (Aldactone)	Potassium-sparing diuretic: promotes loss of sodium and water, but the patient retains potassium!	• Avoid foods high in potassium such as fresh produce. • Use caution with use of salt substitutes, which may contain excess potassium (read labels). • Except for above items, use teaching for diuretics above.[1]

INITIATION OF DIURETIC THERAPY—NURSING INTERVENTIONS   Prior to initiation of diuretic therapy, the nurse must:

- Verify the patient is not allergic to sulfonamides.
- Be alert for any renal or hepatic dysfunction by monitoring BUN, creatinine, and liver function tests (ALT, AST).
- Monitor daily electrolytes (be especially alert to K^+ and Na^+).
- Monitor BP every 2 to 4 hours, being alert to hypotension.
- Prepare to administer isotonic fluid bolus if BP drops too low,<90 mm Hg.
- Be alert to the development of arrhythmias, especially when Aldactone is prescribed (hyperkalemia).
- Dangle patient at bedside before arising and arise slowly to avoid orthostatic hypotension. Monitor and compare three-step BP: taken while lying down, sitting, and standing.
- Be alert to rapid weight loss or gain (i.e., 2–3 lb overnight).

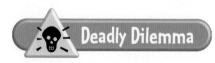

Many diuretics promote loss of calcium, which could cause a life-threatening arrhythmia: Monitor for hypocalcemia! Check Chvostek's sign and Trousseau's sign! Watch for muscle twitching, don't wait for tetany (muscles in a rigid, tight hold) to occur (Figs. 2-2 and 2-3)!

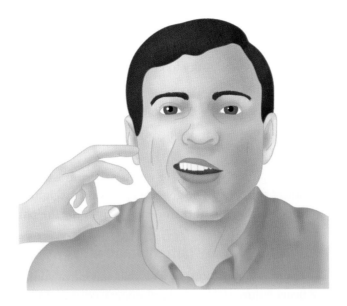

◀ Figure 2-2. Chvostek's Sign. One sign/symptom of hypocalcemia is Chvostek's sign. It is tested by tapping the facial nerve that lies between the area anterior to the earlobe beneath the zygomatic arch and between the zygomatic arch and the outer corner of the mouth. A slight twitching of the lip is considered a positive reaction, but it can elicit a spasm of multiple facial muscles. The extent of the reaction depends on the degree of hypocalcemia the patient is suffering.

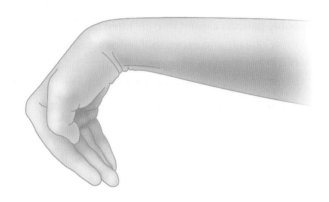

◀ Figure 2-3. Trousseau's Sign. Another sign/symptom of hypocalcemia is Trousseau's sign. To test, a blood pressure cuff is placed on the patient's arm above the elbow and inflated to a pressure greater than the patient's systolic blood pressure and held for 3 minutes. A positive reaction will cause the thumb and fingers to adduct, a flexion of the metacarpophalangeal joints, wrist, and possibly elbow with the fingers held together.

- Monitor effectiveness of the treatment plan; you will be assessing the patient to see if the previous signs and symptoms have decreased or been resolved: such as
  - Patient reports he or she can breathe easier
  - Lungs clearing, decrease in moist rales/crackles
  - Increased SpO_2 >94%
  - Decrease in peripheral edema
  - Flat neck veins, peripheral veins
  - Increased urinary output
  - Decreased weight
  - Decreased abdominal girth (if ascites present)

PATIENT TEACHING   Prior to discharge, the patient must understand the importance of monitoring daily weight, intake and output, and adhering to a sodium-restricted diet. General guidelines for sodium reduction include:

- Avoid all obviously salty foods: salted top crackers, potato chips, pretzels.
- Avoid prepared foods, such as soups, processed meats, and fast foods.
- No added salt at the table: Remove salt shakers!
- Avoid OTC medications because they may contain large amounts of sodium.
- Instruct patients on how to weigh daily and what significant weight changes to report. **The general rule is that weight should be maintained within 2 lb of the normal weight for the patient.**

What can harm my patients and why?

The major complications of FVE that can harm your client are congestive heart failure (CHF) and pulmonary edema. FVE increases cardiac preload, and a healthy heart can compensate for short-term increases in volume. However, increasing the cardiac workload when the heart is weak can lead to acute pulmonary edema, CHF, and possibly death unless prompt and aggressive treatment is instituted.

- Some patients cannot tolerate rapid fluid shifts; they may develop FVE more quickly and experience serious complications related to FVE. This can occur from rapid infusion of intravenous fluids. FVE can be lethal, always use caution when administering IVF to the following patients:
  - Elderly—high-risk population.
  - Pediatric—high-risk population.
  - Cardiac—pre-existing cardiac conditions predispose the patient for heart failure and FVE.
  - Renal—pre-existing cardiac conditions predispose the patient for heart failure and FVE.
- Imaging studies using high osmolality iodinated contrast media (ICM)[2] can also induce pulmonary edema as fluid is pulled rapidly into the vascular space. Low osmolality ICMs are more commonly used in patients that have a higher risk of FVE.
- The patient who becomes hypoxic suddenly will be very apprehensive and frightened. Interventions include:
  - Assess A-B-Cs!
  - Stay with the patient and act quickly to support airway, breathing, and circulation as indicated.
  - Elevate the head of the bed (90 degrees unless contraindicated) to ease the work of breathing and drop the foot of the bed to promote pooling of blood in the lower extremities, keeping it away from the heart.
  - Administer oxygen by mask as indicated to maintain a $SpO_2 > 93\%$.
- Administer diuretics as ordered such as IV furosemide (Lasix) to reduce promote diuresis and decrease circulating blood volume. Morphine sulfate IV push is also often ordered to relieve anxiety and reduce dyspnea. Both of these medications cause vasodilation, which

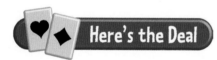

Here's the Deal

Never leave an unstable patient! Stay with the patient, call for help, and notify the primary care physician!

will promote venous pooling and decrease the workload on the heart. An added benefit of morphine is relaxation of smooth muscles of the bronchus, promoting increased air intake.

✛ Fluid volume deficit

What is it?

In fluid volume deficit (FVD), there is not enough fluid in the vascular space. This can result from rapid fluid loss such as hemorrhage or loss of fluid following a burn. It can also result from less obvious causes such as excessive vomiting, diarrhea, NG tube to suction, and thoracentesis. Anytime a patient is losing fluid they are ultimately decreasing the amount of volume in the vascular space.

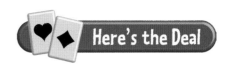

Here's the Deal

Fluid volume deficit can range in severity. For example, mild to moderate *FVD (dehydration)* can occur with diarrhea and/or vomiting caused by an illness (e.g., a stomach virus). On the other hand, the fluid depletion can be severe enough to leave insufficient volume in the vascular space to perfuse vital organs (e.g., major trauma and/or "bleeding out") resulting in *shock*.

Causes and why?

Cause	Why
Gastrointestinal causes	Fluids and electrolytes are lost during vomiting, diarrhea, GI suctioning (NG tube hooked to suction) eating disorders (bulimia).
	Impaired swallowing (e.g., strokes and other neurological disorders), the patient is unable to take in adequate amount of fluids.
	Laxatives can cause abnormal fluid loss if not taken properly.
Diuretics	Excessive excretion of fluid and electrolytes through the kidneys.
Tube feedings	The tube feeding itself is meant to deliver nutrition (vitamins, minerals, calories, etc.), not water. If the patient isn't receiving adequate hydration through an IV, the fluid volume could become depleted. Therefore, the patient should have an order for water administration through the tube to prevent FVD.
Fever	Sweating can cause abnormal fluid loss.
Hemorrhage	Loss of blood volume at a fast rate depletes the vascular volume.
Third spacing	• Blood volume drops when fluid leaves the vascular space and moves into other areas of the body:
	• Ascites—fluid shifts to the peritoneal space.
	• Intestinal obstruction—With intestinal obstruction, the intestinal wall becomes edematous, stretched, and tense (tightness). As a result, the capillaries become permeable and fluid leaks out of the little vessels (vascular space) into the peritoneum. This is called *ascites*. Intestinal obstruction can be caused by things such as fecal impaction or scar tissue from intestinal diseases such as cancer, Crohn's, etc.
	• Hemothorax—blood in the pleural space.
	• Pleural effusion—fluid collects in the pleural space.
	• Fractures—severe fractures lead to bleeding into the tissue.
Vulnerable populations	• Alzheimer's—confused patients lack the ability to respond to thirst; the elderly patient may have decreased thirst perception.
	• Elderly—thirst perception decreases with age.
	• Comatose patients—fluid requirements must be managed by health-care providers because they are unable to care for themselves.
	• Depression—loss of desire for food and water, lack of desire for self-care.

(Continued)

Cause	Why
Endocrine	• DI (diabetes insipidus)—decreased production or secretion of ADH—results in large amounts of dilute urine • Addison's disease • Diabetes mellitus
Skin	• Burns • Excessive sweating without fluid replacement

Source: Created by the author from Reference 1.

Signs and symptoms and why?

The following table shows the signs and symptoms associated with FVD and why they occur.

Signs and symptoms	Why
Acute weight loss	Water weighs about 8 lb/gallon; I liter weight is 2.2 lb or 1 kg. The body loses this weight.
Decreased skin turgor (Fig. 2-4)	Water loss affects the skin's ability to return to its normal position after gently "pinching" the skin. When the skin is slow to return to normal, we say it "tents" (remains up) after gently pinching.
Vital Signs • Decreased blood pressure • Weak and rapid pulse • Decreased CVP (central venous pressure) • Increased respiratory rate • Decreased temperature Postural hypotension (orthostatic hypotension)	Less volume...equals less pressure. Pulse increases to compensate and perfuse the body. Less volume...equals less pressure. Maintain oxygen distribution throughout the body. Compensatory mechanism to conserve fluid because the higher the temperature, the more fluid is lost. Fluid deficit causes BP drop from supine or sitting position to upright position.
Decreased sensorium	Decreased blood pressure leads to decreased brain perfusion.
Sunken eyeballs	Fluid is depleted from the orbital space.
Cool/cold extremities	Peripheral vasoconstriction shunts blood to vital organs and away from extremities.
Thick, sticky respiratory secretions	Low fluid volume leaves secretions depleted of water content.

✔ **Factoid**

Postural hypotension is also known as orthostatic hypotension. It is a decrease in systolic blood pressure of 10 mm Hg or more when changing from a supine to upright position.

(Continued)

Signs and symptoms	Why
Dry, sticky mucous membranes	Decreased fluids cause membrane dryness.
Decreased peripheral pulses	Blood shunted away from extremities; poor tissue perfusion.
Urine: • Oliguria—decreased urinary output • Concentrated urine	Body holding onto what fluid is left.

Source: Created by the author from Reference 1.

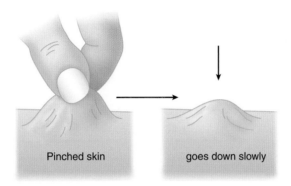

Pinched skin   goes down slowly

◀ Figure 2-4. Decreased Skin Turgor. When testing skin turgor for dehydration, the skin on the sternum and forehead are best, but the skin on the back of the hand, abdomen, and lower arm can be used. The skin is pinched up and held a few seconds in the "tented" position, when released it will snap back into place if turgor is normal. The skin of a person with poor skin turgor will slowly sink back into position.

Testing, testing, testing: FVD

Test	Clinical significance	Nursing care
Increased urine specific gravity	Decreased fluid volume leads to concentrated urine (increased particle content with decreased fluid content). This is also called increased urine specific gravity because the particle to fluid ratio is high.	Ensure all lab work is obtained and properly ordered. Review lab work and report critical values to the physician.
Increased hematocrit	Decreased fluid volume leads to decreased blood plasma (more particles than fluid).	Hypovolemia can range from mild dehydration to shock. Be alert to s/s of shock.

(Continued)

Test	Clinical significance	Nursing care
BUN (blood urea nitrogen)—the liver converts ammonia to urea which is excreted by the kidneys. BUN tells us how the liver and the kidneys are functioning. Renal disease results in inadequate urea excretion. But it can also be elevated in a high protein diet or GI bleeding. It can also be a marker for hydration status—up in dehydration and down in FVE. Significantly low BUN; however, indicates that the liver isn't synthesizing urea from ammonia (a liver problem). High BUN with normal creatinine usually means the uremia is nonrenal (prerenal). BUN is also interpreted along with creatinine in determining renal function. This is called renal function studies. Normal BUN: Adult—10–20 mg/dL (some sources say 5–20 mg/dL). Critical value—↑100 mg/dL—significant renal impairment. BUN/creatinine ratio are usually ordered together. Normal BUN/Cr ratio—10:1. BUN and creatinine are usually ordered together to assess renal function.	Decreased BUN/creatinine ratio. **About BUN (blood urea nitrogen)** Because the kidneys excrete it, the amount reflected in the blood can be an indicator of how well the kidneys are doing. **About Creatinine:** Creatine lives in the skeletal muscle. When metabolized, creatinine is the end product. Creatinine is removed from the circulation and excreted by the kidneys. Serum creatinine rises with impaired renal function. In severe renal impairment, serum creatinine levels will eventually plateau but BUN will continue to rise. Liver function doesn't affect the creatinine enough to be clinically significant like with the BUN. With renal impairment, BUN rises *first*. Creatinine rises *later*.	Remember third spacing from burns and liver disease causing ascites can lead to volume depletion because the volume is leaving the vascular space and settling in other places (i.e., the abdomen). Explain the procedure to the client. Fasting isn't required.
CVP—central venous pressure (see definition above under FVE).	Decreased CVP indicates FVD (low volume).	The critical care nurse monitors hemodynamic status in conjunction with nursing observations.

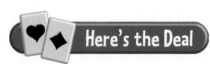

You can't just sit the water pitcher down and say "drink your fluids." Some patients have to be encouraged and you need to be specific about adequate intake. For example, you may say, "I need you to drink this 8-ounce glass of juice and then you need to go back in a reasonable amount of time and make sure you have done it."

Interventions and why?

Depending on the type of fluid that is lost, fluids and electrolytes must be replaced. General guidelines to promote fluid/electrolyte balance include:

- Be alert for diagnoses that can put the patient at risk for developing a fluid volume deficit (FVD). (We want to identify the FVD before it becomes severe and life threatening.)

- Monitor for early signs of FVD such as concentrated urine, dry mucous membranes, decreased capillary refill, poor skin turgor, and confusion. (These are all signs of early FVD.)

- Provide fluids by mouth if the FVD is mild. (Replace fluids).

- Consult with the dietician to establish a hydration plan that is suitable to the patient and includes fluids that they like and those that meet both their fluid and electrolyte needs (establishing a plan and gaining patient input promotes attaining oral fluid replacement goals).
- Intravenous fluid replacement for severe FVD (to replace fluids rapidly).
- Aggressive treatment of the causative illness (i.e., persistent vomiting or diarrhea, polyuria, burns etc.) per physician order to replace lost fluid volume.
- Monitor CVP (the CVP will decrease with FVD because of decreased volume in the vascular space).
- Monitor LOC (FVD can cause mental changes such as confusion, combativeness, decrease LOC, etc.).
- Monitoring hourly urinary output: Urinary output is an indicator of renal perfusion, in severe FVD the kidneys may not be perfused adequately, leading to decreased urine output.
- Monitoring lab reports (electrolytes, urine specific gravity, hematocrit, BUN, creatinine) and relaying critical values to the physician.
- Monitoring vital signs frequently as dictated by patient condition: Vital signs are an indicator of what is happening in the vascular space and the effect on cardiac output.
- Monitoring daily weight: Knowing the patient's customary weight with comparison to the present weight aids in assessment of hydration.
- Monitoring intake and output (to determine fluid replacement needs and ensure adequate replacement is being achieved).

PATIENT TEACHING
- Provide information to the patient and family related to factors that can lead to dehydration.
- Teach the patient and family/caregivers how to measure their intake and output.
- Review medications with the patient focusing on side effects and interactions that can lead to FVD. Identify meds that promote fluid loss (i.e., diuretics).
- Provide instructions related to the identification of early signs and symptoms of FVD (concentrated urine, decreased urine output, dry mucous membranes, skin turgor).
- Teach the patient to identify activities/conditions that predispose to dehydration (excessive sweating, vomiting, diarrhea), and stress the importance of fluid replacement to avoid developing dehydration.
- Recommend reduction of alcohol and caffeine intake as indicated.
- This patient must be taught to weigh herself or himself daily, with a goal of maintaining body weight within 2 lb of normal. Standard guidelines for daily weights include the following:
  - Same time
  - Same scales

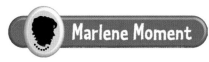

Marlene Moment

Don't make the mistake of putting fluids out of an elderly person's reach and expect her to meet her fluid intake requirements! She may try to get across the room to the bedside table that was moved under the window to get a sip, but then you may have a broken hip or other injury to deal with...this will SCARE the NCLEX©lady.

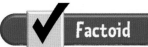

Factoid

Have you ever heard anybody say, "I can't think! My brain is just dried up." So true! FVD affects mental function because of decreased cerebral perfusion.

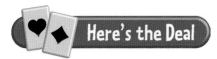

Here's the Deal

Caregivers of cognitively impaired patients and home health aides caring for bedfast patients should be taught that such patients will not report thirst or call for water; therefore, a plan must be developed to prevent FVD in susceptible patient populations. If the patient can swallow without risk of aspiration, teach the caregivers to:
- Keep fresh water readily available and encourage frequent sipping, or administer small amounts of water by syringe into the patient's cheek.
- Use Jell-O, sherbets, and flavored water for variety in pushing oral fluids.
- Small amounts of oral rehydration solutions (CytoMax, Elete, Rehydralyte) may be given to replace electrolyte loss.

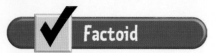

Patients with Addison's disease have adrenal cortical insufficiency and cannot maintain circulating volume because they are losing sodium and water (not enough aldosterone secretion).

- Same clothes
- Void first
- Depending on the severity of the FVD, the most immediate priority is fluid volume replacement therapy to reverse shock and restore perfusion to vital organs. The faster, the better!
  - Raise the patient's legs 30 degrees to quickly accomplish a rapid autoinfusion into systemic circulation from the peripheral venous system (Fig. 2-5)![3]

▶ Figure 2-5. Raising the Patient's Legs. By raising the patient's legs 30 degrees, blood from the lower extremities will rush back into systemic circulation and help perfuse vital organs. (Photo property of Hurst Review Services.)

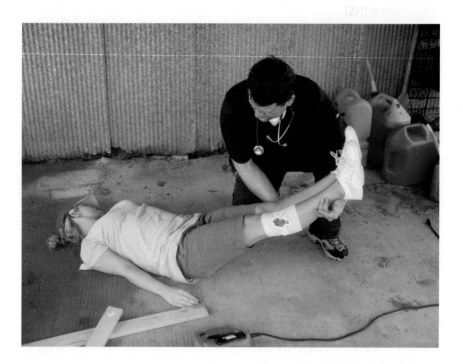

- This can be done while obtaining venous access for a bolus of isotonic intravenous fluid to increase circulating volume.
- If hemorrhage is the cause of FVD/shock natural colloids or synthetic plasma extenders such as dextran or hydroxyethyl starch [HES] solutions[4] may be used for volume replacement while blood is being prepared (type and cross-match).
- Or, depending upon the urgency of the situation, the physician may sign for an emergency transfusion to bypass some of the standard cross-checks.

What can harm my patient?

- Shock
- Kidney failure related to poor volume and decreased perfusion
- Acid–base imbalance
- Cardiac arrhythmias related to electrolyte imbalances
- Reaction to blood transfusion

- Death from total organ failure (depending on the severity)
- If the patient is hemorrhaging, he or she could bleed to death before the volume has been restored with necessary fluids and blood (Table 2-2).[4]

Table 2-2 IV fluid therapy

Tonicity and types IVF	Uses/qualities of fluid	Precautions
Isotonic Solutions: NaCL 0.9%, also called normal saline (NS): - Na⁺ 154 mEq/L - Cl⁻ 154 mEq/L	Isotonic solutions go into the vascular space and stay put! No movement of fluid occurs with balanced (equal) solutions. Isotonic solutions build up vascular volume.	Excessive volumes of NS can lead to volume overload and acidosis owing to the chloride excess. Use caution in the elderly, cardiac patients, and renal patients: risk of overload!
Lactated Ringers (LR) - Na⁺ 130 mEq/L - K⁺ 4 mEq/L Dextrose 5% water - 50 g dextrose - No electrolytes	LR is very similar in concentration of electrolytes to blood plasma (except for magnesium which is lacking), and is wonderful for treating hypovolemia when fluids and electrolytes are lost. D5W is isotonic initially (because of its osmolality), but as soon as the dextrose is metabolized by the cell, free water left behind dilutes remaining fluid becoming hypotonic, which is great if the patient has hypernatremia and needs the blood diluted!	The lactate in LR becomes bicarbonate when metabolized, and can lead to alkalosis if the pH is already high. Contraindicated in renal patients owing to K⁺ content. When dextrose is added to NaCl in any concentration, the solution becomes hypertonic (adding more particles increases osmolality), but when sugars are metabolized, free water dilutes the blood, posing problems with elderly, cardiac, and renal patients because of volume overload. Head-injured patients should not receive D5W because the free water will increase cerebral edema.
Hypotonic Solutions: - 0.45 NaCl (1/2 strength) - 0.33 NaCl - D 2.5% W	Hypotonic solutions are taken up by the cell for hydration to support metabolism. They do not stay in the vascular space, so they don't drive up circulating volume or blood pressure. They provide free water to help the kidneys excrete particles (solutes) in solution.	Excessive volumes of hypotonic solutions can cause large fluid shifts out of the vascular space into the cells leading to cardiovascular collapse and increased ICP.[6]
Hypertonic Solutions: 3% NaCl contains: - Na⁺ 513 mEq/L - Cl⁻ 513 mEq/L 5% NaCl contains: - Na⁺ 855 mEq/L - Cl⁻ 855 mEq/L Dextrose 10% water Dextrose 50% Total parenteral nutrition (TPN) contains dextrose for calories, amino acids for protein, electrolytes, and vitamins as prescribed.	The hypertonicity (increased osmolality) causes a shift of water from the cells into the vascular space, diluting the particles and expanding vascular volume. Excess fluid is removed from the cells, reducing cellular edema. High concentrations of sodium are used when the patient has severe hyponatremia. High concentrations of dextrose are used to prevent or treat hypoglycemia.	Hypertonic solutions are packed with particles, each of which acts like a sponge, pulling water into the vascular space to dilute the particles. These solutions must be administered very slowly to prevent FVE and resultant pulmonary edema.

▶ Figure 2-6. Fluid Movement with Hyper-, Iso-, and Hypo-Tonic Solutions. Water shifts out of the cells with hypertonic solutions into the vascular space. Isotonic solutions stay in the vascular system and do not cause a fluid shift. Hypotonic fluids shift water into the cells.

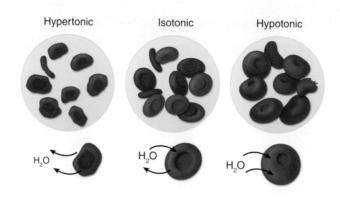

| Hypertonic | Isotonic | Hypotonic |

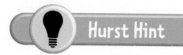

Hurst Hint

- **I**sotonic Solutions stay where **I** put them!
- Hyp**O**tonic Solutions go **O**ut of the vascular space!
- Hyp**E**rtonic Solutions **E**nter the vascular space (Fig. 2-6)!

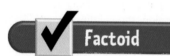

Factoid

When dextrose is added to saline solution or lactated ringers solution, the solution becomes hypertonic (packed with particles/acts like a sponge)! Examples:

- D5LR (contains sugar, sodium, and potassium particles)
- D5NS (contains sugar and sodium particles)
- D5½NS (contains sugar and sodium particles)
- D5¼NS (contains sugar and sodium particles)

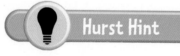

Hurst Hint

Keeping close check on the urine specific gravity is an important part of managing fluid replacement therapy.

Flow rates of IVF vary according to the severity of fluid loss and the body's hemodynamic response to IVF therapy.[7]

ELECTROLYTE IMBALANCES

✚ Hyponatremia

What is it?

Hyponatremia is a serum sodium level <135 mEq/L.[1]

Causes and why?

In hyponatremia, a patient has either lost too much sodium from the vascular space or gained too much water in the vascular space.

The following table shows the causes of hyponatremia related to a loss of sodium from the vascular space, and why these occur.

Causes	Why
Addison's disease (adrenal insufficiency)	Decreased steroids (specifically aldosterone and cortisol). • Decreased aldosterone leads to loss of sodium and water. • Decreased cortisol leads to secretion of ADH, leading to retention of free water. • So the patient is retaining free water and losing sodium at the same time. • Blood becomes diluted and serum sodium decreases.
Loss of GI fluids	Fluids and electrolytes are lost with GI fluids (vomiting, diarrhea, NG suctioning, etc.). The gastric and intestinal mucosa is high in sodium concentrations.
Severe burns and wound drainage	Damaged blood vessels leads to excessive fluid and electrolyte loss.

(Continued)

Causes	Why
Excessive sweating	Not replacing the fluids lost through sweating with the right type of fluid (e.g., not using electrolyte containing sports drinks when playing sports in elevated temperatures).
Diuretics	Along with the loss of fluids, they inhibit the reabsorption of sodium as well.
Low-sodium diet	Not enough sodium in the diet for several months can cause decreased blood levels of sodium.
Vomiting and sweating	Loss of fluids and sodium.

Source: Created by the author from Reference 1.

The following table shows the causes of hyponatremia in relation to gaining too much water in the vascular space, and why these occur.

Causes	Why
Excessive administration of D5W	D5W contains increased amounts of free water, which could dilute the blood, causing the serum sodium to go down.
Too much water with tube feeding	If too much water is administered, the vascular space will become dilute, decreasing the serum sodium.
SIADH	A large amount of water is retained in the vascular space, causing dilution of blood.
Medications: • Oxytocin • Certain tranquilizers • Tap water enemas	Side effect is fluid retention. Side effect is fluid retention. Too much free water decreases the serum sodium.
Psychogenic polydipsia	Patients who are taking medications for psychological/psychiatric problems may experience dry mouth as a side effect of their medications. Excessive free water intake can lead to decreased serum sodium level.
Heart failure	Fluid volume overload with heart failure can lead to decreased serum sodium.
Hyperglycemia	Osmotic gradient causes water to leave the cell into the extracellular fluid which dilutes the serum sodium (water shifts into the vascular space, diluting the sodium level).
Cirrhosis	Water and sodium are both retained because of increased portal pressure. Increased portal pressure leads to increased aldosterone secretion, which leads to sodium and water retention. BUT water is retained in EXCESS of sodium, which leaves the serum sodium diluted.

Hurst Hint

Heart failure, cirrhosis, and nephrosis leave the body in a hypervolemic state.

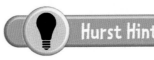

Hurst Hint

Advanced renal disease leaves the tubules of the kidneys unable to respond to ADH. Therefore, sodium and water are lost, leading to a decreased sodium level.

Signs and symptoms and why?

The following signs and symptoms and rationales are associated with hyponatremia.

Signs and symptoms	Why
Lethargy and confusion	Decreased excitability of cell membranes; brain does not function well with low levels of sodium.
Muscle weakness	Decreased excitability of cell membranes.
Decreased deep tendon reflexes (DTRs)	Decreased excitability of cell membranes.
Diarrhea	GI tract motility increases.
Respiratory problems	Late symptom; respiratory muscles become weak and can't function properly.

Source: Created by the author from Reference 1.

Interventions and why?

When sodium imbalances present themselves, the underlying cause must be identified and treated. For example:

- When hypernatremia (dehydration) is caused by diabetes insipidus (DI=not enough ADH), the patient is carefully rehydrated and given DDAVP, a synthetic vasopressin to promote water retention.

- If sodium excess/sodium retention is the problem, a careful history can identify sodium containing medications (prescribed and OTC) that may be discontinued or substituted with low-sodium alternates.

- Hyponatremia can result from either sodium depletion or sodium dilution.

  - If the patient has hyponatremia caused by SIADH (too much ADH), the primary problem is retention of water.

  - Rather than adding sodium, measures can be taken to pull water.

  - This can be accomplished with ultrafiltration (also called Aquapheresis), which can be performed with venous access/antecubital catheter (set up by a dialysis nurse and managed by an intensive care unit [ICU] nurse) to take off up to 4 L/24 hours.[8]

- If the underlying cause of the sodium imbalance is Addison's disease, Florinef (aldosterone) will be prescribed, and the patient will be instructed in daily weights to monitor fluid gain or loss, adjusting medications to keep weight between 2 and 3 lb of normal.

- If the sodium imbalance is severe enough to produce neurologic changes, a treatment plan must be implemented immediately to begin gradual restoration of a normal sodium balance. While corrective measures are underway, the priority nursing intervention is promoting physical safety:

- A-B-Cs first (airway, breathing, and circulation)
- Constant monitoring and protective positioning
- Seizure precautions

- My patient needs sodium: If hyponatremia is severe and neurologic signs are present, a hypertonic sodium (3%, 5%) will be prescribed.
- My patient does not need any more water!
  - Limit fluid to 800 mL/d
  - Administer hypertonic saline (3%, 5%) slowly in the intensive care setting with close monitoring of flow rate and patient response (neurologic status).
  - Monitor serum sodium levels throughout therapy, taking care to avoid overcorrecting or correcting too rapidly.
  - Strict I&O and daily weights (indicated for any patient with a fluid problem)

What can harm my patient and why?

Overhydrated brain cells and cerebral edema:

- Increased ICP
- Seizures
- Coma
- Permanent neurologic damage

PATIENT TEACHING

- If losing sodium and water, replacement with an electrolyte solution is needed, because plain water dilutes existing sodium in the vascular space and causes hyponatremia.
- Add sodium to the diet for Addison's disease (losing sodium and water), and drink electrolyte solution (sports drinks such as Gatorade), especially in warm weather.
- Patients who are retaining sodium and water (Cushing's disease or Cushing's syndrome, hyperaldosteronism/Conn's disease) are taught to limit dietary sodium; usually there is no added sodium.

Cutting edge

Vaprisol (Conivaptan) is a drug released in 2007 for the treatment of hypervolemic hyponatremia such as with SIADH. The drug blocks the effect of ADH on the kidneys, causing water to be excreted. Vaprisol, usually given as an IV bolus of 20 mg and followed by a slow drip, brings the serum sodium back into the normal range as excess water is removed from the vascular space. As vascular volume comes down, sodium level goes up!

✚ Hypernatremia

What is it?

Hypernatremia is serum sodium >145 mEq/L.[1] Hypernatremia is similar to dehydration: There is too much sodium and not enough water in the body.

Causes and why?

The following table details the causes of hypernatremia.

Causes	Why
Administration of IV normal saline without proper water replacement	Too much sodium, not enough water.
Hyperventilation	Exhalation causes water loss, which causes sodium excess.
Watery diarrhea	Fluid loss from the GI tract; water loss causes increased sodium concentration.
Hyperaldosteronism	Retention of large amount of sodium.
Renal failure	Kidneys not able to excrete excess sodium.
Heat stroke	Water loss exceeds sodium loss, causing sodium concentration of the blood.
NPO status	Decreased intake, causing hemoconcentration and increased sodium.
Infection	Fever associated with infection, causing loss of water and concentration of sodium.
Diabetes insipidus	Excess water loss, resulting in sodium concentration.

Source: Created by the author from Reference 1.

Signs and symptoms and why?

The signs and symptoms and corresponding rationales for hypernatremia are listed in the table.

Signs and symptoms	Why
Tachycardia	Heart pumps inadequate fluid trying to ensure tissue and organ perfusion.
Dry, sticky mucous membranes	Decreased saliva.
Thirst	Brain sends signals that fluids are needed to dilute the sodium.
Changes in level of consciousness (LOC)	Increased sodium interferes with brain function.
Decreased heart contractility	Late hypernatremia causes decreased excitability of muscles; high serum sodium decreases the movement of calcium into the cardiac cells, causing decreased contraction and cardiac output.
Seizure	Early hypernatremia causes increased muscle excitability.
Muscle twitching	Early hypernatremia causes increased muscle excitability.
Muscle weakness	Late hypernatremia causes decreased muscle response.
Decreased DTRs	Late hypernatremia causes decreased muscle response.

Source: Created by the author from Reference 1.

Testing, testing, testing: hyponatremia and hypernatremia

Test	Clinical significance	Nursing care and/or interfering factors
Normal adult sodium 136–145 mEq/L Critical value <120 or >160	Sodium lives in the extracellular fluid in greater quantities than any other electrolyte. Very little is found inside the cell. Sodium is responsible for water distribution and extracellular fluid volume. An increase or decrease in sodium causes an increase or decrease water. Low sodium causes water to be drawn into the cells. Increased sodium causes water to be pulled out of the cell. Remember, aldosterone and ADH help control sodium levels by exerting their effect on the kidneys to either retain sodium or excrete it.	Explain procedure to the patient. No fasting is required.

Interventions and why?

The most lethal of all the symptoms are the neurologic effects of hypernatremia or hyponatremia.

- A patient can die from a sodium imbalance, with nothing else being wrong!
- If the sodium imbalance is severe enough to produce neurologic changes, a treatment plan must be implemented immediately to begin gradual restoration of a normal sodium balance.
- While corrective measures are underway, the priority nursing intervention is promoting physical safety:
  - A-B-Cs first (airway, breathing, and circulation)
  - Constant monitoring and protective positioning
  - Seizure precautions
- The patient has too much sodium and not enough water, so he or she needs hemodilution. The patient does NOT need any more sodium!
- The brain cannot tolerate rapid shifts in sodium! Sodium levels must be reduced slowly (no faster than 1 mEq/hour)[6] to avoid cerebral edema, and serum sodium levels must be monitored frequently.
- Restrict sodium and hydrate.
- Dilute the patient with IVF: D5W is good because it makes free water to dilute the sodium, but if polyuria resulting from diabetic ketoacidosis (DKA) is the cause of intravascular dehydration, a hypotonic sodium chloride solution (0.3%) is used.
- Monitor patient neurologic response to therapy: LOC, behavior, pupils, mentation, orientation, following command, muscle strength, and power.
- Daily weight is an excellent indicator of fluid status.
- I&O is always indicated when the patient has a fluid problem.
- Daily labs (serum sodium, hematocrit, potassium, urine specific gravity)

PATIENT TEACHING

- No sodium-containing medications.
- Avoid foods high in sodium.
- Drink plenty of fluids.
- Thirst can be diminished in elderly—teach them to drink a certain *amount*. Do not rely on thirst mechanism.
- In patients with endocrine disorders such as Cushing's, Conn's, SIADH, DI, or diabetes they should monitor and report changes in urine color or output, and signs and symptoms of hypernatremia.
- Teach the elderly or those with endocrine disorders to avoid excessive heat, which leads to heat stroke and hypernatremia.

What can harm my patients and why?

- Seizures
- Acid–base imbalance
- Cardiac arrhythmias
- Permanent brain damage

✛ Hypokalemia

What is it?

Hypokalemia is serum potassium <3.5 mEq/L.[1]

Causes and why?

The following are the causes of hypokalemia:

Causes	Why
Diuretics, thiazide diuretics	Excretes potassium in the urine
Steroids	Retains sodium and water and excretes potassium
GI suction	Removes potassium from the GI tract
Vomiting	Loss of potassium from the GI tract
Diarrhea	Loss of potassium from the GI tract
NPO status; poor oral intake	Not taking in enough potassium
Age	Kidneys lose potassium with age
Cushing's syndrome	Sodium and water are retained, potassium is excreted
Kidney disease	Poor reabsorption of potassium
Alkalosis	Potassium moves into the cell dropping serum potassium
IV insulin	Drives potassium back into the cell, dropping serum potassium

Source: Created by the author from Reference 1.

Signs and symptoms and why?

The signs and symptoms and corresponding rationales for hypokalemia are shown in the following table:

Signs and symptoms	Why
Muscular weakness, cramps, flaccid paralysis	Potassium is needed for skeletal and smooth muscle contraction, nerve impulse conduction, acid–base balance, enzyme action, and cell membrane function.
Hyporeflexia	Muscle cells require potassium for cell membrane excitability.
Life-threatening arrhythmias	Heart cells require potassium for nerve impulse transmission and smooth muscle contraction.
Slow or difficult respirations	Respiratory muscles are weakened.
Weak, irregular pulse	Cardiac muscles are weakened.
Decreased bowel sounds	Hypomotility of GI tract.
ECG changes: ST segment depression; Flat T-wave; inverted T-wave	Potassium is needed for nerve impulse conduction.
Decreased LOC	Potassium is needed for excitability of brain cell membranes.

Source: Created by the author from References 1 and 3.

Interventions and why?

- The top priorities with both hyperkalemia and hypokalemia are monitoring cardiac status, establishing reliable venous access, and having emergency protocols in place in the event of a potentially life-threatening arrhythmia!

- Continuous cardiac monitoring is indicated, because potential lethal cardiac arrhythmias may occur (PVCs, ventricular tachycardia). Potassium replacement therapy will be administered as prescribed, diluted in intravenous fluid, given slowly with a flow rate control pump.

- When the patient has hypokalemia, a careful nursing history will usually reveal the mechanism of potassium loss (Table 2-3). If the patient is taking a cardiac glycoside such as digoxin or Lanoxin, watch for *early* signs of digitalis toxicity (anorexia, nausea, and vomiting) and intervene before the onset of *late* signs (yellow vision, bradycardia, arrhythmias, cardiac arrest).

- My patient needs potassium replacement, and oral supplements are administered if the potassium deficit is mild.

- Oral potassium tastes terrible! Dilute the medicine in juice, and administer with food to reduce GI upset.

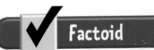

Factoid

Sodium and potassium have an inverse relationship: when one goes up, the other goes down!

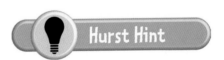

Hurst Hint

Potassium imbalance predisposes to the development of digitalis toxicity! Either hypokalemia or hyperkalemia can predispose to toxicity, but hypokalemia is usually the culprit! Here's my formula: Hypokalemia + Digitalis=Toxicity

- Patients at risk for hypokalemia (those taking thiazide diuretics, Ng suction, patients who are not eating, alcoholics) need a diet rich in potassium (see patient teaching below).
- Alcoholics who are diuresing (alcohol is hypertonic and suppresses ADH) are given information about the health issues associated with alcoholism, and referred to group support therapy (Alcoholics Anonymous).
- During prescribed IVF therapy with potassium containing fluids and with oral potassium administration; monitor urinary output closely because if urinary output decreases, the patient is retaining potassium and may develop hyperkalemia.
- If K^+ loss is the result of vomiting, administer prescribed antiemetic medications/suppositories.
- If K^+ loss is the result of nasogastric suction, monitor serum potassium and notify the physician of potassium levels "trending down" before actual hypokalemia develops.
- Monitor all patients at risk for development of hypokalemia for subjective complaint of muscle weakness or cramping. Don't wait for the development of flaccid paralysis!

PATIENT TEACHING

- Take oral potassium supplements with food to decrease GI irritation.
- Consult with your doctor before beginning any herbal medication.
- Add potassium-rich foods to the diet (see full list below).

Teach patients with compromised renal function to:

- Take the lowest possible dose of NSAIDs, and do not exceed the number of doses per day because of the danger of renal damage.
- Beware of sodium substitutes because even normal usage may lead to excessive potassium ingestion.
- Beware of "low-salt" packaged foods: They contain high potassium!
- Explain the rationale for avoiding salt substitutes: Because of the inability to excrete potassium, toxicity can occur and can stop the heart!
- Patients having Addison's disease (hyperkalemia) and renal failure patients are encouraged to limit dietary potassium (spinach, fennel, kale, mustard greens, brussel sprouts, broccoli, eggplant, cantaloupe, tomatoes, parsley, cucumber, bell pepper, apricots, ginger root, strawberries, avocado, banana, tuna, halibut, cauliflower, kiwi, oranges, potatoes, lima beans, and cabbage).
- Patients having Cushing's disease (hypokalemia) are encouraged to include the above potassium-rich foods in the diet.
- Caution patients taking oral potassium supplement to report any abdominal discomfort, distention, or dark stools immediately because potassium can produce small bowel lesions, which may lead to GI bleeding.

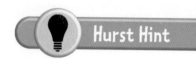

Hurst Hint

When the patient has renal failure, think hyperkalemia!

What can harm my patients and why?

- Increased cardiac irritability.
- Life-threatening arrhythmias.
- My patient is at risk for a lethal arrhythmia and/or sudden cardiac death.

Cutting edge

Hypokalemia is found to occur following trauma, occurring more frequently in younger adults than older adults,[9] who are theorized to have a blunted response to epinephrine. Severity of trauma in this study had previously been correlated with higher levels of epinephrine upon admission to the emergency department, and those patients with significantly high epinephrine also had hypokalemia. A similar epinephrine surge is seen in thyroid storm (thyrotoxicosis) and this also produces hypokalemia induced by Na-K-ATPase, which causes an influx of serum potassium into the cell, necessitating the use of beta blockers for patients in thyroid storm.[10]

Although recovery consists of potassium replacement while being alert to the risk for lethal arrhythmias, attention is focused on risk reduction by a careful review of the patient history and medication reconciliation records. Medications are carefully reviewed and those that reduce serum potassium (thiazide and loop diuretics, penicillin, aminoglycosides) may be re-evaluated in terms of risk versus benefit; however, when hypokalemia is severe enough to cause life-threatening arrhythmias, it is always wise to look for other causes.[10]

✚ Hyperkalemia

What is it?

Hyperkalemia is serum potassium >5 mEq/L.[1]

Causes and why?

The following table details the causes and why of hyperkalemia.

Cause	Why
Renal failure	Kidneys aren't able to excrete potassium.
IV potassium chloride overload	Too much potassium in the IV fluid.
Burns or crushing injuries	Potassium is released when cells rupture.
Tight tourniquets	Red blood cells rupture and release potassium when the tourniquet has been placed too tightly.
Hemolysis of blood sample	Damaged cells in the sample result in a false high reading.
Incorrect blood draws	Drawing blood above the IV (housing potassium) insertion site will cause a false high reading.

(Continued)

Cause	Why
Salt substitutes	Usually made from potassium chloride.
Potassium-sparing diuretics	Retain potassium.
Blood transfusions	Deliver elevated levels of potassium in the transfused blood.
ACE inhibitors	Retain potassium.
Tissue damage	Destroys cells releasing potassium into the blood stream.
Acidosis	Causes serum potassium to increase.
Adrenal insufficiency (Addison's disease)	Causes sodium and water loss and potassium retention.
Chemotherapy	Destroys cells releasing potassium into the blood stream.

Source: Created by the author from Reference 1.

Signs and symptoms and why?

Following are the signs and symptoms and associated rationales of hyperkalemia.

Signs and symptoms	Why
Begins with muscle twitching associated with tingling and burning; progresses to numbness, especially around mouth; proceeds to weakness and flaccid paralysis	Excess potassium interferes with skeletal and smooth muscle contraction, nerve impulse conduction, acid–base balance, enzyme action, and cell membrane function.
Diarrhea	Smooth muscles of the intestines hypercontract, resulting in increased motility.
Cardiac arrhythmia; bradycardia; ECG changes: peaked T wave, flat or no P wave, wide QRS complex; ectopic beats on ECG, leading to complete heart block, asystole, ventricular tachycardia, or ventricular fibrillation	Dysfunctional nerve impulse conduction and smooth muscle contraction.

Source: Created by the author from References 1 and 3.

Testing, testing, testing: hypokalemia and hyperkalemia

Test	Clinical significance	Nursing care and/or interfering factors
Normal serum potassium (adult)—3.5–5 mEq/L Critical value—<2.5 mEq/L	Potassium imbalances can lead to life-threatening cardiac arrhythmias. Note: Calcium gluconate decreases arrhythmias Note: Insulin carries glucose AND potassium into the cell. Be alert for hypokalemia and hypoglycemia when administering IV insulin.	Have the patient keep arm still during venipuncture, because movement of the arm with tourniquet in place can elevate the serum potassium level. Instruct the patient not to open and close the hand while the tourniquet is in place. If the blood sample hemolyzes, the serum potassium level will be increased.

(Continued)

Test	Clinical significance	Nursing care and/or interfering factors
	Kayexalate is given for hyperkalemia by exchanging sodium for potassium in the GI tract	Medications can interfere with the potassium test and cause it to be elevated (antibiotics, potassium sparing diuretics, glucocorticoids, heparin, histamine, mannitol, potassium supplements, salicylates, etc.) or decreased (aminosalicylic acid, potassium wasting diuretics, glucose infusions, insulin, laxatives, lithium carbonate, Kayexalate).
	Review s/s chart for hypokalemia and hyperkalemia	Fasting for the test is not required.
	Increased potassium:	Explain the procedure to the patient.
	Chronic renal failure	Be alert for cardiac arrhythmias with increased or decreased potassium levels.
	Renal tubular acidosis	Patients taking digoxin and diuretics.
	Cushing's syndrome	Dietary intake can affect the potassium level. Excess ingestion of licorice will elevate the urine potassium level.
	Hyperaldosteronism	
	Large intake of licorice	
	Alkalosis	If 24-hour urine—start 24-hour collection after voiding and discarding the urine. Specimen starts at this point. Must keep specimen container with urine on ice or in the refrigerator. Instruct the patient to void prior to bowel movements to prevent contamination of the urine specimen. No toilet paper in the urine specimen. Drink fluids for the whole 24 hours. Void at the end of the 24-hour period and include it in the specimen. After a 24-hour specimen is collected it must be transported as soon as possible to the lab.
	Diuretic therapy	
	Decreased potassium:	
	Dehydration	
	Addison's disease	
	Malnutrition	
	Vomiting	
	Diarrhea	
	Malabsorption	
	Acute renal failure	

Interventions and why?

- The top priorities with both hyperkalemia and hypokalemia are monitoring cardiac status, establishing reliable venous access, and having emergency protocols in place in the event of a potentially life-threatening arrhythmia!

- All of my patients at risk for the development of hyperkalemia need to be closely monitored to detect early symptoms.

- Emergency management of hyperkalemia will include measures to stabilize the heart and lower serum potassium:

  - Administering calcium salts (calcium gluconate or calcium chloride) is the first step to stabilize the heart, reducing the incidence of life-threatening arrhythmias.

- Insulin to drive potassium into the cell, lowering serum potassium.

- Beta agonists (Albuterol) to temporarily lower potassium (4–6 hours) while awaiting hemodialysis.

- Bicarbonate if metabolic acidosis is present to cause a shift of K^+ back into the cell.

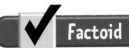

Factoid

Calcium gluconate won't work if the patient is in shock with decreased perfusion to the liver because the gluconate can't be metabolized; therefore, calcium chloride must be used instead.

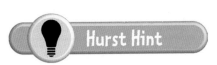

Hurst Hint

Calcium chloride is three times more potent than calcium gluconate, and also causes tissue damage if it extravasates.

- Cation exchange resins and laxatives (Kayexalate): Used for mild hyperkalemia resulting from slow onset of action.
- Hemodialysis to filter and remove excess K^+ from the blood.

Be alert to patients having impaired renal function, elderly patients, any patient with unexplained muscle weakness, and those receiving causative medications (see Table 2-3), especially when used concurrently. Depending on the cause, my patient needs:

- Continuous cardiac monitoring as the potassium imbalance is being corrected.
- Dialysis if the kidneys aren't working.
- Calcium gluconate if ECG changes are present (decreases arrhythmias).
- Glucose and insulin infusion to drive potassium into the cell.
- Accu-Chek (glucose monitoring) to detect hypoglycemia while insulin is being administered.
- Measures to prevent hypoglycemia (such as periodic snacks) during administration of IV insulin.
- Close monitoring of serum potassium levels: The patient can go from hyperkalemia to hypokalemia during the infusion of glucose and insulin.
- Administration of cation exchange agent such as Kayexalate (sodium polystyrene sulfonate), which exchanges Na^+ for K^+ in the GI tract.
- Push fluids (unless contraindicated) during administration of Kayexalate to prevent dehydration/hypernatremia: As the serum potassium comes down, the serum sodium goes up because we are trading one electrolyte for the other.
- When the patient has renal failure: Think hyperkalemia!
- Beware of sodium substitutes, because even normal usage may lead to excessive potassium ingestion.
- Beware of "low-salt" packaged foods: They contain high potassium!
- Explain the rationale for avoiding salt substitutes: Because of inability to excrete potassium, toxicity can occur and can stop the heart!
- Patients having Addison's disease (hyperkalemia) and renal failure patients are encouraged to limit dietary potassium (spinach, fennel, kale, mustard greens, brussel sprouts, broccoli, eggplant, cantaloupe, tomatoes, parsley, cucumber, bell pepper, apricots, ginger root, strawberries, avocado, banana, tuna, halibut, cauliflower, kiwi, oranges, potatoes, lima beans, and cabbage).
- Patients having Cushing's disease (hypokalemia) are encouraged to include the above potassium-rich foods in the diet.

What can harm my patients?

- Cardiac arrhythmias
- Acid–base imbalance
- Muscle paralysis
- Death

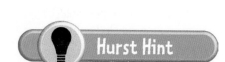

Hurst Hint

Always think HEART first when your patient has a potassium imbalance!

+ Calcium and magnesium imbalances

Let's get the normal stuff straight first!

Calcium is responsible for:

- Building bone and teeth
- Creating nerve impulses
- Muscle contractility

The **sodium potassium pump** (cell membrane) of all cells is responsible for transmitting nerve signals and for nerve function throughout the entire nervous system by maintaining the electrical charge of the cell. The electrical charge is maintained by pumping *sodium out of* the cell and pumping *potassium into* the cell. The **calcium pump** of the cell membrane is important for the function of the nervous system and transmittal of nerve impulses too. It pumps *calcium out* of the cell through calcium channels.

Decreased calcium levels cause the cell membrane to be more permeable to sodium, making the action potential much easier to obtain, or more excitable. High excitability can lead to spontaneous discharging of the nerve, leading to muscle contractions and even tetany. So, to sum it up, calcium leads to neuromuscular excitability.

Cardiac and smooth muscle cells are full of calcium channels, leaving the neuromuscular function of these types of cells very dependent on the transport of calcium across the cell membrane.

Calcium is responsible for the contraction of cardiac, smooth, and skeletal muscle, the transmission of nerve impulses, blood clotting, and much more.

Neurons (nerve cells) are excitable cells and very sensitive to changes in calcium ion concentrations. The nervous system becomes *more* excited when calcium levels fall. The nervous system slows down when calcium levels rise.

Daily intake is approximately 1000 mg/d. Vitamin D enables calcium to be absorbed from the intestines. Only about 350 mg (35%) is actually absorbed. The majority of the rest (of daily calcium intake) is excreted in the feces. Only about 10% is excreted by the kidneys. When calcium is low, the kidneys will reabsorb it to prevent *any* loss. Even slight increases of calcium will trigger the kidneys to increase calcium excretion.

Magnesium is necessary for the following functions:

- Regulation of intracellular enzymes and electrolytes
- DNA synthesis and metabolism of proteins and carbohydrates
- Excitability of cardiac and skeletal muscles at the neuromuscular junction

About half of all magnesium is stored in the bone with the calcium, and a little less than half is inside the cell, leaving low levels, only about 5% as free cations circulating in the blood (1.2–2.1 mEq/L). Like calcium, most of the magnesium is physiologically inactive (bound to proteins).

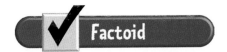

Factoid

Tetany is defined as tetanic contractions of the muscles caused by spontaneous discharges of the nerves. It only takes a 50% reduction of calcium to cause tetany.

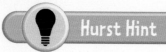

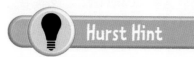

What else do calcium and magnesium have in common?

- MUSCLES! Magnesium and calcium affect neuromuscular excitability.
- Regulating the contraction and relaxation of muscles is critical to maintaining cardiac output, heart rate, and rhythm and respirations.
- Both magnesium and calcium have a sedative effect.
- Too much of either will cause excessive muscle relaxation, which could be life threatening if the heart muscle or the diaphragm becomes flaccid.
- Too little of either calcium or magnesium has the opposite effect, producing tight, rigid muscles.
- When levels of magnesium or calcium are low, PTH stimulates the release of these electrolytes from the bone where they are stored, to raise the blood (serum) level.

✚ Hypermagnesemia and hypercalcemia
What is it?

Serum calcium exceeds 12 mg/dL. Elevated levels of calcium cause the nervous system to become sluggish with decreased reflex activities of the central nervous system. The signs begin to *appear* at around 12 mg/dL, but become very obvious at around 15 mg/dL. At levels above 17 mg/dL calcium phosphate crystals may appear throughout the body (parathyroid poisoning).

> *High* calcium → *Decreased* neuromuscular excitability

- The patient with hypercalcemia has high serum levels of calcium, in excess of 10.5 mg/dL, or levels of ionized calcium exceeding 5.1 mg/dL.
- The serum magnesium is elevated, in excess of the normal range (2.1 mEq/L).
- This patient is overly SEDATED! Magnesium and calcium cause neuromuscular sedation and killer complications result from their sedative action.
- Most of the magnesium is found in the bone and the cells.
- Only a small portion of the magnesium in the body is located in the serum.
- One-third of serum magnesium is bound to protein, and the remainder is ionized (physiologically active).
- Hypermagnesemia is a serum magnesium level >2.1 mEq/L.[1]

Causes and why?

HYPERMAGNESEMIA

Cause	Why
Renal failure	Kidneys are unable to excrete magnesium.
Increased oral or IV intake	Body cannot process excessive magnesium.
Antacids	Many antacids contain a large amount of magnesium, which can build up in the blood making it difficult for the kidneys to excrete the excess.

Source: Created by the author from Reference 1.

HYPERCALCEMIA   The table explores the causes and why of hypercalcemia.

Cause	Why
Hyperparathyroidism	**Primary hyperparathyroidism**—usually caused by a tumor of one of the parathyroid glands. This is more common in women because the parathyroids are stimulated during pregnancy and lactation. Excessive PTH is produced causing the serum calcium to rise as a result of the effect of PTH on the bone, intestines, and kidneys. Note: Primary hyperparathyroidism can cause severe bone disease because of reabsorption, leaving the bone brittle, weak, and easily fractured. X-rays may show where the bone has been eaten away. **Secondary hyperparathyroidism**—PTH is released to compensate for hypocalcemia caused by deficiency of vitamin D or chronic renal disease. In chronic renal disease, the kidneys can't produce the active form of vitamin D. Vitamin D deficiency interrupts absorption of calcium from the intestines. **Primary hyperparathyroidism = hypercalcemic** **Secondary hyperparathyroidism = hypocalcemic**
Bone metastasis	• Many tumors produce PTH. PTH elevates the serum calcium level. • Cancer of the bone, or metastasis to the bone because as bone is destroyed, calcium is released into circulation.
Sarcoidosis	Sarcoidosis may increase vitamin D levels.
Excess vitamin D	Vitamin D promotes calcium absorption.
Immobilization	Calcium leaves the bones and moves into the blood stream (absorption).
Increased calcium intake	Increases serum calcium.
Thiazide diuretics	Cause calcium retention.
Kidney illness	Can cause retention of calcium. Hyperphosphatemia promotes hypocalcemia.
Changes in the blood pH	Acidosis causes less calcium to become bound to protein, thereby increasing ionized serum calcium.[6]

Source: Created by the author from Reference 1.

CAUSES OF HYPOMAGNESEMIA AND HYPERMAGNESEMIA

HypOmagnesemia (not enough magnesium)	HypERmagnesemia (too much magnesium)
Magnesium intake is dependent upon dietary ingestion and absorption. The most frequent "hypo-mag" patient is the alcoholic, and here's why: • Alcohol makes you diurese and Mg^+ is excreted by the kidneys. • Alcohol suppresses the ADH hormone, increasing diuresis. • The alcoholic doesn't like to eat! They prefer to drink instead, and we get magnesium from the foods that we eat, which is why patients having malabsorption syndromes and malnourished patients also develop hypomagnesemia. Other causes of increased magnesium losses include the following: • Increased losses of Mg^+ because of diuretic therapy causing renal excretion. • Chronic diarrhea or laxative abuse: a lot of Mg^+ lives in the intestine! • Prolonged GI suction or vomiting: Mg^+ is a resident of the GI tract!	Hypermagnesemia can happen because of the following: • Chronic renal failure is the most common cause![11] Magnesium is excreted primarily by the kidneys! • If the kidneys aren't working, magnesium levels go up! • Excessive ingestion of magnesium containing medications such as laxatives or antacids. • Excessive administration of IV magnesium in the treatment of pregnancy-induced hypertension (PIH), to stop preterm labor can produce iatrogenic hypermagnesemia.

Signs and symptoms and why?

The following table explores the signs and symptoms and rationales associated with hypermagnesemia.

Signs and symptoms	Why
BP decreases	Magnesium causes vasodilation, which decreases BP.
Facial warmth and flushing	Excess magnesium dilates the capillary beds.
Drowsiness to comatose state depending on severity of imbalance	Excess magnesium acts like a sedative.
Decreased DTRs	Excess magnesium reduces electrical conduction in the muscles, making them sluggish.
Generalized weakness	Excess magnesium reduces electrical conduction in the muscles, making them sluggish.
Decreased respirations to respiratory arrest depending on severity of imbalance	Hypoactive respiratory muscles.
Cardiac changes: decreased pulse; prolonged PR and wide QRS; cardiac arrest	Central nervous depression and smooth muscle relaxation.

Source: Created by the author from Reference 1.

The table lists the signs and symptoms and corresponding rationales of hypercalcemia.

Signs and symptoms of hypercalcemia	Why
Decreased DTRs	Excess calcium causes a sedative effect and decreases tendon reflexes.
Muscle weakness	Excess calcium causes a sedative effect on the peripheral nervous system, weakening the muscles.
Renal calculi (kidney stones)	• Extra calcium and phosphate are absorbed from the intestines. • Calcium is mobilized from the bone. • Leads to increased concentrations of calcium and phosphorus in the urine leading to the formation of crystals.
Pathologic fractures	Vitamin D deficiency or chronic renal disease in which the kidneys can't produce the active form of vitamin D can result in osteomalacia (decreased mineralization of the bones). In this case, the calcium level is **low,** causing increased production of PTH (so you have too little calcium in bone AND blood, related to the deficiency of vitamin D). Bones are brittle because calcium has moved from the bone into the blood.
Central nervous system (CNS) depression: • Lethargy • Coma • Confusion • Behavioral changes	Excess calcium sedates the nervous system.
Early cardiac changes: • Increased P wave • Decreased ST segment • Decreased QT interval • Increased BP • Depressed T waves	Mild hypercalcemia increases cardiac activity.
Late cardiac changes: • Decreased pulse (bradycardia) moving to cardiac arrest • Heart block	Severe hypercalcemia decreases cardiac activity.
Respiratory arrest	Sedated or sluggish respiratory muscles; decreased oxygenation.
Gastrointestinal • Constipation • Decreased bowel sounds (Hypoperistalsis) • Abdominal pain • Peptic ulcer • Decreased appetite	Muscle walls of the GI tract have decreased contractility impairing function.
Increased urine output	Kidneys working to rid of excess calcium, which depletes the vascular space.
Increased clotting	Calcium normally functions to assist with blood clotting. Excess calcium → increased clotting.

Source: Created by the author from Reference 1.

The following table explores the signs and symptoms and related rationales of hypomagnesemia.

Signs and symptoms of hypomagnesemia	Why
Increased neuromuscular irritability	Decreased levels of magnesium can cause neuromuscular irritability.
Seizure	Decreased levels of magnesium can cause neuromuscular hyperactivity.
Hyperactive DTRs	Decreased levels of magnesium can cause neuromuscular hyperactivity.
Laryngeal stridor	The larynx is smooth muscle; if there is not enough magnesium to sedate it, spasms will occur.
+ Chvostek's and Trousseau's signs	Decreased levels of magnesium can cause muscular spasms.
Cardiac changes: arrhythmias; peaked T waves; depressed ST segment; ventricular tachycardia; ventricular fibrillation; irregular heart beat	The heart is a smooth muscle. If there is not enough magnesium to sedate it, impaired nerve conduction and muscle spasms can occur.
Dysphagia	The esophagus is a smooth muscle; if there is not enough magnesium to sedate it, muscle tightness will occur.
Hypertension	Decreased magnesium causes vasoconstriction.
Decreased GI motility	GI muscles contract stalling peristalsis; paralytic ileus may occur.
Changes in LOC	Confusion or psychosis may be caused by central nervous excitability because of decreased magnesium.

Source: Created by the author from Reference 1.

Common signs and symptoms of both

Common symptoms of both hypermagnesemia and hypercalcemia are neuromuscular. (Remember: Magnesium and calcium act like sedatives!)

- Decreased LOC, drowsiness, confusion, lethargy, or impaired memory.
- Slurred speech, impaired ability to articulate words because of weak muscles of mouth and tongue.
- Sluggish, hypoactive reflexes (1+ to absent 0 DTRs).
- Weak, flaccid muscle tone (muscles are sedated).
- Bradycardia, cardiac arrhythmias: Decreased neuromuscular excitability causes changes in electrical conduction of the heart: shorter QT interval, prolonged PR interval, widening of the QRS complex and can lead to heart block, and/or cardiac arrest.
- Hypotension (musculature around vessels becomes weak and dilates).
- Decreased respiratory rate (sedative effect slows everything down).

Testing, testing, testing: hypocalcemia and hypercalcemia[12]

Test	Clinical significance	Nursing care and/or interfering factors
Normal *total* serum calcium (adult)— 9–10.5 mg/dL Normal *ionized* serum calcium (adult)— 4.5–5.6 mg/dL These values tend to be less in elderly patients Tetany occurs around 6 mg/dL 4 mg/dL is lethal	Total serum calcium is the combination of both the ionized (unbound) and nonionized (bound) calcium. About half is bound to the protein albumin and the other half is ionized and physiologically active. Hyperparathyroidism, malignancies, excess vitamin D ingestion, sarcoidosis, and tuberculosis are the most common causes of *hypercalcemia*. Hypoalbuminemia, malnutrition and alcoholism, blood transfusions, intestinal malabsorption, renal failure, rhabdomyolysis, alkalosis, and pancreatitis	If the albumin level is low, the total serum calcium level will be reflected as low. *BUT* this is "pseudohypocalcemia" because the ionized portion will continue to be normal even though the total serum calcium is low. When evaluating the calcium level in the presence of hypoalbuminemia, adjustments have to be made to determine the corrected total serum calcium because the albumin is decreased. A formula can be used to estimate the "corrected calcium" level. However, in critically ill patients the ionized calcium will be directly measured by a special technique rather than estimated with a formula. Remember, the pH determines the level of ionized calcium. If the patient is hypoalbuminemic in the presence of alkalosis, the ionized calcium will decrease because as the pH rises, the ionized calcium level decreases. So, when evaluating the serum calcium levels, one has to consider the albumin level AND the patient's acid–base status. Keeping the tourniquet on too long for venipuncture can increase the serum calcium level in the sample. Explain the procedure to the patient. Fasting is not required for this test alone, but may be part of another test that DOES require fasting. Calcium levels usually peak around 9 p.m. Excess milk ingestion can increase serum calcium levels. Decreased pH causes increased serum calcium level.

Testing, testing, testing: hypomagnesemia and hypermagnesemia

Test	Clinical significance	Nursing care and/or interfering factors
Normal adult serum magnesium—1.3–2.1 mEq/L Critical value <0.5 mEq/L	Most of the body's magnesium is inside the cell, about half of which is inside the bone. Magnesium is bound to ATP (source of energy), so it is extremely important for metabolic processes. Low magnesium can result in cardiac irritability and arrhythmias. Hypermagnesemia slows neuromuscular conduction. Slowed cardiac conduction is manifested as widened PR and QT intervals and wide QRS complex.	Potassium, magnesium, and calcium work together to keep the intracellular charge neutral. Low serum magnesium levels affect the potassium level as a result. Explain procedure to the patient. No fasting required. Leaving a tourniquet on too long can cause hemolysis and affect the level.

Interventions and why?

The A-B-Cs reflect nursing priorities when the patient has a magnesium or calcium imbalance (Table 2-3).

Table 2-3 Priority actions for magnesium/calcium emergencies

A-B-Cs for priority action: hypermagnesemia/hypercalcemia	A-B-Cs for priority action: hypomagnesemia/hypocalcemia
• A—Airway: When there is *excessive* calcium or magnesium, the patient is sedated! Protective positioning is indicated to prevent aspiration of secretions.	• A—Airway: With a *deficiency* of calcium or magnesium, the muscles are rigid and tight (NOT sedated) and the patient could develop swallowing problems, increasing the risk for aspiration. The airway can become obstructed and stridor may occur because of laryngospasm; therefore, a tracheotomy tray should be immediately available at the bedside.
• B—Breathing: Monitor respirations! If a magnesium infusion is in progress, discontinue the medication if respirations drop below 14 and call the doctor! When the patient has *excessive* (hyper) magnesium or calcium, the nurse must be prepared to support ventilation manually with a bag/mask device in the event of respiratory insufficiency or respiratory arrest (muscles sedated) while preparations are underway for endotracheal intubation and mechanical ventilation. Calcium gluconate is the antidote for magnesium toxicity when the diaphragm is too weak (or paralyzed) for effective ventilation.	• B—Breathing: When the patient has a *deficiency* (hypo) of magnesium or calcium, bronchospasm may close off the airway if the larynx becomes rigid and tight, so the nurse must have a tracheotomy tray at the bedside, and notify the doctor immediately if signs of latent tetany are present: positive Chvostek's or Trousseau's sign. If laryngospasm is in progress, an emergency tracheotomy must be performed immediately. A seizure may also be in progress, which will require suction of mucus or blood from the mouth if tongue trauma has occurred.
• C—Circulation: Monitor for arrhythmias! A stat magnesium level may be ordered: 7 mmol/L=cardiotoxic! *Excess* of magnesium or calcium may lead to bradycardia (slowing down the heart, decreasing cardiac output, decreasing electrical conduction through the heart) and cardiac arrest.	• C—Circulation: *Deficit* of magnesium or calcium may lead to arrhythmias secondary to hyperirritability of the heart muscle, and ventricular fibrillation. Notify the rapid response team first (getting immediate help for the patient), and then notify the primary physician.

- Patients with diarrhea are treated promptly, because magnesium is a resident of the GI tract.
- The patient with an ileostomy, who has liquid stool draining continuously, has increased magnesium losses and needs periodic evaluation of serum magnesium.
- Increased dietary sources of magnesium are encouraged: such as summer squash, green beans, and halibut.
- Many foods high in magnesium are hard to digest, or increase peristalsis and are not recommended for the patient with an ileostomy (sesame seeds, flax seeds, pumpkin seeds, celery).
- Known alcoholic patients are encouraged to join an AA 12-step program, and some patients may be given a deterrent to alcohol, such as Antabuse, but they must understand that any alcohol exposure/ingestion will produce a violent reaction. When known alcoholics are admitted to the hospital, a serum magnesium is routinely monitored, and magnesium is administered PRN.

- Patients with hypoparathyroidism need calcium replacement therapy and phosphorus-binding drugs to raise the serum calcium.
- PTH assay is monitored when there is risk of iatrogenic hypocalcemia (thyroidectomy, radical neck, irradiation to the neck).

Calcium

- The patient who has hypercalcemia is at risk for renal calculi and pathologic fractures because of brittle bones.
- Vitamin D supplements, phosphorus, and steroids may be given to lower the serum calcium level.
- Calcitonin may be prescribed to drive calcium back into the bones.
- Forcing fluids (unless contraindicated) is recommended for keeping urine dilute to reduce the incidence of nephrolithiasis.
- The patient should drink enough water to produce 2.5 L of urine per day (24–32 oz is recommended three times daily).
- Treatment for hypercalcemia caused by primary hyperparathyroidism (too much PTH) is surgical removal of some of the parathyroids (parathyroidectomy).
- This surgery may be necessary because of secondary hypocalcemia–producing conditions (such as chronic renal failure) that result in compensatory hyperactivity of the parathyroid glands (too much PTH).
- When this is the case, postoperative hypoparathyroidism is an even greater risk.[8] (Refer to Chapter 10, Metabolic and Endocrine Dysfunction.)
- For this reason, as well as improved renal disease outcomes, a drug that mimics calcium (cinacalcet) has been used as an alternate to surgery to lower serum calcium.[13]

The patient's needs vary according to the underlying cause of the electrolyte imbalance.

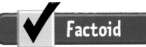

Factoid

When magnesium and calcium are in the presence of each other, they inactivate each other.

Hurst Hint

Calcium gluconate versus calcium chloride: Be sure you know the difference! Don't grab the wrong drug! Calcium gluconate=4.5 mEq calcium, but calcium chloride= 13.6 mEq calcium (three times more potent)!

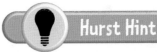

Hurst Hint

When does the NCLEX© lady want you to intervene: early or late? Early, of course! There are fewer patient complications if the doctor is notified before the onset of a code! The rapid response team likes to be notified *before* the patient is clinically dead!

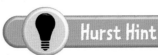

Hurst Hint

IV calcium must be administered slowly, and patients receiving IV calcium must be on a heart monitor. Be alert to widening of the QRS complex.

Causative factors associated with electrolyte imbalances: Mg⁺, Ca⁺	What my patient needs
Hypermagnesemia: Chronic renal failure Excess ingestion of magnesium	• Dialysis if renal failure is the cause of hypermagnesemia. • Volume-expanding IV fluids and diuresis to promote magnesium excretion. • Calcium gluconate administered as antidote to antagonize and inactivate the magnesium. • Monitor for arrhythmias: Be ready to intervene with emergency protocols in the event of a life-threatening arrhythmia.

(Continued)

Causative factors associated with electrolyte imbalances: Mg⁺, Ca⁺	What my patient needs
Hypercalcemia: Hyperparathyroidism (too much PTH) Thiazide diuretics (retain calcium) Immobilization (demineralized bone)	• If the kidneys are working: IVF administration (rapid) to increase urinary excretion of calcium. • Diuretics to aid in excretion and to prevent FVE from rapid IVF. • Calcitonin to drive calcium out of the serum and back into the bones. • Vitamin D to promote uptake and utilization of calcium. • Glucocorticoids to promote excretion of calcium through the GI tract. • Phosphorus-containing laxatives to drive down the calcium. (Remember: Calcium and phosphorus have an inverse relationship.) • Increased dietary phosphorus (protein foods such as beef, fish, pork, chicken). • Cinacalcet HCl (an oral agent) to lower PTH and calcium.[13]
Hypomagnesemia: Alcoholism (diuresing, not eating) Diarrhea (GI excretion of magnesium)	• Antidiarrheal agents to stop GI losses. • Administer magnesium: Check kidney function before and during the infusion. • During magnesium infusion, monitor reflexes (DTRs), hourly urine output, respirations, and blood pressure. • Increase dietary magnesium with foods such as raw spinach, mustard, kale or turnip greens, avocado, white tuna (canned).
Hypocalcemia (Decreased PTH): Hypoparathyroidism may occur as a primary problem, or may follow partial/subtotal parathyroidectomy Radical neck Thyroidectomy	• Calcium gluconate IV slowly (0.5–1 mL/min) for tetany (tonic spasms), seizures or cardiac effects • Correct magnesium deficit if present, otherwise calcium replacement is ineffective. • Phosphorus binding drugs such as Renagel (sevelamer HCl), PhosLo (calcium acetate), and Os-Cal (calcium carbonate) to drive up the serum calcium. For chronic hypocalcemia: • Oral calcium replacement • Vitamin D to increase calcium absorption • Increased dietary calcium

Hurst Hint

Magnesium is excreted primarily by the kidneys.

PATIENT TEACHING   Patient teaching should always be directed toward self-care and monitoring to prevent a recurrence or relapse. Depending upon the cause of the electrolyte imbalance, the following instructions may be applicable:

- Excellent food sources of ALL electrolytes are avocado, low fat yogurt, skim milk, and tuna fish.
- Alcoholics Anonymous 12-step program has documented long-term success.
- Renal patients should NOT take the phosphorus-binding drug Amphojel (aluminum hydroxide gel). Toxicity develops because they cannot excrete the aluminum.
- Vitamin D increases absorption of calcium. Daily unprotected exposure to sun (15 minutes) provides the daily requirement of vitamin D.
- Calcium-rich foods include low-fat yogurt, skim milk, rhubarb, raw collard greens, and cheddar cheese.
- Caution if taking digitalis preparations: Calcium potentiates digoxin effects.
- PTH secretions should decrease after partial parathyroidectomy; however, the calcium level could continue to drop and become too low. Be alert to signs of hypoparathyroidism (hypocalcemia) and notify your doctor immediately if you develop muscle weakness, changes in LOC, or excessive fatigue and sleepiness.
- Exercise daily! Walking (weight bearing) is an excellent way to keep calcium in the bones (and out of the blood).

Cutting edge

When total or partial thyroidectomy is scheduled, perioperative PTH (quick check assay) may be indicated to identify postoperative patients who might be at risk for hypoparathyroidism and resultant hypocalcemia. The results can be a guide to intraoperative autotransplantation of parathyroid tissue, preventing permanent hypoparathyroidism, and can also help the surgeon identify the patients for whom an early discharge would be safe.[14]

✚ Hypocalcemia and hypomagnesemia

Hypomagnesemia is a serum magnesium level below 1.3 mEq/L.[1] The patient with hypomagnesemia and hypocalcemia does not have enough available magnesium or calcium in the blood (serum) to meet normal physiologic needs of the body (magnesium levels <1.2 mEq/L or ionized calcium level <4.6 mg/dL). When magnesium or calcium levels are low, the patient is NOT sedated! Killer complications can happen because of the effect of magnesium or calcium deficits on the muscles! NOT sedated: Muscles become rigid and tight! Could your patient have a seizure? YES! Could your patient have bronchospasm, closing off the airway? YES!

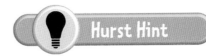

Monitor patient closely during magnesium infusion to prevent magnesium toxicity. Watch for a decrease in these baseline perimeters:
- Deep tendon reflexes
- Hourly urine output
- Respirations
- Blood pressure

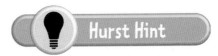

DTRs are the FIRST to go! Stop the magnesium infusion immediately if reflexes are absent!

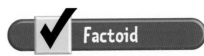

Calcium and phosphorus have an inverse relationship: When one goes up, the other goes down!

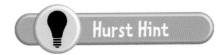

Hypercalcemia=Hypophosphatemia
Hypocalcemia=Hyperphosphatemia

Causes and why?

The table explores the causes and why of hypomagnesemia.

Causes of hypomagnesemia	Why
Diarrhea	Intestines store large amounts of magnesium; diarrhea depletes these stores.
Diuretics	Excretion of magnesium in urine.
Decreased intake	Depletes magnesium stores and does not replenish them.
Chronic alcoholism	Alcoholics are malnourished, which leads to decreased magnesium.
Medications	Some drugs cause increased excretion of magnesium.

Source: Created by the author from Reference 1.

The table explores the causes and why of hypocalcemia.

Cause of hypocalcemia	Why
Hypoparathyroidism—parathyroid glands are not making enough PTH (parathyroid hormone)	In hypoparathyroidism, the parathyroid glands are not making enough PTH. PTH normally controls the serum calcium level by exerting an effect on the bone, kidneys, and intestines. How? The parathyroid glands: • Secrete PTH in response to low serum calcium and pulls calcium from the bone (by causing bone resorption) and puts it in the blood. • Promote reabsorption of calcium from the kidneys. • Cause reabsorption of calcium from the intestines by activating vitamin D. Vitamin D is necessary for the reabsorption of calcium from the intestines. • The result is increased serum calcium. Conversely, when calcium levels are *up,* PTH *decreases,* resulting in no bone resorption; therefore, excess calcium is deposited into the bones rather than being pulled from them. Hypoparathyroidism = decreased PTH and low serum ionized calcium.

(Continued)

Cause of hypocalcemia	Why
Surgery	Parathyroidectomy (because of parathyroid adenoma): Surgical removal of the parathyroid glands halts PTH secretion.
	Radical neck surgery related to cancer (extensive neck surgery)
	• The parathyroids can become damaged and ischemic, or traumatized from radical neck surgery.
	• Damage may be temporary or permanent.
	• If temporary, hypocalcemia will eventually resolve when the parathyroid tissue is healed.
	• If permanent damage occurs, hypocalcemia will be permanent.
	• Radical neck surgery is most likely to cause permanent hypoparathyroidism with permanent hypocalcemia because of the extensiveness of the surgery.
	Thyroidectomy—removable of the thyroid:
	• The parathyroids can be accidentally *removed* OR *damaged* during thyroid removal.
	• Accidental removal is uncommon because thyroidectomy is a less involved surgery than radical neck surgery. Hypocalcemia will be permanent if all of the parathyroid tissue is removed **OR** if damaged parathyroid tissue does not heal and regain function after the surgery.
	• Damaged parathyroid tissue is caused by interruption of the blood supply, causing vascular necrosis to the parathyroids during thyroidectomy.
Thyroid cancer (medullary thyroid carcinoma)	Some thyroid tumors produce the hormone calcitonin. Calcitonin lowers serum calcium.
Kidney disease/renal failure	In kidney disease, vitamin D, which is necessary for calcium reabsorption, is not activated and serum calcium falls.
	In acute renal failure, the kidney is unable to excrete phosphorus; therefore, phosphorus levels rise. Because phosphorus and calcium have an inverse relationship, the calcium level will decrease.

(Continued)

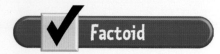

Cause of hypocalcemia	Why
Dietary causes	Insufficient calcium intake: • Inadequate dietary sources of calcium such as dairy products and green leafy vegetables. Insufficient vitamin D intake: • Vitamin D is necessary for the absorption of calcium through the intestines. • Inadequate intake of vitamin D leads to vitamin D deficiency. • Inadequate sunlight leads to vitamin D deficiency because sunlight is necessary for vitamin D absorption. Excessive dietary phosphorus: • Phosphorus binds with calcium leading to decreased absorption.
Vitamin D deficiency	Vitamin D is necessary for the absorption of calcium from the intestines. Inadequate vitamin D leads to inadequate absorption of calcium. Therefore, the parathyroid glands respond by secreting PTH in an attempt to raise the calcium level. So in this case you would see elevated levels of PTH *without* seeing the serum calcium level rise (because it isn't being absorbed from the intestines). This is called *secondary hyperparathyroidism* because the parathyroid is secreting increased amounts of PTH to compensate for hypocalcemia caused by the vitamin D deficiency.
Malabsorption syndromes	Normally, calcium is absorbed from the intestines. Anything that causes decreased intestinal absorption can lead to insufficient quantities of calcium absorption (e.g., pancreatic insufficiency, gastrectomy, Crohn's disease, hepatobiliary disease, etc.).
Diarrhea	Increased excretion of calcium.
Pancreatitis	In pancreatitis, lipase (pancreatic enzyme) is released into soft tissue forming free fatty acids that bind with calcium. In the bound state, it is not available to be used. Steatorrhea resulting from pancreatic insufficiency causes malabsorptive disease, leading to vitamin D deficiency.
Hyperphosphatemia	In renal failure the kidneys are unable to excrete phosphorus. Calcium and phosphorus have an inverse relationship. The higher the serum phosphorus, the lower the serum calcium.

(Continued)

Cause of hypocalcemia	Why
Alkalosis	The pH of plasma will affect how much calcium is ionized (unbound and physiologically active). In alkalosis (increased pH), more calcium becomes bound to protein. The *total* serum calcium in this case doesn't change, but the *ionized* portion of it decreases because more of it is becoming bound to protein. Remember, the ionized portion is physiologically active, so in this case the patient can develop tetany from the decreased ionized calcium even though the total serum calcium is normal! But the pH would be elevated to 7.6 or greater.
Blood transfusions	Citrate solutions are used for storing whole blood. The citrate binds with calcium, making it unavailable for absorption.
Bone metastasis (cancer)	Bone tumors may inhibit bone resorption (calcium leaving the bone and moving into the blood) and increase the deposition of calcium into the bone, leaving decreased serum calcium levels. Note: Thyroid tumors may secrete calcitonin, which causes serum calcium to go down. Calcitonin is an antagonist to calcium.
Alcoholism and hypomagnesemia	Alcoholics are malnourished, so they are deficient in magnesium. Low magnesium leads to decreased PTH release AND poor *response* to PTH, which both lead to hypocalcemia. There are many causes of hypocalcemia in the alcoholic patient, but the magnesium is the most important one.
Medications	Loop diuretics—Lasix Anticonvulsants Blood products buffered with citrate Phosphates Mithramycin Calcitonin Medications that lower the magnesium level EDTA Alcohol Radiographic contrast media—chelate calcium Nicotine Tetracycline Caffeine Cisplatin Corticosteroids Aminoglycosides Isoniazid Aluminum-containing antacids

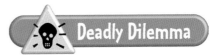

Deadly Dilemma

If the total serum calcium is normal in the presence of an elevated pH at 7.6 or above, check the ionized calcium because tetany can develop!

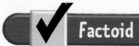

Factoid

Calcium and phosphorus have an inverse relationship. When one is high, the other is low!

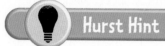

Hurst Hint

Hypocalcemia=Hyperphosphatemia (same clinical findings too!)

Hyperphosphatemia promotes hypocalcemia.

Vitamin D deficiency = *increased* PTH and *low* ionized serum calcium

---

The patient who has a deficiency of magnesium or calcium is NOT sedated! The soothing sedative effect of these electrolytes is gone! Muscles are rigid and tight because of excessive neuromuscular excitability, which produces most of the signs and symptoms of hypomagnesemia and hypocalcemia:

- Changes in LOC: Now the patient is waking up! He or she can be confused, agitated, paranoid, have mood swings, become fearful/combative, or have any variety of mental changes.
- Deep tendon reflexes (DTRs): Hyperactive reflexes (4+/4)
- Rigid, tight muscles: Possible seizure, stridor, and laryngospasm because the larynx is a smooth muscle.
- Highly irritable/excitable muscles: Positive Chvostek's sign, positive Trousseau's sign. Muscles can be stimulated to twitch by tapping over a nerve (Chvostek), or by producing transient hypoxia (such as may be induced by pumping up a blood pressure cuff [Trousseau], causing the muscles to develop spasms).
- Cardiac arrhythmias: Muscles become highly irritable and excitable, and when the heart muscle is irritated, life-threatening arrhythmias can occur!
- Swallowing problems: The esophagus is a smooth muscle, and muscles that are NOT sedated become rigid and tight!

Magnesium excess or deficit

HypOmagnesemia (not enough magnesium)	HypERmagnesemia (too much magnesium)
Magnesium intake is dependent upon dietary ingestion and absorption. The most frequent "hypo-mag" patient is the alcoholic, and here's why: • Alcohol makes you diurese and Mg⁺ is excreted by the kidneys. • Alcohol suppresses the ADH hormone, increasing diuresis. • The alcoholic doesn't like to eat! They prefer to drink instead, and we get magnesium from the foods that we eat, which is why patients having malabsorption syndromes and malnourished patients also develop hypomagnesemia. Other causes of increased magnesium losses include the following: • Increased losses of Mg⁺ because of diuretic therapy causing renal excretion. • Chronic diarrhea or laxative abuse: a lot of Mg⁺ lives in the intestine! • Prolonged GI suction or vomiting: Mg⁺ is a resident of the GI tract!	Hypermagnesemia can happen because of the following: • Chronic renal failure is the most common cause![15] Magnesium is excreted primarily by the kidneys! • If the kidneys aren't working, magnesium levels go up! • Excessive ingestion of magnesium containing medications such as laxatives or antacids. • Excessive administration of IV magnesium in the treatment of pregnancy induced hypertension (PIH), to stop preterm labor can produce iatrogenic hypermagnesemia.

Calcium excess or deficit

Causes of hypocalcemia (not enough calcium in the blood)	Causes of hypercalcemia (too much calcium in the blood)

Hypocalcemia is caused by decreased absorption of dietary calcium:
• Kidney failure reduces the production of an essential kidney chemical (1.25 dihydroxychole-calciferol) needed to convert vitamin D to the active form, which can be used by the body.
• Low serum levels of vitamin D keep calcium from being absorbed from the intestines.
• Not enough PTH (parathormone), which results in decreased serum calcium.
• Changes in the blood pH: alkalosis causes more calcium to become bound to protein, therefore lowering available serum calcium.[6]
	• Hypercalcemia happens when calcium leaves the storage depot in the bones, and is deposited in the blood. Examples of causes are:
	  • Hyperparathyroidism, which produces too much of the hormone, parathormone (PTH).
	  • Thiazide diuretics make you retain calcium.
	  • Immobilization causes demineralization of the bone: When the patient in not bearing weight on long bones, calcium leaves the bone and is released in the serum.
	  • Cancer of the bone, or metastasis to the bone because as bone is destroyed, calcium is released into circulation.
	  • Changes in the blood pH: Acidosis causes less calcium to become bound to protein, therefore increasing ionized serum calcium.[6]

Because excessive magnesium levels are also associated with Addison's disease (Refer to Chapter 10, Endocrine and Metabolic Dysfunction), additional testing may be indicated, such as serum sodium, cortisol, and aldosterone.

Signs and symptoms and why?

Calcium balance is required for the transmission of nerve impulses and muscle contractions. Calcium exerts its effect on the cell membrane to create the nerve stimulus. The nerve stimulus makes the muscle work. The underlying reason for the signs and symptoms of hypocalcemia are the result of *increased* neuromuscular excitability caused by a calcium deficit.

Low calcium → **Increased** neuromuscular excitability

The signs and symptoms and associated rationales of hypocalcemia are listed below.

Signs and symptoms	Why
Muscle cramps	Inadequate calcium causes the muscles to contract because of increased neuromuscular excitability.
Tetany	Inadequate calcium triggers nerve impulses to travel to skeletal muscles because of increased neuromuscular excitability.

(Continued)

Signs and symptoms	Why
Seizures	Increased excitability in the brain
Chvostek's sign	Inadequate calcium causes hyperexcitability of the facial muscles.
Trousseau's sign	Inadequate calcium causes hyperexcitability of the hand muscles.
Carpopedal spam	Tetany of the hand.
Laryngeal spasm	Laryngeal muscles are sensitive to tetanic spasms. When they spasm, respiration is obstructed.Without treatment, laryngeal spasm is the most common cause of death in tetany.
Hyperactive DTRs	Increased neuromuscular excitability leading to hyperactivity of the reflexes.
Cardiac changes: • Arrhythmias • Decreased pulse • Lengthened ST interval • Prolonged QT interval • Decreased myocardial contractility resulting in weak cardiac contractions	Cardiac and smooth muscle cells are full of calcium channels, leaving the neuromuscular function of these types of cells very dependent on the transport of calcium across the cell membrane. The function of the cardiac muscle depends on the availability of calcium. Inadequate calcium causes impaired electrical impulses in the heart caused by increased neuromuscular excitability.
Respiratory arrest	The respiratory muscles are responsible for inhaling and exhaling. Tetanic contractions of the respiratory muscles leave them rigid.
Increased gastric activity	Hyperactivity of the bowel related to increased neuromuscular excitability.

Source: Created by the author from Reference 1.

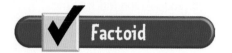

Factoid

Tetany of the hand (carpopedal spasm) will usually occur before tetany of the entire body occurs.

Signs and symptoms of hypomagnesemia and hypocalcemia

• Changes in LOC: Now the patient is waking up! He or she can be confused, agitated, paranoid, have mood swings, become fearful/combative, or have any variety of mental changes.
• Deep tendon reflexes (DTRs): Hyperactive reflexes (4+/4).
• Rigid, tight muscles: Possible seizure, stridor, and laryngospasm because the larynx is a smooth muscle.
• Highly irritable/excitable muscles: Positive Chvostek's sign, positive Trousseau's sign. Muscles can be stimulated to twitch by tapping over a nerve (Chvostek), or by producing transient hypoxia (such as may be induced by pumping up a blood pressure cuff [Trousseau], causing the muscles to develop spasms).
• Cardiac arrhythmias: Muscles become highly irritable and excitable, and when the heart muscle is irritated, life-threatening arrhythmias can occur!
• Swallowing problems: the esophagus is a smooth muscle, and muscles that are NOT sedated become rigid and tight!

What can harm my patient and why?

The most life-threatening events associated with hypermagnesemia and hypercalcemia are cardiac and/or respiratory arrest.

Interventions and why?

The A-B-Cs reflect nursing priorities when the patient has a magnesium or calcium imbalance (see Table 2-3).

Clinical alert

Calcium gluconate versus calcium chloride: Be sure you know the difference! Don't grab the wrong drug! Calcium gluconate=4.5 mEq calcium, but

Calcium chloride=13.6 mEq calcium (three times more potent)!

Testing, testing, testing!

Serum levels of magnesium or calcium are diagnostic of *excesses or deficits* of these electrolytes.

- Phosphorus levels will also be checked (blood test) because calcium and phosphorus have an inverse relationship.
- When serum calcium levels are high, the phosphorus level will be low.
- If serum calcium levels are high because of possible demineralization of bones, a bone density test may be indicated to detect osteoporosis.
- Vitamin D levels are drawn because calcium absorption is dependent upon the presence of vitamin D for normal uptake of calcium by the bones.
- Since renal failure is often present, BUN and creatinine levels may be drawn to evaluate kidney function.

Because excessive magnesium levels are also associated with Addison's disease (refer to Chapter 10, Endocrine and Metabolic Dysfunction), additional testing may be indicated, such as serum sodium, cortisol, and aldosterone.

What do I teach my patient?

Patient teaching should always be directed toward self-care and monitoring to prevent a recurrence or relapse. Depending upon the cause of the electrolyte imbalance, the following instructions may be applicable:

- Excellent food sources of ALL electrolytes are avocado, low-fat yogurt, skim milk, and tuna fish.
- Alcoholics Anonymous 12-step program has documented long-term success.
- Renal patients should NOT take the phosphorus-binding drug, Amphojel (aluminum hydroxide gel): Toxicity develops because they cannot excrete the aluminum.
- Vitamin D increases the absorption of calcium. Daily unprotected exposure to the sun (15 minutes) provides the daily requirement of Vitamin D.

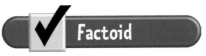

Factoid

When magnesium and calcium are in the presence of each other, they inactivate each other.

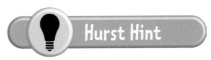

Hurst Hint

When does the NCLEX© lady want you to intervene: early or late? Early, of course! There are fewer patient complications if the doctor is notified before the onset of a code! The rapid response team likes to be notified *before* the patient is clinically dead!

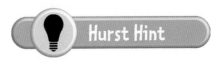

Hurst Hint

IV calcium must be administered slowly, and patients receiving IV calcium must be on a heart monitor. Be alert to widening of the QRS complex.

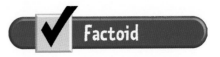

Factoid

Calcium and phosphorus have an inverse relationship. When one is high, the other is low!

- Calcium-rich foods include low-fat yogurt, skim milk, rhubarb, raw collard greens, and cheddar cheese.
- Exercise caution if taking digitalis preparations: Calcium potentiates digoxin effects.
- PTH secretions should decrease after partial parathyroidectomy; however, the calcium level could continue to drop and become too low. Be alert to signs of hypoparathyroidism (hypocalcemia) and notify your doctor immediately if you develop muscle weakness, changes in LOC, or excessive fatigue and sleepiness.
- Exercise daily! Walking (weight-bearing) is an excellent way to keep calcium in the bones (and out of the blood).

What's on the cutting edge?

When total or partial thyroidectomy is scheduled, perioperative PTH (quick check assay) may be indicated to identify postoperative patients who might be at risk for hypoparathyroidism and resultant hypocalcemia. Results can be a guide to intraoperative autotransplantation of parathyroid tissue, preventing permanent hypoparathyroidism, and can also help the surgeon identify patients for whom an early discharge would be safe.[16]

✚ Hypophosphatemia

Let's get the normal stuff straight first!

Phosphorus is:

- An intracellular anion.
- In the serum, the ionized form is the part that is physiologically active.
- Necessary for ATP/energy required to fuel nerve impulses, muscle contractions, and transport of electrolytes.
- A relayer of messages inside the cell.
- Important for the metabolism of carbohydrates, fat, and protein.
- A substance that exists all over the body, but mostly in the muscle cells.
  Phosphorus is important for:
- Red blood cell function
- Muscle function
- Nervous system function
  Important concepts:
- Daily requirements are 800 to 1500 mg per day.
- A healthy diet is sufficient for phosphorus.
- Dietary sources include red meat, fish, poultry, eggs, milk products, and legumes.
- It is absorbed in the jejunum.
- It is excreted mostly by the kidneys; therefore, phosphorus balance is highly dependent on healthy kidneys.

- The kidneys retain phosphorus if intake is insufficient.
- Minimal amounts are excreted in the feces.

What is it?

Hypophosphatemia is serum phosphate that is <3.0 mg/dL.[1]

Causes and why?

Causes fall into three categories:

- Phosphorus moves from extracellular fluid (ECF) to the cell.
- Decreases GI absorption of phosphorus.
- Increases renal excretion.

Causes of hypophosphatemia	Why
Glucose administration (shift from ECF to cell)	Triggers insulin release (which promotes glycolysis), facilitating glucose and phosphorus movement into skeletal muscle cells and liver cells. Usually the decrease will be minimal, but in starving patients the response is exaggerated.
Nutritional recovery syndrome/refeeding syndrome (shift from ECF to cell)	In severe protein-calorie malnutrition (patients with alcoholism, anorexia nervosa, and those unable to eat, such as the elderly), aggressive refeeding with simple carbohydrates without adequate phosphorus can result in hypophosphatemia caused by an influx of phosphorus into the muscle cells. Starvation causes the muscles to be in a state of catabolism (muscle breakdown and cellular depletion of phosphate). With feeding, the muscles return to an anabolic state (capable of tissue building). When TPN (high in glucose) is administered without additional phosphate additives, the muscles return to the anabolic state and phosphorus pours into the cell, which is so severely depleted of phosphorus. The resultant low serum phosphorus level is an identifier as to how depleted the cells are of phosphorus. This is more common with TPN and tube feeding and less common with oral feeding.
Hyperalimentation (shift from ECF to cell)	TPN administration without adequate phosphorus to compensate for the rapid influx of phosphorus into the muscle cells when they return to the anabolic state (capable of tissue building).
Respiratory alkalosis (shift from ECF to cell)	Alkalosis causes phosphate to leave the blood and enter the cell.

(Continued)

Causes of hypophosphatemia	Why
Diabetic ketoacidosis (DKA) (renal excretion)	Cells are starved of glucose and phosphorus. Phosphorus is lost in the urine from osmotic dieresis along with glucose in DKA. Treatment with insulin and IV fluids causes both glucose and phosphorus to re-enter the cell. This causes serum phosphorus to be decreased.
Pharmacologic phosphate binding	Phosphorus binds with aluminum hydroxide, magnesium hydroxide, and aluminum carbonate gels. Aluminum or magnesium based antacids bind to phosphate. If the patient has poor phosphorus intake, the degree of hypophosphatemia will be even greater when using phosphate binding antacids.
Thermal burns	Not well understood but may be related to: • Respiratory alkalosis caused by hyperventilation. • May be lost in urine during dieresis. • When the muscle cells return to the anabolic state, influx of phosphorus into the muscle cells may contribute to the fall of serum phosphorus levels.
Alcoholism	Poor intake. Diarrhea, vomiting. Use of antacids related to GI irritation. Note: Hypophosphatemia can develop in alcoholics in the absence of these causes. It is poorly understood but thought to be related to the ethanol itself, hypomagnesemia, or ketoacidosis.

Hurst Hint

Hypophosphatemia can continue for months in burn patients. The reason for this is poorly understood.

Hypophosphatemia is a serum phosphate concentration below the normal level, which can occur even with a normal total body level of phosphates.

- This may result from redistribution as phosphates shift from the extracellular space to the intracellular space.
- Because of the inverse relationship of phosphorus to calcium, hypophosphatemia is accompanied by hypercalcemia.
- PTH is the main regulator of renal phosphate reabsorption[12]
- Under the influence of PTH, while the renal tubules are reabsorbing calcium and magnesium, they are excreting phosphates.

Three mechanisms account for phosphorus deficit: increased urinary excretion, decreased dietary intake, and redistribution of phosphorus into the cell. The following causes and rationales are related to phosphate deficit:

- Hyperparathyroidism (too much PTH) means excess renal excretion of phosphates.

- Alcoholism causes renal phosphate loss through decreased ADH secretion and diuresis, as well as decreased dietary intake common in alcoholics.
- Respiratory alkalosis caused by redistribution of phosphorus secondary to enhanced uptake by the muscles.[12]
- Diabetic ketoacidosis allows phosphates to more easily enter the cells (leaving the serum) because of an enzymatic action creating a glycolytic pathway.[12]
- Malabsorption syndromes reduce absorption of phosphates from the small intestine.
- Low levels of vitamin D decrease intestinal absorption of phosphorus.
- Use of antacids and drugs that bind phosphorus will lower the serum phosphorus level.

Testing, testing, testing

The following diagnostic tests are evaluated to determine the mechanism of phosphate loss or serum deficit:

- Serum calcium concentration
- Arterial blood gases
- Urinary phosphorus excretion
- Creatinine concentrations, calculating renal phosphate threshold
- Creatinine clearance
- Phosphate clearance
- Serum phosphate
- PTH levels

Signs and symptoms and why?

Hypophosphatemia looks just like hypercalcemia. Signs and symptoms of chronic hypophosphatemia differ from those of acute rapidly falling phosphorus levels, with acute being more severe and life threatening. Patient complaints with chronic phosphorus deficiency include:

- Bone pain
- Weakness
- Demineralization of bone
- Pathologic fractures

Acute symptoms listed below are caused by decreased ATP, and resultant lack of energy within the cells and impaired oxygen delivery to the cells. Clinically, the signs and symptoms of acute hypophosphatemia are neuromuscular:

- Muscle weakness, fatigue
- Numbness, paresthesia
- Dysphagia

- Irritability, confusion
- Decreased cardiac output (weak heart muscle)
- Decreased ventilatory ability (weak respiratory muscles)
- Seizures (cellular hypoxia) and coma

What can harm my patient and why?

Conditions that harm my patient are dependent upon whether hypophosphatemia is acute or chronic.[17] Acute hypophosphatemia can be mild to severe, depending on whether phosphate levels drop slowly or rapidly. Usually mild to moderate hypophosphatemia has few clinical consequences unless the patient is on a ventilator;[12] however, severe acute hypophosphatemia may cause the following serious conditions:

- Rhabdomyolysis (rab-dough-my-OL-i-sis), a condition in which striated muscles break down and disintegrate, and myoglobins from the destroyed muscle tissue are excreted (and can clog up) by the kidneys. Alcoholics are at greater risk for development of rhabdomyolysis, and alcohol also worsens alcoholic myopathy.
- Respiratory failure resulting from muscle weakness and decreased contractability of the diaphragm.
- Hemolysis of red blood cells and anemia because of the decrease in ATP, which is needed to maintain erythrocyte shape and viability. When ATP is depleted, the RBCs have a reduced life span and they lose their ability to change shape as they pass through narrow spaces in microcirculation.[12]
- Heart failure resulting from left ventricular dysfunction secondary to weakening of myocardial muscle fibers.

Unlike acute phosphatemia, which affects muscles, cells, and cellular metabolism, chronic hypophosphatemia results in changes in bone structure and function:

- Demineralization and softening of bone, which seriously impair the ability of the bony skeleton to support the weight of the body.
- Rickets (in children and adolescents), causing bow legs, knock-knees, and deformities of the skull.
- Osteomalacia (softened bones that bend or flatten, causing deformity), affecting mainly the spine, pelvis, and lower extremities.[17]

Any acutely or chronically malnourished patient can develop life-threatening cardiac and respiratory complications as a result of aggressive parenteral refeeding with carbohydrates.[12,18]

- Re-feeding syndrome occurs because insulin release triggers an intracellular shift in phosphate distribution, which coupled with increased urinary phosphate excretion causes serum phosphate levels to drop rapidly.
- Sepsis occurs with TPN because hypophosphatemia impairs leukocyte activity.[12]

Interventions and why?

Phosphorus is best replaced by the oral route, but because hypophosphatemia prolongs intubation/ventilation, IV replacement is warranted.[12]

- Severe hypophosphatemia or rapidly falling phosphorus levels can lead to hemolytic anemia with a compensatory increase in respiratory rate, which can result in the added insult of respiratory alkalosis.

  Hypophosphatemia can also be caused by alkalosis! For this reason, aggressive treatment of severe hypophosphatemia is initiated.

- Dextrose-containing IV fluids are avoided, as these exacerbate hypophosphatemia through the movement of phosphorus into the cells.[12]

- The patient's electrolyte status will determine whether sodium phosphate or potassium phosphate is used for replacement therapy.

- Gradual re-feeding with careful monitoring of susceptible patients can help to avoid the drastic phosphorus shifts that occur with re-feeding syndrome.

  In order to prevent recurrence of hypophosphatemia, a complete patient history and diagnostic work-up is required to find the cause and initiate treatment of the underlying condition.

  Depending upon the severity of hypophosphatemia, endotracheal intubation and mechanical ventilation may be required to support ventilation. When respiratory muscles are weak, the nurse can initiate the following measures to support respiratory effort:

- Elevate the head of the bed.

- Administer prescribed oxygen.

- Support the elbows with pillows to decrease inspiratory effort.

- Monitor respiratory excursion, rate and depth of respirations frequently.

- Monitor oxygenation status using pulse oximeter.

- Be alert to any prescribed medication that may reduce respirations, such as sedatives, hypnotics, barbiturates, and CNS depressants.

  If mechanical ventilation is in progress:

- Administer prescribed IV phosphorus–containing solutions. (Each dose is calculated by weight and administered over 4 to 6 hours per pump.)[12]

- Maintain patency of artificial airway (sterile ET suction).

- Meticulous oral care to reduce bacteria in the mouth.

Clinical Alert

When parenteral feeding is prescribed watch for early signs of hypophosphatemia: apprehension, confusion, and change in LOC!

Because of the risk for development of refeeding syndrome which may be fatal,[18] careful monitoring is required for susceptible patients:

- Any prolonged starvation.

- Critically ill and malnourished.

- Anorexia nervosa.
- Chronic alcohol use.
- Cachexia and wasting (cancer patients).
- Nutritional considerations are based upon the severity of hypophosphatemia and the needs of the patient.
- If the patient is critically ill and receiving specialized nutritional support, weight-based phosphorus dosing algorithms provide guidelines for safe phosphorus IV replacement therapy;[20] otherwise, oral replacement therapy is employed for moderate hypophosphatemia and dietary measures are used for mild hypophosphatemia. Additionally, my patient needs:
  - Phosphate supplements as prescribed (Neutra-Phos or Fleets Phospho-Soda).
  - Monitoring of serum phosphate levels and reporting trends before phosphorus is outside of normal perimeters.
  - Monitoring patient response to TPN or enteral feeds containing phosphates. Watch for behavioral changes and alteration in LOC.
  - Protection from infection: meticulous handwashing, avoidance of cross contamination, avoidance of exposure to infectious agents.

PATIENT TEACHING   The focus of patient teaching is nutrition, preventing infection, and preventing recurrence of hypophosphatemia:

- High protein diet with protein snacks: include organ meats, fish, poultry, nuts, whole grains.
- Avoid contact with persons who have cough/colds; wash hands frequently; avoid crowds.
- Refrain from use of antacids, alcohol, bicarbonates.
- Report bone pain or muscle weakness promptly.

  If the skeleton is demineralized because of chronic hypophosphatemia, the patient with osteomalacia must be taught basic safety measures to prevent falls, because a fracture (especially of the pelvis) can lead to disability and even death in the elderly.

- Remove loose throw rugs.
- Keep night lights on to light pathways.
- Remove wheels from walkers and replace with (cut) tennis balls.
- Install hand rails (interior and exterior) for support on stairways/inclines.
- Use supportive appliances (canes, walkers, braces) as prescribed.
- Lifeline medical alert bracelets or necklaces (with a panic button to call for help in the event of a fall or other emergency) are recommended.

Cutting edge

In addition to the usual causes of hypophosphatemia, some new culprits have been identified: antiviral medications (tenofovir, cidofovir, adefovir dipivoxil) as well as an ingredient in many Chinese herbal medicines, aristocholic acid.[12]

✚ Hyperphosphatemia

What is it?

Moderate hyperphosphatemia is 4.6 to 6.0 mg/dL. Severe hyperphosphatemia is ↑6.0.

Causes and why?

The causes of hyperphosphatemia fall into three categories:

- **Decreased renal excretion:** Hyperphosphatemia most commonly occurs in renal failure because of impaired excretory ability of the kidneys, and phosphates build up in the ECF.
- Phosphorus **leaves the cell** and **enters the ECF.**
- **Increased intake** or increased absorption.

  Additionally

- Hypoparathyroidism is also implicated because PTH is the major regulator of phosphate and this hormone is deficient.
- Overuse of phosphate-containing laxatives can also produce hyperphosphatemia.

Causes of hyperphosphatemia	Why
Renal disease/acute renal failure	When the glomerular filtration rate (GFR) is 25 to 30 mL/min or less in chronic renal disease or acute renal failure, phosphorus is retained and the serum level rises.
Chemotherapy	Chemotherapy destroys cells and releases phosphate into the blood.
High phosphate intake	<ul><li>Cow's milk is high in phosphorus. Infants who drink cow's milk rather than human milk or an appropriate formula may develop hyperphosphatemia.</li><li>Adults who drink large quantities of cow's milk may also develop hyperphosphatemia.</li><li>Too much IV administration of phosphorus.</li><li>Too much oral intake of phosphate substances.</li><li>Phosphate enemas cause absorption of phosphorus from the intestine.</li><li>Overuse of phosphate-containing laxatives.</li><li>Blood transfusions—phosphorus escapes from the blood cells during storage.</li><li>Excess intake of vitamin D—leads to increased phosphorus absorption which combined with renal insufficiency can lead to hyperphosphatemia.</li></ul>
Rhabdomyolysis	Rhabdomyolysis is necrosis of muscle tissue caused by certain illnesses (viruses), trauma, heat stroke, and medications. Muscle necrosis causes release of phosphorus from the destroyed muscle cells.
Endocrine disorders	Hypoparathyroidism—decreased calcium leads to increased phosphorus. Hyperthyroidism—may cause hyperphosphatemia (because of osteoporosis that occurs with hyperthyroidism). Bone contains a tremendous amount of phosphate. Read up on this.

Signs and symptoms and why?

Hyperphosphatemia looks just like **hypocalcemia.** The clinical findings are exactly the same as for hypocalcemia!

Testing, testing, testing: hypophosphatemia and hyperphosphatemia

Test	Clinical significance	Nursing care and/or interfering factors
Normal adult serum phosphorus— 3–4.5 mg/dL Critical value— <1 mg/dL	The phosphorus in the body is in the form of a phosphate. It exists in the inorganic and the organic form. It is the inorganic that we are concerned with. When a phosphorus level is ordered it is "inorganic phosphorus." Most of the inorganic phosphorus is mixed with calcium in the bone, but a small portion of it does exist in the blood (phosphate salt)	Calcium and phosphorus have an inverse relationship. A decrease in one leads to an increase in the other. Laxatives and enemas can increase serum phosphorus levels. Phosphorus enters the cell with glucose, so IV glucose administration or carbohydrate ingestion can lower serum phosphorus levels. Drugs that increase phosphorus include methicillin and excess vitamin D. Drugs that decrease serum phosphorus include antacids and mannitol. Instruct patient about the procedure and the requirements of NPO prior to the test. Patient will be NPO after midnight. The patient may have an order to discontinue IV fluids containing glucose several hours prior to the test. Low serum phosphorus can appear due to a temporary shift into the cells. According to some sources, a more reliable indicator of phosphorus depletion is to measure the urinary phosphorus. Depletion is characterized by a loss of 50–100 mg/day. Don't leave tourniquet on too long because hemolysis may affect the level.

What can harm my patient and why?

Hyperphosphatemia produces the same life-threatening risks as hypocalcemia: Calcium acts like a sedative, and my patient is NOT sedated (refer to Hypocalcemia because complications are similar).

- Tetany (rigid tight muscles in a constant contraction)
- Seizures caused by increased CNS and neuromuscular irritability
- Cardiac arrhythmias caused by highly excitable muscle tissue
- Vascular and soft tissue calcifications due to impaired phosphate excretion

My patient has a very abnormal neuromuscular response because of loss of acetylcholine depression at the myoneural junction, and excessive neuromuscular excitability can lead to these clinical manifestations:

- Mental changes (confusion, hallucinations).
- Muscles are rigid and tight!

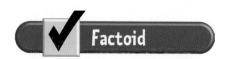
Hyperphosphatemia=Hypocalcemia

- There is high risk for seizure.
- Risk for tetany (continuous tight muscle contraction), which can close the airway secondary to laryngospasm.
- Positive Chvostek's and Trousseau's signs.
- Hyperreflexia (4+ DTRs).
- Hypertension.
- Cardiac dysrhythmias.

Interventions and why?

A-B-C: Protect the airway! A tracheostomy tray must be at the bedside in the event of laryngospasm, which can close off the airway. Due to the risk for cardiac arrhythmias, the patient requires continuous cardiac monitoring. (Refer to treatment for hypocalcemia.)

- Acute hyperphosphatemia may require emergency dialysis (hemodialysis, CRRT [continuous renal replacement therapy], or peritoneal dialysis) to restore electrolyte balance.
- Post-thyroidectomy, immediate tracheotomy and administration of IV calcium gluconate is the standard protocol for treatment of tetany.
- Sedative agents such as pentobarbital may be administered for seizures.
- Parenteral parathormone (PTH) can be administered to treat acute hypoparathyroidism.[6]

If chronic hypoparathyroidism is the cause of hyperphosphatemia, my patient will require:

- A calm, quiet, nonstimulating environment because of increased neuromuscular irritability.
- A high-calcium, low-phosphorus diet.
- Vitamin D oral preparations as prescribed to increase intestinal calcium absorption.
- Phosphorus binding agents as prescribed: Renagel (sevelamer HCl) PhosLo (calcium acetate), Os-Cal (calcium carbonate), or Amphojel (aluminum hydroxide gel) in the absence of renal insufficiency.

Hyperphosphatemia is almost never a problem, because the kidneys are amazing in their ability to excrete excess phosphorus, but renal failure presents a complex balancing act: What goes in has got to come out! Between traditional therapies (above), oral calcimimetics, and dialysis, outcomes are much improved, especially if the patient does his or her part, namely, compliance with low-phosphorus intake between hemodialysis treatments.

Another important consideration in reducing the risk for hyperphosphatemia is changing preoperative bowel preparation. Phosphate salts have been traditionally used, but changing to polyethylene glycol agents for bowel cleansing can avoid the incidence of hyperphosphatemic acidosis and other severe electrolyte imbalance induced by the traditional phosphate salts.[20]

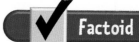

Factoid

The effect of hypocalcemia on mental function and stability can produce safety issues: A confused, disoriented patient requires more frequent assessments and structured environmental controls.

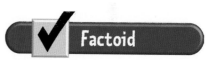

Factoid

Renal patients become toxic if given the phosphorus-binding agent Amphojel (aluminum hydroxide gel) because they can't excrete the aluminum. Don't give it!

PATIENT TEACHING In addition to patient teaching indicated for hypocalcemia, the patient must be taught the signs and symptoms of hyperphosphatemia (the same clinical picture as hypocalcemia) to insure that he or she is knowledgeable and will report noticeable signs and symptoms that may signal recurrence:

- Confusion or other mental changes
- Tense, tight muscles
- Difficulty swallowing
- Heart palpitations

Teach the patient with chronic hyperphosphatemia:

- High calcium, low phosphorus diet (raising serum calcium lowers phosphorus) for long-term therapy.

Teach the renal patient:

- Not to use OTC antacids which may contain aluminum
- Between times for dialysis, to avoid foods or drinks containing phosphorus: milk, milk products, egg yolk, spinach
- To avoid phosphorus-containing laxatives

Cutting edge

Chronic renal patients on maintenance hemodialysis (MDH) are currently prescribed dietary restriction of phosphorus despite the many phosphorus-binding drugs currently on the market.[21] A later study has determined that renal patients on MDH actually have a higher death rate with protein restriction because of the low serum albumin, and generally poor nutrition! Rather than withholding dietary protein to lower serum phosphorus, it is better to eliminate highly processed fast foods and convenience foods from the diet, and utilize the low phosphorus foods that are being marketed especially for renal patients.[22]

Outcomes with patients having chronic renal failure are improved with the use of oral calcimimetics when compared to traditional therapies (vitamin D, steroids, phosphate binders).[13,12]

PRACTICE QUESTIONS

1. The patient with fluid volume excess is found sitting straight up in bed with labored respirations, saying, "I can't get my breath." Which first action by the nurse will provide the most immediate benefit to the patient?

A. Dangle the patient's legs over the side of the bed and call for help.

B. Auscultate anterior and posterior lung fields bilaterally and notify the doctor of moist rales.

C. Call respiratory therapy to the room stat to bring an oxygen mask.

D. Administer PRN morphine 2 mg IVP via existing venous access device.

2. While administering IV Lasix to a patient who has been receiving large doses of furosemide over several days, the nurse notes that the patient's eyelid is twitching. Which next action by the nurse is most appropriate?

A. Stop the IVP furosemide and check the patient's blood pressure.

B. Complete the IVP administration of furosemide at a slower rate.

C. Hold the remaining medication and check for Trousseau's sign.

D. While completing the IVP, question the patient about any previous tendency for eyelid spasm.

3. When the patient is in FVD/shock which of the following signs/symptoms most definitely forewarn of impending renal failure? Select all that apply:

A. Sustained hypotension <90 mm Hg

B. Tachycardia >140 beats/min

C. Cold, clammy skin

D. Dyspnea and air hunger

4. When the patient has a diagnosis of hyponatremia accompanied by neurologic changes, which of the following IV fluid orders would the nurse question? Select all that apply:

A. Dextrose 5% water (D5W)

B. Sodium chloride 3%

C. NS 0.9% with KCl 40 mEq

D. Sodium chloride 0.5%

5. An elderly, bedfast patient receiving G-tube feeding at home is transported to the emergency department after onset of behavioral changes and hallucinations. Which nursing action is priority while diagnostic testing is underway?

A. Seizure precautions

B. Monitor for signs of ICP

C. Orient to time, place, and person

D. Obtain vital signs q 15 minutes

6. After receiving a bowel prep followed by a diagnostic procedure using radiopaque dye, acute renal failure develops. While in the oliguric phase, the patient develops a decreased LOC, muscle weakness, bradycardia, and hypoactive reflexes. Which next nursing assessment is the priority?

A. The hourly urine output

B. The blood pressure

C. The respiratory rate

D. The pupillary reaction to light

7. Which of the following is the priority nursing assessment post-para-thyroidectomy?

   A. Heart rate

   B. Blood pressure

   C. Chvostek's sign

   D. Respiratory rate

8. After being convinced to seek treatment, a suicidal hemodialysis patient comes to the ED after missing two hemodialysis treatments. Which next nursing action is the priority?

   A. Monitor the BP.

   B. Weigh the patient.

   C. Notify the dialysis nurse.

   D. Place the patient on a heart monitor.

   E. Schedule a mental health consult.

9. The patient has serum potassium of 6.2 during the early hours after an extensive burn. Which physician order would the nurse question?

   A. Insulin and glucose IV

   B. Calcium gluconate IV

   C. Albuterol updraft (nebulized)

   D. Lasix IV (loop diuretic)

10. A patient receiving IVF containing KCl complains of burning at the site, and the nurse notes slight red streaking up the affected vein. Which next nursing action is most appropriate?

   A. Stop the infusion and call the doctor.

   B. Elevate the affected arm on a pillow.

   C. Apply a warm compress above the site.

   D. Advise the patient that this reaction is normal.

References

1. Hurst M. *Pharmacology in a Nutshell. Hurst Review's NCLEX-RN Review*. New York: McGraw-Hill Medical; 2008.

2. Getter HB. Contrast-media-induced pulmonary edema. *Action Stat* 2002.

3. Maizel J, Airapetan N, Lome E, et al. Diagnosis of central hypovolemia by using passive leg raising. *Int Care Med 33*(7):1133–1138, 2007.

4. Boldt J, Suttner S. Plasma substitutes. *Minerva Anesthesiol 71*(12):741–758, 2005.

5. Boldt J. Do plasma substitutes have additional properties beyond correcting volume deficits? *Shock 25*(2):103–116, 2006.

6. Crowley SD, Gurley SB, Oliverio M, et al. Distinct roles for the kidney and systemic tissues in blood pressure regulation by the renin-angiotensin system. *J Clin Invest* 115(4):1092–1099, 2005.

7. Smeltzer SC, Bare BG, Hinkle JL, Cheever KH. *Brunner & Suddarth's Textbook of Medical-Surgical Nursing.* 11th ed. Philadelphia: Lippincott Williams & Wilkins; 2008.

8. Suhayda R, Walton JC. Preventing and managing dehydration. *Med-Surg Nursing* 11(6):267–278, 2002.

9. Peterangelo M. Incorporating Aquapheresis into the hospital setting: A practical approach. *Progr Cardiovasc Nurs* 23:168–172, 2008.

10. Beal AL, Deuser WE, Beilman GJ. A role for epinephrine in post-traumatic hypokalemia. *Shock* 27(4):358–363, 2007.

11. MiyashitaY, Monden T, Yamamoto K, et al. Ventricular fibrillation due to severe hypokalemia induced by steroid treatment in a patient with thyrotoxic periodic paralysis. *Int Med* 45:11–13, 2006.

12. Miller SJ. Death resulting from overzealous total parenteral nutrition: The refeeding syndrome revisited. *Nutr Clin Pract* 23(2):166–171, 2008.

13. Mittendorf EA, Merlino JI, McHenry CR. Post-parathyroidectomy hypocalcemia: Incidence, risk factors and management. *Am Surg* 70(2):114–119, 2008.

14. De Francisco AL. New strategies for the treatment of hyperparathyroidism incorporating calcimimetics. *Expert Opin Pharmacother* 9(5):795–811, 2008.

15. Barczynski M, Cichon S, Konturek A, Cichon W. Applicability of intraoperative parathyroid hormone assay during total thyroidectomy as a guide for the surgeon to selective parathyroid tissue auto-transplantation.*World J Surg* 32(5):822–828, 2008.

16. Sitara D, Kim S, Razzaque MS, et al. Genetic evidence of serum phosphate-independent functions of FGF-23 on bone. *PLoS Genet* 4(8):100–154, 2008.

17. Amanzadeh J, Reilly RF Jr. Hypophosphatemia: An evidence-based approach to its clinical consequences and management. *Nat Clin Pract Nephrol* 2(3):136–148, 2006.

18. Brown C, Dickerson RN, Morgan LM, et al. A new graduated dosing regimen for phosphorus replacement in patients receiving nutritional support. *J Parent Ent Nutr* 30(3):209–214, 2006.

19. Ezri T, Lerner E, Muggia-Sullam M, et al. Phosphate salt bowel preparation regimens alter perioperative acid–base and electrolyte balance. *Can J Anesthes* 53:153–158, 2006.

20. Porth CM. *Pathophysiology: Concepts of Altered Health States.* 7th ed. Philadelphia: Lippincott Williams & Wilkins; 2007.

21. Hurst M. *A Critical Thinking and Application NCLEX Review.* Brookhaven, MS: Hurst Review Services; 2008.

22. Pagana KD, Pagana TJ. *Mosby's Diagnostic and Laboratory Test Reference.* 5th ed. St. Louis: Mosby; 2001.

23. Agraharkar M, Workeneh BT, Fahlen M. Hypermagnesemia. *MedScape's Emedicine.* Updated May 16, 2006.

24. Hurst M. Fluids and electrolytes. In: Hurst M. *Hurst Review's NCLEX-RN Review.* New York: McGraw-Hill Medical; 2008.

25. Blackburn GL. Salt shakedown. DASH diet beats salt restriction at lowering blood pressure. *Health News 8*(12):5, 2005.

26. Scisney-Matlock M, Glazewski L, McClerking C, Kachorek L. Development and evaluation of DASH diet tailored messages for hypertension treatment. *Appl Nurs Res 19*(2):78–87, 2006.

27. King M. Shock. In: Hurst M. HurstReview's Pathophysiology Review. New York: McGraw-Hill, 2008.

28. Sakai H, Sato A, Takeoka S,Tsuchida E. Rheological properties of hemoglobin vesicles (artificial oxygen carriers) suspended in a series of plasma-substitute solutions. *Langmuir 23*(15):8121–8128, 2007.

29. http://www.medscape.com/medLine/abstract/17567054. Accessed December 28, 2008.

30. Huether SE. Fluids and electrolytes, acids and bases. In: Hueher SE, McCance KL, eds. *Understanding Pathophysiology.* 3rd ed. St. Louis: Mosby; 2004, pp. 105–126.

31. Uribarri J. Phosphorus homeostasis in normal health and in chronic kidney disease patients with special emphasis on dietary phosphorus intake. *Semin Dial 20*(4):295–301, 2007.

32. Shinaberger CS, Greenland S, Kopple JD, et al. Is controlling phosphorus by decreasing dietary protein intake beneficial or harmful in persons with chronic kidney disease? *Am J Clin Nutr 88*:1511–1518, 2008.

33. Sood MM, Sood AR, Richardson R. Emergency management and commonly encountered outpatient scenarios in patients with hyperkalemia. *Mayo Clinic Proc 82*(12):1553–1561, 2007.

34. Elmahi N, Noor M, Mehra S. Hypokalemia and thyrotoxicosis in a patient with quadriplegia. *Hosp Phys 43(2)*:43–48, 2007.

35. Woywodt A, Herrmann A, Haller H, Haubitz M. Severe hypokalemia: Is one reason enough? *Nephrol Dial Transplant* 19(11):2914–2917, 2004.

36. Venes D, ed. Chloride. In: *Taber's Cyclopedic Medical Dictionary.* 19th ed. New York: FA Davis; 2007.

37. Miller BF, Keane CB. In: O'Toole M, ed. *Miller-Keane Encyclopedia and Dictionary of Medicine, Nursing and Allied Health.* 5th ed. Philadelphia: Saunders; 1992.

38. Mathews KD, Stark JE. Hyperchloremic, normal anion-gap, metabolic acidosis due to topiramate. *American Journal of Health-System Pharmacy.* Posted 10/07/08. Accessed 01/16/09.

39. George-Gay B, Chernecky CC. *Clinical Medical Surgical Nursing: A Decision-Making Reference.* Philadelphia: Saunders; 2002.

3 Acid–Base Imbalances

OBJECTIVES

In this chapter you will review:

- The role of electrolytes, renal, and respiratory systems in maintaining and responding to acid–base balance.
- The difference between metabolic and respiratory disorders.
- Primary medical-surgical and clinical events which initiate acid–base imbalance.
- The body's compensatory response to acute and chronic alterations in pH.
- Treatment modalities for restoration of acid–base balance.

Let's get the normal stuff straight first!
See Figure 3-1.

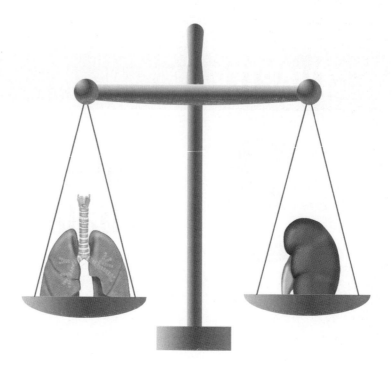

▶ Figure 3-1. Scales. The kidneys and lungs help keep the body's pH in balance.

Hydrogen is a proton that is released from a hydrogen atom. Molecules that have hydrogen *atoms* that *release* hydrogen *ions* are called **acids.** The concentration of hydrogen in the body is very small BUT it is responsible for every cell function, and it has to be kept under tight control. Its concentration in relationship to bicarbonate is 20:1 (20 parts bicarbonate to 1 part acid); therefore, even a small change (increase or decrease) in the hydrogen content is clinically significant. Keeping the hydrogen under control is done by **chemical buffers** and by excreting carbon dioxide and other waste products. A base can accept a hydrogen ion so HCO_3^- (bicarbonate) accepts (or combines with) hydrogen (H^+) to form $H_2CO_3^-$ (carbonic acid). An acid donates hydrogen ions. So H_2CO_3 (carbonic acid) can give up a hydrogen ion to form HCO_3 (bicarbonate) which is a **base.** The acid and base are two of those **"chemical buffers"** that are quickly able to accept and release hydrogen ions in order to keep a stable acid–base balance (normal pH). pH is the measurement of how many hydrogen ions are in the blood. Normal pH is 7.35 to 7.45. BUT, when things go wrong, two major organs will kick in to set things straight, the **kidneys** and the **lungs.** The **lungs** have a powerful and quick buffering ability by blowing off excess CO_2 to decrease the acidity of the blood until the kidneys kick in and do their part. The **lungs** are responsible for removing carbon dioxide from the body. **Carbon dioxide** (CO_2) is the "gas" that forms carbonic acid (H_2CO_3) when dissolved in water. CO_2 is constantly being formed inside the cell from cellular metabolism. Remember, a base (bicarbonate) can accept a hydrogen ion so HCO_3 (bicarbonate) accepts (or combines with) hydrogen (H^+) to form H_2CO_3

(carbonic acid). This leads to the production of CO_2 (carbon dioxide, a "gas") through the process of cellular metabolism, which is then removed from the body by the lungs. Then it diffuses from inside the cell to the blood. The blood takes it to the lungs, where it diffuses into the alveoli. The lungs then remove it from the body through exhalation. When hydrogen is above normal, the respiratory system is stimulated. This is why we say breathing is CO_2 dependent and not O_2 dependent. CO_2 is a powerful stimulant for respiration! The kidneys produce **HCO_3^- (bicarbonate)** whose responsibility is to *buffer* H^+ (hydrogen). Remember, HCO_3 (bicarbonate) accepts H^+ to form H_2CO_3 (carbonic acid). It leads to the production of an acid, CO_2 (carbon dioxide, a "gas") through the process of cellular metabolism, which is then removed from the body by the lungs. The kidneys excrete very little hydrogen (about 1%). If the kidneys fail, it could take days to develop an acid–base imbalance. On the other hand, if the lungs shut down, it would take minutes to develop and acid–base imbalance because they are removing CO_2 from the body with every breath. Remember the lungs have a very powerful and rapid buffering ability. The kidneys excrete HCO_3 (base) in the urine, removing it from the blood. They also excrete H^+ in the urine, removing acid from the blood. Acid–base imbalances are either **respiratory** or **metabolic.** Respiratory acid–base imbalances affect the carbonic acid concentrations. Metabolic acid–base imbalances affect bicarbonate. Therefore, acidosis will either be caused by an *increase* in carbonic acid which is controlled by the lungs, or a *decrease* in bicarbonate, which is controlled by the kidneys. On the other hand, alkalosis will either be caused by a *decrease* in carbonic acid or an increase in bicarbonate.

✤ Metabolic acidosis

See Figure 3-2.

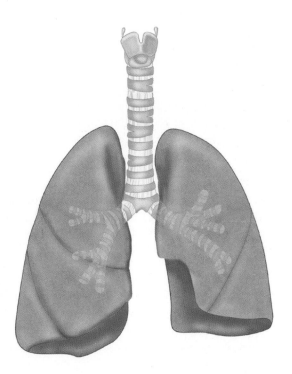

◀ Figure 3-2. Lungs. The lungs compensate for the imbalance during metabolic acidosis by increasing respirations and "blowing off" CO_2.

What is it?

Metabolic acidosis is an acid–base imbalance characterized by a deficit of base and increased concentration of fixed acids with a low pH (pH <7.35).

Metabolic acidosis is a decrease in the base "bicarbonate" resulting in a low pH (increased hydrogen concentration). To compensate, the lungs will increase the respirations and blow off excess CO_2 and the kidneys (if able to) will add new bicarbonate back to the blood.

Compensatory Mechanism

The compensatory mechanism for metabolic acidosis is increased respirations to eliminate CO_2 (acid) from the body via the lungs.

Causes and why?

Causes	Why
Accumulation of acids other than carbonic acids in the body. For example: • Acidic poisoning from acetylsalicylics (aspirin and aspirin-containing medications) • Ethylene glycol • Methyl alcohol • Accidental poisoning from certain household cleaners and antirust compounds	• Ingested acidic substances can raise the acidity of the blood leading to acidosis. • Salicylates cause an overproduction of organic acids. • Ethylene glycol is metabolized into glycolic and oxalic acid. • Methanol is converted to formaldehyde and formic acid.
Severe diarrhea (most common)	GI secretions contain large amounts of bicarbonate. Severe diarrhea results in losing large amounts of bicarbonate into the feces. The effects of severe diarrhea on small children are very serious, including possible death.
Vomiting	Vomiting from the stomach normally causes a loss of *acid*. However, when contents from deeper in the GI tract are lost during vomiting, bicarbonate is lost and leads to acidosis.
Renal disease/renal failure	The kidneys can't excrete excess hydrogen from the body and they can't add bicarbonate back to the blood. Note: When acidosis is caused by something other than renal impairment, *healthy* kidneys will compensate. If renal impairment is the reason for the metabolic acidosis, they obviously can't compensate.
Diabetic ketoacidosis (DKA)	When insulin production is insufficient to carry glucose into the cell, it stays in the blood, resulting in high blood glucose. Glucose is necessary for normal cellular metabolism and the production of energy. When glucose is unavailable to the cell for metabolism, metabolism is accomplished by the breakdown of fat for energy instead of glucose. Ketones are a by-product of fat metabolism (lipolysis). Fat is broken down into free fatty acids, which are converted to ketones in the liver. Ketones are **acids.** The kidneys will compensate by excreting large amounts of acidic urine. The lungs will compensate by increasing respirations and blowing off CO_2.

(Continued)

Causes	Why
Starvation leading to ketoacidosis	When the body breaks down fat for energy, ketones (acids) are produced. This type of acidosis tends to be less severe than in diabetic or alcoholic ketoacidosis.
Alcoholic ketoacidosis	This can lead to ketones in the blood similar to DKA.
Lactic acidosis caused by: • Overwhelming infection • Critical illness • Shock/trauma (including burns)	Accumulation of lactic acid significantly reduces the pH. Lactic acidosis is the result of anaerobic metabolism owing to a lack of intracellular oxygen. This is seen in very sick patients, such as those with cardiopulmonary problems, and overwhelming infections, such as sepsis. Anaerobic metabolism yields lactic acid *and* hydrogen ions. Together, they are known as *lactic acid.*
Hyperthyroidism (thyrotoxicosis)	The overactive thyroid gland causes an extremely elevated metabolism, resulting in cell breakdown/destruction (catabolism). This in turn results in the release of acids.

Signs and symptoms and why?

Some signs and symptoms are manifestations of *compensation* of the acid–base imbalance. There will also be signs and symptoms related to the *cause* of the imbalance, which would be far too numerous to list here.

Signs and symptoms	Why
Hyperkalemia—elevated serum potassium Hyperkalemia begins with muscle twitching and proceeds to weakness and flaccid paralysis in the more severe form.	Acid–base abnormalities can cause changes in the distribution of K^+. In **acute** acidosis, hydrogen ions have an inhibitory effect on the sodium-potassium ATPase pump. This leads to decreased cellular uptake of potassium (hyperkalemia). So an increase in H^+ leads to a decreased cellular uptake of K^+ resulting in increased serum K^+ levels.
Headache, confusion, lethargy	
Increased respirations	
Nausea and vomiting	
Peripheral vasodilatation with warm flushed skin	
Decreased cardiac output when pH of <7.1	

Testing, testing, testing

When acid builds up in the body, acidosis occurs and pH goes down. When too much bicarbonate (base) is lost from the body, this leaves the body too acidic, again causing acidosis.

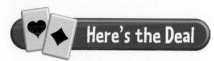

Before we look at ABGs, let's get our terminology straight:

- pH measures hydrogen ion concentration.
- P_{CO_2} measures partial pressure of carbon dioxide.
- P_{O_2} measures partial pressure of oxygen.
- HCO_3 measures bicarbonate level.
- ABG means these blood gases are ARTERIAL (ouch!).

Table 3-1 ABGs in acute and chronic metabolic acidosis

Normal ABG values arterial blood	Acute metabolic acidosis	Chronic metabolic acidosis
pH 7.35–7.45	7.22 (acidosis)	7.4 (normal)
P_{aCO_2} 35–45 mm Hg	40 mm Hg (normal)	32 mm Hg (low)
P_{aO_2} 80–100 mm Hg	92 mm Hg (normal)	94 mm Hg (normal)
HCO_3 22–26 mEq/L	23 mEq < loss HCO_3	34 mEq/L > gain HCO_3
Base excess/deficit ± 2 mEq/L	–5 (significant deficit)	+12 (significant excess)
Oxygen saturation >94%	93%	94%

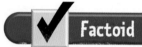

Always manually hold pressure at the arterial site after blood is drawn for ABGs!

- Arterial blood gases are measured. Depending upon whether the metabolic acidosis is acute or chronic, the gases will reflect the body's compensatory response to move the pH toward the normal range (7.35–7.45). Typical ABGs reflect acute metabolic acidosis and are evaluated in Table 3-1.
- Anion gap is calculated from serum electrolytes (Na^+, possibly K^+).
- Urine chloride levels determine the underlying cause of the metabolic acidosis.
- Serum glucose (to detect hyperglycemia).
- BUN and creatinine to detect renal dysfunction.

Signs and symptoms and why?

The pH must be at least partially corrected before you can expect the cardiac output to come up; when there is severe acidemia the heart cannot pump effectively.

- Lactated Ringer's (LR) solution will be helpful in raising the pH because the liver will convert the lactate to bicarbonate.
- IV bicarbonate may be prescribed (based on ABGs) to neutralize excess acid.

In addition to administration of prescribed IVF and bicarbonate, the nurse must closely monitor the patient, and document even subtle respiratory, cardiac, and neurologic changes to evaluate effectiveness of the treatment. Any sign of deterioration of the patient's condition is to be reported immediately.

While the patient is still acutely ill, ongoing monitoring will include:

- Respiratory rate, depth, and exertion
- Pulse oximetry to measure oxygen saturation (hypoxia may accompany acidosis)
- A focused assessment of cardiac output (Refer to Chapter 4, Cardiovascular dysfunction)
- A focused neurological assessment: LOC, reflexes, muscular coordination.
- 24-Hour intake and output
- Frequent vital signs, especially while the patient is unstable (refer to Chapter 2, Vital Sign Guidelines Related to Frequency)
- Monitoring the IV site of bicarbonate (if prescribed) for local redness or irritation, checking frequently for extravasation
- Monitoring the patient's response to LR or Hartmann's solution if prescribed

PATIENT TEACHING   After correcting the underlying condition that precipitated metabolic acidosis, the patient needs focused teaching to reduce the risk for recurrence and recognize early warning signs before acidosis can develop. Depending on the specific cause of the event, teaching may address these issues:

- The importance of maintaining euglycemia through diet, exercise, and insulin, stressing the health benefits of compliance.
- The importance of regular dialysis, as well as a low-potassium diet between treatments.
- The necessity of prompt treatment of infections before they become widespread and systemic.
- Pneumonia (pneumococcal) vaccine/flu shots for susceptible individuals (age >65, chronic heart and lung disorders, kidney failure, sickle cell disease, immune-compromised persons).
- Dietary teaching is focused toward reducing sodium chloride and increasing dietary potassium, planning daily intake to balance alkali-rich foods (vegetables/fruits) with acid producing foods (meat/grains).[1]

What can harm my patient and why?

The patient who is in metabolic acidosis has complications of the initiating medical condition plus the acid–base imbalance. Harm to my patient in metabolic acidosis will come from hypoperfusion, electrolyte imbalance, and base deficit, which can cause:

- Life-threatening arrhythmias
- Cardiac arrest
- Multisystem organ failure (see Chapter 5)
- Coma
- Death

Cutting edge?

There may be more occult (hidden) lactic acidosis in hospitalized patients than we realize! When people don't do well after surgery or major insults to the system, and aren't healing/recovering within the expected time frame, hypoperfusion should be suspected and halted before it leads.

✛ Respiratory acidosis

What is it?

Respiratory acidosis is a buildup of H^+ in the blood caused by abnormalities of respiration, resulting in a decreased pH. Normally, the lungs have a powerful buffering ability by blowing off excess CO_2 to prevent acid build up in the blood, but when the lungs are sick, the CO_2 (an acid) builds up. Remember, when acidosis is caused by an *increase in CO_2*, it is respiratory acidosis (pH <7.35, Pco_2 >45 mm Hg).

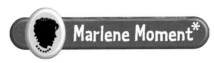

Marlene Moment*

Okay, don't freak out! Let's just look at one item at a time, and don't try to make this hard either:

- The pH tells you whether the patient is too acid, normal, or too alkaline. Always determine this first.
- Next, look at the primary cause of the imbalance: which of these values is messed up in relation to the pH? The CO_2? No, it's normal in acute acidosis. The HCO_3? Yup ... just look at it! If the bicarbonate is messed up, then we must have a kidney problem, meaning this is metabolic acidosis.
- And since the Po_2 is normal, obviously this is an acute situation because the lungs haven't started trying to help yet by blowing off some of that acidic CO_2. They need at least two hours to really kick in for us to see changes on the ABGs.
- The base deficit shows that the bicarbonate is being used up trying to neutralize the acid, and the kidneys haven't had time yet to start reabsorbing bicarbonate or excreting hydrogen.

*Note that when metabolic acidosis is a chronic condition, the ABGs look different, showing that compensation is effective (Table 3-2). The problem chemical (Bicarb → Kidney → Metabolic) is moving the same direction as the compensator (CO_2 → Lungs) and both numbers are going the same direction (7.4 is up from 7.2, and 34 is up from 23)! That's how compensation looks!

▶ Figure 3-3. The kidneys are responsible for the compensatory action during respiratory acidosis.

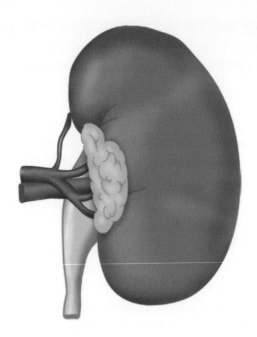

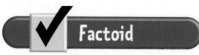

Factoid

Administering sodium bicarbonate can be very dangerous, because it can actually intensify acidosis because of changes at the cellular level (changes that are way over my head). Sodium bicarbonate should be used only as a quick, temporary fix for increased acid levels (to buy some time), while hopefully somebody can figure out what the problem is, and fix it!

 Here's the Deal

Sodium bicarbonate should only be given according to specific ABG values, rather than generously (and sometimes indiscriminately) as we used to do in the past during code situations.

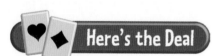 **Here's the Deal**

If you're giving bicarbonate, be SURE to flush the line before and after with normal saline. If there is any bicarbonate in the line, it will precipitate out and turn to cement (just kidding, but you get the picture) in the patient's vascular space.

The patient's needs vary depending on the underlying cause of the metabolic acidosis. Specific implementations are directed toward improving oxygenation/perfusion status, restoring fluid and electrolyte balance, and treating DKA, sepsis, trauma, or renal failure.

Compensatory Mechanism

The kidneys will compensate, but they react much slower than the lungs in their buffering ability. To compensate, they put base bicarbonate back into the blood by reabsorbing the filtered bicarbonate and producing new bicarbonate. The rise in HCO_3^- helps offset the rise in CO_2 and returns the pH to normal.

Causes and why?

Causes	Why
Medications such as sedatives, hypnotics, and narcotics	Can decrease the respiratory rate and cause CO_2 retention.
Excessive alcohol ingestion	Sedative effect leads to decreased respirations and CO_2 retention.
Altered deep breathing associated with things like postoperative pain or fractured ribs	Postoperative surgical pain (especially abdominal) or from fractured ribs leads to shallow breathing and CO_2 retention.
Hypoventilation	• Conditions such as myasthenia gravis, and Guillain-Barré syndrome cause weak muscles, and can lead to altered gas exchange and retention of CO_2. • Obesity contributes to hypoventilation, especially if in a compromised state of health. • Abdominal binders and/or dressings postoperatively can lead to hypoventilation. • Postoperative pain. • Fractured ribs (pain!). • Ascites (related to cirrhosis).

(Continued)

Causes	Why
Brain trauma (medulla) brain stem?	Decreased respiratory rate.
High-flow O_2 in chronic lung disease	In healthy individuals, CO_2 is the stimulus for respiration. But in people with chronic lung disease, the CO_2 *remains* elevated because of impaired lung function and altered gas exchange. CO_2 loses the effect on respiration it once had because the respiratory center becomes desensitized to the CO_2. The drive for breathing in these people is decreased $PaCO_2$ (hypoxemia). Administration of high-flow O_2 can be dangerous because it can reduce the stimulus to breathe.
Any pulmonary problem: • Emphysema • Chronic bronchitis • Bronchial pneumonia • Pneumonia • Asthma • Cystic fibrosis • Pulmonary edema • Pulmonary embolism • Airway obstruction • Foreign body aspiration • Atelectasis • Pneumothorax, hemothorax • Respiratory arrest/cardiac arrest • Respiratory distress syndrome • Laryngospasm • Improper settings on the ventilator	Any respiratory problem, if it's bad enough, can lead to CO_2 retention! Impaired lung function causes impaired gas exchange, inability to blow off CO_2, retention of CO_2, and eventually acidosis.

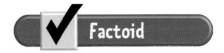

The typical American diet contributes to acid–base imbalance in that sodium chloride is consumed in excess, coupled with a potassium deficit, to lactic acidosis. Clinical researchers have already figured this out! Increased blood lactate levels are an important warning sign in surgical patients.

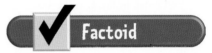

Hypercapnia is an increase of CO_2 > 45.

Signs and symptoms and why?

Signs and symptoms	why
Feeling full in the head, altered LOC, confusion	$PaCO_2$ causes vasodilatation with increased cerebral blood flow, particularly if the CO_2 level reaches 60 mm Hg or greater
Dizziness, palpitations/arrhythmias restlessness, hypotension, and tachycardia	Hyperkalemia, hypoxia, vasodilatation leading to low blood pressure with compensatory increase in heart rate to perfuse vital organs
Acidic urine	Excretion of H^+—kidneys are compensating
Warm skin	Vasodilatation
Decreased muscle tone, decreased DTR	Increased H+, hyperkalemia, hypercalcemia (calcium?)

(Continued)

Signs and symptoms	why
Hyperkalemia (with **acute** acidosis)	Acid–base abnormalities can cause changes in the distribution of K^+
	In **acute** acidosis, hydrogen ions have an inhibitory effect on the sodium-potassium ATPase pump. This leads to decreased cellular uptake of potassium (hyperkalemia).
	So an increase in H^+ leads to a decreased cellular uptake of K^+, resulting in increased serum K^+ levels

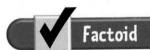

If the bicarbonate falls, the acidosis is metabolic acidosis. If the CO_2 rises, the acidosis is respiratory acidosis.

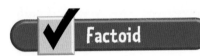

Anything that causes slow or shallow breathing (hypoventilation) can lead to retention of CO_2 and respiratory acidosis.

- ABGs reveal a high $Paco_2$ (>45 mm Hg) and a low pH (<7.35).
- Drug screen may be indicated if drug overdose is suspected.
- Chest X-ray may reveal broken ribs or a collapsed lung (pneumothorax, hemothorax) or pulmonary edema with lung fluid.
- Serum electrolytes (potassium, calcium especially important).
- Serum lactate always elevates with tissue hypoperfusion when anaerobic metabolism takes over and leaves behind the acidic by-product lactic acid.

Testing, testing, testing

See Table 3-2.

Table 3-2   ABGs in respiratory acidosis

Normal ABG values arterial blood	Acute respiratory acidosis	Chronic respiratory acidosis
pH 7.35–7.45	7.28 (low)	7.4 (normal)
$Paco_2$ 35–45 mm Hg	60 mm Hg (high)	40 mm Hg (normal)
Pao_2 80–100 mm Hg	79 mm Hg (low)	94 mm Hg (normal)
HCO_3 22–26 mEq/L	24 mEq (normal)	34 mEq/L > gain HCO_3
Base excess/deficit ± 2 mEq/L	–2 (significant deficit)	+6 (significant excess)
Oxygen saturation >94%	93%	94%

Signs and symptoms and why?

A-B-Cs are priority! Because ventilation is inadequate, measures must be promptly implemented to improve ventilation. Bronchospasm can be relaxed with bronchodilators.

- Pulmonary embolus can be "busted up" with thrombolysis and anticoagulant therapy.
- Intubation may be necessary with upper torso burns where permeable vessels have leaked and edema fluid is closing off the airway.
- Percussion, vibration, and suction may be used to clear secretions from the pulmonary tree.
- Antibiotics are indicated for lung infections to eradicate the causative microorganisms.
- Endotracheal intubation with mechanical ventilation if less invasive measures cannot immediately restore adequate respirations.

Adequate hydration (by mouth and parenteral therapy as prescribed) to liquefy thick pulmonary secretions.

- Turn, cough, deep breathe, and instruct in use of incentive spirometer to exhale excess CO_2.
- Supplemental oxygen as prescribed.
- Monitoring vital signs and oxygen saturation.
- Monitoring ABGs and serum electrolytes.

PATIENT TEACHING   Patient teaching is specific to the underlying cause of respiratory acidosis. For example:

- Patients with sleep apnea are instructed in the use of continuous positive airway pressure (CPAP) machines.
- Surgical patients are taught the importance of incentive spirometry to fully ventilate the lungs, especially after analgesia.
- Chronic lung patients are taught to keep oxygen flow low, even if short of breath because of possibly depressing the stimulus to breathe.
- Asthma patients are taught the importance of self-monitoring and strict adherence to the prescribed medications.

What can harm my patient and why?

Respiratory acidosis can be caused by many different conditions; therefore, the complications will be different based on the underlying problem. However, all respiratory acidosis left unchecked will result in:

- Respiratory arrest
- Cardiac arrhythmias
- Shock

✚ Metabolic alkalosis

What is it?

Metabolic alkalosis is an excess of the **base bicarbonate**. The compensatory mechanism is decreased respirations in order to increase CO_2 (acid) in the blood.

Causes and why?

Causes	Why
Prolonged vomiting	Loss of acid from the stomach. The result is **base bicarbonate excess.**
Gastric suctioning (eg, NG tube to suction)	Loss of acid from the stomach. The result is **base bicarbonate excess.**
Ingestion of bicarbonate (eg, baking soda, Alka-Seltzer, antacids)	**Base bicarbonate excess.**

(Continued)

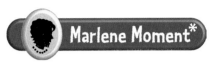

Marlene Moment*

Now don't freak out! You did fine on the other ABGs, and you will get this one too. Remember ... the first thing we look at is the pH to see if the patient is in acidosis or alkalosis (or normal):

- The pH tells you whether the patient is too acidic, normal, or too alkaline. Always determine this first. Do you see the acidosis? 7.28 is hard to miss!
- Next, look at the primary cause of the imbalance: which of these values is messed up in relation to the pH, which is high? The HCO_3? No, it's normal in acute acidosis because nothing is wrong with the kidneys. The CO_2? Yup ... just look at it! If the carbon dioxide is messed up, then we must have a lung problem, meaning this is respiratory acidosis.
- Because the HCO_3 is normal, obviously this is an acute situation for the reason that the kidneys haven't started trying to help yet by retaining/conserving bicarbonate (HCO_3).
- It takes at least two days for the kidneys to really kick in before you see changes on the ABGs.
- The base deficit shows that the bicarbonate is being used up trying to neutralize the acid, and the kidneys haven't had time yet to start reabsorbing more bicarbonate or excreting hydrogen.
- Did you notice the Pao_2? Now our patient is hypoxic!

*Note that when respiratory acidosis is a chronic condition, the ABGs look different, showing that compensation is effective (see Table 3-2). The problem chemical (Respiratory = Lung → CO_2 →) is moving in the same direction as the compensator (HCO_3 → Kidneys). The pH 7.40 has moved UP from pH 7.28. The compensator chemical HCO_3 34 mEq has moved UP from 24 mEq, showing that there is more bicarbonate now to neutralize all that lung acid! That's how compensation looks!

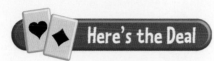

Just because compensation occurs in respiratory acidosis does not mean that the primary cause of the problem is being corrected. It just means that the kidneys are working overtime trying to stay on top of things, cranking out more bicarbonate to neutralize all that acid the lungs can't seem to get rid of! The underlying problem must be corrected simultaneously with the acidosis.

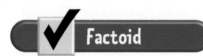

When CO_2 is UP the O_2 is DOWN.

Respiratory insufficiency is always the root cause of respiratory acidosis. My patient needs a plan of care that will enhance cellular respiration to correct the immediate underlying problem.

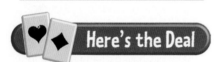

With reversal of acidosis the accompanying hyperkalemia, hypercalcemia may also be resolved; however, electrolytes are monitored closely, along with ABGs.

Factoid

Aldosterone (mineralocorticoid) is the most important hormone in the body that regulates K^+ balance.

Causes	Why
Conn's syndrome (excessive aldosterone secretion)	Aldosterone stimulates the kidneys to secrete H^+. When the kidneys secrete H+, they reabsorb HCO_3^- and add it back to the blood. Adding the bicarbonate back to the blood leads to alkalosis. **How does this work?** To understand this concept, you have to know that *normally* when the kidneys need to reabsorb bicarbonate and put it back in the blood, they have to secrete H^+ first. So when aldosterone (excessive) tells the kidneys to secrete H^+, their natural response is to do it and then reabsorb HCO_3^- and add it back to the blood. The difference here is that the kidneys are responding to a pathophysiologic condition (hyperaldosteronism) rather than being a normal compensatory response in the regulation of acid–base balance. The result is **base bicarbonate excess.** Conversely, if the kidneys were responding as a normal compensatory response, it would have restored the pH, but instead it caused alkalosis because the kidneys were responding to the *aldosterone* and not the blood pH.
Profound potassium depletion (<2.0 mEq/L) Potassium-depleting diuretics (thiazides, furosemide, ethacrynic acid)	Hypokalemia causes the kidneys to conserve K+ and increase H^+ secretion. When the kidneys secrete H^+, they reabsorb bicarbonate and add it back to the blood. The result is **base bicarbonate excess.** Note: Plasma K^+ concentration leads to changes in H^+ secretion, which in turn can affect acid–base status.
Cushing's syndrome	Excess glucocorticoid production leads to hypokalemia. Remember, profound hypokalemia can lead to alkalosis as stated above. The result is **base bicarbonate excess.**
Administration of $NaHCO_3$ during CPR	**Base bicarbonate excess** **Note:** Cessation of breathing leads to retention of CO_2 leading to acidosis. Addition of bicarbonate restores the blood pH, but excessive administration can lead to alkalosis.

Signs and symptoms and why?

The patient is alkalotic and the problem is not the lungs. Something is metabolically wrong, and the lungs will try to compensate for the problem.

Metabolic alkalosis (high pH = excess base bicarbonate or hydrogen deficit) causes the following neuromuscular signs and symptoms once the body compensates for the acid–base imbalance. (Refer to Table 3-1 for a comparison of metabolic acidosis and metabolic alkalosis and the "whys.") These are the "biggies":

- Highly irritable, excitable muscle cells.
- Tetany (muscles contract in a constant, tight hold).
- Hyperreflexia (4 + DTRs).
- Muscles become weak, and begin twitching and cramping.

Signs and symptoms	Why
Urine alkaline	Decreased ability of the failing kidney to excrete hydrogen ions.
Hyperkalemia	When excess hydrogen ions move out of the vascular space into the cell, the K^+ moves out of the cell, into the serum.
	Addison's disease causes K^+ to be retained and NaCl excreted.
Weak, flaccid muscles Decreased DTRs	Caused by hypercalcemia, which has a sedative effect on muscles.
Cardiac arrhythmias Cardiac arrest	Caused by hyperkalemia. Peaked T wave.

Testing, testing, testing

See Table 3-3.

- Serum electrolytes: NaCl, K^+, Ca^+.
- Serum lactate (indicator of lactic acid caused by hypoperfusion).
- ABGs will reflect base excess.

Table 3-3   ABGs acute and chronic metabolic alkalosis

Normal ABG values arterial blood	Acute metabolic alkalosis (no compensation)	Chronic metabolic alkalosis (lungs compensate)
pH 7.35–7.45	7.46 (alkalosis)	7.40 (normal)
$Paco_2$ 35–45 mm Hg	42 mm Hg (normal)	32 mm Hg (low)
Pao_2 80–100 mm Hg	93 mm Hg (normal)	93 mm Hg (normal)
HCO_3 22–26 mEq/L	28 mEq (high)	28 mEq/L (high)
Base excess/deficit ± 2 mEq/L	+12 (significant excess)	+12 (significant excess)
Oxygen saturation >94%	93% (no hypoxia)	94% (no hypoxia)

Okay, now don't go crazy! We'll look at each item and it's going to make sense, so you just look at the numbers and we will figure this out together:

- The pH tells you whether the patient is too acid, normal, or too alkaline. Always determine this first. Do you see the alkalosis?

- Next, look at the primary cause of the imbalance. Which of these values is messed up in relation to the pH, which is high? The CO_2? No, it's normal in acute alkalosis because nothing is wrong with the lungs. The HCO_3? Yup … just look at it! If the bicarbonate is messed up, then we must have a kidney problem, meaning this is metabolic alkalosis.

- Now, because the PO_2 is normal, obviously this is an acute situation because the lungs haven't started trying to help yet by retaining/conserving some of that acidic CO_2. They need at least two hours to really kick in for us to see changes on the ABGs.

- The base excess shows that the bicarbonate is being used up trying to neutralize the acid, and the kidneys haven't had time yet to start reabsorbing bicarbonate or excreting hydrogen.

Note that when metabolic acidosis is a chronic condition, the ABGs look different, showing that compensation is effective (see Table 3-2). The problem chemical (Metabolic = Kidney → Bicarb →) is moving the same direction as the compensator (CO_2 → Lungs) and both numbers are going in the same direction (pH 7.40 is down from 7.46 and $PaCO_2$ of 32 is down from 42) showing that the CO_2 is being used up as it combines with water in the plasma to make carbonic acid to offset excess bicarbonate! That's how compensation looks!

Signs and symptoms and why?

If the muscles of respiration and the heart are depressed by the HYPOs: hypokalemia and hypocalcemia, cardiorespiratory support may be indicated.

The kidneys will not be able to excrete the excess base until the chloride deficit is corrected. Here are the priority interventions:

- NaCl (isotonic) IVF to replace chloride losses via vomiting, suction, or diuresis.

- IVF with KCL if replacement therapy is indicated because of hyperaldosteronism or diuresis.

- Seizure precautions until hypocalcemia is resolved.

- Ventilator and tracheostomy tray in readiness in anticipation of tetany.

Nursing interventions will focus on the initiating event or condition and problems resulting from metabolic alkalosis:

- Monitor ABGs, watching for compensation by the lungs.

- Monitor serum electrolytes and urine chloride to evaluate the effectiveness of treatment.

- Monitor for developments such as ileus. Peristalsis is decreased by the depressant action of hypokalemia and hypocalcemia on the muscle layer of the bowel.

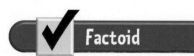

Factoid

H_2O (water) + CO_2 (carbon dioxide) = H_2CO_3 (carbonic acid)
Plasma water plus carbon dioxide = carbonic acid

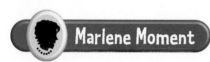

Marlene Moment

Let's give a round of applause to the lungs for taking care of our little bicarbonate problem by mixing up a recipe of carbonic acid! And just think, the only other ingredient was water!

- Withhold oral intake and notify the doctor if bowel sounds are absent.
- Monitor oxygen saturation and clinical evidence of hypoventilation.
- Monitor cardiac output (for a focused assessment see Chapter 4).
- Continuous cardiac monitoring to detect possible arrhythmias.

PATIENT TEACHING   Patient teaching will be directed toward the condition or causation of the metabolic alkalosis:

- Teach patients that oral antacids have a systemic effect, and that they are not to take them indiscriminately.
- Patients on thiazide and loop diuretics who are also on a low-sodium diet should be encouraged to eat small amounts of "real" salt (sodium plus chloride) in addition to herbal seasonings because chloride depletion enhances bicarbonate resorption, which increases alkalinity.
- Teach patients the dangers of using baking soda (bicarbonate) for indigestion, or overuse of OTC preparations (such as Alka-Seltzer).
- Include a good source of potassium and calcium in the diet on a daily basis.
- If you are a licorice lover, don't overdo it because it causes sodium and water retention, and potassium loss, which could lead to recurrence of alkalosis.
- Caution dialysis patients not to miss treatments, and to maintain a low-potassium diet between treatments.

What can harm my patient and why?

The brain does not like it one little bit when the pH is messed up! The neuromuscular and cardiac events that lead to a high morbidity rate are:

- Tetany
- Seizures
- Life-threatening arrhythmias

Harm can also be manifested by electrolyte imbalance (hypocalcemia and hypokalemia) and resultant muscle weakness:

- Decreased cardiac output
- Cardiac arrest
- Respiratory arrest

✚ Respiratory alkalosis

Respiratory alkalosis is not as common as respiratory acidosis, but it will be easier for you to spot because the primary symptom is visible and obvious.

Let's get the normal stuff straight!

The lungs are the organs that are responsible of clearing the blood of carbon dioxide: That's their job! When the lungs fall down on the job, P_{CO_2} builds up in the blood. The only way that P_{CO_2} can leave the body is through exhalation, made possible by healthy lungs.

| Bicarbonate-chloride exchange | Sodium and chloride follow each other, and the kidney reabsorbs these electrolytes together. When blood volume is low from vomiting with resultant chloride depletion, the kidney reabsorbs more bicarbonate to compensate for chloride loss. Excess bicarbonate coupled with low a chloride level causes hypochloremic alkalosis. The opposite occurs with hyperchloremic acidosis: The drop in pH occurs because of decreased bicarbonate reabsorption in response to increased chlorides owing to a buildup of acidic chlorine salts. |

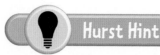

Opposites attract:
LOW blood K^+ means HIGH pH number (alkalosis)
HIGH blood K^+ means LOW on pH number (acidosis)

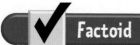

Hyperventilation causes low CO_2 (carbon dioxide) levels, which decrease the plasma levels of H_2CO_3 (carbonic acid).

What is it?

Respiratory alkalosis describes an acid–base imbalance in which the P_{CO_2} is low (<35 mm Hg) and the pH is high (>7.45). Depending on the cause of the underlying problem, respiratory alkalosis may be acute or may be present as a chronic problem.

Causes and why?

Acute respiratory alkalosis is usually related to rapid decrease in P_{CO_2} caused by hyperventilation. There are also some "non-lung" as well as some "sick lung" problems that cause the lungs to respond with fast breathing because the respiratory center is stimulated.

Marlene Moment

The recipe for carbonic acid (H_2CO_3) calls for water (H_2O) plus CO_2. If I'm all out of carbon dioxide, obviously I can't cook up any carbonic acid!

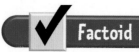

Fast respirations = Low carbon dioxide. The faster you breathe, the more CO_2 is blown off.

Causes	Why
• Anxiety • Severe pain • Panic attack • Aspirin overdose (early phase) • Acute respiratory distress syndrome (early phase) • Ventilator rate settings turned up too high • Hypoxemia • High altitudes • Gram-negative bacteria producing sepsis (early phase)	A rapid increase in respirations will result in excess CO_2 being exhaled and lead to respiratory alkalosis.
Conditions that result in long-standing hypocapnia will cause chronic respiratory alkalosis: • Anemia • Brain tumor • Impaired hepatic function	Decreased oxygen combining power and hypoxia, which causes increased respirations. Causes intracranial pressure changes. Leads to increased levels of ammonia.

Signs and symptoms and why?

Respiratory alkalosis signs and symptoms	Why
Hyperventilation	Increased rate of respirations (causes loss of O_2 acid) leading to a base (alkaline) excess.
Alkaline urine	Kidneys attempt to compensate by excreting bicarbonate ions.
Neurologic changes: Light headedness Vertigo Syncope	Hypocapnia causes vessels in the brain to vasoconstrict, reducing cerebral blood flow.
Tachycardia	Hypocapnia activates medullary receptors to increase heart rate.
Hypokalemia	When hydrogen moves out of the cell and into the serum to reduce alkalinity, potassium moves into the cell, reducing serum K^+.
Hypocalcemia: My patient is NOT sedated. Muscles are hyperirritable: muscle twitching, cramps, and spasms Tingling, and numbness of fingers and toes; 4+ DTRs (hyperreflexia) Positive Trousseau Positive Chvostek Tetany Convulsions	Calcium acts like a neuromuscular sedative, and my patient doesn't have enough of it! Cause of symptoms is neuromuscular irritability.
Cardiac arrhythmias	Caused by hypokalemia.

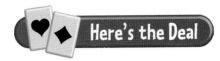

This is the last set of ABGs that you have to evaluate, so hang in there! We always look at the same things in the same order to keep from getting confused:

- First, what is the pH? Well, duh, 7.56 is obviously high (plus it says so on the report above). Alkalosis is the problem, but is it respiratory or metabolic? Let's find out!

- Second, look at the primary cause of the imbalance. Which of these values is messed up in relation to the low pH? The carbon dioxide or the bicarbonate? Because the CO_2 is low but the bicarbonate is normal, obviously the lungs are causing the problem! Bingo! Respiratory alkalosis!

- Now, because the HCO_3 is normal, obviously this is an acute situation for the reason that the kidneys haven't started trying to help yet by retaining/conserving bicarbonate (HCO_3). They need at least two days to really kick in before we see changes on the ABGs.

- The base excess shows that the bicarbonate is not being used to neutralize acid, because there IS none to neutralize. The patient is blowing off the acid and bicarbonate is not needed! The kidneys haven't had time yet to start excreting the excess bicarbonate.

Testing, testing, testing

Depending upon whether the respiratory alkalosis is acute or chronic, the gases reflect the body's compensatory response to move the pH toward the normal range (7.35–7.45). Typical ABGs will look like this for acute respiratory alkalosis (Table 3-4).

Table 3-4   Acute and chronic respiratory alkalosis

Normal ABG values arterial blood	Acute respiratory alkalosis	Chronic respiratory alkalosis
pH 7.35–7.45	7.56 (high)	7.4 (normal)
$Paco_2$ 35–45 mm Hg	32 mm Hg (low)	40 mm Hg (normal)
Pao_2 80–100 mm Hg	93 mm Hg (normal)	94 mm Hg (normal)
HCO_3 22–26 mEq/L	25 mEq (normal)	22 mEq/L > gain HCO_3
Base excess/deficit ±2 mEq/L	+6 mEq (significant excess)	–2 (low normal)
Oxygen saturation >94%	93%	93%

Note that when respiratory alkalosis is a chronic condition (eg, long-standing anemia), the ABGs look different, showing that compensation is effective (see Table 3-2). The problem chemical (Respiratory → Lung → CO_2 →) is moving in the same direction as the compensator HCO_3 → Kidneys. The pH 7.56 has moved DOWN to pH 7. The compensator chemical HCO_3 25 mEq has moved DOWN to 22 mEq.

- The bicarbonate deficit shows that there is less bicarbonate now because it is being used up neutralizing excess lung acid! That's how compensation looks!

Signs and symptoms and why?

See Figure 3-4.

▶ Figure 3-4. Paper Bag Breathing. One way to help a patient who is hyperventilating (breathing too fast and shallow) is to have him or her breathe into a paper bag. The patient will rebreathe his or her own CO_2 and help to maintain proper acid–base balance.

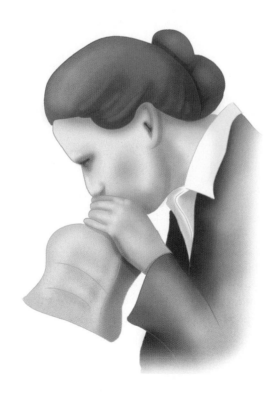

My patient needs to stop breathing so fast, or shallow! My patient needs to take some nice deep, slow breaths. How can we make this happen?

- If the problem is hysteria causing my patient to breathe really fast, you should have the patient cup a paper bag around the top, placed snugly against the lips to rebreathe his or her own CO_2.
- Sedation may also be given to depress the respiratory center in the brain, thereby slowing respirations.

In addition to treating the cause of the acid–base imbalance, the immediate treatment for hypochloremic alkalosis (related to severe, persistent vomiting—see bicarbonate-sodium exchange) is to:

- Administer sodium chloride to rehydrate.
- Replace the sodium and chloride (based on serum electrolytes and hematocrit).
- Hold the patient NPO and treat the cause of vomiting.
- If the patient has an artificial airway with mechanical ventilation in progress, the rate setting and the tidal volume will be reevaluated.

PATIENT TEACHING Patient teaching is based on the underlying cause of the respiratory alkalosis. The teaching varies according to specific causative conditions. Many times patient teaching can reduce fear and anxiety (with subsequent tachypnea) by providing factual information to replace myths or unfounded fears.

What can harm my patient and why?

What harms your patient will be totally related to the underlying cause of respiratory alkalosis. For example, if an aspirin overdose is implicated, you would expect specific complications for this event. So, focus on the cause of the acid–base imbalance, but always be on the lookout for the most life-threatening complications:

- Seizures
- Arrhythmias

Cutting edge

It is well known that psychological tension in the preoperative period is related to anxiety and fear of the unknown. A Japanese study of women awaiting total hysterectomy used saliva samples to measure salivary chromogranin A as an index of the degree of preoperative psychological tension. Chromogranin A levels were measured before and after premedication with either butorphanol (Stadol) or midazolam (Versed), while the control group received no premedication. Lower chromogranin A levels (less psychological tension) were found in the group premedicated with midazolam.

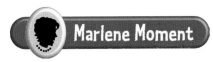 **Marlene Moment**

I don't want you to get all crazy or anything, but there is something I need to tell you. In the real world when you are a real nurse (RN), you will see ABGs that don't fit the guidelines we've been using, and here's why: There can be problems with *both* the lungs and the kidneys! This represents mixed respiratory and metabolic acidosis. It looks weird, but remember, I told you so! If you can't make any sense out of the ABGs, then it must be "mixed" because the ABGs don't fit the rules.

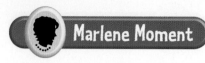
Marlene Moment

The prom queen (PQ) is sitting atop the back seat of a convertible when the driver hits a speed bump and she slides off the back. A hysterical PQ is scooped up and brought to the emergency room, dropping sequins everywhere. The PQ is fine, but she has "road rash" and her dress is ruined. Her friends in the waiting room are not faring so well. They're breathing hard and fast and dropping expensive cell phones because of muscle spasms. Should you tell them to all go home? (In about three days, their kidneys will kick in.) Tell them to go finish off that keg of booze in the trunk of the convertible? (After all, alcohol IS a central nervous system depressant!) No! Give them all a paper bag, and instruct them to re-breathe!

The underlying cause of hyperventilation (sepsis, heat stroke, hypochloremia, etc.) must be identified and treatment must be initiated promptly.

- Maintain NPO as long as nausea/vomiting persist.
- Administer parenteral, rectal, or topical (wrist band) antiemetics as prescribed.
- Administer antipyretic medications to lower the fever, and the rate of respirations.
- Obtain stat culture and sensitivity and initiate prescribed broad-spectrum IVPB antibiotics promptly.
- Monitor and report changes in ABGs promptly.

PRACTICE QUESTIONS

1. Which finding from the ABGs would the nurse expect to find when a patient has been unable to eat because of protracted vomiting?

   A. Elevated Po_2

   B. Elevated HCO_3

   C. Decreased Pco_2

   D. Decreased HCO_3

2. An outpatient who completed the prescribed bowel prep Fleets laxatives and enemas (Phospho-Soda) received Valium 5 mg IV prior to a colonoscopy. Upon return from an uncomplicated procedure, the patient is lethargic and difficult to fully arouse. Which next nursing assessment is the priority?

   A. Palpate her abdomen and check for firmness or tenderness.

   B. Auscultate bowel sounds and check for rebound tenderness.

   C. Collaborate with the physician for administration of Romazicon.

   D. Turn her on her side, while assessing for tense, tight musculature.

3. An obese surgical patient has been requesting (and receiving) frequent PRN narcotics for pain control, but the abdominal binder (recently applied) seems to be helping, because you have not heard a peep from her since the last PRN narcotic injection. Upon entering the room, you find that she is sleeping soundly. Which next nursing action is the priority?

   A. Wake her up and make her use the incentive spirometer.

   B. Tiptoe back out, and document that analgesia has been effective.

   C. Check the oxygen saturation (finger nail bed probe) noting SaO_2.

   D. Awaken her and question her to determine LOC and orientation.

4. A surgical patient is making an uneventful recovery (no bleeding, no infection, and stable vital signs), but just doesn't feel well: general malaise, dull headache, anorexia and nausea, weakness and fatigue. Which nursing action would be of the most benefit to this patient?

   A. Notify the hospital pharmacist that a possible drug reaction is in progress.

   B. Alert the infection control officer that an occult infection will require nasal and blood smears.

   C. Collaborate with the surgeon to have blood drawn for serum lactate level immediately.

   D. Update the nursing care plan with a nursing order for assisted ambulation in the hall qid.

5. The patient with chronic respiratory acidosis should be monitored closely for which electrolyte imbalance?

　A. Hypocalcemia

　B. Hyperkalemia

　C. Hypomagnesemia

　D. Hyperphosphatemia

6. A chronic lung patient is given morphine sulfate in the emergency department (ED) for acute abdominal pain, prior to admitting the patient to the med-surg unit. Which nursing assessment should be reported to the physician immediately?

　A. A 10 mm Hg drop in blood pressure since transfer from the ED.

　B. Quiet, slow, rhythmic respirations 12 to 14 range (counted while sleeping).

　C. Pink nail beds, rosy cheeks, and tip of nose with nasal oxygen at 2 L/min.

　D. Skin is warm and slightly moist, with tenting present on back of hands.

7. Arterial blood gases reflect a pH of 7.28, PCO_2 of 50, and HCO_3 of 24. To which of the following patients would these ABGs most likely belong?

　A. Type 1 diabetic with blood glucose of 546 mg/dL.

　B. Highly anxious with a panic attack and hyperventilation in progress.

　C. Alzheimer's with recent overdose of aspirin related to arthritic pain.

　D. Postop with gastric suction, nauseated and vomiting around the NG tube.

8. The patient has hyperkalemia and hypercalcemia after having been on a restrictive diet intended to promote weight loss. Which of the following acid–base imbalances would be expected to accompany this electrolyte imbalance?

　A. Metabolic acidosis

　B. Metabolic alkalosis

　C. Respiratory acidosis

　D. Respiratory alkalosis

9. The head-injured patient has increased ICP and neurologic symptoms of headache, decreased LOC, decreased DTRs, and blurred vision. Stat ABGs are most likely to reveal:

　A. Metabolic acidosis

　B. Respiratory acidosis

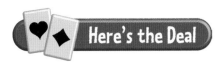

Here's the Deal

Sometimes, respiratory alkalosis is medically induced to reduce intracranial pressure. The patient is mechanically hyperventilated to vasoconstrict blood vessels in the brain, thereby lowering the ICP.

ABGs are monitored at frequent intervals throughout therapeutic respiratory alkalosis.

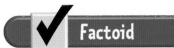

Factoid

Respiratory problems cause changes in the PCO_2 (dissolved CO_2 in the blood).

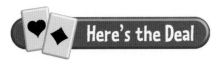

Here's the Deal

The cranium (skull) is a rigid compartment that contains neural tissue, blood, and cerebrospinal fluid. These three components comprise 100% of what is inside the cranium. If blood flow increases or the brain swells, something has to "give" because your head can't hold more than 100% of anything. There isn't room for more!

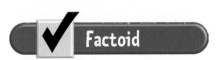

Factoid

Acidosis causes peripheral vasoconstriction and cerebral vasodilatation to increase incoming blood flow to the brain.

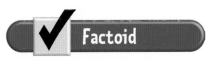

Factoid

Alkalosis causes peripheral vasodilatation and cerebral vasoconstriction to decrease incoming blood flow to the brain.

C. Metabolic alkalosis

D. Respiratory alkalosis

10. A patient with an acid–base imbalance is intubated and has been mechanically ventilated for several days. An indwelling catheter is draining freely, but the nurse notes that the patient's urine has now become acidic. These findings should be interpreted as:

   A. Bad, because now the patient has developed respiratory acidosis.

   B. Good, because the kidneys are compensating for respiratory acidosis.

   C. Odd, because acidic urine is unrelated to ventilator respiratory support.

   D. Helpful, because acidic urine will help reduce UTI secondary to the Foley.

References

1. Vormann J, Remer T. Dietary, metabolic, physiologic and disease-related aspects of acid-base balance. *J Nutr* 138:413S–414S, 2008.

2. Meregalli A, Oliveira R, Friedman G. Occult hypoperfusion is associated with increased mortality in hemodynamically stable, high-risk, surgical patients. Medscape. From *Critical Care*. Posted April 5, 2004. Accessed January 20, 2009.

3. Porth CM. *Pathophysiology: Concepts of Altered Health States*. 7th ed. Philadelphia: Lippincott Williams & Wilkins; 2007.

4. Moviat M, Terpstra AM, Ruitenbeek W, et al. Contribution of various metabolites to the unmeasured anions in critically ill patients with metabolic acidosis. *Crit Care Med* 36(3):752–758, 2008.

5. Hurst M. *Hurst Review's Pathophysiology Review*. New York: McGraw Hill; 2008.

6. Nicks BA, McGinnis HD, Borron SW, Megarbane B. Lactic Acidosis. http://emedicine.medscape.com/article/768159-overview. Updated April 9, 2008. Accessed February 10, 2009.

6a. Mathews KD, Stark JE. Hyperchloremic, normal anion-gap, metabolic acidosis due to topiramate. Medscape Nurses, From *American Journal of Health-System Pharmacy*. Posted October 7, 2008. Accessed January 16, 2009.

7. Clancy J, McVicar A. Intermediate and long term regulation of acid-base homeostasis. *Br J Nurs* 16(17):1076–1079, 2007.

8. Vormann J, Remer T. Dietary, metabolic, physiologic and disease-related aspects of acid-base balance. *J Nutr* 138:413S–414S, 2008.

9. Meregalli A, Oliveira R, Friedman G. Occult hypoperfusion is associated with increased mortality in hemodynamically stable, high-risk, surgical patients. Medscape, From *Critical Care*. Posted April 5, 2004. Accessed January 20, 2009.

10. Pagana KD, Pagana TJ. *Mosby's Diagnostic and Laboratory Test Reference.* 6th ed. St. Louis: Mosby; 2003.

11. Hurst M. *Finally Understanding Fluids and Electrolytes.* [Audio CD-ROM]. Baltimore: Lippincott Williams & Wilkins; 2004.

12. Hurst M. Fluids and electrolytes. In: Hurst M, ed. *Hurst Review's NCLEX-RN Review.* New York: McGraw-Hill Medical; 2008.

13. Smeltzer SC, Bare BG, Hinkle JL, Cheever KH. *Brunner & Suddarth's Textbook of Medical-Surgical Nursing.* 11th ed. Philadelphia: Lippincott Williams & Wilkins; 2008.

14. Liu KD, Matthay MA. Advances in critical care for the nephrologists: Acute lung injury/ARDS. *Clin J Am Soc Nephrol* 3:578–586, 2008.

15. Cartotto R, Walia G, Ellis S, Fowler R. Oscillation after inhalation: High frequency oscillatory ventilation in burn patients with the acute respiratory distress syndrome and co-existing smoke inhalation injury. *J Burn Care Res* 30(1):119–127, 2009.

16. Obara S, Iwama H. Assessment of psychological tension after pre-medication by measurement of chromogranin A. *J Clin Anesthesiol* 17(7):554–557, 2005.

17. Ezri T, Lerner E, Muggia-Sullam M, et al. Phosphate salt bowel preparation regimens alter perioperative acid-base and electrolyte balance. *Can J Anesthes* 53:153–158, 2006.

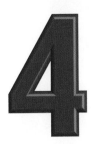

CHAPTER

4 Cardiovascular Disorders

OBJECTIVES

Probably the most common disability from all medical-surgical diseases is associated with cardiac dysfunction. In this chapter, nursing care related to cardiovascular dysfunction will focus on patient teaching for risk reduction and health maintenance in an effort to avoid disabling conditions associated with structural heart damage, and amputations secondary to vascular insufficiency. Medical management and good nursing care can be of great benefit, but you will learn that the patient has to do his or her part too!

In this chapter you will review:

- Selected pathophysiology associated with cardiovascular dysfunction.
- The body's compensatory response to cardiovascular dysfunction.
- The effects of cardiovascular dysfunction related to priority needs of oxygenation, circulation, and physical safety.
- The key concepts and priorities associated with cardiovascular nursing care.
- Treatment modalities and nursing care to promote restoration of optimal cardiovascular function.
- The technologic advances that improve the quality of life and reduce threat to life when the cardiovascular system fails or is compromised.
- The impact of age, nutritional status, lifestyle choices, genetics, and comorbidities that alter heart health.
- Nursing measures to create and maintain a safe, effective care environment for the patient experiencing cardiovascular dysfunction.
- Components of a teaching plan to enhance self-care monitoring for the patient recovering from a cardiovascular dysfunction.

Let's get the normal stuff straight first!
See Figure 4-1.

▶ Figure 4-1. Anatomy of the Heart. The heart is the center of the cardiovascular system and is comprised of four separate chambers. (Reproduced from Hurst M. *Hurst Reviews: Pathophysiology Review.* New York: McGraw-Hill; 2008.)

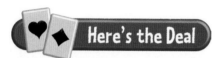

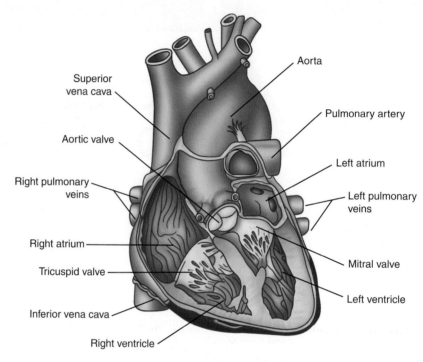

To the best of its ability, the heart will try to maintain adequate blood flow and oxygen delivery to the cardiac cells at all times and in exchange the heart makes the "all or none" promise. Let me explain this "all or none" law of the heart: The heart will give 100% with every heart beat, doing the absolute best that it can under the existing conditions with each and every heart beat for your entire life (and maybe somebody else's, too, if you designate "organ donor" on your driver's license). Who else could make this kind of promise? NO ONE! This plan was set up during organogenesis (the beginning of a new little organ, the embryonic heart) when the coronary arteries branched right off the little embryonic aorta. Greedy from the start! "I'll get my blood flow FIRST!" Before the brain (carotid and vertebral arteries), before the lungs (pulmonary circulation), and before the kidneys (renal arteries)! Henceforth, we will call these *vital organs* the "Big Four."

The heart is a muscle, but unlike any other in the body, the cardiac muscle cells that make up the cardiac tissue have rhythmicity, automaticity, an electrical energy system with its own generator (pacemaker), electrical pathways (conduction system), and a physical energy plant (blood flow with branches throughout the heart) that is ALL its own, and not shared. That sounds a bit stingy, but the heart has to have all of these, in good working order and sufficient quantities to fill the big job of moving oxygenated blood from the lungs forward to the entire body, beating nonstop 24 × 7!

Here are the rules:

- If there is ever limited blood flow, as in the event of shock, peripheral vasoconstriction immediately begins to shift blood flow to these vital organs.

- If that shift cannot adequately supply all four vital organs, guess who gets voted off the island first? You guessed it! The low man on the totem pole! I should say men, because they are twins: the kidneys!

- After that, the lungs begin to try to compete with the brain for their fair share, and the heart is still grabbing its blood flow as it leaves the left ventricle, with those little secret doors opening right off the base of the aorta into the right and left coronary arteries, which are so named because they encircle the heart like a crown (coronation of the king … me! the heart).

- The brain EEG can be flat as a pancake, and the heart is still ticking away (providing that you have kept it healthy). Relevant "normal stuff" is included with each topic.

✛ Hypertension

What is it?

The first stage of hypertension, called "prehypertension," is defined as a systolic blood pressure of 120 to 139 mm Hg, and a diastolic blood pressure of 80 to 89 mm Hg.

- Treatment begun at the onset of early-stage prehypertension can prevent predictable complications of hypertension.

- A consistently elevated blood pressure >140/90 defines actual hypertension in adults.

- The blood pressure must be properly monitored (sitting down, cuff of correct size, in correct position) on two or more separate occasions.

Causes and why?

Hypertension is caused by a narrowing of the body's smaller arteries (arterioles), causing blood to put excessive pressure against the vessel walls. There are three categories of problems that can cause hypertension.

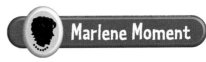

Marlene Moment

You and your heart established a relationship a long time ago when you were just an embryo, and your little primitive heart was in the center of your body and bigger than you, back when you looked like ET (the famous extraterrestrial movie star)!

That relation was a marriage of sorts with the same promise, "Till death do us part." And guess who is going to have to KILL you if you don't take good care of your life mate?

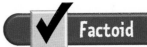

Factoid

Resistant hypertension is defined as persistent systolic blood pressure in excess of 160 mm Hg despite a regime of three antihypertensive medications. This term can also be applied to blood pressure that is controlled, but requires four or more medications for effectiveness.

Causes	Why
• Excessive sodium intake • Volume retention from kidney disease or hypothyroidism • Excessive aldosterone production (Cushing's disease = too many of all the steroids, and Conn's disease = hyperaldosteronism only) causing increased sodium and water retention	Circulatory volume overload Remember! More volume, more pressure!
• Cardiovascular disease • Chronic renal failure • Pheochromocytoma • Coarctation of the aorta	Vasospasm and vasoconstriction: smaller diameter = increased pressure. This is always true, whether in regard to a syringe (3 mL size versus 60 mL size), a water hose (the high pressure in a tiny hose versus low pressure in a large hose), or blood vessels.

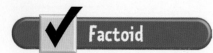

Hypertension has been called "the silent killer" because it can go undetected for years as it causes damage to the cardiovascular system.

Signs and symptoms and why?

High blood pressure usually has no symptoms. The only way to detect high blood pressure is to have your blood pressure taken. Accelerated hypertension may cause retinal changes that can be detected on funduscopic exam (visualizing the retina with an ophthalmoscope), such as retinal edema.

Testing, testing, testing

Standard laboratory tests are performed before beginning any treatment plan for hypertension:

- Hematocrit
- Serum electrolytes (potassium, sodium, and calcium)
- Urinalysis
- Fasting blood glucose
- Fasting lipid profile (HDLs, LDLs, triglycerides)
- EKG (ECG)

  Additional tests to determine renal response to hypertension are:
- Urinary albumin excretion/24-hour urine protein (Remember that albumin is a large molecule that is only excreted when there is damage to the glomerulus.)
- Albumin/creatinine ratio
- Creatinine clearance
- Renin level

Signs and symptoms and why?

Different "first" interventions are indicated according to the stage and severity of hypertension.

✚ Prehypertension

Prehypertension has to be detected, and treatment (including lifestyle modifications) must be initiated. A thorough health history begins the process of identifying contributing health issues that are causative factors for hypertension. Lifestyle and dietary practices, height/weight, and blood pressure readings provide the basis for discussing short-term goals and measures for reaching the target blood pressure established by the health care provider.

When health care providers show empathy and make sure that clinic visits are associated with positive experiences and words of encouragement and support, the patient is more apt to make strides in recovery and/or risk reduction. It has been determined that patients are more compliant with the treatment plan if they have confidence and trust in the health care provider (Table 4-1).

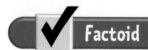

Medication alone will not cure hypertension. Additional interventions and lifestyle changes are required!

Table 4-1 Combined antihypertensive medications

Combination Drugs (abbreviations) Angiotensin converting enzyme = ACE Calcium channel blocker = CCB Angiotensin receptor blocker = ARB Hydrochlorothiazide = HCTZ	Therapeutic action	Nursing implications and patient teaching
ACE inhibitors PLUS CCB: • Amlodipine/benazepril, hydrochloride (Lotrel) • Enalapril maleate/felodipine (Lexxel) • Trandolapril/verapamil (Tarka)	ACE inhibitor blocks conversion of angiotensin I to angiotensin II, halting the powerful vasoconstrictor effect of angiotensin II. Added action of CCB causes systemic and peripheral vasodilation as well as coronary artery dilation. Has effect of lowering BP and improving blood flow and oxygen to the myocardium. Because CCB inhibits calcium ion influx into muscles, it has an antiarrhythmic effect also.	For ACE inhibitor: Monitor serum electrolytes and fluid status before and during therapy: Hold medication and notify health care provider for hypokalemia or hyponatremia. Monitor for excessive hypotension. Teach patient and/or family proper technique for BP monitoring. Refer to urologist if impotence is a concern. Danger of angioedema, which could close airway: Notify health care provider immediately for any facial swelling, or difficulty swallowing or breathing! Teach the patient that periodic blood tests are necessary (WBC and diff) to check for neutropenia (low neutrophils). Notify the health care provider at the first sign of any infection! For CCB: Monitor EKG, watching for prolonged PR interval and bradycardia.
ACE inhibitors PLUS diuretics: • Benazepril/hydrochlorothiazide (Lotensin HCT) • Captopril/hydrochlorothiazide (Capozide) • Lisinopril/hydrochlorothiazide (Prinzide) • Quinapril HCl/hydrochlorothiazide (Accuretic)	ACE inhibitor blocks conversion of angiotensin I to the powerful vasoconstrictor angiotensin II. They also reduce aldosterone levels. Antihypertensive effects from thiazide diuretic results from loss of sodium and water, and possibly reduced peripheral vascular resistance with dilation of arterioles. Captopril has an added bonus of decreasing the progression of diabetic neuropathy!	Monitor serum electrolytes and fluid status before and during therapy: Hold medication and notify the health care provider for hypokalemia or hyponatremia. Monitor for excessive hypotension. Teach the patient and/or family proper technique for BP monitoring. Refer to urologist if impotence is a concern. There is a danger of angioedema, which could close the airway: Notify the health care provider immediately for any facial swelling, or difficulty swallowing or breathing! Teach the patient that periodic blood tests are necessary (WBC and diff) to check for neutropenia (low neutrophils). Notify the health care provider at the first sign of any infection!

(Continued)

Table 4-1   Combined antihypertensive medications (*Continued*)

Combination Drugs (abbreviations) Angiotensin converting enzyme = ACE Calcium channel blocker = CCB Angiotensin receptor blocker = ARB Hydrochlorothiazide = HCTZ	Therapeutic action	Nursing implications and patient teaching
ARBs PLUS diuretics (hydrochlorothiazide = HCTZ): • Candesartan cilexetil/HCTZ (Atacand HCT) • Eprosartan mesylate/HCTZ (Teveten HCT) • Losartan potassium/ HCTZ (Hyzaar) • Telmisartan/HCTZ (Diovan HCT)	ARB blocks the vasoconstrictor and aldosterone effects of angiotensin II at receptor sites in vascular smooth muscle and the adrenal glands for a net effect of lowering blood pressure. Coupled with a thiazide diuretic, the added antihypertensive effects result from loss of sodium and water. Peripheral vascular resistance may also be decreased as arterioles dilate.	Monitor fluid status and correct volume depletion before beginning therapy. Check renal function before and during therapy. Caution the patient that NSAIDs decrease the antihypertensive effect. Angioedema is more common if the patient had previous swelling from an ACE inhibitor. If so, notify the health care provider for any facial edema, dysphagia, or dyspnea. Orthostatic hypotension can occur, so caution the patient to avoid: • Alcohol • Standing for long periods • Hot weather • Vigorous exercise Advise patients to change positions slowly, and sit down if feeling dizzy.
Beta-blocker PLUS diuretic: • Atenolol/chlorthalidone (Tenoretic) • Metoprolol tartrate/HCTZ (Lopressor HCT) • Propranolol LA/HCTZ (Inderide)	Beta-blocker blocks stimulation of beta 1 (myocardial) and beta 2 (pulmonary and vascular) receptor sites to decrease the heart rate, blood pressure, and myocardial contractility. Thiazide diuretics promote loss of sodium and water to lower circulating volume, which produces an additive antihypertensive effect.	Caution the patient to never abruptly stop taking a beta-blocker! Life-threatening hypertensive crisis, arrhythmias, or myocardial ischemia can occur. Advise the patient to refill medication before weekends, holidays, and travel to avoid interruption of daily dosing. An extra written prescription can be kept for emergencies. Monitor effects of beta-blocker on cardiac output: count pulse, and effectively self-monitor blood pressure. Caution the patient to make position changes slowly because of possible orthostatic hypotension. Advise that fatigue, weakness, and drowsiness may resolve after a time of adjustment to the medication. Listen to concerns about sexuality because of impotence and decreased libido, and advise the patient to seek a GU referral if indicated.

(Continued)

Table 4-1 Combined antihypertensive medications (*Continued*)

Combination Drugs (abbreviations) Angiotensin converting enzyme = ACE Calcium channel blocker = CCB Angiotensin receptor blocker = ARB Hydrochlorothiazide = HCTZ	Therapeutic action	Nursing implications and patient teaching
Centrally acting drug PLUS diuretic: • Methyldopa/hydrochlorothiazide (Aldoril) • Reserpine/chlorothiazide (Diupres) • Reserpine/hydrochlorothiazide (Hydropres)	Centrally acting drugs act on the central nervous system to stimulate alpha-adrenergic receptors, producing reduction of sympathetic outflow to heart, kidneys, and blood vessels, lowering blood pressure and peripheral vascular resistance. Thiazide diuretic adds effect of sodium and water loss, reducing blood volume and blood pressure, and may produce dilation of arterioles to reduce peripheral vascular resistance.	Monitor electrolytes: Thiazides promote loss of sodium, chloride, potassium, magnesium, and bicarbonate. Caution patients that centrally acting antihypertensives interact with NSAIDs to decrease effectiveness. An adverse effect of methyldopa is drug-induced hepatitis and myocarditis. Monitor AST (6–12 weeks after beginning therapy, then every 6 months). Caution the patient to notify the health care provider about any unexplained fever. Caution the patient to avoid other central nervous system depressants (eg, alcohol) because of their additive effect (sedation, decreased mental acuity, and depression). Refer the patient to a urologist if impotence is bothersome.
Diuretic PLUS diuretic: • Amiloride HCL/HCTZ (Moduretic) • Spironolactone/HCTZ (Aldactone) • Triamterene/HCTZ (Dyazide, Maxzide)	Potassium-sparing diuretics (amiloride, spironolactone, triamterene) promote mild diuresis while conserving potassium. HCTZ increases excretion of sodium and water in the distal tubule and also promotes excretion of chloride, potassium, magnesium, and bicarbonate.	HCTZ and triamterene both cause photosensitivity: Caution patients to wear sunscreen. Monitor serum electrolytes before and during therapy: Hold medication and notify the health care provider for hypokalemia or hyperkalemia. Advise patients to avoid salt substitutes that are high in potassium. Caution the patient that NSAIDs may decrease the antihypertensive effect of the medication. Instruct the patient and/or family in the correct technique for monitoring weekly BP and daily weights.

PATIENT TEACHING   Effective management of hypertension requires patient compliance, if he or she is to meet the mutually agreed upon blood pressure goals. In terms of self-care practices, some patients actually don't know what to do, and others know and then don't do what they should more than 50% of the time![1] The following lifestyle modifications recommended by the American Heart Association (news release April 7, 2008) are the focus of patient teaching:

• Weight reduction

• Regular exercise

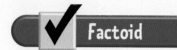

- Sodium restriction
- Stress management
- Discontinuing smoking
- Reducing alcohol consumption
- Avoiding OTCs that raise blood pressure (especially NSAIDs)

What can harm my patient and why?

Organs having the highest oxygen demand (heart and brain) and very vascular organs (kidneys and retina) are targets of damage from hypertension.

- High blood pressure damages peripheral blood vessels as well as vital organs (heart, brain, and kidneys).
- Continuous high pressure inside vessels can lead to cardiovascular disease owing to the development of atheromatous plaques.
- Plaques narrow the lumen of blood vessels and lead to a heart attack (AMI) or can rupture and bleed, which could lead to a thrombus casing a heart attack or stroke.
- Small arterioles in the brain can also rupture from the pressure, causing a hemorrhagic stroke.[2]

Cardiac afterload is increased by hypertension, causing the heart to work harder in an effort to eject blood against this higher pressure.

- The heart enlarges as a direct result of the added workload, tachycardia, and injury to the cardiac muscle fibers.
- Once injured, the muscle fibers try to repair themselves, and remodeling permanently alters the chambers and functional capacity of the heart.

Damage doesn't happen immediately, but after months or years of hypertension, bad things begin to happen to target organs:

- Coronary artery disease (CAD)
- Heart failure
- Kidney failure
- Stroke (cerebrovascular accident, CVA)
- Retinopathy and blindness

  Hypertensive crisis is a medical emergency because if the severely high pressure is not effectively relieved the patient may die from an intracranial bleed, stroke, or heart failure. It's time to go to the intensive care unit (ICU), where an arterial line will be inserted for continuous blood pressure monitoring while vasoactive medications/antihypertensives can be classified as:

- ACE inhibitors
- Angiotensin receptor blockers
- Beta-blockers
- Calcium channel blockers (see Pharmacology in a nutshell, Table 2-14).

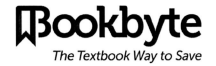
The Textbook Way to Save

SHIP TO:
Angel Chavez
5530 Olvera Ave
San Diego,Ca 92114
US
Total Items: 1
Green

SHIPPED FROM:
Bookbyte.com
2800 Pringle Road SE
Salem, OR 97302

3

YOUR SHIPMENT METHOD:
Standard

Hello Angel Chavez,

Here is your **Order #7611811** from Bookbyte which is also **Order #107-9321660-0829832** from Amazon.com Market.

TITLE: Hurst Reviews Medical-Surgical Nursing Review, by Hurst
SKU: 104007958
INVENTORY LOCATION: G-13-4-4

CONDITION: Good Used
DESCRIPTION: Disc(s) Included; Has minor wear and/or markings.

Thanks for ordering from Bookbyte! We appreciate your business.

If necessary, you may return any book for any reason within 14 days of delivery. For additional information and instructions, check out our complete Return Policy on our website.

RENTED YOUR BOOKS? HERE'S OUR SIMPLE RETURN PROCESS:

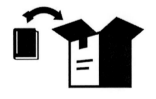
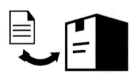

Print your shipping label
from your account page.

Place your books
in any box.

Shipping label goes
on the box.

Drop-off box at nearest
FedEx location.

Hypertension can be classified as a medical emergency when there is an immediate threat of heart attack or stroke, or a medical urgency when the patient has a nosebleed or severe headache.

- In both instances blood pressure exceeds 180/120. Prompt lowering of the blood pressure to the 140/90 range is required to prevent damage to vital organs (heart, brain, and kidneys).

- Hypertensive crisis is a medical emergency with threat to vital organs, and is usually treated in an intensive care setting with capabilities for hemodynamic monitoring, cardiac monitoring, and continuous blood pressure monitoring per arterial line.

The medication and the route (intravenous) are selected because of their immediate effect. Examples are:

- Sodium nitroprusside (Nipride, Nitropress)
- Nitroglycerin (Nitro-Bid, Tridil)
- Nicardipine (Cardene)

For medically urgent hypertension, fast-acting oral agents may be used, usually in the emergency room setting. The drugs may include:

- Beta-adrenergic blocking agents such as labetalol (Normodyne, Trandate)
- Angiotensin-converting enzyme (ACE) inhibitors such as captopril (Capoten)
- Alpha$_2$ agonists such as clonidine (Catapres)

After stabilizing the medically urgent hypertension, the patient is evaluated as to the cause of hypertensive crisis. The patient could be poorly controlled or hypertension could be resistant to treatment.

✚ Coronary artery disease

Let's get the normal stuff straight!

The blood passing through the heart chambers only comes in contact with the endocardium, and does not reach the myocardium. The heart muscle is dependent on sufficient blood supply if it is to efficiently perform the job of pumping blood throughout the body. In order to contract normally, the muscle also needs oxygen, glucose, amino acids, and the proper ratio of potassium, sodium, and calcium. The heart muscle gets its blood supply from arteries that start in the aorta and run on the surface of the heart, known as the coronary arteries. These arteries operate under different "rules" than other vessels in the body. When all other vessels are clamping down (vasoconstricting) in response to shock or decreased circulating volume, the coronary arteries actually vasodilate to get more oxygenated blood to the heart muscle (Fig. 4-2)!

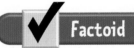

Factoid

The myocardium requires adequate blood flow at all times, and if the heart doesn't get the necessary blood flow, there is only one message it can send: PAIN.

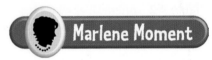

Marlene Moment

If you are not giving your heart enough oxygen-rich blood flow, you are going to be in a world of hurt. The coronary vessels are going to "put the squeeze" on you big time! It's called angina.

▶ Figure 4-2. Coronary Arteries. The coronary arteries provide the blood supply to the heart's tissues.

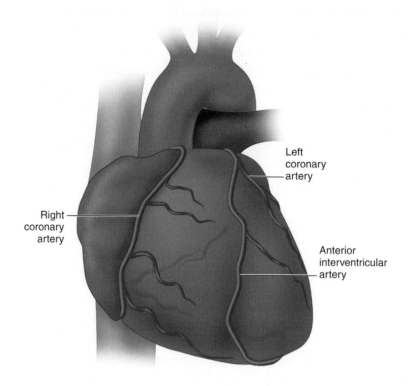

Norepinephrine causes the vasculature of the body to vasoconstrict, in order to raise blood pressure, but because the coronary arteries are highly reactive to adrenergic stimulation, norepinephrine causes vasodilatation in coronary vasculature.[3]

Vessel walls are lined with endothelial cells to keep blood cells zipping through lickety-split. There are also built in, antithrombotic, anti-inflammatory, and antiproliferation properties to keep them that way (no junk building up) (Table 4-2).

Table 4-2   Arterial map of coronary blood flow

Coronary artery	Area supplied with oxygen
Main left coronary artery (LCA) (called the "widow maker")	Supplies both the anterior and the lateral walls of the left ventricle
Right coronary artery (RCA)	Supplies the posterior surface (back wall) of the right ventricle of the heart and lower portion of the left ventricle
Left anterior descending artery (LAD)	Supplies the majority of the anterior wall of the left ventricle
Left circumflex artery (LCA)	Supplies the back wall of the left ventricle
Posterior descending artery (PCD)	Supplies the inferior wall of the heart to the apex and the ventricular septum

What is it?

Coronary artery disease (CAD) develops over time as fatty plaques (atheromas) build up and narrow the coronary arteries, reducing the amount of blood flow going to the heart muscle. As stenosis (narrowing) of a coronary artery increases, it is less able to supply enough blood to the heart muscle, especially under conditions of stress, heavy exertion, or exercise.

Coronary artery disease is said to occur when at least one major coronary artery has sufficient disease process to be 50% occluded;[4] however, symptoms do not usually occur until the coronary vessel has become at least 70% occluded with well-established inflammatory changes inside the vessel (the endothelial surface).[5] These inflammatory changes actually reduce the protective function of nitric oxide that is produced by a healthy endothelium (Fig. 4-3).

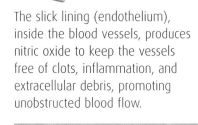

Here's the Deal

The slick lining (endothelium), inside the blood vessels, produces nitric oxide to keep the vessels free of clots, inflammation, and extracellular debris, promoting unobstructed blood flow.

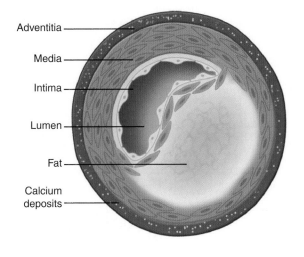

Adventitia
Media
Intima
Lumen
Fat
Calcium deposits

◀ Figure 4-3. Progression of Atheroma Development. As the atheromas develop the lumen of the vessel narrows.

Stage 1 = Foam cell invades surface lining of vessels (tunica intima)
Stage 2 = Fatty streak (earliest lesion) appears in the vessel
Stage 3 = Fibrous plaque forms
Stage 4 = Vessels grow into the well-established plaque
Stage 5 = Plaque ruptures and bleeds, forming clots and producing scarring

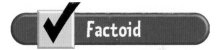

Factoid

When there is not enough oxygen/blood flow into the heart muscle, the muscle starts to suffer/hurt from ischemia (lack of oxygen).

Causes and why?

A number of variables contribute to the formation of plaques in coronary arteries. Increased risks for CAD and coronary heart disease (CHD) are associated with certain other conditions: diabetes, hypertension, familial hyperlipidemia, hypercholesterolemia, chronic renal disease, and autoimmune disorders such as rheumatoid arthritis, as well as central obesity.

Most cardiovascular risk factors can be modified by diet, exercise, medications, and lifestyle choices, which can compensate in part for those few nonmodifiable risk factors (see Table 4-2). For example, a diabetic woman has a three to five times greater risk for death from CHD compared to three times the risk for men, but if tight glucose control can be maintained, the risk becomes almost like that of the general population.[6,7]

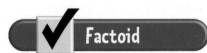

Criteria for determining central obesity uses the waist-to-hip ratio, and others consider ethnicity, but generally a waist circumference greater than 35 inches in women or 40 inches in men is considered central obesity. Metabolic syndrome increases the risk for development of CHD because of its propensity for triggering inflammatory and prothrombotic mediators in blood vessels.

Inflammatory changes in the endothelium reduce production of the normally protective function of nitric oxide.

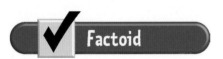

Damaged vessels lose the ability to heal themselves!

![Factoid]

Deposits of fats and sugar destroy blood vessels (Table 4-3).

Metabolic syndrome, a rapidly escalating health problem in the United States, is defined as the presence of three or more of the following:

- Hypertension
- Elevated serum triglycerides
- Low levels of HDLs (high density lipoproteins)
- Elevated serum glucose
- Central obesity (increased waist circumference)[8]

Metabolic syndrome can lead to cardiovascular disease and premature death, especially in women. Different combinations of the components of metabolic syndrome result in varying degrees of risk, the greatest being when all five components are present.[9] The addition of nicotine dependency accelerates cardiovascular disease.

Table 4-3 Nonmodifiable and modifiable risk factors

Nonmodifiable	
Risk factor	**Why**
Age	The longer we live, the more time we have to develop plaques.
Gender	Men are at an increased risk, but women approach the same risk after menopause.
	It was thought that estrogen had a cardioprotective property, although current research does not support this theory. At this time it is not clear why postmenopausal women are at an increased risk for having an MI.
Heredity	Some families are just really good at making plaque in their coronary arteries.
Modifiable	
Risk factor	**Why**
Hyperglycemia	High glucose levels damage vessels.
Hypertension	Anything that damages the endothelial lining speeds up hardening of the arteries. Hypertension damages the endothelial lining of the vessels.
Hyperlipidemia	Diets high in fat lead to increased levels of LDL (the bad cholesterol). This speeds up hardening of the arteries.
Cigarette smoking	Increases LDL and decreases HDL, thereby increasing fatty streaks in the vessels. Nicotine is a powerful vasoconstrictor that decreases blood flow to the heart and carbon monoxide, further decreasing myocardial oxygen delivery because of the displacement of oxygen molecules.
Sedentary lifestyle	Inactivity increases LDL levels and decreases HDL (the good cholesterol).

(Continued)

Table 4-3 Nonmodifiable and modifiable risk factors (*Continued*)

	Modifiable
Risk factor	**Why**
Hypertensive lifestyle	A lifestyle filled with stressors accompanied by ineffective coping mechanisms can cause an elevation in blood pressure.
Abdominal/visceral obesity	Increased adipose tissue, especially around the midsection of the body, has been linked to increased risk for developing CAD.
Hypothyroidism	People with hypothyroidism tend to have hyperlipidemia, thereby putting them at risk for CAD.

Testing, testing, testing

There are a variety of tests that are utilized to assess the risk of CAD and CHD. These tests are also used as assessment tools for other disease processes, some of which are risk factors for CAD and CHD (Table 4-4).[10]

Table 4-4 Tests to assess risk for CAD and CHD

- Total cholesterol
- High density cholesterol
- Triglycerides
- Apolipoprotein B
- Lipoprotein (a)
- Fibrinogen
- C-reactive protein
- Homocysteine
- Insulin, fasting

Lipid profile testing is commonly conducted to identify patients at risk for CAD. This profile evaluates cholesterol, high density lipoproteins (HDLs), low density lipoproteins (LDLs), and triglycerides (Table 4-5).[10]

Table 4-5 Laboratory tests: lipid profile

Laboratory test	Indication	Normal range
Cholesterol	Used to determine risk for CAD and to evaluate hyperlipidemia	<200 mg/dL
High density lipoproteins (HDLs)	An accurate predictor of heart disease and useful for monitoring effectiveness of therapy for hyperlipidemia	Male: >45 mg/dL Female: >55 mg/dL
Low density lipoproteins (LDLs)	An accurate predictor of heart disease and useful for monitoring effectiveness of therapy for hyperlipidemia	60–180 mg/dL
Triglycerides	Identifies risk of developing CAD and CHD	Male: 40–160 mg/dL Female: 35–135 mg/dL

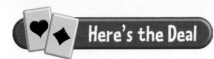

A person can't change his or her hereditary or the genetic predisposition for a certain type of body build or the family tendency to develop diabetes, hypertension, or hyperlipidemia. However, risk reduction and disease processes each can be changed through early recognition, diagnosis, and medical management. A low-sodium diet, stress management, weight loss, exercise, diuretics, and antihypertensive medications can convert hypertension into normotension. Diet, exercise, oral hypoglycemics, or insulin can all work together to produce euglycemia.

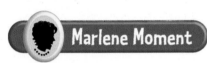

The male gender has been considered the highest risk for CVD, but women are rapidly making strides toward increasing the number who develop CVD. In fact, more women die from CVD than from breast cancer,[12] so it boils down to this: You can't do anything about your family or your age, but all the other things can be fixed (Table 4-3)!

Laboratory testing also plays an important role in identifying and defining metabolic syndrome and the criterions are:

- Low levels of high density lipoprotein (HDL) <40 mg/dL in men, <50 mg/dL in women
- Serum glucose >100 mg/dL
- Elevated serum triglycerides >150 mg/dL

Additional laboratory testing to identify the initiation and progression of metabolic syndrome are C-reactive protein (CRP), homocysteine levels (Hcy), and vitamin D levels. Homocysteine is derived from amino acids of animal protein and increases with low serum levels: Folate, B_6, B_{12}, and riboflavin. C-reactive protein (CRP), a serum marker for systemic inflammation, is now considered a major risk factor marker for metabolic syndrome and cardiovascular disease (CVD).[11]

Interventions

Nurses are instrumental in helping patients to see the benefits and make health decisions to enjoy a high quality of life. The nurse serves as a motivator, helping patients set realistic goals, giving encouragement and support along the way. This is an especially important role with the newly diagnosed CAD patient. Compliance, with the treatment plan, is fundamental in maintaining health and preventing further complications (Table 4-6).

Table 4-6 Key nursing interventions for the CAD patient

- Provide patient teaching related to diet modification (low fat, high fiber), proper exercise, and medication regimen.
- Educate the patient and family related to signs and symptoms of disease progression such as angina and myocardial infarction.
- Prepare the patient and family for scheduled tests.
- Emphasize the importance of keeping appointments for follow-up monitoring.
- Provide emotional support related to adjusting to a chronic medical condition.

If after a trial period (usually 4–6 months) of faithful adherence to a low-fat/high-fiber diet, regular exercise, and a weight loss program, the patient fails to respond adequately, and serum triglycerides (LDLs >100 mg/dL) remain high and HDL levels remain low (<40 mg/dL men, <50 mg/dL women), antilipidemic medications may be added to the treatment plan.

Pharmacology in a nutshell

Table 4-7 Lipid-lowering agents

Drug/trade name	Action	Side effects/adverse effects
The bile acid resins (cholestyramine): Questran Cuemid Prevalite	Works in the intestine to bind bile acids, making them insoluble so they will be excreted, forcing the liver to use up serum cholesterol to make new bile acid! Lowers serum cholesterol and LDLs. Does not significantly raise HDLs or decrease triglycerides.	Causes constipation. Long-term use may cause decreased levels of fat soluble vitamins (A-D-E-K) and folic acid. Powder is nasty tasting! Mix with juice or applesauce. Don't put in carbonated beverages because it will foam over the top of the glass!
The nicotinic acids (niacin, B$_3$): Niacin Niacor Nicobid	Works on the liver to reduce synthesis of lipoproteins and stimulates lipid metabolism, thereby reducing LDLs.	Flushing because of peripheral vasodilation. Possible hepatic dysfunction: Monitor liver enzymes.
The statins (also known as 3-hydroxy 3-methylglutaryl coenzyme A reductase inhibitors): Lipitor (atorvastatin) Zocor (simvastatin) (lovastatin) (pravastatin)	Works in the liver to block cholesterol synthesis, excreted primarily in bile. Acts early in the synthesis pathway, inhibiting the enzyme necessary to make cholesterol. Lowers LDL and total cholesterol levels to significantly reduce progression of CAD, reducing deaths and heart attacks.	Possible hepatic dysfunction: Monitor liver enzymes. Avoid alcohol use, as this increases hepatotoxicity! WARNING: Not to be combined with clofibrate or niacin; causes rhabdomyolysis (breakdown of striated muscle, such as skeletal and cardiac muscles) and renal failure because the myoglobins (muscle proteins) are excreted by the kidneys and can cause clogging!
The fibrates (fibric acid): Atromid-S (clofibrate)	Inhibits liver synthesis of cholesterol in the early stage to reduce cholesterol levels.	Can cause hepatic tumors and gall stones (cholelithiasis). Fetal damage if pregnancy occurs. Not to be used in patients with liver or renal dysfunction, as these drugs are metabolized by the liver and excreted primarily in the urine.

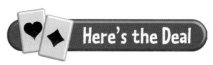

Here's the Deal

Other little known risk factors that predispose someone to CAD are vitamin D deficiency and chronic periodontitis. Periodontitis (a gum disease) is a major cause of tooth loss caused by long-term accumulation of bacteria in pockets around the teeth.[13] A long-range study by the Boston University Goldman School of Dental Medicine has coupled periodontitis with CAD, showing that men >60 years with no other risk factors except for being edentulous (having no teeth) and younger men <60 years with chronic periodontitis, had an increased incidence of CAD.[10] A long range study of men with vitamin D deficiency (independent of other cardiovascular risk factors), found a 2½ times greater likelihood for cardiovascular events than men whose vitamin D levels were in the lower range of normal.[14]

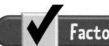

Factoid

The patient with CAD is at risk for psychosocial harm as well:

- It's normal to experience fear with chest pain, but pathologic fear can range from a mild level to a crippling condition.
- Once CAD is diagnosed, the patient may assume the cardiac cripple role, afraid that any physical exertion will bring on the pain.

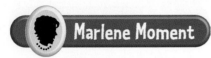

Marlene Moment

Too many trips to the burger joint and sitting playing video games means having to take lipid-lowering agents to control your cholesterol.

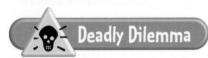

Marlene Moment

Don't get too upset with Granny, some families are just better at making cholesterol than others. Heredity plays a major role in cholesterol levels. Granny could live on green beans and still need lipid-lowering agents (Table 4-7).

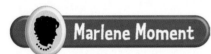

Deadly Dilemma

WARNING: The fibrates are not to be combined with statins because they can cause muscle damage and renal failure!

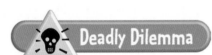

Deadly Dilemma

It is very dangerous to self-medicate in an attempt to lower serum lipids. When taking a drug history, nurses should be alert to any over-the-counter health supplements/vitamins the patient may be taking concurrently with prescribed antilipidemics.

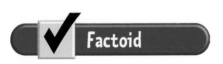

Factoid

Not all forms of angina are related to atheromas and atherosclerosis.

▶ **Critical Labs**

LDLs should be <100 mg/dL

HDLs (men) should be >40 mg/dL

HDLs (women) should be >50 mg/dL

✛ Angina

What is it?

Angina pectoris is chest pain that occurs when there is inadequate oxygenated blood flow to the heart muscle. This condition is usually related to CAD, but can be caused by coronary spasm or any condition that creates increased oxygen demand on the myocardium when the blood/oxygen supply is deficient. CAD develops over time as fatty plaques (atheromas) build up and narrow the coronary arteries, reducing the amount of blood flow going to the heart muscle. As stenosis (narrowing) of a coronary artery increases, it is less able to supply enough blood to the heart muscle, especially under conditions of stress, heavy exertion, or exercise.

Causes and why?

Just like arm muscles that begin to hurt if you lift too much, or legs that hurt when you run too fast, the heart muscle will ache if it doesn't get adequate blood supply. Stable angina caused by myocardial ischemia is temporary, transient, and totally reversible in the early stages when the pain is predictable and manageable.

Signs and symptoms and why?

Refer to Table 4-8 for characteristics of chronic stable angina.

Table 4-8 Signs and symptoms of stable angina

Characteristics of chronic stable angina	Rationale/underlying pathophysiology
Predictable chest pain brought on by exertion or some stressor that increases the heart rate.	The demand for myocardial oxygen EXCEEDS the available supply. Anaerobic metabolism begins in the heart muscle and lactic acid accumulates.
Pain is relieved by rest or nitroglycerin.	Rest creates a lower demand for oxygen. Nitroglycerin vasodilates coronary vessels to deliver more oxygen directly to the heart muscle.
Pain is temporary, transient, and reversible.	No permanent damage occurs to the heart muscle from ischemia.

(Continued)

Table 4-8 *Signs and symptoms of stable angina (Continued)*

Characteristics of chronic stable angina	Rationale/underlying pathophysiology
The location of pain may be: • Under breastbone (substernal) • Behind breast bone (retrosternal) • If it radiates, the pain will radiate upward to the neck, jaw, shoulder, or either arm. • Sometimes the pain is felt in the back or abdomen (not typical).	The pain message from the heart muscle is transmitted to cardiac nerves and upper thoracic posterior roots, giving rise to shoulder and arm pain.

When assessing chest pain associated with angina, the nurse will question the patient about the characteristics of the pain: location, quality, and description of the pain. Patients usually report the quality of the pain as mild to moderate, and the nurse will ask for a number, using the pain rating scale (0–10). When describing the character of the anginal pain, the patient may use terms such as, "tightness, heaviness, or squeezing," while rubbing the center of the chest.

Testing, testing, testing

When a patient presents with undiagnosed chest pain, a typical first step is to rule out myocardial infarction (MI). Typically, four lab tests are evaluated to determine the presence (or absence) of myocardial injury:

• Total creatinine kinase (CK), which comes from brain tissue (BB), skeletal muscle (MM), or cardiac tissue (MB).

• CK-MB, the isoenzyme of CK (above), which is an indicator of MI.

• Troponin I or T, both of which come from injured cardiac muscle.

• Myoglobin, which is an indicator specific to cardiac muscle.

If these biomarkers are within the normal range and the EKG is negative for myocardial ischemia or injury, the patient with stable angina will undergo further testing using the following "least invasive first" rules:

• EKG: During the anginal episode if possible (totally noninvasive). Ischemic heart muscle tissue will have difficulty repolarizing, and the T wave will sag, dip, or become completely inverted.

• (24-hour) Holter monitor: Use this for ambulatory EKG monitoring while the patient keeps a diary of the day's activity (totally noninvasive). The memory tape is replayed and correlated with the log of patient activities to identify any abnormalities brought on by activities of daily living. Hopefully the monitor might "catch" an episode of chest pain with resultant T-wave changes.

• Stress testing: (Exercise EKG = 12-lead EKG done on the treadmill or during medication-induced tachycardia. This test is minimally invasive if an injection is given for chemical stress testing). A perfectly normal

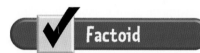
Factoid

Denial can hurt my patient because it leads to a delay in seeking health care.

• The pain from angina is a warning, which could lead to worsening of symptoms and cardiac status if ignored.

• Angina can lead to acute coronary syndrome (ACS).

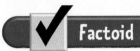

Factoid

Exercise normally causes the heart vessels to dilate, getting more blood flow to the heart muscle when needed. People who can't exercise on a treadmill get a medication (eg, Persantine or dipyridamole) to simulate the vasodilating effect of exercise.

Hurst Hint

The patient must be monitored constantly during the stress test and a reliable IV access device must be in place in the event that emergency medications are required.

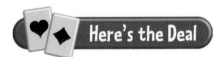

Here's the Deal

Abruptly increasing the need for oxygen with exercise stress testing may trigger angina or the onset of an acute MI, because diseased coronary vessels cannot meet the added demand for oxygen.

resting EKG may show changes in the T wave (representing the repolarization/resting phase of the myocardium) during the stress of exercise. This change depicts ischemia, giving proof that the nonstressed heart muscle received adequate oxygen at rest, but during exercise, when the heart requires more oxygen, there is a lack of adequate oxygenation. This test is terminated immediately upon onset of chest pain.

- Myocardial perfusion imaging (only invasive for IV injection of the isotope): Usually performed in conjunction with the exercise stress test. An injection of thallium or Cardiolite (radioactive isotopes) is given while the heart is responding to the stress of exercise, with an accelerated heart rate and increased oxygen demand. A scintillation camera shows a picture of how the radionuclide is distributed in the heart muscle. Initial results: Cold spots (if present) show areas of decreased or absent myocardial perfusion. These are called "cold" because no warm blood is flowing into the area of heart muscle that is not being perfused under stress. The scary picture looks like a black hole superimposed on a red heart over the area of myocardial tissue that is not receiving adequate blood flow.

  A later scintigram (scan) of the resting heart, with a normal heart rate may show recovery, as blood flow returns into the area of the cold spot (called a stress defect), previously lacking blood flow. If the cold spot is still visible with rest, this is called a fixed defect, which is much worse than a reversible stress defect, because no blood flow is being transported into the area regardless of activity or rest. Necrotic (dead) tissue doesn't take up blood, so the isotope does not spread out in this tissue!

- Coronary angiography and cardiac catheterization: This invasive procedure is performed first. It involves threading a long, thin tube (a catheter) through an artery or vein in the leg or arm into the heart. Once this has been done, dye is injected into the heart and X-rays are taken as blood flows through the coronary arteries, helping to identify areas of narrowing (stenosis) of the coronary arteries (Table 4-9).

Testing, testing, testing

See Table 4-9.

Table 4-9 Nursing implications associated with diagnostic tests

Diagnostic test	Patient instructions: preprocedure and postprocedure	Potential complications and priority monitoring
EKG (ECG): Records the electrical activity of the heart picked up by electrodes placed over the chest. A 12-lead "picture" of the waveforms (PQRST) of the heart to detect arrhythmias, myocardial ischemia, injury, or necrosis. Amplitude of waveforms (high voltage) is associated with hypertrophy. Measurements of intervals can detect conduction blocks.	Have patient remove watch and lie very still to reduce movement artifact. Wearing a button-up shirt will help in the placement of electrodes, and women must remove bra.	No complications: noninvasive. Make haste. This should be initiated within 10 minutes of arrival in the emergency department.[15] Notify health care provider immediately upon recognition of injury on EKG. Remove electrodes and wipe away conduction gel.

(Continued)

Table 4-9 Nursing implications associated with diagnostic tests (*Continued*)

Diagnostic test	Patient instructions: preprocedure and postprocedure	Potential complications and priority monitoring
Exercise stress test: Cardiac rhythm is monitored while the patient is physically active (treadmill, stationary bike, or arm weights) and the heart rate is accelerated to a target zone. If the patient is physically unable to exercise (ie, amputee or severely disabled) the heart rate is accelerated with a medication (Persantine stress test) and then reversed after the test.	Wear comfortable shoes and a front-buttoned shirt to facilitate electrode placement. Immediately report the first onset of any chest discomfort (pressure, tightness, pain) or heavy feeling in chest or arms, as this will terminate the test. Blood pressure and heart rate are monitored throughout the test per facility policy.	Can induce angina or precipitate an MI. Monitor for chest pain/arrhythmias. An IV access is needed in the event emergency medications must be administered. The patient must be stable with return of heart rate and blood pressure to normal range before discharge.
Myocardial perfusion imaging: Usually performed in conjunction with the exercise stress test. A radionuclide such as thallium (TI 201) or technetium (Tc99m) is injected IV where it will be carried via the blood to the heart muscle, to identify zones where perfusion is poor during stress.	Reassure the patient that he or she will not be radioactive, and that the IV injection of the radionuclide used is not harmful. After the first image is complete, the patient is instructed not to smoke, ingest any caffeine, or eat anything "heavy," and to rest comfortably for several hours before returning for the second imaging with a resting heart rate.	The patient must be stable with the return of heart rate and blood pressure to normal range before discharge.
Cardiac catheterization with coronary angiography	Collaborate with health care provider about discontinuing any of the following medications prior to this invasive procedure: blood thinners such as Coumadin (warfarin) or antiplatelet medicines such as aspirin or Plavix. NPO for 6–8 hours. Mark pulses and obtain baseline circulation check. Evaluate renal function prior to test because the dye used is excreted through the kidneys. Warn about the feeling of warmth as the dye circulates, and possible palpitations.	Watch for arrhythmias as the catheter (a foreign body) approaches the heart. Have a crash cart with defibrillator readily available. The catheter could dislodge a piece of plaque or a blood clot and cause an acute MI. The catheter could puncture the heart or blood vessel. Hemorrhage and hematoma at the access site are the most common complications. Monitor the extremity distal to the puncture site for adequate circulation. Have the patient lie flat (no more than 10–15 degrees if elevated), with leg straight for 6–8 hours after manual compression or 2 hours after insertion of a vascular closure device (VCD). Check those 5 Ps and impress on the patient the importance of reporting ANY pain as soon as possible (see Case in Point below).
Coronary angiography: Provides information about the size and distribution of coronary vessels and the extent of stenosis or obstruction of the vessels.	Question patient about allergy to shellfish or iodine.	Monitor for allergy to the dye. Force fluids to flush out the dye! Recognize the potential risk for acute renal failure, secondary to the nephrotoxic dye.

Hurst Hint

Reducing the number of venipunctures are important because at the time of admission, it is not yet known if these symptoms are the result of an acute MI, which would necessitate antithrombotic or "clot-busting" therapy.

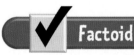

Factoid

Prophylactic use of nitroglycerin improves work performance.

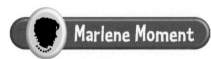

Marlene Moment

Oxygen!! The heart uses chest pain to get my attention and send the message to me that my heart needs increased oxygen via coronary blood flow. A lack of oxygen is the problem, and nitroglycerin is the "anti-ischemic" answer, because vasodilating coronary arteries brings more blood flow and oxygen into the heart muscle.

Hurst Hint

Always keep the old supply of nitroglycerin (just in case) until the new prescription is obtained.

Interventions

Implement the emergency chest pain protocol, which may include:

- Place the client in a reclining (45-degree elevation) position.
- Apply oxygen per nasal cannula.
- Attach chest electrodes for cardiac monitoring.
- Obtain a stat 12-lead EKG.
- Establish an IV line for venous access and obtain a blood specimen from IV access if possible.

Pharmacology in a nutshell

Sublingual (SL) nitroglycerin is used for immediate relief of anginal pain, and all patients with angina should receive teaching about how and when to take sublingual nitroglycerin as well as importance of proper storage and refill dates (Table 4-10).

Table 4-10   Nitroglycerin self-administration

Action	Rationale
Take the smallest amount necessary to relieve chest pain.	Tolerance to the drug can build up! For example, initially chest pain is relieved by one tablet SL, then two tabs are required for relief, then three, four, or five are required. This is an example of how tolerance develops. Tolerance is easily broken by stopping the SL tabs for a short time while using an alternate medication.
Keep only a day's supply of "nitro" with you each day, leaving the rest in a cool, dry place in the original brown glass bottle with the lid tight. Carry nitro in a purse or in an outside breast pocket (but not in pockets close to the groin area).	Nitroglycerin is very volatile and is easily destroyed by time/age, heat, air, moisture, or light. (This is also why you can't carry nitroglycerin in your pants pocket: Heat from the groin area will render it useless. (Think about it! Coins that have been in your pocket are warm, aren't they?)
Refill nitroglycerin every 6 months and then discard the old supply.	Keeping a fresh supply ensures potency of the drug. When you need nitroglycerin, you want it to work, don't you?
Never swallow SL tablets (and don't swallow your saliva either) until pain is relieved or 2 minutes have passed.	If tablet or saliva (containing dissolved nitroglycerin) is swallowed, it will not get out of the stomach and into circulation for 30 minutes. When you need nitroglycerin, you need it NOW!

PATIENT TEACHING See Table 4-11.

Table 4-11 Guidelines for living with chronic stable angina

Avoid all forms of nicotine.	• No transdermal nicotine patches or nicotine gum (this is the same as smoking). • No breathing second-hand smoke. • Seek proven cessation methods, such as aversion therapy or AHA Fresh Start Program.
Avoid exposure to extremes of temperature.	• Avoid exposure to cold (dress warmly) or stay inside for bitter cold. • Avoid breathing cold air (wrap a scarf over nose and mouth). • Keep cool in hot weather (wear hats, light clothing). • Heat wave: Stay inside under air conditioning.
Avoid OTCs and self-medicating.	• Ask health care provider before taking any medications that increase the heart rate and oxygen requirements of the heart, such as diet pills or nasal decongestants.
Eat sensibly.	• Low fat, high fiber, plant-based (fruits and vegetables) diet with polyunsaturated fats. • Avoid overeating. • Avoid excess caffeine.
Regular daily activities.	• Promptly discontinue any activity that produces chest pain, shortness of breath, or fatigue. • Avoid sudden bursts of intense activity. • Avoid isometric exercise (anything that makes the muscles squeeze and tense up).
Exercise.	• Check with health care provider before beginning an exercise plan. • Establish and maintain a regular pattern of exercise.
Use SL nitroglycerin for immediate treatment of anginal episodes.	• Carry nitroglycerin at all times. • Take one tablet (SL: do not swallow) every 5 minutes for up to three doses. • If unrelieved or if pain is severe or different, have someone drive you to the nearest emergency room or call 911 after the first dose!
Stress	• Decrease stress level and manage response to stressors.

The most important life-saving thing that you can teach your patient is how to differentiate "normal" (stable) angina from ACS in progress, and what to do. Here's how to KNOW and when to GO:
• Pain lasts longer than 15 minutes.
• Pain is more intense than usual (severe).
• Pain is accompanied by nausea, vomiting, shortness of breath, or sweating.
• Call 911 or have someone drive you to the nearest ER if chest pain is unusual or different.

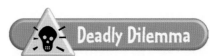
Deadly Dilemma

Don't wait! Call 911 for severe chest pain accompanied by other symptoms (dyspnea, diaphoresis, or nausea/vomiting)!

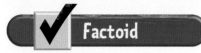

Patient teaching regarding the meaning of pain is crucial to the rehabilitation process. Many patients have the misconception that each anginal episode represents further heart damage. Patients who are living with angina need a sound knowledge base for monitoring daily symptoms and making decisions about when to seek emergency assistance. Use those therapeutic communication skills that you learned in fundamentals to determine what the pain means to the patient, and how it has changed his or her life.

Measures to increase the oxygen supply to the myocardial tissue will include three classifications of drugs; the nitrates, beta-adrenergic blockers, and calcium channel blockers (see Pharmacology in a nutshell).

The first step the patient has to make is the most difficult. After receiving information about angina, the cause and nature of the disease, as well as the possible deadly progression to heart attack, decisions must be made.

- The decision to stop smoking is a difficult one, especially when nicotine addiction is strong.
- Even nonsmokers must make hard decisions for change, including healthy diet, regular exercise, and stress management.
- Decisions have to be made about how to handle stressors, and whether that hard-driving high-stress job is worth keeping.
- Referrals are indicated for smoking cessation programs, stress management workshops, and clinics; dietary consults, and consults to psychologists/CAD support groups, or weight management programs.
- None of the above referrals will produce any improvements in the course of angina pectoris until the patient makes the decision that change is needed, and puts forth the effort to make the necessary lifestyle changes.

✚ Acute coronary syndrome

What is it?

The heart muscle requires sufficient oxygen to perform the work of keeping blood moving in a forward motion. In the presence of an adequate oxygen supply, this work is accomplished through aerobic metabolism, with waste products of working muscles constantly being removed from tissues with circulating blood. When blood flow is suddenly cut off or is chronically and critically insufficient, there is a switch from normal aerobic to anaerobic metabolism and lactic acid builds up. As hypoxic cells become increasingly permeable, histamines, bradykinins, and specific cardiac enzymes are released that further stimulate nerve fibers in the myocardium, sending pain signals to the central nervous system.[16]

Acute coronary syndrome (ACS) is a term that has three presentations: unstable angina, non ST-elevation myocardial infarction (NSTEMI), and ST-elevation MI (STEMI).

Unlike *stable* angina, unstable angina is more severe pain that is unpredictable, occurring with increasing frequency and lasting longer with less of a trigger (exertion or stress), even occurring during rest or

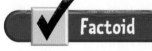

sleep.[17] An acute and severe shortage of oxygen (ischemia) to the heart muscle causes irreversible changes in the muscle cells and myocardial necrosis. This is caused by obstructed coronary blood flow impairing the ability of the left ventricle to maintain cardiac output.

Myocardial infarctions (MIs) are named according to their appearance on the EKG (either NSTEMI or STEMI), their location, and surface area involved. For example (see Table 4-1) the MI may be anterior, posterior, or lateral (in terms of location), and the surface area can be transmural, subendocardial, or intramural.

Causes and why?

With unstable angina and both presentations of myocardial infarction, underlying CAD is present (Table 4-12; Fig. 4-4; also see Table 4-6).

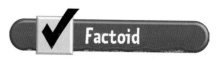

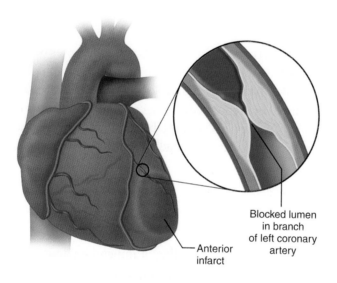

◄ Figure 4-4. Myocardial Infarction. A heart afflicted by myocardial infarction.

Table 4-12 What causes ACS and why?

Cause of acute coronary syndrome (ACS)	Rationale (why)
Sudden blockage of a coronary artery	Occlusion can be caused by: • A blood clot forming on the rough, porous surface of an ulcerated atheromatous plaque • Atheromatous debris (junk) • A crack in the endothelium and the fibrous "cap" is extruded (poked out) to block the vessel lumen
Bleeding with clot formation into or underneath an atherosclerotic plaque	• Small vessels growing into the plaque rupture and bleed into the plaque, enlarging the size of the plaque to occlude the lumen. • The plaque itself-can rupture, bleed, and form a clot.[12]

(Continued)

Table 4-12 What causes ACS and why? (*Continued*)

Cause of acute coronary syndrome (ACS)	Rationale (why)
Arterial occlusion caused by spasm.	Spasms can occur: • In the vicinity and/or adjacent to atheromatous plaques owing to irritation/inflammation of vessel walls • As a result of cocaine use • As a response to Prinzmetal's angina
Sudden greatly increased, undue and/or unaccustomed myocardial oxygen requirement.	May be caused by activities such as: • Shoveling snow in –10°F. • Playing a "grudge" tennis match in 110°F. • Snorting cocaine. All of the above greatly increase myocardial oxygen consumption (and need). The diseased coronary arteries with very narrow lumens are unable to deliver adequate blood flow to the heart muscle and severe ischemia develops, which leads to necrosis if the duration exceeds 20 minutes.

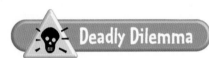

Cocaine has very powerful effects on the cardiovascular system: Sympathetic stimulation makes the heart beat faster and more forcefully, thereby increasing myocardial oxygen demand. While cocaine is working on the heart muscle, peripheral vessels are constricting and raising the blood pressure. Increasing workload on the heart adds an even greater need for oxygen, but at the same time cocaine is constricting the coronary arteries! Arterial spasm can cause a heart attack even with coronary vessels free of atheromas, so cocaine users with any degree of atherosclerosis are asking for a heart attack!

Regardless of how the coronary vessel becomes occluded, the end result will be the same! When a part of the heart totally loses its blood supply, that portion of the muscle dies. This is called a heart attack, a myocardial infarction (MI), or a coronary occlusion. Heart attacks don't just happen, they evolve. Unstable angina is a heart attack in progress because a small vessel is already occluded or partially occluded.

Signs and symptoms and why?

The patient may display the classic textbook picture of an acute MI:

• Crushing substernal chest pain, unrelieved by rest or nitroglycerin.

• Anxiety with morbid feeling of impending doom.

• Dyspnea or shortness of breath is common.

• Heart is racing, and palpations may be felt.

• Skin is cold and clammy, with diaphoresis (perspiring heavily).

• The patient may be unable to move or call for help.

These symptoms are hard to ignore or deny, and the patient would welcome an ambulance with sirens blaring … anything to get some help! In reality, here's the more common picture of how heart attacks happen over days or weeks:

• Mild symptoms come and go; therefore, they are easy to deny or attribute to other causes such as indigestion, or "that pizza I ate."

• Because symptoms subside spontaneously, the person said or thought, "Well, I sure am glad that wasn't a heart attack."

• In actuality, the heart attack was evolving all along, with ACS in progress (Table 4-13).

Table 4-13 Acute coronary syndrome (ACS) signs and symptoms

Typical ACS symptoms	Cause
Chest pain (radiates upward)	Extreme narrowing of coronary vessels owing to atherosclerosis, or rupture of a plaque with a blood clot to occlude the vessel dramatically reduces or cuts off oxygen supply to a portion of the heart muscle. Lactic acid from anaerobic metabolism creates the pain.
Tachycardia	A damaged heart muscle cannot pump as efficiently. Falling cardiac output (CO) activates sympathetic stimulation to increase the heart rate in effort to raise the CO. Sympathetic stimulation also results from pain and anxiety.
Anxiety	Crushing chest pain is accompanied by an impending sense of doom, which triggers fight or flight mechanisms with all systems on "red alert." Psychological unrest produces the anxiety response.
Arrhythmias	Caused by extreme irritability of the ischemic heart muscle adjacent to the infarct. May also be caused by damage to the conduction system in or near the zone of infarction or injury.
Nausea, vomiting	Anytime the CO drops suddenly, blood flow is shunted away from gastrointestinal circulation (nonvital organs). Reflex nausea and vomiting may also occur in response to severe pain.
Diaphoresis (sweating)	Sympathetic stimulation activates the sweat glands.[16]
Cool extremities	Caused by peripheral vasoconstriction in an effort to shunt blood to vital organs when CO drops.
Shortness of breath	Decreased CO secondary to the necrosis of a portion of myocardium results in decreased lung perfusion.

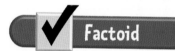

It is important to know that symptoms differ in character, intensity, location, and general presentation, because it is well documented that the more severe the symptoms, the greater the urgency and the more intensive and aggressive the treatment. Many elderly and diabetic patients have been diagnosed with an MI, yet none of the typical symptoms were present. This atypical presentation is known as a "silent" MI. The elderly patient will more typically experience a change in level of consciousness or a behavioral change as a result of decreased CO because the damaged myocardium cannot pump as efficiently with an area of nonfunctional necrosis.

There are a wide range of symptoms across different populations. Gender, age, and comorbidity (other disease conditions occurring simultaneously) affect the intensity and location of symptoms.

Elderly and/or diabetic patients may have a "silent" MI (no symptoms). There are differences among men and women in regard to symptoms reported when ACS is in progress:

- Women have prodromal (before the actual onset of disease) symptoms of unusual fatigue, altered sleep patterns, and shortness of breath.
- When women do actually experience chest pain (57%) it is reported as being "mild," and they hesitate to use the word pain to describe chest sensations.[19]
- Women complain more of epigastric discomfort, fullness, or indigestion.
- Male patients more often present with the classic signs and at least some form of chest pain.
- Diabetics and elderly patients are less likely to have chest pain. They report such complaints as back pain, indigestion, nausea/vomiting, and unusual fatigue and weakness.

Testing, testing, testing

The EKG is the best initial diagnostic test to evaluate chest pain, and the gold standard calls for it to be obtained within 10 minutes of arrival.

- The waveforms seen on the EKG will either show an obvious injury current, reflected by elevation of the ST segment (STEMI).
- Waveforms may show ST segment depression, flat or inverted T waves characteristic of unstable angina (partially blocked vessels) as well as completely blocked small coronary vessels (NSTEMI).

If the facility has a central lab, the standard is for stat labs to be accomplished within 30 minutes. Essential diagnostic tests include stat:

- 12-Lead EKG to identify waveforms for diagnosis of myocardial injury (ST segment elevation) or ischemia (ST segment depression). Nonspecific changes, flat or inverted T-wave changes can also warn of impending infarction. Arrhythmias or conduction defects caused by ischemia/injury can also be present.
- Troponin I, Troponin T: (two highly specific cardiac biomarkers: "I" and "T") proteins found in cardiac muscle cells, that are highly specific for cardiac muscle cell injury. These biomarkers rise within a few hours of injury and remain elevated for 1 to 3 weeks (which is helpful when patients delay seeking treatment for chest pain).
- Cardiac enzyme (total CK) is fractionated to separate the three creatinine kinase isoenzymes: CK-BB comes from brain tissue, CK-MM comes from skeletal muscle tissue, and the CK-MB comes from heart muscle cells. The presence of CK-MB >4% indicates damage to cardiac muscle cells.
- Myoglobin: rises as early as 1 to 2 hours after onset of myocardial necrosis; although not cardiac specific, a negative result means that chest pain is not cardiac in origin.

Factoid

The main difference between an STEMI and an NSTEMI is whether the occluded coronary vessel is large or small and whether the occlusion was sudden or gradual.

▶ **Critical Lab**

Troponin T (normal <0.2 ng/mL)
Troponin I (normal <0.03 ng/mL)

▶ **Critical Lab**

CK-MB (normal 0%–4%)
(This percent is of total CK.)

With both types of acute MI, there are zones around the central area of infarction (dead tissue). Around the area of dead tissue is a zone of tissue that is dying or injured. Quick action is required to save the injured tissue and prevent the necrotic area from becoming larger, thereby limiting the size of the infarction by improving blood flow and oxygenation into the area. The outermost zone is the ischemic area, in which the tissue is hurting (and possibly dying) because of lack of oxygen.

Testing, testing testing

You know the routine testing for chest pain to detect the presence of myocardial injury:

- Stat EKG (within 10 minutes of arrival)
- CK (total) and CK-MB (specific to heart muscle)
- Troponin
- Myoglobin

When all these initial tests (EKG, biomarkers, and myoglobin) are negative, does this mean the patient is ready for discharge? No! A heart attack could be in progress, or this could be the warning that saves a life by initiating early intervention! While the patient is in a safe environment (either intensive care or cardiac step down with telemetry monitoring), be alert to possible arrhythmias. The EKG and cardiac biomarkers will be repeated (serial EKGs and biomarkers), after which negative findings indicate a need for further diagnostic testing (see Table 4-3) such as:

- Exercise stress testing
- Myocardial perfusion imaging with a radionuclide (ie, thallium)
- Echocardiogram to evaluate ventricular wall motion and effectiveness
- 3 D computed tomography (CT) angiography (similar to regular angiography) with the advantage of being noninvasive except for IV injection of iodinated contrast media
- Cardiac catheterization with coronary angiography to visualize any narrowing of coronary vessels

What can harm my patient?

Let's talk about arrhythmias first!

✛ Arrhythmias

Arrhythmias can be classified according to whether the rhythm is fast or slow, and whether the QRS complex is narrow or wide. Narrow QRS complex rhythms originate above the ventricles, and wide QRS complex rhythms originate in the ventricles. Whether the rate is fast (tachyarrhythmias) or slow (bradyarrhythmias), narrow complex or wide complex, any combination of arrhythmias can appreciably drop the CO.

In order to know what's wrong with your patient, you must be able to recognize the following on the monitor strip:

- Deviations from normal cardiac conduction
- Heart rates (tachycardias, bradycardias)
- Appearances of waveforms (PQRST)
- Intervals (PR interval, QRS interval, ST segment and QT interval)

In order to know what you are looking at when you are evaluating rhythm strips, you must first:

- Understand cardiac conduction.
- Be able to recognize normal waveforms.

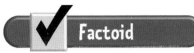

- Sudden cardiac death can occur at any moment after an acute MI, resulting from a fatal arrhythmia, usually ventricular fibrillation.
- The insult to the pump because of nonfunctional necrotic tissue can cause a dramatic drop in CO, leading to other big killers—cardiogenic shock and pulmonary edema, both of which are caused by a failing heart.
- Cardiac tamponade, seen with transmural infarctions, allows seepage of fluid (pericardial effusion) into the pericardial sac.

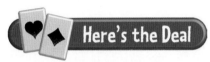

A transmural infarction leaves a full thickness of necrotic myocardium. Through the process of phagocytosis, the necrotic tissue is cleared away, leaving the ventricular wall very thin and cardiac rupture can occur. Blood seeping from the heart into the pericardial sac will compress the heart and prevent filling of the chambers.

- Patients surviving a heart attack can be left with a damaged heart muscle, and varying degrees of angina and heart failure.[20]

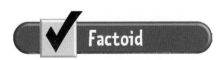

Arrhythmias are no big deal until they mess with your CO!

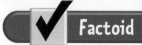

Factoid

Cardiac Output (CO) = Stroke Volume (SV) × Heart Beats per Minute

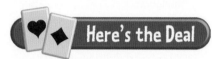

Here's the Deal

Cardiac output (measured in liters) is the volume of blood that is ejected from the heart each minute.

Abrupt changes in the heart rate can drop the CO significantly. If the CO drops suddenly, the body will think it is in shock, and a set of compensatory mechanisms will immediately become activated to raise the blood pressure.

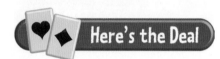

Here's the Deal

A very fast heart rate (>140) shortens the period of diastole and thereby reduces ventricular filling time, dropping the stroke volume, and subsequently dropping the CO.

▶ Figure 4-5. An ECG strip.

Hurst Hint

When the EKG paper rolls off the EKG machine or the monitor, the markings on the paper horizontally denote time: One large square represents 0.2 seconds, and each of the five little squares (inside of the large squares) each represent 0.04 seconds. Every 15 large squares equal 3 seconds in time, so a 6-second strip represents 30 large squares.

- Understand what normal waveforms mean.
- Know how to accurately measure intervals.

Let's get the normal stuff straight first!

Define time

The waveforms of one normal PQRST represents one cardiac cycle that should generate one palpable heart beat.

Normal cardiac conduction begins at the SA node, which sits atop the right atria, set on a rate of 60 to 100, and under autonomic control of the sympathetic nervous system.

Electrical conduction travels along conduction pathways:

- From the SA node across Bachmann's bundle across the walls of both atria.
- To the AV node where the electrical impulse pauses slightly (0.12–0.20 seconds), allowing ventricles to stay relaxed (diastole) long enough to fill properly.
- Then electricity spreads quickly across the bundle of His, down both bundle branches (going to the right and left ventricle).
- Terminating in the Purkinje fibers, which connect with the myometrial muscle fibers, and stimulate synchronous contraction of the ventricular muscle (right and left).

When the ventricular muscle responds electrically, it is said to depolarize, which should produce contraction of the ventricular muscle (Fig. 4-5).

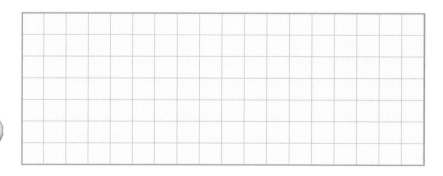

Ask yourself these five questions (above) as you evaluate the following cardiac rhythm strips (Table 4-14), looking at the "rules" for each rhythm.

Table 4-14 Rhythm strips/characteristics/treatment

Cardiac rhythm strip (6 second strip compressed to 3 inches)	Characteristic waveforms and measurements	Indicated treatment
Sinus rhythms: The sinus node is the pace-maker of the heart and initi-ates these rhythms: Normal sinus rhythm (Fig. 4-6)	Rate: 60–100 bpm Rhythm: regular Conduction: 1:1 (meaning that for every one P wave, there is one QRS) PR interval: 0.12–0.20 QRS interval: 0.8–0.11 • A normal QRS must always be <0.12, which is three small squares! • 0.12 or more is too wide! • ≥0.12 is a branch block or a rhythm originating from the ventricle.	Everything is normal, but you still have to check your patient, because what you see (waveforms on the paper) is only the electrical event. The electrical event (PQRST) must be accompa-nied by a mechanical event (the heart beat). So, if this cardiac rhythm is generat-ing a pulse, no treatment is indicated.

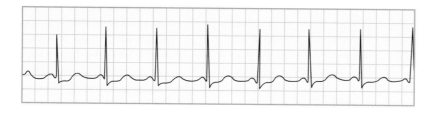

◀ Figure 4-6. Normal Sinus.

Sinus arrhythmia (Fig. 4-7)	Rate: 60–100 bpm Rhythm: irregular (bold)* Conduction: 1:1 PR interval: 0.12–0.20 QRS interval: 0.8–0.11[27]	No treatment is necessary because this rhythm is a vari-ation of normal. The slight R to R irregularity is usually associated with respirations.

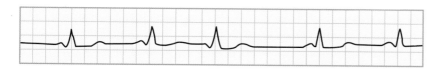

◀ Figure 4-7. Sinus Arrhythmia

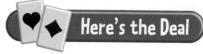

Here's the Deal

When calculating the heart rate from a 6-second rhythm strip, you can count the number of R spikes (the first upright wave-form after the P wave, usually tall and nar-row) and multiply × 10. (6 seconds × 10 = 60 sec/1 min heart rate). Fast and easy for an approximate heart rate! You can also use the "box" method to calculate rate. Count the number of large squares between two R spikes and use the follow-ing guideline for an approximate heart rate:

Sinus bradycar-dia (Fig. 4-8)	Rate: <60 bpm Rhythm: regular Conduction: 1:1 PR interval: 0.12–0.20 QRS interval: 0.8–0.11	Everything is normal, except the rate is too slow, so what's wrong with my patient? I have to go to the bedside to find out: Perform a focused cardiac assessment! First, call the per-son's name to see if he or she will arouse and respond appropriately.

(Continued)

(Continued)

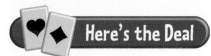

Here's the Deal

- Rhythm must be regular to use this method!
- Line up R spike on a heavy line of BIG boxes and count the number of boxes between R to R intervals.
- 1 box = 300 heart rate
- 2 boxes = 150 heart rate
- 3 boxes = 100 heart rate
- 4 boxes = 75 heart rate
- 5 boxes = 60 heart rate
- 6 boxes = 50 heart rate

If you want a more accurate heart rate, count the number of small squares between regular R spikes and divide this number into 1500.

When evaluating arrhythmias, there are basically only five things you need to evaluate to determine what is wrong with your patient! Ask yourself these five questions:

- What is the rate? Brady? Tachy? Normal range?
- Is the rhythm regular or irregular?
- Is there one (and only one) normal upright P wave in front of every QRS? 1:1 conduction?
- Is conduction normal from the SA node to the AV node: Is PR interval 0.12 to 0.20?
- Is conduction normal through the bundle branches? Are the QRS intervals wide (0.12 or greater) or narrow (0.11 or less)? If the QRS is 0.12 (three small squares or greater) this is too wide, but if everything else is normal, it tells you that there is bundle branch block.

▶ Figure 4-8. Sinus Bradycardia

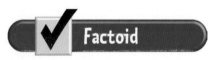

Factoid

Any heart rhythm or extra beats that have a wide QRS (≥0.12) is originating in the ventricles (not normal).

▶ Figure 4-9. Sinus Tachycardia.

Table 4-14   Rhythm strips/characteristics/treatment (*Continued*)

Cardiac rhythm strip (6 second strip compressed to 3 inches)	Characteristic waveforms and measurements	Indicated treatment
		Continue to assess for adequacy of CO. No treatment is indicated unless the patient is having symptoms related to decreased perfusion secondary to decreased CO.
		If CO is dropping and the patient is symptomatic, IV atropine (a vagolytic drug) is used to speed up the heart rate.
		If the bradycardia is resulting from abnormal conduction through the ventricles (ie, a complete heart block) a transcutaneous or transvenous pacemaker may be needed if atropine is not effective. The patient may need a permanent, implanted pacemaker if a third-degree heart block is causing the symptomatic bradycardia.

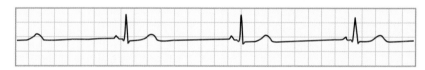

| Sinus tachycardia (Fig. 4-9) | Rate: >100 bpm
Rhythm: regular
Conduction: 1:1
PR interval: 0.12–0.20
QRS interval: 0.8–0.10 | The rate is too fast. Assess your patient and see if pain or fever is causing the rate to be too fast, if so administer analgesia or antipyretic (treat the cause). Perform a focused cardiac assessment to see how your patient is tolerating this arrhythmia.

Notify the health care provider for any sign of decreased perfusion and decreased CO. |

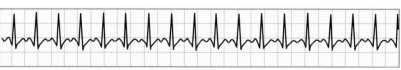

(*Continued*)

Table 4-14   Rhythm strips/characteristics/treatment (*Continued*)

Cardiac rhythm strip (6 second strip compressed to 3 inches)	Characteristic waveforms and measurements	Indicated treatment
Atrial rhythms and ectopics (Fig. 4-10) Sinus rhythm with PACs	Always look at the under-lying rhythm first and see if it is regular. Extra beats that come early (prema-ture) interrupt the normal regular rhythm. Look to see if the QRS on the extra beat is wide or narrow. Narrow QRS means that the beat originated above the ventricle, and is com-ing from the SA node or AV node. Look for a P wave on the early beat. If one is pres-ent, this is a PAC.	Any piece of atrial tissue can become hyper-irritable, and depolarize (electrically fire) automatically, before the SA node initiates the next nor-mal beat. Here's what to do: • Advise your patient to reduce intake of caffeine or alcohol. • Discuss ways that stress might be reduced. • Provide resources to assist with smoking cessation.

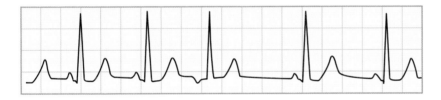

◄ Figure 4-10. Sinus Rhythm with PACS.

PSVT (Fig. 4-11)	Rate: fast PR interval: not measur-able because PSVT (*parox-ysmal* means sudden onset) supraventricular tachycardia is so fast that if a P wave is present, you cannot see it, because the P wave will be buried in the preceding T wave.	Assess your patient immedi-ately to see how he or she is tolerating this fast rhythm. Usually the patient will say his or her heart is pounding like a jackhammer, and will feel breathless and dizzy with "fluttering" in the chest. The heart is beating so fast, that the cardiac output drops sec-ondary to decreased diastole and decreased ventricular fill-ing. If your patient is stable, here's what to do: • Wash his or her face with a cold washcloth. • Instruct the patient to bear down, grunt. These interventions will stim-ulate the vagus nerve and slow the heart rate.

(*Continued*)

Table 4-14 Rhythm strips/characteristics/treatment (*Continued*)

Cardiac rhythm strip (6 second strip compressed to 3 inches)	Characteristic waveforms and measurements	Indicated treatment
		Medications (adenosine) may be indicated to chemically correct the heart if Valsalva maneuvers are unsuccessful, but if the patient is unstable (hypertensive or having chest pain or other symptoms), ACLS protocols call for synchronized low-voltage shock.

▶ Figure 4-11. Paroxysmal Supraventricular Tachycardia. (PSVT)

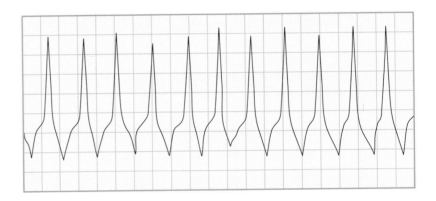

| PAT (Fig. 4-12) | Rate: 160–220 A more peaked P wave is visible in front of each narrow QRS and the PR interval is normal. Paroxysmal atrial tachycardia has a sudden onset. | Paroxysmal atrial tachycardia (PAT) is a fast supra- (above) ventricular tachycardia, but the difference is you can see the P waves because the waveforms are more spread out. Valsalva maneuvers and medications (below) are helpful to abolish the atrial pacemaker, allowing the sinus node to take over with a slower rhythm. |

▶ Figure 4-12. Paroxysmal Atrial Tachycardia (PAT).

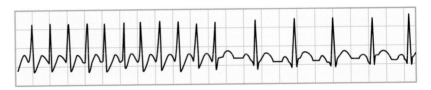

(*Continued*)

Table 4-14 Rhythm strips/characteristics/treatment (*Continued*)

Cardiac rhythm strip (6 second strip compressed to 3 inches)	Characteristic waveforms and measurements	Indicated treatment
Atrial flutter (Fig. 4-13)	Atrial rate: 220–350. Ventricular rate: Could be normal, fast, or slow, depending on how many flutter waves are in front of each QRS. Flutter waves (rather than normal P waves) precede each narrow QRS. The AV node tries to protect the ventricles against fast rates, and will selectively block one, two, or more of the flutter waves, giving rise to a variable block, 2:1, 3:1, or 4:1 QRS. Flutter waves have a "sawtooth" appearance.	Atrial cells are depolarizing all over throughout the atrial walls, and medications can be used to stop the abnormal depolarizations: • Beta-blockers • Calcium channel blocker (verapamil) Followed by guanidine, procainamide, flecainide, or amiodarone to prevent recurrence. If the patient has a fast rhythm, is unresponsive to medications or becomes unstable, synchronized cardioversion can be used to depolarize the heart, stopping all abnormal conduction, which allows the SA node to take over again.

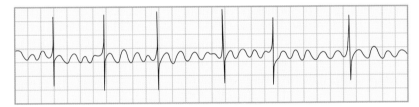

◀ Figure 4-13. Atrial Flutter.

Atrial fibrillation (A-Fib) (Fig. 4-14)	Atrial rate: 400–600 Cardiac cells in the atria are depolarizing so rapidly that the atria can no longer contract with depolarizations, but instead quivers (fibrillation). P waves: none visible, only fibrillatory waves are visible. Rhythm: always irregular.	Afib can be controlled (<100 ventricular rate) or uncontrolled (fast: >100). Determine how your patient is tolerating the rhythm change and notify the health care provider. New A-Fib that lasts longer than 48 hours may cause the patient to develop clots along the walls of the atria, which are now quivering rather than contracting and squeezing down to empty the atria.

(*Continued*)

Table 4-14   Rhythm strips/characteristics/treatment (*Continued*)

Cardiac rhythm strip (6 second strip compressed to 3 inches)	Characteristic waveforms and measurements	Indicated treatment
		The CO drops 25%–30% because the atrial kick is lost when the atria start quivering instead of forcefully contracting. Loss of atrial kick means that the ventricles do not fill adequately with blood.

▶ Figure 4-14. Atrial Fibrillation.

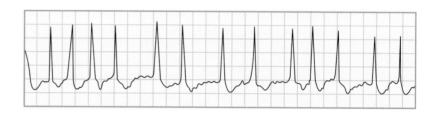

| Junctional rhythms and ectopics (Fig. 4-15) Sinus with PJC | Rules for sinus rhythm:* Everything is normal, except that the regular rhythm is interrupted with premature beats, which have a narrow QRS. There may be no P wave in front of the QRS, or the P wave could be upside down or behind the QRS, on the T wave. | Extra beats with a narrow QRS coming from the AV node. The patient is usually asymptomatic and no treatment is needed for occasional early junctional contractions. |

▶ Figure 4-15. Sinus Rhythm with PJC.

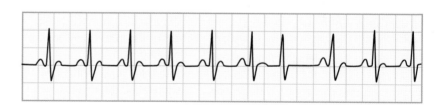

| Upper junctional rhythm (Fig. 4-16) | Rate: 40–60 Rhythm: regular PR interval: P wave is in front of the QRS and upside-down (inverted). | If the AV node has control of the rhythm, something has happened to the SA node! The faster pacemaker always takes over, and because the slower AV junction is in charge, you have to wonder, "Where is the sinus node?" |

(*Continued*)

Table 4-14   Rhythm strips/characteristics/treatment (*Continued*)

Cardiac rhythm strip (6 second strip compressed to 3 inches)	Characteristic waveforms and measurements	Indicated treatment
		A junctional escape rhythm is a lifesaving rhythm if the SA node is in the area of ischemia, injury, or necrosis after a heart attack. Watch the patient closely, and notify the health care provider! The AV node is not as dependable as the SA node! Assess to see if the patient is asymptomatic: Not all patients can tolerate the decrease in CO because of the slow rhythm.

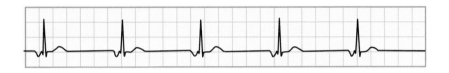

◀ Figure 4-16. Upper Junctional Rhythm.

Mid-junctional rhythm (Fig. 4-17)	Rate: 40–60 Rhythm: regular The narrow QRS does not have a P wave in front! No P waves are visible. PR interval: not measurable if there is no P wave!	The atria are being depolarized simultaneously with the ventricles, and the P wave is hidden in the middle of the QRS. If the AV junction is the fastest pacemaker, your patient may be in trouble because the heart rate could be a significant bradycardia, in the lower range (40 bpm). Assess to see how well your patient is perfusing and call the health care provider!

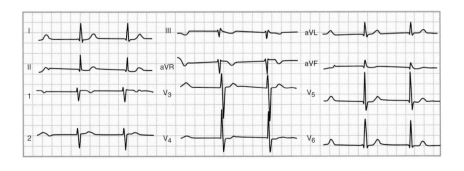

◀ Figure 4-17. Mid-junctional Rhythm.

(*Continued*)

Table 4-14   Rhythm strips/characteristics/treatment (*Continued*)

Cardiac rhythm strip (6 second strip compressed to 3 inches)	Characteristic waveforms and measurements	Indicated treatment
Lower junctional rhythm (Fig. 4-18)	Rate: 40–60 QRS: Narrow (<0.12) P waves: behind the QRS	The atria are being depolarized after the ventricles, rather than before, which is weird! But this slow rhythm can drop the CO and notify the health care provider.

▶ Figure 4-18. Lower Junctional Rhythm.

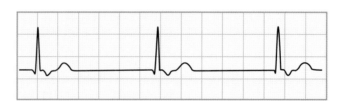

| Junctional escape rhythm (Fig. 4-19) | Rate: 40–60
QRS: narrow (<0.12)
Normal looking sinus rhythm may be interrupted with junctional beats coming (not early) in the cardiac cycle. | Escape beats are never (early) premature! This will help you differentiate between PJCs and junctional escape beats.
The lower pacemaker is trying to help increase the heart rate when you see narrow complex beats with P waves coming before (inverted) or behind the QRS. Notify the health care provider immediately. |

▶ Figure 4-19. Junctional Escape Rhythm.

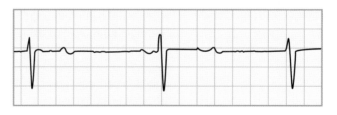

(*Continued*)

Table 4-14   Rhythm strips/characteristics/treatment (*Continued*)

Cardiac rhythm strip (6 second strip compressed to 3 inches)	Characteristic waveforms and measurements	Indicated treatment
Atrioventricular (AV) blocks: First-degree heart block (Fig. 4-20)	Rate: normal Rhythm: regular Conduction 1:1 (one P wave per QRS) PR interval: prolonged >0.20	Check medications that the patient is receiving to see if any of the prescribed drugs (eg, antiarrhythmics) act to slow conduction through the AV node. For example, if a lidocaine drip is infusing, this may be the cause of the pro-longed conduction. If this is a new block, hold any poten-tially offending medication and notify the health care provider.

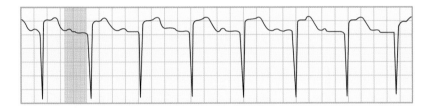

◀ Figure 4-20. First-Degree Heart Block.

Second-degree heart block (Fig. 4-21) Mobitz 1 called Wenckebach	PR intervals are changing: PR gets longer, and longer, and longest, until a P wave is finally dropped! Then the pattern starts over again!	Not dangerous. Run a rhythm strip and document on the chart.

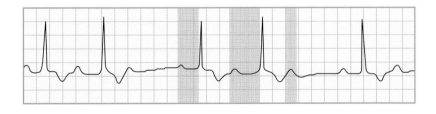

◀ Figure 4-21. Second-Degree Heart Block Type 1.

Second-degree heart block[22] type 2 (Fig. 4-22)	Rate: normal or slow, depending on how many P waves are blocked. Rhythm: could be irregular if it is a variable block.	This rhythm is dangerous! It can rapidly progress to a complete (third-degree block).

(*Continued*)

Table 4-14   Rhythm strips/characteristics/treatment (*Continued*)

Cardiac rhythm strip (6 second strip compressed to 3 inches)	Characteristic waveforms and measurements	Indicated treatment
	Two or more P waves before the QRS. PR interval uniform, not changing. The PR interval always constant, could be normal or prolonged, but will always be the same for the P wave closest to the QRS. Conduction: more than one P wave per QRS. Could be 2:1, 3:1, or 4:1.	Notify the health care provider immediately, and keep the crash cart with the transcutaneous pacemaker nearby! If the rate is really slow and the patient is symptomatic, atropine (vagolytic drug) can be given per ACLS protocol to increase the heart rate.

▶ Figure 4-22 Second-Degree Heart Block Type 2

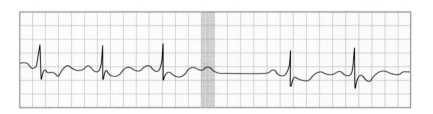

Third-degree heart block (Fig. 4-23)	There is complete dissociation between atrial and ventricular activity: P waves are regular PR intervals grossly different … none are the same. There is no relationship of P waves to the QRS. The atria and ventricles are beating independently of each other.	Notify the health care provider immediately. If the rate is slow and the patient is symptomatic, ACLS protocol calls for atropine to speed up the rate. Have the transcutaneous pacemaker available! The health care provider may insert a temporary transvenous pacemaker, and if the rhythm persists, a permanent pacemaker may be indicated.

▶ Figure 4-23 Third-Degree Heart Block.

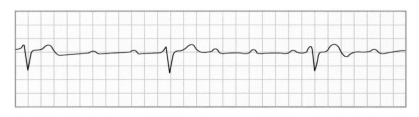

(*Continued*)

Table 4-14 Rhythm strips/characteristics/treatment (*Continued*)

Cardiac rhythm strip (6 second strip compressed to 3 inches)	Characteristic waveforms and measurements	Indicated treatment
Ventricular rhythms and ectopics (Fig. 4-24) Ventricular tachycardia	Rate: 140–200 P waves: none visible QRS: wide, uniform Rhythm: regular	Can occur spontaneously without warning, but is usually started by a PVC hitting on a vulnerable spot in the cardiac cycle. The ST segment and the top of the T wave are places where the electrical stimuli cannot be conducted because the heart muscle has not fully repolarized (not ready yet, to receive another beat). V-Tach can be stable or unstable. If the patient is alert, oriented, warm, and dry with good circulation and a good blood pressure, these medications can be given to convert the rhythm back to a sinus rhythm: • Lidocaine • Amiodarone If the patient is unstable (having chest pain, not perfusing well, hypotensive) call the code team and prepare to synchronize and cardiovert with low voltage electricity.

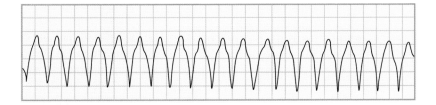

◀ Figure 4-24. Ventricular Tachycardia.

Clinical alert!

V-tachycardia can rapidly deteriorate to ventricular fibrillation.

(*Continued*)

Table 4-14   Rhythm strips/characteristics/treatment (*Continued*)

Cardiac rhythm strip (6 second strip compressed to 3 inches)	Characteristic waveforms and measurements	Indicated treatment
Ventricular fibrillation (V-Fib) (Fig. 4-25)	Rate: none Rhythm: chaotic P waves: none QRS: none	Check your patient immediately. If he or she is awake and talking, this is not vfib! Maybe the electrodes are loose or off, the patient could be scratching over the electrodes, or conduction jelly has dried up! Never shock somebody who is awake and talking to you! If the patient is nonresponsive, lifeless, and pulseless, immediate defibrillation is necessary.

▶ Figure 4-25 Ventricular Fibrillation.

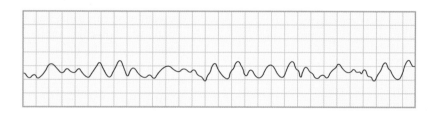

Ventricular escape (Fig. 4-26)	Rate: 20–40 Rhythm: regular sinus. The rhythm is supplemented with wide ventricular beats to raise the heart rate. PR interval: normal for the beats coming from the sinus node. QRS: wide (coming from a site in the ventricle)	Escape rhythms are always lifesaving. Even though these wide, funny looking beats are ventricular, they do not come early; rather, they come late in the cycle, and therefore do not meet the criteria for PVCs. Do NOT give medications to stop these supplemental beats, because they are helping to maintain the CO. You will drop the rate and drop the CO if medications are given to suppress these beats.

▶ Figure 4-26 Ventricular Escape.

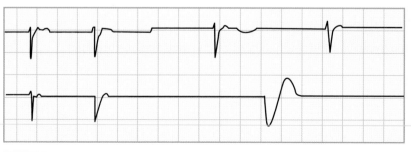

(Continued)

Table 4-14   Rhythm strips/characteristics/treatment (*Continued*)

Cardiac rhythm strip (6 second strip compressed to 3 inches)	Characteristic waveforms and measurements	Indicated treatment
Idioventricular rhythm (Fig. 4-27)	Rate: 20–40 Rhythm: regular P waves: none QRS: wide >12	Called a "dying heart" or an agonal rhythm. If the ventricles are in control of the rhythm, the higher pacemakers (SA node and AV node) are gone! The patient is dying and resuscitative efforts may be terminated per order of the attending physician. Concern is directed toward family members in preparation for imminent demise.

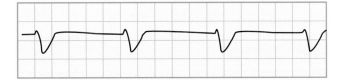

◀ Figure 4-27. Idioventricular Rhythm.

| Pulseless electrical activity (PEA) (Fig. 4-28) | Nothing can look wrong on the rhythm strip or monitor. NSR is depicted, but PEA can look like anything except:
• V-Fib
• V-Tach
• Asystole | When electricity is present and the patient has an identifiable cardiac rhythm but no heart beat can be palpated or auscultated, you must quickly find the cause of the electromechanical dysfunction and take aggressive steps to correct the problem!
Look for 5 "Hs" and 2 "Ts":
• Hypoxia (always first)
• Hypokalemia
• Hyperkalemia
• Hypothermia
• Hypovolemia
• Tension pneumothorax
• Tamponade |

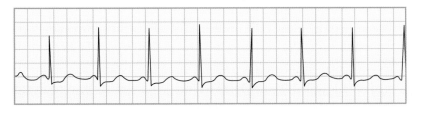

◀ Figure 4-28. Pulseless Electrical Activity

*See rules for sinus rhythm.
*This is not a life-threatening arrhythmia, but increasing PACs could forewarn of a PSVT or PAT.

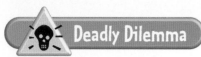

Deadly Dilemma

PVCs that are chained (hooked together) and occur at least three in a row are actually a short burst of ventricular tachycardia. Even if this converts back to the original rhythm spontaneously, it forewarns of increasing ventricular irritability, and it may not stop the next time! Shorts bursts of ventricular tachycardia can become sustained ventricular tachycardia. Use medication protocols (lidocaine, amiodarone) to stop PVCs in their tracks when you count more than five per minute, or PVCs that are coupled, paired, or chained.

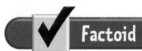

Factoid

An unresponsive, pulseless (clinically dead) patient can have a great rhythm on the monitor! This rhythm is called pulseless electrical activity (PEA).

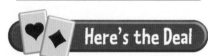

Here's the Deal

Family members call you to the room because Paw-Paw won't wake up. Upon entering the room you note that Paw-Paw is unresponsive, lifeless, and pulseless, but a normal sinus rhythm is clearly visible, marching across the bedside monitor screen. What should you do first? Shut off the monitor? The family members will think you just killed Paw-Paw! (But then you can turn the monitor on again, and they will think you brought Paw-Paw back to life: You go girl!) NO! You better call a code and start CPR while you try to figure out "What's wrong with my patient?" You can't reverse the pulseless electrical activity because the heart cannot respond (mechanically) unless you first figure out the problem and fix it!

> **Always assume hypoxia first!**

✚ Sudden cardiac death

Lethal arrhythmias can occur after an acute MI because the injured and ischemic zones surrounding the area of infarction are highly irritable due to hypoxia.

Populations at risk for sudden cardiac death (SCD) post-myocardial infarction are smokers (not necessarily snuff dippers)[23] and persons who have a reduction in left ventricular ejection fraction(<40%).

What is it and why?

Myocardial cells within the zones surrounding the central area of necrosis behave differently, depolarizing spontaneously all throughout the affected area due to ischemia and injury. Because ventricular fibrillation can occur at any time after an acute MI, the slogan "better safe than sorry" encourages all persons experiencing chest pain to check it out with a visit to the local emergency department.

Causes and why?

Many patients for whom early defibrillation has been unsuccessful may arrive at the emergency department with CPR and ACLS protocols in progress.CPR may be stopped and the lifeless, pulseless patient is pronounced dead by the emergency physician. Those patients (arriving alive) for whom circulation has been restored, may be hemodynamically unstable and are classified as high risk and need aggressive interventions to accomplish reperfusion/revascularization.

In cardiogenic shock, the heart can hardly perfuse itself (perfusion deficit), so how can it possibly carry on an effective pumping function? It cannot! And when the pump fails to keep blood moving forward, it backs up into the lungs, culminating in pulmonary edema and certain death without prompt, aggressive intervention.

Interventions

A portable, hands-free defibrillator, called an automated (or semiautomated) electronic defibrillator (AED) and designed for prehospital use, saves lives!

- AEDs have been placed in stadiums, gymnasiums, airplanes, and many public places where people gather for various activities.
- The push of a button (ON) activates voice instructions to apply electrodes, allowing the device to monitor and interpret the heart rhythm.
- If ventricular fibrillation is present, up to three initial shocks are delivered after a verbal "stand clear" warning to hopefully restore a cardiac rhythm that will provide perfusion to vital organs.

Implantable cardiac defibrillators (ICD) are indicated for high-risk patients[24] who are prone to ventricular arrhythmias. Even though the

ICDs are lifesaving, they can alter the quality of life with frequent discharges of electricity to convert the heart back to a normal rhythm.

Primary prevention of SCD is accomplished through myocardial salvage by early revascularization after MI, and early primary care to reduce left ventricular remodeling after MI and with heart failure.

Not all of the patients who come to the emergency department with chest pain will be diagnosed with a cardiac problem; however, until proved differently, a heart attack must be assumed to be in progress until ruled out. This means that all patients with complaints of chest pain must be rapidly evaluated and treated according to guidelines set forth by The American College of Cardiology and the American Heart Association Evidence-Based Recommendations.[25]

- Because the patient is at high risk for arrhythmias after acute MI, the patient must be immediately connected to a cardiac monitor with a bedside nurse who is skilled in interpreting heart rhythm tracings and protocols for immediate action in the event of an arrhythmia that compromises CO. Here are general guidelines for immediate nursing care:

  - Provide oxygen because myocardial injury and hypoxia cause irritability, giving rise to arrhythmias.

  - Afford continuous cardiac monitoring (with high and low rate alarms set).

  - Maintain reliable venous access (routinely check placement and check site for infiltration or local inflammation).

  - Administer antiarrhythmic medications as prescribed for PVCs >5/min, or coupled or chained PVCs.

  - If the patient is a candidate for a clot buster (reperfusion therapy), two antecubital venous access sites are established, and blood is drawn for stat labs to minimize the number of venipunctures (see Table 4-8).

What does the nurse look for to evaluate the effect of an arrhythmia on the cardiac output? You must determine whether the heart is functioning well enough to perfuse vital organs! Go immediately to the bedside, and don't forget to take the blood pressure machine or a cuff and stethoscope. This immediate focused cardiac assessment should include:

- LOC: Is the brain being perfused? Change in LOC, mental confusion, slow, sluggish responses (lethargy), difficulty in arousing, decreased mentation, inappropriate responses, or memory loss indicate poor perfusion.

- Skin: Cold and clammy? Vasoconstriction to shunt blood to vital organs.

- Nail bed color and capillary refill: Cyanosis and sluggish blood return.

- SaO_2: Should be >92%, but cold clammy hands and ears don't give a good read.

- StO_2: Measures tissue oxygenation.

- Chest pain: Poor perfusion to heart muscle.

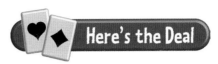

Here's the Deal

The heart monitor may show a fast, slow, or normal heart rate with NO pulse! That's bad! The patient can be having any one or more of seven reversible problems causing a condition known as PEA. You and the code team have to figure out what is wrong, and FAST!

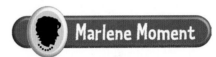

Marlene Moment

If I'm going to be given a clot buster after my MI, don't send a student nurse to start my IV! (No offense, please.) The most highly skilled staff member should perform the venipuncture to reduce bleeding and hematoma formation at the site while a clot buster is on board! One clean stick is optimal: no digging, no redirecting the cutting edge on the needle, or puncturing vessels! Any tissue trauma will cause hematoma and bleeding.

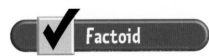

Factoid

- When the patient is having an arrhythmia, perform an immediate "focused" cardiac assessment, to determine how the patient is tolerating the change in heart rhythm.

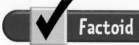

Factoid

Knowing signs and symptoms will help you to get all of your assessment and evaluation questions right: assessments (symptoms present) or evaluation (signs and symptoms gone—resolved) if treatment has been effective.

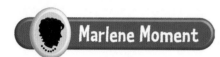

Marlene Moment

If you intervene to save my heart muscle, use aggressive efforts to salvage my brain too!

- Vital signs: Tachycardia and low systolic BP indicate decreased CO.
- Urinary output (UO): Decreased UO means decreased renal perfusion.
- Lung sounds: Shortness of breath, wet sounds, crackles, and moist rales mean decreased CO, backflow of blood into the lungs, and/or decreased lung perfusion.
- Heart sounds: The presence of S3 or S4 gallops or murmurs.
- Peripheral pulses: Decreased, weak volume (remember the rule: less volume, less pressure).

Cutting edge

Many MI patients survive cardiac arrest and subsequent PCI, and are never in a coma because of neurologic damage. Hypothermia is being used to save the brain during such periods of ischemia. When the patient remains unresponsive, induced hypothermia (cooled to a core body temperature of 33ºC for 24 hours) has improved outcomes in sudden clinical death, with survivors recovering to return to work![26]

The American Heart Association has established protocols for Advanced Cardiac Life Support (ACLS), so that the nurse can begin life-saving interventions immediately upon recognition of a life-threatening arrhythmia.

Immediately upon recognition and verification, the following three lethal arrhythmias always warrant emergency response:

- Asystole (Fig. 4-29)

▶ Figure 4-29. Asystole.

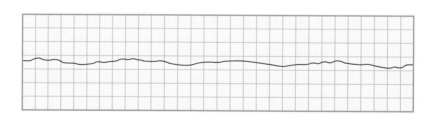

- Ventricular fibrillation (Fig. 4-30)

▶ Figure 4-30. Ventricular Fibrillation.

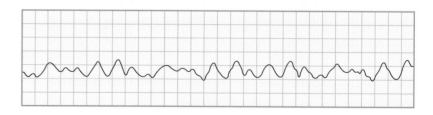

- Pulseless ventricular tachycardia (or V-tach, with a pulse that can rapidly become pulseless or can deteriorate into V-Fib) (Fig. 4-31)

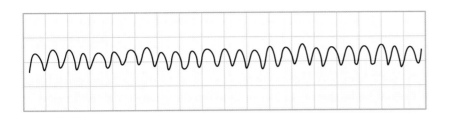

◀ Figure 4-31. Pulseless Ventricular Tachycardia.

When the patient has ventricular fibrillation or pulseless ventricular tachycardia, here's what to do:

● For V-Fib: Call a code and get the defibrillator! The patient needs immediate defibrillation and a supportive team response.

● For unstable V-Tach: The rule is to use electricity to convert arrhythmias when the patient is unstable (signs of falling CO: hypotension, chest pain, etc.) rather than relying upon IV medications that may not be circulated.

● If the patient is stable (asymptomatic): Ventricular arrhythmias can be treated with medications such as lidocaine or amiodarone.

● Implement established protocols: Generally ACLS protocols are in place in hospitals, with emergency protocols in place and laminated guidelines hanging from the crash cart.

The first thing to do is to identify patients who are at risk and assess them very closely for early cardiac decomposition: the earlier, the better, before you have to roll out the ventilator or the intra-aortic balloon pump.

✚ Cardiogenic shock

What is it?

Cardiogenic shock can be a killer complication following acute MI (Table 4-15). Cardiogenic shock happens because of severely diminished CO (acute heart failure), which can occur as a result of:

● Damaged heart muscle (following acute MI)

● Poor ventricular filling (from any reason)

● Poor outflow because the damaged left ventricle can't contract efficiently

● Ventricular arrhythmias

Our bodies are optimized to maintain circulating volume, and when the damaged heart muscle can no longer maintain a systolic blood pressure, compensatory mechanisms are activated by the central nervous system. Here's what happens:

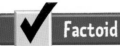

Factoid

V-Fib, V-Tach, and asystole are always "big deal" arrhythmias because the cardiac output is minimal (V-Tach with a pulse) or absent (pulseless V-Tach, V-Fib, and asystole).

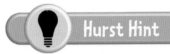

Hurst Hint

Never delay defibrillation when V-Fib occurs!

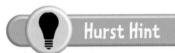

Hurst Hint

Remember the old adage, "An ounce of prevention is worth a ton of cure?" Well, there may not be a cure when the condition has progressed to late-stage cardiogenic shock, heart failure, or pulmonary edema. The mortality rate rises significantly (80%)[27] with these complications.

Monitor clinical parameters and notify the health care provider when you note early signs of a falling CO.

Perform a focused cardiac assessment at frequent intervals (see previous bulleted list of assessments).

Arterial lines provide a continuous blood pressure and are ideal for monitoring minute-by-minute changes in the systolic blood pressure, and evaluating the pulse pressure, because changes can happen very fast!

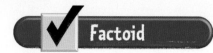

Falling systolic blood pressure = falling CO.

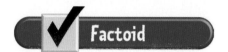

Shock kills kidneys first! Then all other vital organs follow if shock is not corrected!

- At the onset of cardiogenic shock, the drop in CO reflected by a low systolic blood pressure triggers systemic vasoconstriction to raise the blood pressure.
- As cardiogenic shock progresses, the heart is unable to adequately perfuse all body organs, so available blood flow is diverted to the vital organs (heart, lungs, brain, and kidneys) necessary to maintain life.
- If all four of these organs cannot be adequately perfused, the kidneys will be the first of the vital organs to be dropped from the "essential" list, and after only 20 minutes of poor perfusion, acute renal failure can result.
- When cardiogenic shock follows acute MI, it is apparent that the damaged heart muscle cannot eject blood forward, and myocardial perfusion decreases as well. The already damaged heart muscle, now ischemic, can no longer maintain effective function and the heart begins to beat erratically, even further dropping CO.

Table 4-15   Signs and symptoms of cardiogenic shock

Signs and symptoms	Why
Tachycardia	Caused by sympathetic stimulation in an effort to improve CO and coronary blood flow, but actually decreases both, because the faster heart rate increases oxygen demand and ischemia of the heart muscle. Coronary vessels are perfused during diastole, and tachycardia reduces diastole.
Hypotension	Systolic pressure falls because the damaged heart muscle cannot effectively eject blood from its chambers.
Cool, ashen skin	Vasoconstriction secondary to sympathetic stimulation brings less blood flow, warmth, and color into the skin surface.
Diaphoresis	Sympathetic stimulation activates the sweat glands.
Cyanosis of lips and nail beds	Stagnation of blood in the capillary bed after available oxygen is extracted.

Source: Table from *Hurst Pathophysiology Review* with permission (M.F. King, contributing author).

In cardiogenic shock, the heart has failed so miserably because of the perfusion deficit and loss of functional (working) heart muscle, that the left ventricle can no longer keep blood moving forward.

- Systolic failure results in a dramatic drop in CO, and the heart "votes ITSELF-off the island," as myocardial perfusion decreases.

- The heart can't keep up with the workload and is overwhelmed by the tachycardia and the never-ending preload (volume) coming into the heart as well as the afterload, which the heart has to work against in order to eject blood out of the heart.

- You've got to "unload" this patient fast, and get some intensive hemodynamic support in place, such as an intra-aortic balloon pump.

- Anything that increases the amount of blood returning to the right side of the heart (eg, FVE or tachycardia) will increase preload, and consequently increase the workload of the heart.

- Any factor that decreases the volume of blood returning to the right side of the heart will decrease preload, reducing the workload on the heart.

- When the vascular system vasodilates, blood pools in the extremities (increasing venous capacitance), so less blood returns to the right side of the heart (less preload).

- Diuresis causes the patient to excrete fluid, so there is less volume returning to the right side of the heart to be pumped forward; therefore, preload is decreased.

- Medications that reduce preload do so through the mechanism of diuresis and/or vasodilation.

It is always a good thing to decrease the workload on a heart patient![28]

- The greater the systemic vascular resistance (SVR), the greater the workload on the heart. Imagine trying to push open a door against a heavy wind! Will the door be easy to open? I don't think so!

- High blood pressure is like that heavy wind, making it very hard for the left ventricle to pump blood out into systemic circulation against that strong pressure.

- Anything that vasodilates arteries will make it easier for the left ventricle to eject blood out into systemic circulation, as there is less pressure to pump against.

Again, it is always a good thing to decrease the workload on a heart patient!

✛ Pulmonary edema

When cardiogenic shock (perfusion deficit to the heart muscle) occurs, it is primarily because of left ventricular failure; and when the left ventricle fails, blood backs up into pulmonary circulation. Because oxygen cannot diffuse through water, the patient is hypoxic. As the heart muscle becomes more hypoxic, the pump is even less effective (Table 4-16).[29]

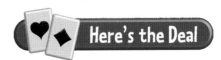

Preload refers to the volume of blood sloshing into the right side of the heart, stretching the chambers with a workload of volume that must be moved forward to the lungs. Imagine blowing up a balloon and stretching it with a volume of air pressure! Get the picture?

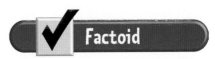

Preload is all about volume returning to the right side of the heart! More volume = more pressure = more preload!

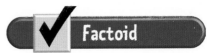

Afterload refers to the resistance out in the blood vessels (aorta and peripheral arteries) that the left side of the heart has to overcome in order to eject blood out of the heart.

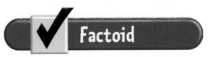

Fight or flight hormones (sympathetic stimulation: epinephrine/ norepinephrine) raise the blood pressure and the heart rate. Would this be good for your heart patient? No!

Table 4-16   Signs and symptoms and why?

Sudden onset of breathlessness	Lung water seeps into the space surrounding the alveolus, hindering diffusion of oxygen.
Severe hypoxia: • Early hypoxia manifested by restlessness/anxiety and tachycardia • Late hypoxia with cyanosis and bradycardia	Oxygen cannot diffuse through water. The alveoli are under water! The heart initially speeds up trying to get what little available oxygenated blood, there is, to the cells. Not being able to get enough air is very frightening to patients, and the sympathetic nervous system kicks in to the fight or flight mode. As hypoxia progresses, deoxygenated blood is visible as cyanosis of the lips, ear lobes, fingers, and nail beds, and the hypoxic heart begins to slow down as the myocardium and body systems decompensate.
Productive cough with pink frothy sputum	Fluid from the vascular space (plasma water) pours into the alveoli and mingles with oxygen to produce frothy expectorations.
Decreasing systolic blood pressure	Reflects decreasing CO. Less blood is moving forward into circulation because the failing ventricle allows backflow into the lungs.
Cool, pale skin	Left ventricular failure causes a fall in CO, triggering peripheral vasoconstriction and decreased perfusion to nonvital organs. The scant blood flow leaving the left side of the heart has to be shunted to vital organs.

Interventions

The nurse must perform rapid triage! A physician evaluation and EKG must take place within 10 minutes! The patient having chest pain does not take a number and sit in the waiting room, nor at the registration desk fumbling through a billfold trying to find insurance cards!

- A fatal arrhythmia can occur at any time without warning.
- The patient must be observed and monitored with a defibrillator immediately accessible.
- Unstable patients are immediately placed on bed rest in an upright position with supplemental oxygen while IV access, cardiac monitoring, vital signs, critical lab work (troponin, CK-MB, myoglobin), and stat EKG are being obtained.

When a heart attack is in progress, the goal is to restore blood flow to the heart muscle as soon as possible, minimizing necrosis and limiting the size of the infarction. Knowing that treatment guidelines call for antiplatelet, antithrombotic medications and anticipating reperfusion or revascularization procedures, all carrying a risk for hemorrhage, the nurse must ask the right questions for a nursing history relevant to bleeding. These questions can be asked while other nursing activities are in progress:

- Can you take aspirin without any major GI intolerance or allergy?
- Have you had any significant bleeding, such as from a peptic ulcer?
- Have you had any black stools? Are you vomiting blood?
- Are you predisposed to bleeding easily from minor cuts or after brushing your teeth?
- Have you had any acute abnormal bleeding in the last month?
- Have you had any major surgery in the last six weeks?

- Have you ever had a hemorrhagic stroke (bleeding into your brain)?
- Have you ever had severe high blood pressure, not controlled with medicine?
- Has anyone ever told you that your platelets were low (<100,000 mm)?

> The goal is to salvage the heart muscle (as much as possible) by restoring blood flow ASAP!

Whether the patient will receive early conservative treatment (noninvasive) or early invasive intervention, the immediate goal is to relieve ischemia and pain while monitoring the EKG monitor for arrhythmias. Here's how:

- Bed rest in a semi-Fowler's position to reduce the workload on the heart and improve cardiac output.
- Supplemental oxygen therapy using pulse oximeter to evaluate effectiveness.
- ASA 160- to 325-mg tablet, chew and swallow with a sip of water to reduce platelet aggregation and "stickiness," limiting the size of the clot blocking the coronary artery.
- Nitroglycerin 0.4 mg sublingual tablet or spray initially to reduce preload and afterload and dilate coronary arteries, getting more oxygenated blood flow into the myocardium. May be followed as an IV infusion in the first 48 hours after unstable angina/NSTEMI for ischemic chest pain, heart failure, or hypertension.[30]
- Morphine sulfate IV, titrated for pain unrelieved by nitroglycerin. Added effects are reduced anxiety, reduced cardiac work load through the vasodilating effect, to pool and trap blood in the extremities, away from the heart and enhanced oxygenation caused by bronchial dilation.

MONA (morphine, oxygen, nitroglycerin, aspirin) meets the MI patient at the door to initiate treatment, and then friends "Beta" and "ACE" drop in to see if they can help!

- Beta-blockers: To reduce cardiac workload, by blocking sympathetic response, especially in patients with ongoing chest pain.
- ACE (angiotensin-converting enzyme) inhibitors: Especially helpful when the left ventricular is impaired and not contracting well as a result of damaged muscle, or the patient has persistent hypertension not corrected by the nitroglycerin or beta-blocker.

Cutting Edge

In previous years, the STEMI (visible injury current) was the heart attack presentation that was treated aggressively, but currently both NSTEMI as well as high-risk unstable angina are being treated with the same sense of urgency: ACS is a heart attack in progress! Based on risk scores using evidence from clinical trials, emergency physicians take into consideration age, history, and clinical findings to make decisions, utilizing the appropriate guidelines for management of patients with angina/NSTEMI.[30]

Hurst Hint

There are four absolute contraindications for hemolysis (clot busting). Remember 2 + 2 = 4.

Two things in the head (a tumor or a bleed) and two things in the belly (internal bleeding or suspected aortic dissection)! 2 + 2 = 4 means: clot busting not 4 you![28]

Factoid

Before administering IV nitroglycerin, always question the patient about use of Viagra (sildenafil) within the last 24 hours; Cialis (tadalafil), or Levitra (vardenafil) in the past 48 hours!

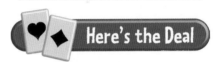

Here's the Deal

IV nitroglycerin is contraindicated with the above male enhancement drugs, as it may cause an unsafe drop in blood pressure and CO.

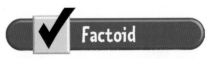

Factoid

When a heart attack is in progress: "Time is muscle."

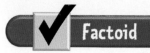

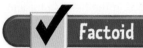

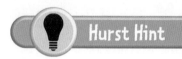

In particular, deaths are reduced significantly in patients with unstable angina or NSTEMI who receive a GP IIb–IIIa inhibitor within 24 hours of admission.

General Interventions for Acute Coronary Syndrome

When acute MI is in progress, protocols are in place so that patients can receive the following medications:

- Oxygen (yes, oxygen is classified as a drug)
- Antiplatelet/antithrombotic drug therapy
- Nitroglycerin, morphine sulfate
- A beta-blocker and possibly an ACE inhibitor

The physician-prescribed plan for recovery is individualized for each patient, depending on risk factors (from history and physical exam) for MI and SCD. Here are general guidelines:

- When the patient has unstable angina or NSTEMI with low risk for MI or death, the initial treatment plan will be early conservative treatment consisting of antiplatelet drug therapy, which can be used sequentially or concurrently with anticoagulants and thrombolytic agents.
- Generally, low-risk patients will undergo treadmill stress testing at some point after stabilization to determine a need for further intervention.
- If clinical findings (eg, compromised CO as evident by hypotension, murmurs, gallops, rales, or ventricular arrhythmias) indicate an acute problem with the unstable patient in immediate danger, a more aggressive plan will be implemented.
- The high-risk plan includes the same antiplatelet, anticoagulant, anti-ischemic therapy plus thrombolysis (clot busting) or a diagnostic cardiac catheterization with coronary angiography (see Table 4-3), and PCI (percutaneous intervention) or CABG (coronary artery bypass graft) as indicated within 24–48 hours.

Table 4-17   ACS drug therapy

Anti-platelet drugs: keeps platelets from clumping up and sticking together.

- Platelet aggregation inhibitors: Aspirin, clopidogrel (Plavix), cilostazol (Pletal), ticlopidine (Ticlid)
- GB llb–lll inhibitors: eptifibatide (Integrilin), tirofiban (Aggrastat), abciximab* (ReoPro)
- Platelet adhesion inhibitor: dipyridamole (Persantine IV, Apo-Dipyridamole, Novo-Dipiradol, Dipridacot)

Antithrombotic drugs: to achieve anticoagulation, reduce extension of clot/reocclusion.

- Heparin (unfractionated) blocks thrombin formation, increasing action of antithrombin. It has a very short half-life and is easily reversed, which is important if open heart surgery (CABG) is considered.
- Heparinoids (low molecular weight): enoxaparin (Lovenox), danaparoid (Orgaran) have longer lasting effects, giving more sustained anticoagulation.
- Bivalirudin (Angiomax) inhibits thrombin by binding to its receptor sites; prevents conversion of fibrinogen to fibrin, inhibits platelet adhesion and aggregation. Has a very predictable half-life of 25 minutes with normal renal function.[31]

(Continued)

Table 4-17 ACS drug therapy (*Continued*)

Anti-ischemic drugs improve oxygenation to maintain O_2 saturation >93%.
- Oxygen
- Nitroglycerin: Nitrostat, NitroQuick, Nitro-Bid IV, Nitrolingual (spray)

When the patient has an STEMI (visible ST segment elevation), blood flow into the heart muscle must be quickly re-established. Interventions may take place:

- In the emergency department with coronary reperfusion (clot busting)
- In the cath lab with percutaneous intervention (PCI with stent)
- In the operating room for revascularization with coronary artery bypass graft (CABG)

With any of the aforementioned interventions, time is of the essence and must be accomplished as soon as possible because heart muscle is dying while the clock ticks away.

Clot busting is indicated if the facility does not have capability of performing percutaneous coronary intervention (PCI) or cannot safely transfer a patient within 60 minutes. PCIs are the preferred method of opening up blood flow when one or two vessels are involved. The door to cath lab time should be <90 minutes.[28]

Multivessel disease (three or more) will require CABG for revascularization.

PCI is accomplished with local anesthesia, usually at the groin, where a catheter and guidewire is introduced through a sheath advanced to the aorta and from there, into the coronary artery that is blocked. Contrast media identify the narrowed artery and the coronary intervention of choice is then performed: percutaneous transluminal coronary angioplasty (PTCA), laser angioplasty, or atherectomy (removal of the plaque) followed by placement of a stent to hold the artery open. The catheter is removed through the sheath (introducer) and the sheath stays in place until such time as safe removal can be accomplished.

After any invasive procedure for restoring coronary blood flow, or providing ventricular support, the nurse must monitor the patient frequently, and always be on the alert for possible complications. Refer to the following table for complications related to specific procedures and nursing interventions.

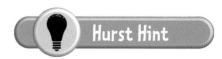

Better watch for signs of hypoxemia and HYPOTENSION.

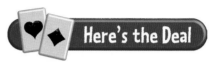

The window of opportunity for (clot-busting) thrombolysis of a coronary artery is 6 to 8 hours, after which time the patient is no longer a candidate for hemolysis because the risk of intervention at this late stage outweighs the benefits.

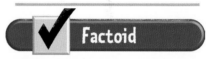

A word about vascular closure devices (VCDs) versus manual pressure to promote hemostasis after cardiac catheterization! Older studies with a small sample size indicated that not only were VCDs only marginally effective, they actually caused more vascular complications such as hematoma, bleeding, arteriovenous fistula, and pseudoaneurysm.[32]

Newer studies with larger sample sizes (one study of 21,841 consecutive cardiac catheterizations),[33] attribute improved physician skill and institutional experience, smaller sheath size, and improvements in the devices themselves with improved outcomes. Newer studies show VCDs to have comparable or fewer vascular complications compared with manual compression. Three VCDs in particular (Angio-Seal, VasoSeal, and Perclose) were associated with a lower risk for vascular complications.[34]

The major complication during PCI is MI, and the most commonly occurring complication following PCI is bleeding complications.[35]

Table 4-18   Complications postinvasive procedures and nursing care

Clot busting (fibrinolysis) with fibrinolytic agents such as: • TPA (tissue plasminogen activator) • TNKase • Retavase • Streptokinase Anticoagulants are used during and after reperfusion/revascularization procedures to prevent reocclusion. These agents also carry a risk for overt or covert bleeding. Major complication: Hemorrhage Other complications: • Allergy with streptokinase • Failed hemolysis or reocclusion	Watch for reperfusion arrhythmias and monitor CO: • Perform a focused cardiac assessment for signs of decreased perfusion. • Monitor vital signs for <CO. Watch for bleeding: • Monitor urine for hematuria. • Monitor stools for melena (black tarry feces). • Monitor expectorations for blood from gums, mouth, throat, or lungs. • Examine any emesis for blood. Take bleeding precautions: • There should be no IM injections. • Hold pressure after venipunctures. • Use soft toothbrushes. • Use an electric razor for shaving. • Avoid all trauma. Monitor lab results: • PT (ProTime) • Fibrinogen level • aPTT (activated partial thromboplastin time) • HCT (hematocrit)
Intra-Aortic Balloon Pump (IABP), which has or requires: • Helium-filled polyurethane balloon • Console with counterpulsation pump attached to the catheter • Femoral artery access Potential complications with IABP: • Massive arterial hemorrhage if accidentally pulled out of femoral artery! • Acute limb ischemia, which could lead to amputation. • Rupture of the balloon and gas embolism, which could lead to death. • Thrombus formation/embolism with prolonged delay of counter-pulsations can occur during change of helium tank or mechanical malfunction. • Vascular problems such as aortic dissection, accidental perforation of an artery, arteriovenous fistula, or compartment syndrome.[36] This seems like a huge list of really bad possible complications, but the benefit to the patient is tremendous when the left ventricle cannot sustain adequate circulation. Most common complications are vascular (not life threatening) and can be resolved by removing the catheter and using the other (contralateral) leg if IABP must be continued.[33]	Perioperative nurses set up and activate the IABP when the patient fails to wean from the cardiopulmonary bypass, but this is a procedure that requires specific technical instruction. The following interventions focus on the nurse who is providing care to a patient in cardiogenic shock, or one who is being supported (kept alive) while awaiting a heart transplant or ventricular assist device. In order to save life and limb, the nurse must be able to pick up on complications early. Here's what you do: • Frequently monitor the patient's response to IABP therapy by performing a focused assessment of CO plus evaluating measures of hemodynamics such as CVP, pulmonary capillary wedge pressure (PWP). • Frequently check the machine and never turn off alarms! If an alarm sounds, always check the patient first, and then look at the machine. • Always have a spare tank of helium immediately available, and another pump console in case of a malfunction requiring a fast switch/swap! • Be prepared to manually deflate and inflate the balloon while a skilled person is swapping tanks or pumps to prevent clotting around a deflated balloon. • Watch for blood in the driveline (from the machine) or the catheter (from the patient) which means the balloon has ruptured.[37] • Keep the affected leg straight (no hip flexion) and frequently monitor peripheral circulation (7 Ps below).

(Continued)

Table 4-18 Complications postinvasive procedures and nursing care (*Continued*)

Procedures requiring femoral access site (at the groin) involving a catheter/sheath with concurrent antithrombin, antiplatelet therapy (see Table 4-10) such as:
• IABP
• Cardiac catheterization
• PCI
Studies show that there is an increased mortality rate with a major femoral bleed that requires blood transfusion.[38]
	Receive report from cath lab or OR, taking note of any complications during the procedure and usage of mechanical compression devices or vessel closure device.
	
	Recognize patients at higher risk for complications and observe groin area more closely for hemorrhage, hematoma, and vascular problems:
	
	Advanced age
	
	Elevated systolic BP[39]
	
	Monitor peripheral perfusion hourly for 6 Ps (plus one more) and compare "sheath" leg to the other leg:
	
	   Pulseless
	
	   Pain
	
	   Pallor
	
	   Paresthesia
	
	   Paralysis
	
	   Poikilothermy (pronounced POY- kilo-thermie) is a huge word to say the extremity is cold!
	
	   Press: blanch nail beds and see if you get capillary refill.
	
	Before the sheath is pulled:
	• Aspirate the sheath using a 10-mL syringe to check for the presence of blood clots.
	• Be ready to fluid bolus NS (make sure you have venous access) and manually compress PRN hemorrhage.
	• A second nurse on standby to monitor the patient as the sheath is pulled.
	• Note the type of anticoagulant used and time discontinued: two hours required after bivalirudin (Angiomax) and heparin (UF) must be past peak.[31]
	• Monitor lab: ACT (activated clotting time) usually 150–200 seconds is safe when heparin is used. (normal ACT = 70–120 seconds).
	
	After the sheath is pulled:
	
	Apply continuous pressure to the site for 10–20 minutes.
	
	Monitor vital signs every 3–5 minutes.
	• Apply dressing when bleeding stops.
	• Elevate HOB slightly, no more than 30 degrees.[33]
	• Keep affected leg straight and still (sand bags/trochanter rolls may be needed as well as frequent reminders).
	• Bed rest is mandated for 2–6 hours if there are no complications.
	• Examine the site for bleeding, swelling, and hematoma formation.
	
	The above guidelines are compiled from best current practices, but nursing is changing as technology changes, so here is the Hurst rule: Always follow established hospital protocols and policies.

(Continued)

Table 4-18 *Complications postinvasive procedures and nursing care (Continued)*

Coronary artery bypass graft (CABG) can be performed on or off the cardiopulmonary bypass machine.

"On pump" carries additional risks because the patient's blood has been in contact with the machine:

- Systemic inflammatory response syndrome (SIRS)
- Stroke
- Cognitive changes
- Renal failure
- Micro emboli
- Blood clotting problems

Both "on pump" and "off pump" increase risk of heart problems such as:

- Tachyarrhythmias such as atrial fibrillation (A-Fib) common on second or third postoperative day
- Bradycardias and heart block during the first several hours after surgery
- Increased stroke risk if A-Fib occurs
- Ventricular arrhythmias usually early postoperative because of surgical manipulation of the heart, hypothermia during surgery, electrolyte imbalance and ischemia
- Acidosis
- Pericardial effusion, which could cause cardiac tamponade

Both "on pump" and 'off pump' patients have respiratory problems such as:

- Atelectasis (collapsed, airless alveoli) caused by hypoventilation
- Pulmonary edema caused by volume overload during surgery
- Pleural effusion (fluid collecting in the pleural space) caused by bleeding where the graft artery (usually internal mammary artery) was taken
- Ventilator-associated pneumonia

Monitor the patient for development of systemic inflammatory response:

- Evaluate lab reports, WBC, CRP
- Monitor temperature frequently
- Notify physician of abnormal values and fever

Monitor for stroke and cognitive changes:

- Can patient follow command?
- Is smile/facial expression symmetric?
- Equality of muscle strength and power? (hand grips, pushing against resistance with feet)
- Altered speech pattern or slurring?

Monitor for renal failure:

- Question patient about signs that toxins are being retained:
  - Fatigue, no energy
  - Nausea, vomiting
  - Headache
- Note and report elevations of BUN or creatinine.
- Evaluate the 24-hour record and compare to previous graphics looking for trends in weight gain, increasing BP, and decreasing urine output.

Monitor for blood clotting problems:

- Observe for bruising, petechiae.
- Evaluate blood clotting studies such as PT, aPTT, activated clotting time.
- Observe urine and stools for blood.

Be alert for signs of cardiac tamponade:

- Jugular vein distention
- Hypotension
- Muffled heart sounds
- Increasing CVP
- Decreasing systolic BP

Report abnormal findings promptly and prepare for needle aspiration if tamponade confirmed by CT or echocardiogram.

Monitor for pulmonary problems:

- Auscultate lung fields (anterior and posterior) to detect rales or areas of atelectasis.
- Use sterile technique for endotracheal suction and watch for changes in color and consistency of respiratory secretions.
- Monitor temperature frequently, remembering that immune-suppressed patients (and those on steroids) will not spike a temperature, so low-grade elevations may be a red flag.
- Obtain sputum specimens as ordered for culture and sensitivity.
- Watch for increasing areas of dullness on percussion across the sternum, which can warn of an increasing pericardial effusion that precedes tamponade.

*If any of the above Ps are present, notify the physician and increase frequency of observations as changes in the limb can occur rapidly.[40]

Cutting Edge

Advances in noninvasive coronary artery imaging using magnetic resonance angiography (MRA) and multidetector computed tomography angiography[41] (MDCTA) provide great images of coronary vessels, demonstrating narrowing of arteries with pictures like those of regular angiography.

After an MI, the heart is in a weakened state because the area of necrosis will be cleared away by phagocytes, leaving once functional muscle tissue a matrix of scar tissue.

- Areas of noncontractile myocardium do not help with the pumping action of the heart.

- If the area of necrosis occurred in the region of conduction pathways, the patient could be left with various forms of heart blocks, a common one being a bundle branch block.

- When the ventricles are not beating in synchrony (together) as a result of one ventricle depolarizing (contracting) sooner than the other, the CO and the ejection fraction (percent of blood emptied from the ventricle during systole) decreases.

- The patient may be left with varying degrees of heart failure and angina.[42]

Regardless of age, patients can benefit from cardiac rehab after having a heart attack.

Studies following patients after acute MI have shown that even though there is a higher mortality rate in the elderly population (>75), they have higher quality of living with fewer symptoms than younger patients. A number of patients across the age spectrum will continue to experience angina after a heart attack. These data support the need for strategies to systematically assess and treat symptoms after acute MI.[38]

- Sudden cardiac death (SCD) can occur at any moment after an acute MI, resulting from a fatal arrhythmia, usually ventricular fibrillation.

- The insult to the pump caused by nonfunctional necrotic tissue can cause a dramatic drop in CO, leading to other big killers: cardiogenic shock and pulmonary edema, both of which are caused by a failing heart.

- Cardiac tamponade, seen with transmural infarctions that allow seepage of fluid (pericardial effusion) into the pericardial sac.

- Patients surviving the heart attack can be left with a damaged heart muscle, and varying degrees of angina and heart failure.[1]

✛ Heart Failure

What is it?

Heart failure is a condition that occurs when the heart function is so compromised that the pump can no longer keep blood moving in a forward motion through the heart. The heart cannot keep up with the workload and failure produces higher than normal pressures within the chambers of the heart, overstretching the muscular walls, weakening the heart's ability to contract.

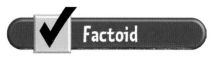

Factoid

Heart attacks can happen during PCI because blood flow is obstructed during PCI, while the balloon is inflated. This can lead to chest pain or arrhythmias, the catheter could dislodge a plaque or clot, or a clot could form around the catheter. Antiplatelets and anticoagulants are given before, during, and after this procedure to reduce the incidence of these complications, with stents to stabilize the vessel, holding it open after PCI.

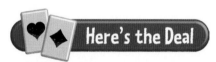

Here's the Deal

A transmural infarction leaves a full thickness of necrotic myocardium. Through the process of phagocytosis, the necrotic tissue is cleared away, leaving the ventricular wall very thin and cardiac rupture can occur. Blood seeping from the heart into the pericardial sac will compress the heart and prevent filling of the chambers.

- When the right side of the heart is overwhelmed with incoming blood flow, and cannot effectively move this volume forward, venous pressure increases in systemic circulation and fluid begins to leak out to create enlarged organs, edema, and ascites.
- When the left side of the heart fails, pressure increases and blood backs up to produce respiratory signs and symptoms.
- The increased workload on the heart triggers the renin angiotensin aldosterone system (RAAS).
- The stress hormones epinephrine and norepinephrine are released, which rather than actually helping the problem, create more problems. Under the influence of epinephrine and norepinephrine, the heart is beating faster with greater contractile strength (increasing the workload on a heart that is already overloaded), against more resistance caused by the peripheral vasoconstriction effect of catecholamines.
- Cardiac muscle fibers (myofibrils) become damaged because of the stress of increased preload and afterload.
- Damaged myofibrils attempt to repair themselves, but the repair process called "remodeling" results in grossly abnormal muscle mass and ventricular chambers because of the poorly functioning myofibrils.
- More stress and more damage results in more remodeling and increasingly severe heart failure.[20]

Heart failure is classified and grouped into four stages of disease, according to risk assessment and severity of symptoms:

- Stages A is at risk for heart failure,
- Stage B is pre-heart failure, and
- Stages C and D have varying degrees of severity of symptoms.

This is different from the New York Heart Association (NYHA) functional classification, which describes what the patient with heart disease is functionally able to do. Patients are classified as stage 1 through 4.

The stages of heart failure are used as a guide to treatment protocols and are listed below:

- Stage A: Patients do not currently have any heart damage or symptoms, but because of pre-existing conditions (atherosclerosis, diabetes, metabolic syndrome, hypertension and obesity, and exposure to cardiotoxins) are at high risk for developing heart failure.
- Stage B: Patients have structural heart disease, but do not display signs or symptoms of heart failure yet. This could include persons with damage from an MI, asymptomatic valvular heart disease, or left ventricular hypertrophy with a low ejection fraction.
- Stage C: Patients have structural heart disease (remodeling) and have current or prior symptoms of heart failure.
- Stage D: End-stage heart disease patients have symptoms at rest therefore home care cannot be maintained without specialized interventions.

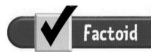

Factoid

The New York Heart Association has developed a grading system for CHF related to the disability associated with each class. There are four classes. NYHA Class 1 carries the least disability, and Class 4 has the worst incapacitation.

What causes it and why?

Heart failure is a commonly occurring complication following acute MI or prolonged ischemic heart disease that damages the heart muscle. Heart failure can also be caused by:

- Cardiomyopathy (any cause)
- Chronic tachycardia (untreated hyperthyroidism)
- Pulmonary hypertension (acute or chronic)
- Congenital heart disease
- Acquired valvular disease, rheumatoid heart disease (RHD) = endocarditis
- Myocarditis (viruses attacking the heart muscle)
- Longstanding systemic hypertension (years of increased afterload)
- CAD with chronic ischemia
- Replacement of myocardial muscle fibers with scar tissue (damage of any cause)
- Infiltration of myocardial muscle fibers with foreign material (eg, iron deposits from hemochromatosis) or any other matter that will cause the muscle to be stiff and lose its flexibility

Any condition that damages the heart muscle will interfere with the ability of the heart to keep blood moving in a forward motion. There are various forms of cardiomyopathy:

- Iatrogenic (physician/treatment-induced) such that can occur with cancer chemotherapy (anthracyclines and trastuzumab) or ionizing radiation over the chest wall
- Inherited (familial, genetic) condition called hypertrophic cardiomyopathy, which produces overgrowth (hypertrophy) and fibrosis (muscle scarring), ischemia, and mitral regurgitation

Remember!

Exercise extreme caution when giving IV fluids to these patients:

- Elderly
- Pediatric
- Cardiac
- Renal

Signs and symptoms and why?

Systolic heart failure describes a failing left side of the heart that cannot contract effectively to eject a sufficient volume of blood forward.

- When left ventricular function cannot be maintained to move oxygenated blood forward, the CO drops.
- Left ventricular failure leads to high pressure in the capillary bed surrounding the alveoli, which causes fluid to leak into the alveolus.
- Because oxygen cannot diffuse through water, obviously the patient becomes hypoxic.

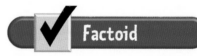

Factoid

Any acute fluid gain in susceptible persons (elderly, pediatric, renal, and cardiac patients) can overload the heart causing heart failure!

Diastolic failure is a term that describes a right sided heart condition whereby the ventricles cannot relax and fill properly with blood. Right sided heart failure caused by high pressure in the lungs secondary to obstruction is called cor pulmonale (Table 4-19).

Table 4-19   Contrasting systolic and diastolic heart failure signs and symptoms

Systolic failure: The heart cannot contract and eject.	Diastolic failure: The heart cannot relax and fill.
Pulmonary congestion: moist crackles (rales) heard on auscultation.	Peripheral and dependent edema due to pooling of blood in the lower extremities. Increasing pressure in the vascular space owing to FVE exceeds pressure in the tissues and fluid leaks out of the vascular space causing pitting edema. Fluid leaks into the abdominal cavity causing ascites.
Dyspnea, complaints of shortness of breath with minimal activity. Breathless wakening at night (nocturnal dyspnea) and orthopnea (having to sit erect to breathe).	Enlarged liver creating abdominal discomfort and tenderness owing to increased venous pressure and backflow of blood.
Cough may be nonproductive initially, becoming productive as lung water increases with pink frothy sputum.	Ascites caused by increased pressure in the vascular space, causing fluid to leak into the peritoneal space.

Symptoms common to both systolic and diastolic heart failure

Tachycardia

What can harm my patient and why?

The patient in heart failure is at risk for pulmonary edema, because:

- The weakened heart muscle and/or faulty valve(s) is/are unable to keep blood flowing in a forward motion.
- As the failing pump beats faster over time (tachycardia) trying to keep up with the fluid load, the heart enlarges because it is working overtime.

The patient in heart failure is at risk for ACS because:

- The enlarged heart outgrows its blood supply and becomes ischemic.
- With sustained tachycardia, the myocardial cells are working harder and demanding more oxygen, yet with a falling CO, even less oxygen is available.

The patient in heart failure is at risk for chronic leg ulcers and deep vein thrombosis (DVT) because:

- Venostasis occurs because of increased venous pressure causing fluid to leak out into peripheral tissue. Sitting long periods with legs dependent owing to fatigue and activity intolerance contribute to dependent edema.

Atrial fibrillation (common with heart failure) results from irritable cells in the atria of the heart that begin to "fire" (depolarize) spontaneously, causing a fast heart rate that "outruns" the SA node to take over the rhythm of the heart. When the atria are just quivering instead of physically contracting, blood clots can form along the wall of the atria. The intramural thrombi can be showered into circulation.

Testing, testing, testing

Laboratory testing usually includes routine labs plus a general metabolic panel to check for predisposing factors (eg, diabetes) or malfunction in other vital organs because of poor perfusion (chronic or acute). This workup is comprehensive because when the heart fails, other organs follow suit. Admission labs usually include:

- CBC (complete blood count)
- Urinalysis
- Serum electrolytes, including magnesium and calcium
- Fasting lipid panel
- Fasting serum glucose and glycohemoglobin
- Serum creatinine
- Thyroid profile
- Liver function tests
- Ferritin level (if hemochromatosis is suspected)
- BNP (brain type natriuretic peptide)

The BNP is a protein that is stored primarily in the ventricular myocardial tissue. When diastolic pressures rise (increasing the stretch of the ventricle), BNP is released. This happens when the ventricle is stressed, occurring with ventricular hypertrophy, hypertension, or heart failure. Elevated BNP levels in combination with clinical evaluation can help diagnose heart failure, but should not be used alone to confirm or exclude a diagnosis of heart failure.[43]

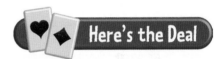

Here's the Deal

Some cardiovascular drugs interfere with the BNP test results: beta-blockers, calcium antagonists, diuretics, digitalis, glycosides, and vasodilators. Consult with the health care provider to see if any of these drugs should be withheld for 24 hours before a BNP level is drawn.[44]

Biomarkers for myocardial damage may be prescribed if the clinical evaluation suggests that the heart failure may be due to ACS.

> ▶ **Critical Values**
>
> BNP > 100 = Ventricular Stress

Radiologic studies

Radiologic studies may include one or more of the following:

- Chest X-ray to detect enlarged heart, dilated chambers, pulmonary infiltrates
- Echocardiogram: noninvasive ultrasound to detect any abnormalities of cardiac size, shapes, and motion; can determine ejection fraction and myocardial ischemia when performed with a stress test.
- Transesophageal echocardiogram (TEE) is used the same way as echocardiogram (above), but the ultrasound gets pictures from inside the esophagus, which gives a better, sharper image, especially when the patient has large breasts or a lot of muscle mass.

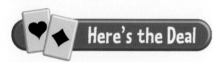

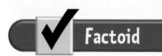

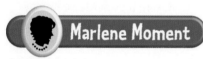

Clinical Alert

TEE may be hazardous to your health if you have dysphagia or have had radiation to your chest because the probe has to be swallowed.

- Computed tomography (CT) also called computed axial tomography (CAT), and electron beam computed tomography (EBCT) is a super-fast scanning technique to identify congenital heart lesions, evaluate muscle mass of the ventricles, chamber volumes, CO, and ejection fraction.[45]

- Multiple gated acquisition (MUGA) scan looks at the left ventricle to compare function at rest and with activity; images allow for evaluation of wall motion and ejection fraction. This test is also called equilibrium radionuclide angiocardiography (ERNA).

- Magnetic resonance imaging (MRI) can reveal problems with the heart muscle, great vessels, pericardium, and valves.

Interventions

Because heart failure patients have problems with fluid volume excess, they need:

- Bed rest in a Fowler's position.

- Low-sodium diet (varies from no added salt to 1–2 g sodium restriction).

- Daily weight (same time, same scales, same clothes, and void first). The goal is to keep weight between 2–3 lb of normal.

- 24-hour intake and output.

- Compression stockings as prescribed to prevent trapping of venous blood predisposing to DVT formation and dependent edema.

- Monitor for shortness of breath (a subjective complaint) by counting respirations, making note of any halting speech patterns, and observing any respiratory effort such as use of accessory muscles and flared nares.

- Administer medications to block neurohormonal stress hormones (RAAS).

- Administer antiplatelet therapy when atrial fibrillation complicates heart failure.

- Administer heart failure specific unloading drugs such as angiotensin receptor blocking agents (ARBs: the "sartans").

Interventions

NUTRITION/FLUID BALANCE My patient needs to know the necessity of keeping an accurate record of daily weights:

- Same time (usually first thing in the morning after voiding)

- Same scales

- Same clothes

- Void first (so you don't include the weight of a bladder full of urine)

My patient needs to know how to grocery shop and prepare low-sodium meals:

- Shop the parameter of the grocery store: Don't even go down that cookie and chip isle: There is nothing there that you can have (well, maybe graham crackers)!

- Buy canned vegetables packed in water only (not water and salt), fresh or frozen vegetables.

- Avoid all prepared foods (ready to eat) and/or processed foods such as canned meats, sausage, and bacon.

- No added salt is the rule for a 2-g (2000 mg) daily sodium allowance. This means buying crackers with unsalted tops and throwing out the salt shaker.

MEDICATIONS   See Table 4-20.

Table 4-20   Pharmacologic therapy for heart failure

Drug classification/ name	Drug action/use	Nursing implications and patient teaching

Diuretics:
Examples of thiazide diuretics:
• Chlorothiazide (Diuril)
• Hydrochlorothiazide (HydroDIURIL, Esidrix)
• Chlorthalidone (Hygroton)
Examples of Loop diuretics:
• Lasix (furosemide)
• Bumex (bumetanide)
Potassium sparing diuretics:
• Amiloride (Midamor)
• Triamterene (Dyrenium)
Aldosterone receptor blocker:
• Spironolactone (Aldactone)
• Eplerenone (Inspra)
	Diuresis reduces preload and afterload. Loop diuretics block reassertion of sodium and chloride, while increasing renal excretion of water.
	
	Aldactone and Inspra inhibit aldosterone binding and have diuretic effects as they promote loss of sodium and water but cause the patient to retain K⁺.
		Administer IVP Lasix slowly: 40 mg over 1–2 minutes to avoid sudden hypotension and ototoxicity, can cause permanent irreversible nerve deafness.
		Give IVP Bumex slowly at a rate of 0.5–1 mg over 2 minutes.
		• Daily weight
		• I&O
		• Caution patient to make position changes slowly to avoid orthostatic hypotension and dizziness.
		• Monitor "three-step" BP and record.
		• Monitor serum K⁺ levels.
		• With aldosterone antagonists caution patients to:
		  • Avoid NSAIDs, as this can lead to hyperkalemia and worsening renal status.
		  • Avoid salt substitutes, which may be high in K⁺.
		  • Report diarrhea or other dehydration states, which increase K⁺ levels.

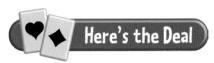

Here's the Deal

When patients are chronically short of breath, it feels "normal" for them. Ask your patient to repeat a sentence (10 syllables or more), such as, "I'm going to town today to buy some eggs." Paw-Paw will probably say it this way, "I'm going (gasp) to town (gasp) today to (gasp) buy some (gasp) eggs." Then after auscultation of the chest, you will report to the health care provider and document: Moist rales mid-scapular area bilaterally; Respirations appear labored with use of accessory muscles. Halting speech noted, yet denies shortness of breath.

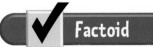

Factoid

Concentration makes numbers go UP!

(Continued)

Table 4-20   Pharmacologic therapy for heart failure (*Continued*)

Drug classification/ name	Drug action/use	Nursing implications and patient teaching
Angiotensin-converting enzyme (ACE) inhibitors: (the "-prils"): • Enalapril (Vasotec) • Fosinopril (Monopril) • Lisinopril (Zestril) • Captopril (Capoten) • Ramipril (Altace) • Quinapril (Accupril) • Moexipril (Univasc)	Selectively suppresses the renin-angiotensin-aldosterone system and inhibits ACE (angio-tensin-converting enzyme), preventing the conversion of angiotensin I to angiotensin II (potent vasoconstrictor): Has antihypertensive action owing to systemic vasodilation to decrease preload and afterload in heart failure.	Use cautiously if there is a history of angioedema: can cause a big tongue that can block the airway! Commonly used with diuretics; watch for hypotension; monitor blood pressure and hold medicine if systolic is <90 mm Hg. Consider fluid bolus for excessive hypotension. If given with K⁺ sparing diuretic, monitor serum K⁺ (can lead to hyperkalemia). Dose is decreased with renal impairment: monitor BUN, creatinine, urine protein. Monitor WBC and differential periodically for patients with renal disease or collagen disease. Hold the drug if neutrophil count is <1000.
Angiotensin II receptor–blocking agent (ARBs): The "-sartans": • Candesartan (Atacand, Atacand HCT) • Eprosartan (Teveten) • Irbesartan (Avalide, Avapro) • Losartan (Cozaar, Hyzaar) • Tasosartan (Verdia) • Telmisartan (Micardis) • Valsartan (Diovan, Diovan HCT)	Angiotensin is a hormone that causes blood vessels to constrict and has aldosterone-producing effects that increase sodium and water retention. These effects (vaso-constriction, and fluid and sodium retention) result in high blood pressure and increased workload on the heart. ARBs prevent angiotensin from working, thereby lowering blood pressure, which means decreased workload for a failing heart. ARBs decrease the strain on the heart and promote vasodilatation and diuresis to: • Reduce preload and afterload • Reduce cardiac workload • Decrease serum Na⁺ • Improve CO • Decrease pulmonary congestion	During initiation there is a risk for orthostatic hypotension. "three-step" BP should be monitored: • Lying down • Sitting • Standing Excreted in urine and feces (via bile). Monitor for adverse effects and side effects: • Renal failure (monitor output and creatinine). • Drug-induced hepatitis (monitor liver enzymes). • Hyperkalemia (monitor serum K⁺). • Hypotension (monitor I&O, daily weight, BP).

(Continued)

Table 4-20 Pharmacologic therapy for heart failure (*Continued*)

Drug classification/ name	Drug action/use	Nursing implications and patient teaching
Beta-blockers (the "-O-lols): • Propranolol (Inderal) • Atenolol (Tenormin) • Carvedilol (Coreg) • Labetalol (Trandate) • Metoprolol (Lopressor, Toprol) • Nadolol (Corgard)	When we are nervous, frightened, or physically active, our bodies produce adrenalin. Adrenalin makes the heart beat faster and harder and constricts the blood vessels, which makes our blood pressure shoot up. Adrenalin works by attaching to structures called beta receptors on the muscle cells of the heart. Beta-blockers are used to stop adrenalin from hooking on to these receptors. Blocking the receptors (and preventing adrenalin from working) slows the pulse and lowers blood pressure. This makes it easier for the heart to work.	Reduced cardiac workload is a desired effect of the beta-blockers; however, the decreased contractile force of the myocardium may decrease the ability of the failing myocardial muscle fibers to keep blood moving forward! Monitor your heart failure patient for: • Exertional dyspnea or fatigue • Moist rales • JVD • Weight gain and edema • Gallops: S3, S4
Digitalis glycosides: Example: Digoxin (Lanoxin) Digoxin is not a first-line drug, but is supported for use in late, symptomatic heart failure with structural changes (Stage C). Having no new data or evidence since 2001 guidelines regarding value/usefulness, it is believed that in terms of risk/benefit, other agents such as aldosterone blockers may be of greater benefit with less risk/ toxicity.[43]	This very old drug has a positive ionotropic effect directly on the heart muscle fibers to strengthen the force of contraction. Atrial fibrillation with loss of the atrial kick reduces CO, and the digitalis effect of increased contractile force helps to compensate for this loss. Conduction is delayed through the AV node to decrease the heart rate. There is a risk for toxicity, especially in the presence of electrolyte imbalance, especially hypokalemia. Diuresis results from an improved CO, which increases renal perfusion.	Monitor serum electrolytes closely, being especially alert to hypokalemia, which can precipitate digitalis toxicity! Prior to administering digitalis preparations: • Count apical pulse and record. • Hold the drug if HR <60 and notify health care provider. Teach the patient to report early signs of toxicity: • Anorexia • Nausea/vomiting • Visual changes (may be a yellow/green tint) Bradycardia and arrhythmias are late signs of toxicity. Therapeutic blood levels of digoxin are: 0.5–2 ng/mL. Anything >2 is TOXIC!

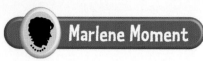

Marlene Moment

Don't overdo it!! Start out slow and gradually increase activity tolerance. Listen to your body! If unusual weakness, fatigue, or shortness of breath occurs, this is the signal to rest! Learning how to pace oneself is paramount.

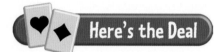

Here's the Deal

Paw-Paw can still mow the yard with his riding lawn mower, just not all at once. Paw-Paw has learned to pace himself. He mows the front yard early in the morning when it is cool, goes inside to rest under the air conditioning during the heat of the day, and then finishes the back yard late in the evening when the sun has gone down. Paw-Paw also knows that fatigue is a warning sign that means "I have overdone it" and it is time to rest!

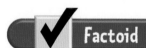

Factoid

Frequent hospitalizations for heart failure have a negative impact on quality of life! We need to do something!

Clinical alert

Normal digoxin level = 0.5–2 ng/mL
  Toxic digoxin level = >2.0 ng/mL

INVASIVE PROCEDURES If during hospitalization, there has been any device inserted into artery/vein (radial artery line for blood pressure measurements), cardiac catheterization, IABP for hemodynamic support (Table 4-11), and/or use of X-ray dye, my patient needs to know that delayed complications can occur, and he or she should be diligent in self-monitoring:

- Immediately report any pain, numbness, and tingling, or color or temperature changes in the affected extremity.
- If bleeding occurs at the site, hold manual pressure 1 in above the puncture site and call 911.
- Watch urinary output as this is a good indicator of kidney function. Report decreasing urinary output and weight gain >2–3 lb.
- Report malaise (just generally feeling bad), fatigue (no energy), headache, nausea, vomiting, as these may be signs that toxins are building up, which could result from renal failure (use of nephrotoxic dyes).

Fluid volume excess and pulmonary congestion are the two main reasons that patients with heart failure require hospitalization.[46] Here are the facts:

- Most patients were getting sick for days or weeks before they actually began having signs and symptoms.
- By the time that patients with heart failure (Class 3 and 4) get to the hospital and high pulmonary wedge pressures are recorded, they have an average of 10 lb of extra fluid and they are in trouble, requiring hospitalization.
- Patients with heart failure (Class 3 and 4) are often short of breath and cough an average of three days before hospitalization, so proactive monitoring makes really good sense.
- Pulmonary congestion doesn't just happen overnight, it begins as left ventricular dysfunction that can't keep blood moving forward, and causes the following chain of events:
  - Pressure builds up first in the left ventricle and (going backward) increases the left atrial pressure.
  - Pressure in the pulmonary vascular bed increases (backing up from the left atria), and this pressure is transmitted to the pulmonary artery, then to the right atria and ventricle.
  - Finally the patient is symptomatic with dyspnea, jugular venous distention, and all the symptoms of decompensation.
  - So here we go again, back to the ICU! Only this time my patient may not wean off the ventilator!

Lastly, the patient with longstanding heart failure, who has chronically inadequate CO and decreased perfusion to vital organs (heart, brain, lungs, kidneys) can develop multisystem organ failure.

✚ Pulmonary edema

If hemodynamic monitoring is in place, pressure readings provide objective indicators that the patient is going into left ventricular failure well before the patient crashes and drowns in his own lung fluid. Measures can be in place to support the failing heart and hopefully avoid fluid volume excess. If this technology is unavailable, you have to be alert to subtle objective and subjective signs.

CASE IN POINT An acute MI patient calls the nurse, complaining of feeling slightly short of breath. He is in a normal sinus rhythm, but heart rate has increased from 88 to 100 beats/min and the systolic blood pressure is elevated 20 mm Hg from the last reading. Lung fields are clear, so the nurse reassures the patient and administers an anxiolytic medication (Valium 1–2 mg IVP prn). The patient is resting comfortably at last check before reporting off at 7 p.m. The next day the nurse finds this patient's bed empty, and a chest film on the view box shows a total white out: All lung tissue is underwater!

Clinical alert

Always be alarmed when the patient with heart failure complains of shortness of breath plus symptoms of restless and tachycardia: Think hypoxia first!

As soon as the early signs of pulmonary edema are recognized the health care provider is to be notified stat, and if hemodynamic monitoring is in place these "other vital signs" can alert you to increasing ventricular and pulmonary artery pressures before the patient is symptomatic.

The patient in pulmonary edema requires the following actions stat:

- Immediately position the patient (to improve cardiac output) with legs dependent (so blood pools in lower extremities away from the heart).
- Titrate oxygen (nasal cannula is best initially because the patient struggling for air may resist a mask) to achieve saturation levels >92% (hopefully).
- Administer morphine (drug of choice) which not only relieves pain and anxiety but also causes vasodilation and reduction of the workload on the heart (decrease blood return to the heart).
- Administer diuretics (Lasix, Bumex) to reduce circulating volume quickly. (IV Lasix begins to work in 2 minutes.)

Monitor patient for worsening of symptoms (air hunger with frothy pink spittle), which could culminate in the development of "full-blown" pulmonary edema! Hemodynamic monitoring, indicated for such critically ill patients, uses invasive direct pressure monitoring systems and is usually managed in critical care units.

- A Swan-Ganz catheter (triple lumen central line) is inserted through the femoral vein (antecubital or external jugular sites could also be used), guided to the vena cava and advanced into the right atrium, and connected to a pressure monitoring system for measurement of central venous pressure (CVP).

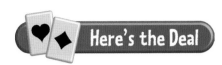

When a patient has longstanding atrial fibrillation, blood clots form on the inside surface of the atria. It would be hazardous to convert this patient from A-Fib into a sinus rhythm, because in doing so, when the walls of the atria contract forcefully after the long period of quivering, the force of the atria squeezing down can shower little blood clots into systemic circulation. (Not good!)

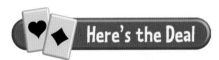

The worst case scenario of left-sided heart failure is pulmonary edema.

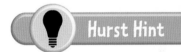

Restlessness and tachycardia: always think hypoxia first!

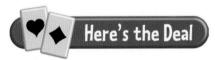

As long as hydrostatic capillary pressure in the vascular space ≤18 mm Hg, fluid will stay in the vascular space, but at pressures 22 to 25 mm Hg, fluid moves out around the alveoli (not yet inside the alveoli, where you can hear air moving over fluid), but putting a layer of water between the alveoli and the capillary bed, so your patient will experience shortness of breath in advance of moist rales that can be auscultated.

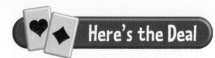

Here's the Deal

The patient (above) who took a Valium-induced nap did not have a chance for early intervention because he awakened in pulmonary edema. Who knows? Maybe if the nurse had notified the health care provider of the patient's subjective complaint, a stat portable chest x-ray could have seen the fluid surrounding the alveolus before it poured in up to both clavicles, drowning the patient, who would have benefited more from the prn Lasix order than from the Valium.

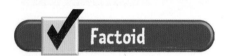

Factoid

Decreasing CVP = Fluid Volume Deficit = Decreased Preload
Increasing CVP = Fluid Volume Excess = Increased Preload

- Rising CVP readings warn of increasing fluid volume (increased preload) and decreasing CVP reflects decreasing preload, commonly associated with hypovolemia.

- Central venous pressure readings can detect the beginning of pulmonary or developing shock before the patient even has symptoms, allowing for early management of these critical conditions.

The pulmonary monitoring system is preferred (over CVP) when left heart failure is suspected or diagnosed.

- A pulmonary artery (PA) catheter requires a large vein (jugular, subclavian, or femoral).

- After insertion, the catheter is directed into the right heart (where the proximal lumen opens), advanced through the tricuspid valve and positioned in the pulmonary artery.

- Cables are connected to a monitoring system for obtaining pulmonary pressures.

- The pulmonary catheter has an inflatable balloon at the tip that, when inflated at intervals (ever so briefly) allows for measurement of pulmonary "wedge" pressures (so called because the inflated balloon is "wedged" in place when inflated).

- The balloon sensor detects back pressure exerted on the balloon, making a waveform seen on the bedside monitor that can be translated into a number.

- Rising PWP readings mean rising pressure in the lungs.

Both of these invasive catheters provide data for evaluating left ventricular function (cardiac output), and are used for managing fluid volume status in unstable patients. The more sophisticated pulmonary artery catheter has other specialized capabilities (cardiac pacing) and thermistor ports for measuring cardiac output, monitoring CVP (through proximal lumen in right atrium), measuring systolic and diastolic pulmonary artery pressures, as well as measuring pulmonary and systemic vascular resistance.[45]

Clinical alert

NEVER use any triple lumen central line for administration of fluids or medications without positive X-ray confirmation first!

The complications that can occur with pulmonary artery PA catheters include:

- Infection occurring because an invasive line is in the heart.

- Air embolus caused by negative pressure sucking air in through a break in the connection (as occurs with changing lines).

- Pulmonary artery rupture caused by trauma of a foreign body (also guidewire used for insertion).

- Cardiac arrhythmias caused by irritability as the foreign body approaches the heart.

- An inflated balloon obstructs blood flow into the lung and can cause a pulmonary infarction if the balloon is not quickly deflated (within seconds) of obtaining the pressure reading.
- Thrombi (and emboli) can occur if the catheter is not flushed adequately (heparinized solution under pressure).

Clinical alert

Care of PA catheters require specialized instruction and practice and are managed in critical care units by critical care nurses. This is NOT to be attempted by a new nurse!

An arterial line may be inserted (a tiny catheter is usually inserted into the radial artery) enables the nurse to monitor blood pressures continuously.

- Prior to insertion, an Allen's test must be performed to determine if arterial blood flow into the hand is adequate.
- If when both arteries are compressed, the hand is pale (no arterial circulation). It would be hazardous to occlude the artery with a catheter.
- When continuous intra-arterial blood pressure monitoring is accomplished, it allows for minute-by-minute evaluation of the cardiac output.
- Auscultate all lung fields, remembering that posterior rales develop first.
- Maintain bed rest in a Fowler's position with pillows for elbow support to make breathing easier.
- Titrate (adjust to achieve a desired response) oxygen flow rate to maintain acceptable oxygen saturation levels.
- Administer "unloading drugs" (see pulmonary edema: Pharmacology in a nutshell).

INVASIVE PROCEDURES If during hospitalization, there has been any device inserted into the artery/vein, such as radial artery line for blood pressure measurements, cardiac catheterization, IABP for hemodynamic support (see Table 4-11), and/or use of X-ray dye, my patient needs to know that delayed complications can occur, and he or she should be diligent in self-monitoring:

- Immediately report any pain, numbness, and tingling, color, or temperature changes in the affected extremity.
- If bleeding occurs at the site, hold manual pressure 1 in above the puncture site and call 911.
- Watch urinary output, as this is a good indicator of kidney function. Report decreasing urinary output and weight gain >2 to 3 lb.
- Report malaise (just generally feeling bad), fatigue (no energy), headache, nausea, and vomiting, because these may be signs that toxins are building up, which could be caused by renal failure (use of nephrotoxic dyes).

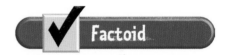

The systolic pressure directly reflects the cardiac output!

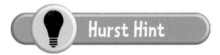

Restlessness and tachycardia: Always think hypoxia first!

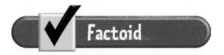

Bed rest induces diuresis.

Pulmonary congestion doesn't just happen overnight, it begins as left ventricular dysfunction that can't keep blood moving forward causing the following chain of events:

- Pressure builds up first in the left ventricle and (going backward) increases the left atrial pressure.

- Pressure in the pulmonary vascular bed increases (backing up from the left atria), and this pressure is transmitted to the pulmonary artery, and then to the right atria and ventricle.

- Finally the patient is symptomatic with dyspnea, jugular venous distention, and all the symptoms of decompensation.

- So here we go again, back to the ICU! Only this time my patient may not wean off the ventilator!

IMPLANTABLE HEMODYNAMIC MONITORING DEVICE[45]   Even small increases in fluid volume status may have a huge impact on heart failure patients, causing symptomatic cardiac decompensation. The implantable hemodynamic monitoring device has a dual function: a sensor in the left atrium to measure left atrial pressure, body temperature, and an intracardiac electrogram, with a patient advisory monitor (PAM).

- PAM is very smart! "She" has software that tells the patient what to do, based on the real-time left atrial pressure that the sensor picks up!

- The patient's cardiologist programs the prescription algorithm into the software.

- Then based on the patient's fluid status, PAM tells the patient to take medication, hold medication, or when to measure pressures and call the doctor.

The name of one such device is the Heart POD, which allows for readjustment of medications without daily communication with the physician. For example, if left atrial pressure is rising, PAM may tell the patient to take an extra Lasix 40 mg today (based on the order programmed into the database by the patient's cardiologist), therefore creating pulmonary congestion (and another hospital admission).

Patients with implantable defibrillators who have repeated runs of ventricular fibrillation can experience "electrical storm" when the programmed electrical stimuli fires repeatedly. Catheter ablation (going straight to the irritable spot in the ventricle that keeps triggering V-Fib) has been successful in preventing sudden death from electrical storm.[47]

THE THREE Rs: RECOVERY, RISK REDUCTION, AND REHAB   The ACC/AHA Guidelines (2005) spell out recommendations for treatment for heart failure according to staging degree and severity of heart failure (HF) symptoms:

Stage A: At risk for HF but without any structural damage or symptoms of HF. Treatment goals include lifestyle modifications and therapies for risk reduction, such as:

- Measures to cease illicit drug use and alcohol intake; referrals to addiction centers, counseling, support groups.

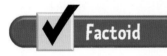

Factoid

Electricity, when applied to the irritable spot, can halt an electrical storm. Ablation also decreases electrical storm.

- Measures to promote smoking cessation (drugs such as Wellbutrin or Chantix), aversion therapy programs, American Heart Fresh Start program, and group support.
- Recognition, diagnosis, and control of metabolic syndrome: treatment for lipid disorders, protocols for management of diabetes, weight loss, exercise program, and treatment for hypertensive disorders (depending on the cause). Recommended pharmacologic interventions for vascular disease are ACE inhibitors and ARBs.[44]

✛ Inflammatory/infectious cardiac diseases

Let's get the normal stuff straight!

The heart is the center of the vascular space, and is continuous with the vascular space. The triple layered pericardial sac encloses the heart and the base of the great vessels. Normally a small amount of fluid (15–50 mL) reduces friction between the inner parietal and visceral layers of the pericardium.[48] The heart (like the blood vessels) is comprised of three layers:

- The epicardium (the serous membrane that lines the outer pericardial sac)
- The myocardium (the middle muscular layer that does the work)
- The endocardium (the inside slick lining that is continuous with the vessels)

Inflammation and/or infection can affect any of the three layers of the heart, all of which present some commonalities, with specific differences in causation, symptoms, and treatment. Let's start with the outermost layer first!

What is it?

Any time tissue is traumatized or infected, our body's immunologic system activates the inflammatory process to protect (wall off the invader), heal (clear away the damaged/necrotic tissue with phagocytosis), and repair (fibroblasts to the rescue forming scar tissue). The hallmark signs of inflammation are:

- Redness (hyperemia as more blood flow and WBCs rush to the area)
- Local heat (increased blood to the area and metabolism produce heat)
- Swelling (edema because of fluid leaving damaged, permeable capillaries)
- Pain (pressure on nerve endings in the area because of edema and damaged tissue)
- Loss of function (a swollen, inflamed, stiff with edema, damaged body part just does not perform its normal function very well!)

✛ Pericarditis

What is it?

Pericarditis is inflammation of the fibrous sac surrounding the heart, and can be caused by a number of diseases, conditions, toxins, or pathogens. When infection is present, the organism may be bacterial, viral, fungal, or tubercular; however, the one pathogen that really loves the heart (and kidney) is strep!

Causes and why?

Pericarditis can result as a complication of acute myocardial infarction (Dressler's syndrome), or can be precipitated by any mechanical/surgical trauma to the heart (instrumentation, heart surgery).[49]

Pericarditis can also result as a direct result of infection: viruses, bacteria, fungi could occur following acute myocardial infarction. Autoimmune conditions such as rheumatic fever, rheumatoid arthritis, or systemic lupus erythematosus (SLE) are known causes of pericarditis.[50] Pericarditis may also occur as a complication of a number of other disease conditions because circulating toxins can trigger inflammatory processes. There are several forms of pericarditis, depending on the cause:

* Acute pericarditis is caused by infection with a virus, bacteria, or fungus—usually in the lungs (example tuberculosis, TB) and upper respiratory tract (eg, strep throat).
* If the pericarditis is caused by bacteria, it is called bacterial or purulent pericarditis.
* Neoplastic pericarditis (neoplasms, cancer).
* Idiopathic pericarditis (unknown cause).
* Uremic pericarditis can occur because of a buildup of toxins in the blood secondary to renal failure.[48]

Signs and symptoms

Acute pericarditis: signs and symptoms and why?

Signs and symptoms	Why
Pericardial friction rub (scratchy, grating like sound heard in systole and diastole)	Inflammation of the inner and outermost lining of the pericardial sac causes scarring and roughening. The scraping together of the inner and outermost layers produce a sound called a friction rub. It can best be heard at the apex of the heart.
Dysphagia (difficulty swallowing)	The fluid around the heart can place pressure on the nerve endings supplying the esophagus.
Chest pain: worsens with inspiration and decreases when the client leans forward; can radiate to neck, shoulders, chest, and arms	Inflammatory process stimulates the pain receptors in the heart. Leaning forward takes some of the pressure off the pleural tissue.

Source: Created by the author from References 4, 5, and 6.

The patient with pericarditis has low-grade intermittent fever and feels sick. Pericardial friction rub can be detected in about half of the patients, and can be easily missed because it could be intermittent or so soft that it goes undetected.

The most common symptom of acute pericarditis is pain over the heart or pain behind the heart. The pain is different from any other presentation of chest pain:

* The quality of this chest pain is described as sharp and stabbing.
* Onset may be either sudden or gradual.

- The pain may radiate to the back, neck, left shoulder, or arm.
- Movement or breathing in deeply aggravates the pain.
- Pain is most severe when the patient is lying down.
- Pain is intensified by coughing or swallowing.
- Pain is relieved when the patient sits up and leans forward.
- Patients can present with acute abdominal pain, but this is not the normal presentation.

Other commonly associated signs and symptoms include dyspnea, cough, and dysphagia. If pericarditis is a complication of tuberculosis, the patient will have all of the above symptoms plus some unique TB signs as well:

- Fever
- Night sweats
- Weight loss

Testing, testing, testing

Any time a patient has chest pain, EKG, cardiac enzymes, and troponin levels and myoglobin are all first-line tests to rule out possible myocardial infarction. The EKG will show a peculiar pattern: The ST segment is elevated above the baseline like an acute MI; however, the ST segment shows a slurring, concave pattern (like a dip) suggestive of pericarditis. BNP or Doppler tissue imaging may be ordered to rule out constrictive cardiomyopathy because this condition can mimic pericarditis.[51]

Depending on the suspected cause of pericarditis, other tests may be ordered (Fig. 4-32):

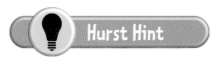

Hurst Hint

To auscultate a pericardial friction rub, position the patient to get the heart in close proximity to the chest wall: sitting up and leaning forward. Have the patient hold his or her breath (or listen after exhaling), not breathing during auscultation. Listen with the diaphragm of the stethoscope and notify the physician ASAP if you hear a grating scratchy sound like leather surfaces rubbing together.

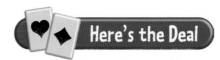

Here's the Deal

If a pericardial friction rub is present and pericardial effusion is confirmed with echocardiography, a focused cardiac assessment at frequent intervals is necessary to monitor cardiac output while preparations are being made for performing a pericardiocentesis (see Cardiac Tamponade) with a priority on aftercare.

◄ Figure 4-32. Pericarditis ECG Changes.

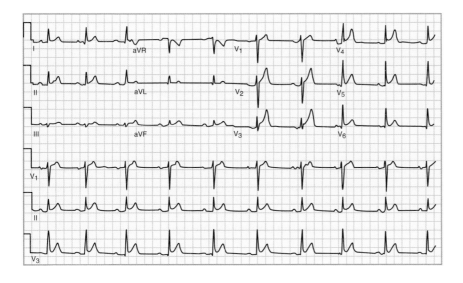

- Complete blood count (CBC)
- Blood culture and sensitivity
- Inflammatory markers: C-reactive protein, erythrocyte sedimentation rate

If a pericardial friction rub is auscultated during physical examination of the patient, a stat bedside echocardiogram will be performed to detect the presence of a pericardial effusion.

Interventions

Just like any condition, the patient with pericarditis can be mildly ill or severely compromised. If the patient is stable (good cardiac output, no myocardial ischemia, MI ruled out, no significant pericardial effusion) outpatient treatment may be a possibility with home self-care (see Patient Teaching below).

The treatment plan will include pathogen-specific antibiotic therapy, anti-inflammatory agents, and analgesia.

- Pericardiocentesis is indicated to relieve pericardial effusion when cardiac output is threatened.
- Tachypnea and tachycardia will be managed with bed rest and supplemental oxygen.

Treatment plans differ based on the specific cause of the pericarditis and resultant pericardial effusion. For example, if the pericardial effusion is caused by breast cancer or lung cancer, intrapericardial treatment of neoplastic pericarditis with cisplatin may be indicated to prevent recurring pericardial effusion.

- If autoimmune conditions are implicated, low-dose corticosteroids may be given for a period of time and then slowly tapered off. Prednisone has proved effective in treating recurrent pericarditis.[52]
- Referral for rheumatology consult is indicated if pericarditis is related to a possible autoimmune response.
- Patients can gradually resume normal activities when pain and fever resolve, but must understand that pain may continue for several months.
- Follow-up visits, and compliance with the treatment plan is important for recovery.
- Any worsening of symptoms must be reported immediately rather than awaiting the next scheduled office visit.

Nursing care of the hospitalized patient includes:

- Monitor lab results and report deviations from normal.
- Position for comfort: upright with pillows behind the back to tilt the chest forward or orthopneic position (leaning over pillow padded overbed table).
- Monitor pain level, having patient to rate pain on scale of 1 to 10.
- Administer prescribed nonsteroidal anti-inflammatory drugs (NSAIDs) to reduce inflammation and pain.
- Administer prescribed oral analgesics prn: codeine, hydrocodone, etc.
- Notify physician for unrelieved or severe pain.

- For infective pericarditis: Obtain cultures first (from blood or aspirated pericardial fluid)! Then administer prescribed anti-infectives (broad-spectrum antibiotics until culture reports are obtained, then antibiotics or antifungals as ordered).
- For uremic pericarditis, monitor patient response to dialysis.

PATIENT TEACHING   Self-care and monitoring are the priority following pericardiocentesis and during recovery from pericarditis. Teach the patient to:

- Take and record the patient's temperature daily (a calendar works nicely).
- Restrict activity to reduce pain and decrease cardiac oxygen demand, avoiding all vigorous activity.
- Take oral analgesics at the onset of pain for optimal results.
- Continue antibiotics and anti-inflammatory agents as prescribed.
- Notify the physician immediately for worsening of symptoms or unrelieved pain.

What can harm my patient?

- Cardiac tamponade
- Pericardial effusion
- Infection

✚ Myocarditis

What is it?

Myocarditis is inflammation (see five hallmark signs above) of the muscle layer of the heart that can be triggered by acute infections. Myocarditis is rare and usually mild but can be deadly if untreated.[48]

Causes and why?

Myocarditis is caused by a number of organisms as well as cardiotoxic chemicals and drugs. General agents and conditions known to cause myocarditis are:

- Pathogens: bacteria, fungus, virus
- Cardiotoxic drugs or chemicals
- Autoimmune response (eg, SLE)[50]
- Tropical diseases (usually parasitic)

    When the myocardium is invaded by pathogens or exposed to toxic drugs/chemicals, the body's inflammatory response is activated. The inflammatory process in the muscle tissue leads to changes in the myocytes: fibrosis, scarring, and reduced blood flow.

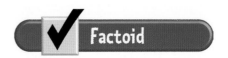

Factoid

Most common viruses causing myocarditis are coxsackievirus and adenovirus!

Signs and symptoms

Signs and symptoms	Why
Fever	Normal response to infection. Some bacteria and fungi cannot survive in an environment with an elevated temperature.
Splenomegaly: The spleen is an important immune system organ.	The spleen is working overtime to protect immunity; this causes hypertrophy.
Petechia	Tiny spots caused by hemorrhaging under the skin. The microemboli and septic emboli can shower any organ, including the skin, leading to clotting followed by bleeding.
Hematuria	Microemboli and septic emboli can shower any organ, especially the glomeruli, leading to clotting followed by bleeding.
Cardiac murmurs	Vegetation on the valve prevents the valve from closing properly, resulting in a murmur.
Pleuritic pain	Microemboli and septic emboli can shower any organ, including the lungs. The inflammatory response kicks in. Tissue edema occurs and places pressure on nerve endings. This pleuritic pain may be present during inspiration or expiration.
Fatigue, weakness	Vegetation on the mitral valve prevents proper closure of the valve, causing backward flow during systole, which eventually leads to heart failure. This causes fatigue and weakness.
Late signs include signs and symptoms of left-sided heart failure: Nocturnal dyspnea; S 3; pink, frothy sputum; cough; crackles; orthopnea; tachycardia; restlessness; JVD; hepatomegaly; ascites; peripheral edema; pulmonary edema.	Infection and/or clot formation on the mitral or aortic valves can lead to left-sided heart failure.

Source: Created by the author from References 4, 5, and 6.

Testing, testing, testing

The following diagnostic tests can help differentiate myocarditis from other cardiac conditions:

* Lab studies: Creatinine kinase may be elevated because of muscle injury. The sedimentation rate and WBCs increase because of the inflammatory process.

* The EKG may show arrhythmias and/or heart block as well as ST segment and T-wave changes. Myocarditis is reflected by the small QRS (low voltage) and transitory Q-wave development.[48]

* The echocardiogram may show decreased contractility of the heart muscle and changes in the size of chambers and valve dysfunction.

* The chest X-ray may show evidence of heart failure: enlarged heart and pulmonary infiltrates.

* The endomyocardial biopsy provides a definite diagnosis if the sample (obtained via cardiac catheterization) actually gets into a portion of muscle tissue with damage. Endomyocardial biopsy can be hit or miss because the myocardial disease is patchy rather than widespread.

Interventions

If the patient develops heart failure the priority nursing goals are to decrease preload and afterload immediately! Bed rest, I&O and daily weights, low-sodium diet, and administration of unloading medications are standard nursing interventions (see the section on heart failure and Pharmacology in a nutshell).

Arrhythmias and cardiac failure can be killers, so supportive treatment for myocarditis is a priority! The following nursing interventions are promptly initiated:

- Bed rest in a Semi-Fowler's position to decrease the workload on the heart and improve cardiac output
- Continuous cardiac monitoring, being alert to development of arrhythmias and using established protocols (ACLS) for prompt treatment of "big deal" arrhythmias
- Pulse oximeter to monitor oxygen saturation levels
- Supplemental oxygenation as needed
- Ionotropic agents intravenously (eg, dobutamine) to improve cardiac output if heart failure becomes apparent
- Measures to promote safety and prevent trauma if anticoagulation is prescribed (refer to Table 2-11 for bleeding precautions)

Clinical alert

If digoxin is prescribed, monitor for toxicity. Myocarditis increases sensitivity to digoxin!

PATIENT TEACHING   When the patient develops varying degrees of heart failure after myocarditis, the priorities for teaching include self-care and monitoring, maintaining fluid/electrolyte balance, nutrition, medications, rest, and activity. Refer to heart failure teaching. Instruct the patient to notify his or her physician immediately if any of the signs of recurring failure occur:

- Weigh daily and report a gain in excess of 2 to 3 lb.
- Ankle, pretibial edema: Press and see if fingertips make "pitting."
- Shortness of breath or awakening at night coughing.
- Unusual fatigue with little or no exertion.
- Mental confusion.

After the patient is stable, a referral may be made to a rheumatologist for diagnostic workup and treatment of autoimmune disorders if indicated.

If heart failure develops, unloading medications are added to the treatment plan, such as ACE inhibitors, diuretics. The patient is evaluated for progression of the disease with use of invasive and noninvasive modalities (see heart failure: Testing, testing, testing), and if resultant cardiomyopathy causes the ejection fraction to fall below 35%, with worsening cardiac decompensation, a heart transplant may be the last available option.[48]

✚ Endocarditis (infective endocarditis)

See Figure 4-33.

▶ Figure 4-33. Endocarditis. Endocarditis involves the inflammation and infection of the heart's lining, including all internal structures.

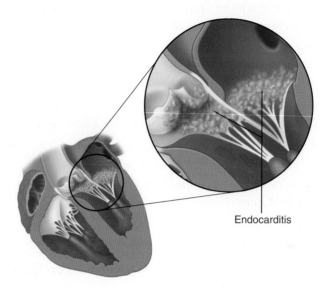

Endocarditis

What is it?

Inflammation and infection of the lining of the heart is very serious because endocarditis involves all the internal structures of the heart (the septum, valves, chordae tendineae, and chambers).

- The infection results in dense vegetative clusters made up of platelets, fibrin, cellular debris, and microorganisms that cling to the lining and internal structures of the heart, with tiny clumps becoming emboli.
- Damage to the endothelium can lead to erosion, thrombi, and abscesses, and destruction of valves and underlying structures.

Causes and why?

Prior to aggressive treatment of streptococcus, rheumatic fever was a common cause of endocarditis, primarily affecting the mitral valve between the left atria and ventricle. In this era when a sore throat is cultured and treated aggressively, rheumatic fever now accounts for less than one third of all endocarditis.[48]

With endocarditis, the most common bacterial infections are *Streptococcus viridans* or *Staphylococcus aureus*. Other bacteria, viruses (adeno- and coxsackie-), and funguses (*Candida albicans*) are also implicated.

Signs and symptoms and why?

Signs and symptoms	Why
Fever	Normal response to infection. Some bacteria and fungi cannot survive in an environment with an elevated temperature.
Splenomegaly: The spleen is an important immune system organ.	The spleen is working overtime to protect immunity; this causes hypertrophy.
Petechia	Tiny spots caused by hemorrhaging under the skin. The microemboli and septic emboli can shower any organ, including the skin, and leading to clotting followed by bleeding.
Hematuria	Microemboli and septic emboli can shower any organ, especially the glomeruli, leading to clotting followed by bleeding.
Cardiac murmurs	Vegetation on the valve prevents the valve from closing properly resulting in a murmur.
Pleuritic pain	Microemboli and septic emboli can shower any organ, including the lungs. The inflammatory response kicks in. Tissue edema occurs and places pressure on nerve endings. This pleuritic pain may be present during inspiration or expiration.
Fatigue; weakness	Vegetation on the mitral valve prevents proper closure of the valve causing backward flow during systole, which eventually leads to heart failure. This causes fatigue and weakness.
Late signs include signs and symptoms of left-sided heart failure: nocturnal dyspnea; S 3; pink, frothy sputum; cough; crackles; orthopnea; tachycardia; restlessness; JVD; hepatomegaly; ascites; peripheral edema; pulmonary edema	Infection and/or clot formation on the mitral or aortic valves can lead to left-sided heart failure.

Source: Created by the author from References 4, 5, and 6.

The patient feels bad and looks sick! The patient may complain of nonspecific ailments such as back, neck, leg aches, and joint pain. Chills and fever are reported, as well as fatigue, anorexia, and weight loss. Physical findings reveal the following:

- A systolic murmur, heard best at the apex of the heart
- Pale conjunctiva (look inside lower lid) and mucus membranes are dotted with petechiae
- Red or purple macular lesions (flat, round, non tender) on palms and soles (called Janeway lesions)
- Tender, red raised tiny solid lesions (Osler nodules) on fingertips and toes, with tiny reddish brown hemorrhagic streaks under the nail beds

The conjunctival and skin lesions are thrombotic complications of endocarditis, and the new murmur is because the nodular endocardial vegetation has shortened the chordae tendinea, which don't allow the cusp of the valve to close properly.

Testing, testing, testing

A routine CBC and urinalysis reveal the first clues:

* White blood cells: elevated (consistent with infection)
* Red blood cells: decreased (consistent with anemia)
* Urinalysis: microscopic hematuria and proteinuria

Diagnostic findings specific to inflammatory/infectious disorders provide definitive clues:

* Elevated sed-rate, C-reactive protein
* Positive rheumatoid factor
* Two separate blood cultures, positive for bacteria

Echocardiography (all types) provides an actual picture of the vegetative growths and thrombi that adhere to the internal structures of the heart as well as disruption of a prosthetic valve:

* Echocardiogram or TTE (transthoracic echocardiogram).
* TEE (transesophageal echocardiogram) gets in closer without the disadvantage of having to visualize the heart through all the artifact of body/breast tissue (especially helpful with obese patients).

Interventions

If the patient is in respiratory distress because of a pulmonary infiltrate or pulmonary infarction, immediate problems are the result of ineffective gas exchange and perfusion deficit!

During the acute phase of endocarditis, the patient is at risk for perfusion deficits (caused by the microemboli) and impaired gas exchange caused by lung fluid (secondary to valvular dysfunction). Here's what to do:

* Place the patient on immediate bed rest to reduce oxygen demand.
* Position the patient upright for optimal chest expansion and cardiac output.
* Position legs dependent (hanging down) to trap blood in the periphery, away from the heart if lung fluid is severe.
* Administer supplemental oxygen.
* Implement dependent orders to reduce preload (see acute pulmonary edema).

Monitor the patient for signs of organ damage or failure owing to systemic emboli:

* Stroke: Check LOC, ability to follow command, unilateral facial droop, and grip.
* Heart: As about chest pain, watch for arrhythmias, look for changes in pulse and blood pressure.
* Kidney: Check urine output, monitor for hematuria, and proteinuria.
* Spleen: Use gentle percussion to determine enlargement, be alert to tenderness in the upper left quadrant.
* Lungs: Auscultate anterior and posterior, being alert to any area of atelectasis.

Deadly Dilemma

Emboli are killers! So is pulmonary edema! So which one of these two very dangerous patient problems would be priority? Is it circulation (emboli) or breathing (pulmonary edema)? If your lungs are full of water, visible as frothy pink spittle with every breath, are you going to worry about where the clot in your leg is going to stop, or will you quick get the patient up in the bed, dangle his legs over the side to trap blood out in the extremities and get some IV Lasix on board? Yes, breathing is still a priority, even if a heart attack for a stroke happens. You work on the breathing first!! (Review stat actions for pulmonary edema earlier in this chapter!)

Hurst Hint

Here's how to tackle priority questions when both seem equally important: Ask yourself, "Which one will kill my patient first?" and then use your A-B-Cs.

Notify the physician stat for any indication of systemic or peripheral perfusion defect.

After immediate attention to the A-B-Cs, the next priority is managing the infectious process, beginning the prescribed antibiotic as soon as possible after the blood cultures are obtained. IV antibiotics must be given on time to maintain high blood levels of the drug, and will be continued for a prolonged time (up to 6 weeks) to totally eradicate all the bacteria embedded in the dense vegetative patches inside the heart. Continuing care includes the following:

- Monitor temperature, administering prescribed antipyretics prn.
- Maintain bed rest (any forceful, fast heart beat may shower tiny clots into circulation).
- Hydrate the patient to decrease blood viscosity and keep blood flowing freely so microemboli can't hang out and attract more cells, getting bigger and more dangerous.
- Monitor peripheral perfusion by doing vascular checks: the 7 Ps.
- Monitor perfusion to vital organs by auscultating the lungs and evaluating oxygenation status, being alert to changes in LOC (brain) and questioning the patient about subjective symptoms of chest pain or dyspnea.
- Monitor bowel sounds, asking about any abdominal pain (mesenteric and GI circulation).
- Administer unloading drugs (see Pharmacology in a nutshell, heart failure) and cardiac isotopes as prescribed.

PATIENT TEACHING   The patient must be made aware of the nature and course of this infection; otherwise, he or she may be alarmed when the fever continues for weeks (which may occur), and after recovery, may not understand the lifelong implications of having had endocarditis. The endocarditis survivor is at high risk for repeat infections, especially if valvular damage has occurred. If emergency valve replacement surgery was necessary because of life-threatening pulmonary edema/heart failure, the patient has a high risk for valve reinfection. Activity restrictions, medications, and signs and symptoms of infection, which are usual topics for discharge teaching, are an even greater priority for the patient recovering from endocarditis. While providing emotional support, the nurse explores creative coping strategies for offsetting the psychosocial aspects of a prolonged recovery.

In addition, the nurse must teach the high-risk patient to:

- Tell all health care providers about the high-risk status for developing endocarditis (including the dentist and urologist).
- Maintain meticulous oral hygiene, using a soft toothbrush so as not to cause additional injury. Use a dental Waterpik to cleanse any pockets if gums have receded from teeth, because bacteria love to hide in pockets, just waiting for a chance to get into the blood.
- Maintain meticulous personal cleanliness and hygiene, and be especially alert to ways that fecal contamination could lead to urinary tract

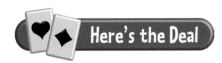

Here's the Deal

Strange as it seems, anticoagulation is not routinely prescribed for endocarditis (unless the patient was already taking an anticoagulant), because the risk of an intracranial bleed outweighs the benefit of anticoagulation.[48]

infections. (For example, women should always wipe front to back to avoid bringing *Escherichia coli* forward to the urethra.)

- Women are instructed that IUDs are not an option for birth control because of mucosal trauma leading to a portal for entry of bacteria.

The revised ACC/AHA guidelines recommend routine endocarditis prophylaxis for the following:

- Patients who have had previous endocarditis

- Patients who have prosthetic valves or prosthetic material to repair their valves

- Patients with congenital heart disease, unrepaired cyanotic congenital heart disease, any palliative shunts, or conduits used for repair of congenital heart disease.

- Anything foreign in the heart, such as prosthetic patches or prosthetic devices, because these inhibit endothelialization at the site, providing a portal of entry.

- All cardiac transplant patients who have any valve regurgitation owing to a valve that is not structurally functional.[53]

The above high-risk persons have underlying cardiac conditions that mandate prophylaxis prior to any invasive dental procedures involving manipulation or perforation of oral tissue, gingival tissue (gums), or the (periapical) tooth root.[53]

Surgical interventions may be necessary for debridement of vegetative masses, closure of abscesses or masses, or valve repair or replacement, which will improve the prognosis when the patient has severely damaged valves. Autograft (best for aortic valve), prosthetic, or biological valves may be used.

The risk for a recurring infection is great, and patients may require home health services for continuing intravenous administration of IV antibiotics. Once the patient begins to feel better it may be difficult to accept activity restrictions and continuing care until full recovery, requiring reinforcement of patient and family education. Patient teaching regarding antibiotic prophylaxis and measures to avoid infections is reinforced.

Once fever has subsided and blood cultures are negative, the patient will be re-evaluated for residual damage and activity tolerance. A graduated return to normal activities is advised while monitoring for activity tolerance.

What can harm my patient and why?

Half of the patients who have endocarditis will develop a blood clot that becomes an embolus[48] whose final destination could be the heart (AMI), the brain (stroke), the lungs (PE), or other places (spleen, bowel, extremities) that could be catastrophic. The patient's risk for thromboembolism begins to drop after the first two weeks, which is the time of greatest risk. The endothelial injury triggers the blood clotting cascade in the heart where little thrombi form and cling to internal structures before being showered out into circulation.

Here's the Deal

Identifying the organism and eradicating the body of infection is the cornerstone for recovery. Monitoring for the development of life-threatening complications is paramount, and immediate interventions are indicated at the earliest onset.

Once the heart valves become damaged from endocarditis, they cannot close properly. Now the patient is at risk for development of heart failure and pulmonary edema because dysfunctional valves allow blood to flow backward into the lung, rather than forward into systemic circulation.

✦ Cardiac valve dysfunction

Let's get the normal stuff straight first!

Normal, healthy heart valves swing open to allow blood to flow through in a forward direction and then snap tightly shut again.

- The valves are synchronized to open and close in the same rhythm as the cardiac cycle.
- When the heart contracts (systole), valves open and during relaxation (diastole), valves close.
- This opening and closing of the valves creates the characteristic "lub–dub" sound of the heartbeat.
- The four heart valves are like doors between the chambers of the heart and their purpose is to keep blood from flowing in the wrong direction as blood moves through the chambers of the heart.
- When valves don't work properly, blood can go backward instead of forward.
- If a valve is narrowed and does not open fully (called *stenosis*), less blood moves through the "doorway."
- If the valve doesn't close tightly, blood can leak backward (regurgitation).
- Both stenosis and regurgitation require the heart to work harder to maintain perfusion to body organs.
- Over time, the overworked heart muscle can fail, allowing blood to back up into the lungs (pulmonary edema).

Causes and why?

A number of conditions can occur to alter cardiac valves structurally, so they do not close properly, becoming leaky:

- Genetic (inborn) structural problems with the valves
- Infection or endocarditis (which scar and damage valves)
- Degenerative conditions (anything that causes the heart to lose its ability to perform well)
- Aging

Signs and symptoms

When heart valve trouble is present, the patient will report symptoms similar to early heart failure, such as:

- Supine dyspnea: Problems in breathing when lying down
- Exertional dyspnea: Wheezing, coughing, shortness of breath with activity

- Paroxysmal nocturnal dyspnea: Night-time awakening with coughing and shortness of breath
- Weakness, fatigue, no energy
- Vertigo: Dizzy spells, fainting
- Edema: Swollen ankles or feet
- Chest pain or pressure
- New or worsening murmurs: Valves don't close properly
- Poor exercise tolerance: Easily fatigues, or tachycardia/shortness of breath
- Paroxysmal nocturnal dyspnea (PND)

When the patient has mitral valve prolapse (MVP), the two "flaps" of the mitral valve don't close properly and the floppy valve billows out in the wrong direction and looks "floppy."

When heart valve trouble is present, the patient will report symptoms similar to early heart failure, such as:

- Supine dyspnea: Problems breathing when lying down
- Exertional dyspnea: Wheezing, coughing, shortness of breath with activity
- Paroxysmal nocturnal dyspnea: Night-time awakening with coughing and shortness of breath
- Weakness, fatigue, no energy
- Vertigo: Dizzy spells, fainting
- Edema: Swollen ankles or feet
- Chest pain or pressure
- New or worsening murmurs: Valves don't close properly
- Poor exercise tolerance: Easily fatigues, or tachycardia/shortness of breath
- Paroxysmal nocturnal dyspnea (PND)

Patients are advised to report the following warning signs immediately:

- Palpitations
- Shortness of breath
- Chest pain
- Dizziness
- Fainting

Testing, testing, testing

Tests to diagnose valve conditions include:

- Echocardiogram
- EKG
- Chest X-ray
- Cardiac catheterization

Interventions

Because of the possibility of the above complications of valvular heart disease, the nurse monitors:

- Oxygen saturation levels (SaO_2)
- Telemetry heart rhythm being alert to arrhythmias
- Vital signs, comparing to baseline
- Heart and lung sounds for murmurs, gallops, rales
- Peripheral pulses for volume/tissue perfusion
- Objective and subjective complaints signaling heart failure

Patients are treated conservatively, and are monitored closely for any worsening of symptoms that could suggest mitral regurgitation, which would require more aggressive treatment.

Based on the patient condition and the type of the defect, valves may be surgically repaired using biological or prosthetic material. When defective valves must be replaced, patients are apprised of the risks and benefits of various types of valves.

- Mechanical (artificial) valves last significantly longer (average, 30 years) than biological valves (from animals or human donors), but they require lifelong anticoagulation because of increased risk for blood clots.
- Biological (tissue) valves do not increase the risk of blood clots, so anticoagulation is not required.
- Obviously, a woman of childbearing age who desires pregnancy would decline an artificial valve because anticoagulation is not compatible with pregnancy.
- Because biological valves require periodic surgical replacement when they begin to wear out, the childbearing woman could opt for the artificial valve after her family is complete.

Follow-up visits may include periodic echocardiograms to visualize the mechanical valve or prosthetic repair to make sure there is complete closure of the valve with no leakage.

What can harm my patient and why?

The endocardium is ripe for infection when there is damage (congenital or acquired) to the valves or other internal structures, or prosthetic valves.

- When these conditions are present, organisms (particularly *Streptococcus viridans*) will go straight to the site and adhere to the endothelium, while other organisms adhere to tiny clots that form after injury to the endothelial surface.
- Platelet-fibrin thrombi that form at the site can become emboli and travel to other parts of the body.

The major patient problems associated with valvular dysfunction are:

- Bacterial invasion causing endocarditis

- Heart failure
- Pulmonary edema (mitral regurgitation)

Because valvular heart disease increases risk of bacterial endocarditis, the AHA Prevention of Infective Endocarditis Committee recommends prophylactic antibiotics before dental or any invasive medical procedures that could introduce bacteria into the blood stream. It is reasonable that infections in the high-risk patient have to be treated and eradicated before any invasive examinations are performed (eg, cystoscopic exam or other endoscopic exams of the GU or GI tract).[53]

✚ Cardiac tamponade

Let's get the normal stuff straight!

The heart in positioned in the center of the chest, within a space called the *mediastinum,* having a lung nestled on each side. The rigid rib cage expands with inspiration as the lungs inflate (getting bigger), encroaching upon the space housing the heart.

The pericardial sac enclosing the heart consists of three layers:

- The outermost layer is the *fibrous pericardium.*
- The serous membrane lining underneath called the *parietal pericardium.*
- The innermost serous membrane, on top of the heart muscle, is called the *visceral pericardium* or the *epicardium* (literally, *upon the heart*).

Between the two serous layers is a potential space called the *pericardial cavity.* Serous fluid bathes these two membranous layers to reduce friction as the heart beats. The chambers of the heart are flexible and distensible, so that as blood flows in they stretch and fill with blood during diastole.

What is it?

Cardiac tamponade is a condition that results from a pericardial effusion (fluid or blood collecting in the pericardial space), which can compress (squeeze) the heart as fluid in the sac surrounding the heart accumulates. When the heart is being squeezed from the outside, the inside chambers cannot fill with blood. If blood cannot get into the heart, the cardiac output drops, and may quickly become nonexistent. Cardiac tamponade is a medical emergency, and without prompt recognition and emergency intervention, death may ensue (Fig. 4-34).

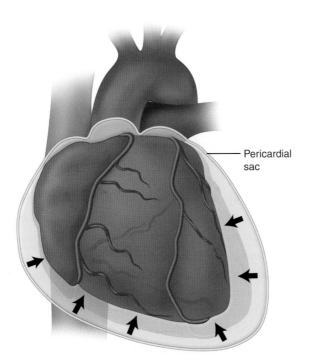

Pericardial sac

Causes and why?

Cardiac tamponade can result from any condition that produces a pericardial effusion with a volume of fluid pressure sufficient to squeeze the heart and prevent filling during diastole. The following are examples of such conditions:

- Myocardial rupture after a transmural myocardial infarction or lightning strike
- Trauma to the heart (stabbing, gunshot, blunt impact, or invasive cardiac procedures)
- Perforation of the heart or great vessels during invasive procedures (eg, cardiac catheterization or insertion of central lines)
- Infectious conditions of the heart producing exudates that could collect in the pericardial sac
- Connective tissue/collagen diseases (eg, vasculitis, rheumatoid arthritis, systemic lupus erythematosus, or rheumatic fever) in which serous fluid or inflammatory exudates collect in the pericardial sac

Patients at risk for cardiac tamponade:

- Trauma (blunt trauma or stab wound to the chest)
- Infection (any pericarditis)
- Cancer (metastasis)
- Heart surgery (CABG, valve replacement, etc)

Iatrogenic causes (physician or treatment induced):

- Central line placement
- Pacemaker insertion
- Cardiac catheterization[19,49]

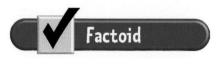

The three most common causes of cardiac tamponade are:

- Pericarditis
- Cancer
- Uremia[48]

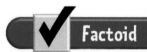

Pulsus paradoxus describes a systolic blood pressure that is lower on respiratory inspiration by at least 10 mm Hg. *Pulsus* (from Latin word for *beating*) means pulse, and a paradox is something that seems untrue or contradictory but proves to be real.

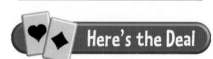

A paradoxical pulse is detected by monitoring blood pressure readings during the respiratory cycle. For example, when the patient breathes in (lungs inflated/crowding mediastinal space) the blood pressure may be 100 systolic, but when the patient breathes out (whew ... lungs get smaller/more room in the thorax, now the heart can refill better), the blood pressure comes back up to 120 systolic.

The right atrium is the most common site of perforation from catheter placement. Perforation, as well as direct catheter infusion of fluids, can cause tamponade.

Clinical alert

Never use a central line without positive X-ray confirmation of placement first!

Catheter misplacement may not result in an immediate tamponade. There could be a delay of hours to days when there is a slow leak of fluids into the pericardial space.

Our bodies are optimized to maintain circulating volume, so when the cardiac output drops, no matter what the reason, the body feels like it's in shock and a set of compensatory mechanisms kicks in to try to maintain circulating volume and blood pressure. Depending on how quickly the fluid accumulates in the pericardial sac and how well the patient is compensating, the signs and symptoms of gradually worsening pericardial effusion (stuff leaking out into the sac) could be overlooked or attributed to other causes. The heart has finally decompensated when symptoms of cardiac tamponade appear. When the nurse performs a focused cardiac assessment, the patient will display signs of decreased perfusion to organs, which reflect the falling cardiac output:

- Brain: decreased LOC, alteration in mentation, anxious, restless, or lethargy
- Heart: rapid, weak peripheral pulses, fluctuations in blood pressure (pulsus paradoxus) with decreased arterial pressure, and narrowing pulse pressure

When the patient in ICU has a radial artery line for continuous monitoring of blood pressure, it is easy to stand at the bedside and watch for changes in the blood pressure related to respirations. When your med-surg or telemetry patient has blood pressure readings which seem to be false or illogical (a paradox), you'd better check it out!

Be on the lookout for pulsus paradoxus for patients at high risk for cardiac tamponade:

- Lungs: shortness of breath, dyspnea, orthopnea
- Kidneys: decreased urine output
- Skin: cold, clammy, diaphoresis, pallor, and/or cyanosis

Cardiac tamponade can be suspected by a unique set of clinical signs and symptoms, called "Beck's triad." These three signs (seen together = triad) occur only with cardiac tamponade:

- Jugular vein distention (JVD) in the presence of clear lung fields
- Muffled or distant heart sounds
- Hypotension

These signs may be subtle for a slow pericardial effusion (even when the patient has a large amount of accumulated fluid), but an immediate life-threatening situation can develop following a small but rapid bleed/effusion into the pericardial sac because the body does not have time to compensate and the cardiac output falls dramatically.

Testing, testing, testing

When cardiac tamponade is suspected, it is urgent that diagnostic measures be implemented as quickly as possible, before compression of the heart causes a hemodynamic crash! The following tests are prescribed:

- Computed tomography (CT) may be the initial diagnostic test if the patient signs are nonspecific and the clinical findings are vague. The technician injecting the contrast media will pick up the first clue when the dye does not inject easily, and backs up into the azygos vein. Findings may show that the inferior vena cava (IVC) is enlarged, which happens because blood flow continues to come in to the right heart, but because of cardiac compression, the back pressure in the venous system distends the vena cava.[54]

- Computed tomography coronary angiography can definitely diagnose cardiac tamponade as evidenced by findings of compression of the coronary arteries, because these arteries supplying the heart muscle are on the outside of the heart and will show compression in advance of the cardiac chambers.

- Transthoracic echocardiogram is the gold standard when tamponade is suspected because this ultrasound procedure allows for real-time visualization of the chambers of the heart and specifically can show up any pericardial fluid around the heart,[54] in addition to giving a clue as to the type of the fluid.[54]

- Chest X-ray may be a routine.

Interventions

Notify the physician at the very onset of symptoms, before the patient has time to crash! If the tamponade results from a slow bleed into the pericardial sac, the patient will bleed and compensate, bleed and compensate. This may result in a large tamponade with relatively few symptoms. However, a small bleed occurring rapidly may produce cardiac decompensation and the cardiac output will fall quickly. Prepare the patient for immediate pericardiocentesis:

- Obtain pre-procedural vital signs.
- Obtain hemodynamic pressure measurements if available.
- Place the patient on continuous heart monitoring.
- Ensure reliable peripheral IV line (preferably 18-gauge) is in place in the event that fluids, blood or blood products, or emergency medications must be administered.
- Have crash cart supplies and a defibrillator available if needed for emergency resuscitation.
- Assemble equipment: sterile gloves, a sterile needle attached to a 50-mL sterile syringe with a three-way stopcock, and sterile occlusive dressing material to cover the puncture site.
- Ultrasound imaging is used to guide the needle into place as it is slowly advanced into the fluid pocket.
- Position patient upright (40–60 degrees) to bring the heart closer to the chest wall, so the needle can better reach the sac.

- Postprocedural vital signs and monitoring cardiac output every 15 minutes until stable.

After decompression of the cardiac tamponade, the patient will immediately feel a sense of relief from the pressure, but he or she still needs me (the nurse) at the bedside to closely monitor cardiac output and perfusion to vital organs (see Focused Cardiac Assessment). Patient assessments are in order to evaluate the effectiveness of the pericardiocentesis! Watch for these signs that indicate improved cardiac output:

- Increasing systolic blood pressure
- Decreasing CVP or PWP
- Strong palpable pulses
- Absence of JVD
- Eupnea
- Stable pulse and blood pressure (not bouncing around)
- Clearly audible heart sounds (no longer muffled)

Notify physician for any subtle changes in patient condition. After needle aspiration, is it possible that the trauma from the cutting edge of the needle could cause even more seepage into the pericardial sac? Can another tamponade develop? Yes!

- Closely monitor BP, pulse, and respirations.
- Monitor pulse oximeter and administer oxygen prn.
- Hold any anticoagulant medication until resumed by the physician.
- Position the patient Semi-Fowler's (to increase cardiac output).
- Monitor for cardiac arrhythmias and/or chest pain.
- Allay fear and anxiety by explaining all procedures and give reports of good blood pressure, color, and pulse, being optimistic, yet truthful.

PATIENT TEACHING   The problem should be thoroughly resolved by discharge; however, depending on the cause of the tamponade, the patient should seek re-entry into the health care system for any evidence of a repeat performance:

- Feeling of chest pressure/fullness
- Any chest pain: diffuse, localized, or vague
- Signs of decreasing cardiac output such as racing heart, unusual fatigue, pale, cool, moist skin, or shortness of breath

A pericardiocentesis may be performed as a single lifesaving event, or the fluid/exudates may continue to build and require further intervention depending on the cause.

- Frequent ultrasounds or CTs may be performed to detect fluid that may be accumulating in the pericardial sac.
- If a large pocket of fluid was identified with radiology, a small catheter may be left in place to drain fluid.
- Surgery may be performed if a fluid-secreting tumor is present or an open pericardiotomy is required for additional removal of fluid/blood.

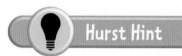

Hurst Hint

Never leave an unstable patient! Stay at the bedside constantly until the blood pressure comes back up and is producing good perfusion.

- Anti-infective therapy may be indicated if the exudate is a result of infection.
- Fluid samples are sent to the laboratory for analysis and culture and sensitivity.

The patient is assisted to gradually resume self-care activities of daily living in a monitored setting with assistance as needed. Activity tolerance is assessed and short-term goals are set to encourage gradually progressive activity.

What can harm my patient?

Cardiac tamponade is a form of circulatory shock, and the patient can decompensate quickly. Obstructive shock occurs when blood cannot be ejected from the left ventricle into systemic circulation because the heart is being compressed.[55]

✚ Peripheral vascular disease
Let's get the normal stuff straight!

Blood vessels carry blood away from the heart (arteries) and back to the heart (veins). Both types of vessels have three layers, each having its own function:

- The tunica intima (slick endothelial lining inside blood vessels that allows blood cells to zip along unobstructed)
- The tunica media (middle layer of smooth muscle that responds to CNS stimulation and/or medications by vasoconstricting or vasodilating)
- The tunica adventitia (the protective outermost fibroelastic layer surrounding blood vessels)

✚ Buerger's disease
What is it?

Buerger's disease is an inflammatory condition that affects small and medium-sized blood vessels and nerves of the extremities. The term *thromboangiitis obliterans* fully describes what happens to arteries and veins exposed to chronic inflammation and irritation:

- Vessels are obliterated after becoming occluded with clots.[56]
- The disease affects all three layers of the vessel wall and is therefore classified as vasculitis.[57]

Causes and why?

The exact cause is unknown, with literature supporting autoimmune theory and genetic mutation of prothrombin. The disease is definitely linked to all forms of nicotine:

- Cigarettes
- Smokeless tobacco

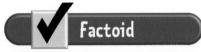

Arteries carry oxygenated blood and veins carry deoxygenated blood.

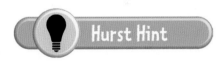

Never pick an oxygen answer when you have a vein problem! You know that just doesn't go together!

- Nicotine patches
- Second-hand smoke

Young men (20–40 years) who have a history of long-term heavy smoking are primarily affected. Smoking causes vasoconstriction and triggers endothelial dysfunction and formation of thrombi.[6]

Signs and symptoms

The lower extremities are most commonly affected, but in rare cases the upper extremities and viscera can be involved. When blood flow to the extremities is diminished, the patient will complain of the following subjective experiences:

- Painful intermittent claudication (spasmodic cramping) with walking occurs because of anaerobic metabolism (no oxygen available), which leaves behind lactic acid that causes tissue pain.
- Unpleasant indicators of nerve damage (paresthesias) such as numbness, tingling, stinging, or burning sensations.
- Feet and legs tire easily.

Absent or diminished pulses may be accompanied by positional color changes, tissue damage, and necrosis:

- Red, hot, and tingling: dependent rubor (reddish-blue discoloration when hanging the extremity down)
- White: Cadaver pallor occurs when the extremity is elevated since arterial blood (already insufficient) does not travel uphill very well.
- Blue nail beds and tissue: Cyanosis is caused by lack of oxygen.
- As the disease progresses, leg ulcers develop because of poor circulation.
- Leg ulcers progress to necrosis and gangrene.

Lack of oxygen and nourishment to the cells leads to atrophy of muscles, loss of hair follicles, and changes to the nails (thick and brittle).

✚ Raynaud's disease

What is it?

Raynaud's disease occurs mainly in young women and affects primarily the fingers, but less commonly may affect toes as well.

Causes and why?

Vessel spasm occurs in small arteries and arterioles and an exaggerated vasomotor response (vasoconstriction) can be elicited by exposure to cold or strong emotions.

Signs and symptoms

The patient reports episodes of varying frequency, duration, and severity of vessel spasms, which affect both hands. This red, white, and blue

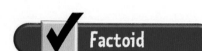

Factoid

The claudication in the arch of the foot is an early sign of Buerger's disease.[57]

disease (very patriotic) is readily visible and occurs in the following sequence:

- Red: Blood rushes back into the tissues (hyperemia) when the spasm ends.
- White: Vasospasm cuts off arterial blood flow to produce pallor.
- Blue: Tissues are hypoxic and become cyanotic.

Lack of oxygen and nutrients to the digits results in ulcerations and gangrene.

Raynaud's phenomenon is the exact same set of signs and symptoms and complications without the disease, and commonly occurs with the use of certain agents or patients having connective tissue disease, such as:

- Scleroderma
- Systemic lupus erythematosus (SLE)
- Sjögren's syndrome
- Chemotherapy agents
- Exposure to chemicals such as vinyl chloride[58]

Peripheral vascular disease is diagnosed using the following means:

- Lab tests: The erythrocyte sedimentation rate (ESR, or sed-rate) tests for inflammation by measuring how quickly RBCs fall to the bottom of a test tube. Rapidly descending cells indicate an inflammatory process in the body and the sed-rate is elevated.

- Allen's test: This is used to detect arterial insufficiency in the hand. Use the thumbs to occlude the radial and ulnar arteries of the patient's hand. The patient is instructed to open the hand (palm up) and the examiner releases pressure from one artery and observes for blood flow into the hand. The procedure is repeated with the other artery. It detects radial/ulnar arterial insufficiency.[57]

- Angiography (radiographic visualization of vessels using radiopaque dye) reveals the absence of atheroma/atherosclerotic plaques, and the site of arterial occlusions[57] with "corkscrew" collateral vessels.[59]

- Ankle-brachial index (ABI) test: Systolic blood pressures are taken and recorded for each arm and a hand-held Doppler is used to measure systolic pressure in each ankle (two readings per foot, on inner medial aspect and outer lateral aspect). The index (ratio) is calculated by dividing the highest of the ankle systolic pressures for each foot by the highest of the arm pressures. Vascular diseases that produce narrowing of arteries and limited blood flow will cause ankle systolic pressures that are lower than the brachial pressure. The ratio (index) will be 1.0 for normal healthy peripheral vessels, which means that arm and ankle pressures are the same with no limited ankle blood flow. The lower the index, the less blood flow is moving through that vessel, representing greater vascular insufficiency.

- CW (continuous wave) Doppler flow studies allow the examiner to hear blood flow through the vessels.

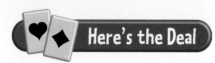

Here's the Deal

Stop smoking!! Even minimal smoking (1–2 cigarettes/day) or exposure to passive smoke will keep the disease active and render any treatment ineffective. The only means of stopping disease progression is total smoking cessation.[59] Referral to a smoking cessation clinic/addiction center is indicated.

- Exercise testing on a treadmill detects claudication with walking.
- In duplex ultrasonography, the velocity of blood flow is measured using color flow techniques to evaluate flow to distant vessels.

Interventions

The patient needs improved blood flow to the distal extremities. This can be accomplished by the following interventions:

- Maintain a comfortably warm room.
- Check patient alignment and positioning frequently, especially during sleep when a hand could become compressed between pillow and cheek.
- Ensure adequate hydration, keeping water available at the bedside.
- Provide fluids in a container with handle or an insulated container.
- Keep a nightlight on and the pathway free of articles that cause a stubbed toe.
- Administer prescribed vasodilator medications (to relax smooth muscles), adrenergic blocking agents (to block the vasoconstrictive effect of catecholamines), and calcium channel blockers.
- Instruct the patient to hang his or her legs over the bedside for nighttime pain if a sleep chair (legs dependent) is unavailable.

In order to evaluate the effectiveness of treatments, the nurse will perform ongoing assessments:

- Monitor ABI (see guidelines above) and record.
- Inspect and assess distal extremities for adequate perfusion (7 Ps).
- Urge the patient to report pain promptly and evaluate on pain scale of 1 to 10, administering prescribed analgesia prn.
- Rest pain or severe pain indicates critical tissue ischemia and bed rest is mandated.[59]

Local wound management may involve hydrotherapy or debridement with wet to dry dressings, application of topical antimicrobial agents, dressings, medicated "boots," and nutritional support (TPN, supplements) in addition to a diet high in protein, calories, and vitamin C, with three meals and three high-quality snacks.

PATIENT TEACHING The goals are to make lifestyle modifications to reduce progression of the disease and prevent complications of ulceration, necrosis, and amputation. Family members and significant others should be included in the teaching plan. This helps to build a support system and hopefully enhance compliance. The patient should be taught how to avoid injury:

- Apply pressure to itchy areas rather than scratching or rubbing.
- Wear protective shoes with smooth inside edges, seams, and insoles.
- There should be no lotions, powders, or moisture between the toes at any time.

- Do not use harsh chemicals on the hands or feet.
- Do not walk barefoot at home or at the beach!
- Do not bite nails! Have nails trimmed straight across by a podiatrist.
- Exercise caution when using knives, needles, or other sharp objects.
- Use gloves and padded garden tools rather than digging with hands.

The patient should be taught to avoid anything that causes vasoconstriction, with instructions for the following:

- No tobacco or nicotine in any form or use and no exposure to second-hand smoke.
- Avoid emotional upset and stress (epinephrine/norepinephrine surge).
- Use meditation, biofeedback, music, journaling, diversion, or other preferred methods for stress management.
- Do not use medications that contain vasoconstrictive agents, such as OTC cold medications, ergotamine preparations for migraine headaches (eg, Cafergot/Wigraine).
- Bathe in warm (never hot) water (which causes vasoconstriction).
- Avoid exposure to cold or lowering of core body temperature (which lowers skin temperature and triggers a vessel spasm).
- Turn off air conditioning and dress warmly indoors.
- Wear thick socks and mittens to bed during cold weather.
- Wear oven mitts when picking up frozen foods.
- Use tongs for icing glasses.
- Carry insulated gloves to the grocery when shopping for frozen foods or ice cream.

The patient should be taught to avoid anything that may cause vascular compression with instructions for the following:

- Do not cross legs, or wear tight jeans or other constrictive garments.
- No prolonged sitting, flexed at the hip! Get up and walk around at frequent intervals!
- No prolonged standing still! Walk in place while waiting if standing in a line.
- Do not wear garters, elastic in the sleeves of a blouse, or socks with elastic bands.

New possibilities for treatment may include cannabinoids or endothelin receptors to block sympathetic effects and gene or cell-based therapy to support formation of new healthy vessels. A selective cannabinoid receptor antagonist, rimonabant, is being used to help patients stop smoking. New collateral vessels became evident about the site of DNA injection (vascular endothelial growth factor = VEGF) in five of seven patients who received VEGF. Intramedullary Kirschner wire insertion has also stimulated new growth of collateral vessels. Other therapies, such as epidural spinal cord stimulation, are being tested and some have demonstrated effectiveness.[59]

Flare ups of pain will continue to recur if the patient continues to smoke, and ulcerations will not heal until the patient stops smoking. The choice of smoking versus amputation is presented to the patient.[57] Once necrosis or gangrene is present, the only treatment is amputation. The following treatment modalities have been used with no additional harm; some with more promising results than others:

- Sympathectomy per laparoscopy has met with good results.[59]
- Bypass graft surgery. This is often ineffective for the reason that there isn't much to bypass because vessels are small with distal involvement and no target vessels.[60]
- Hyperbaric oxygen therapy.
- Bier's block (regional anesthesia using lidocaine and guanethidine).

The following medications are being prescribed and evaluated for improved blood flow in patients with Raynaud's disease:

- Losartan (Cozaar), an antihypertensive drug
- Iloprost (Caverject) and alprostadil (Edex), which are prostaglandin drugs[61]
- Ticlopidine (Ticlid) an antithrombotic drug
- Gingko biloba, an herbal remedy[60]

Based on individual needs and/or condition (severity of arterial insufficiency) the patient may be advised and/or assisted to:

- Continue total cessation of smoking as well as all forms of nicotine usage.
- Avoid any activities or events that may induce mechanical or thermal trauma.
- Create a stress management plan.
- Exercise as prescribed (usually walking to activate the venous pump) to the point of claudication, using pain as the signal to rest.

Onset of rest pain or severe pain unrelieved by rest is the indicator to seek re-entry into the health care system immediately.

The chair-cane is a lightweight device that transforms from a single-footed cane with a curved hand handle, into a three-footed stool for resting when claudication occurs.

What can harm my patient and why?

Continuing to smoke (or use any form of nicotine) will cause progression of the disease.[62]

- Wounds do not heal well when circulation is compromised.
- Gangrene may occur with both forms of peripheral vascular disease and will require amputation of black, lifeless fingers, toes, feet, and legs.
- Intermittent claudication has a negative impact on functional ability, mobility, and psychological well-being.[63]
- Amputation produces disfigurement resulting in body image changes and disability, which diminish the quality of life.

PRACTICE QUESTIONS

1. The nurse is collecting data from a woman with CAD. Which of the following findings are components of the clustered symptoms called *metabolic syndrome*, which promotes coronary artery disease? Select all that apply:

   A. Blood pressure 146/90

   B. Blood glucose >116 mg/dL

   C. LDL serum levels 38 mg/dL

   D. HDL serum levels 62 mg/dL

   E. Waist measurement of 38 inches

2. Which patient teaching is a priority when a calcium channel blocker such as amlodipine (Norvasc) is prescribed for treatment of angina?

   A. Avoid eating grapefruit or drinking grapefruit juice.

   B. Rest at frequent intervals in a semireclining position.

   C. Take at bedtime because the drug may cause fatigue and drowsiness.

   D. Do not take sublingual nitroglycerin in conjunction with amlodipine.

3. After completion of a teaching/learning session, which statement by the patient would indicate a need for further teaching regarding medications for management of angina?

   A. "I will monitor my heart rate daily while taking atenolol (Tenormin)."

   B. "B-complex vitamins work together with Lipitor (atorvastatin) to help keep blood vessels healthy."

   C. "I will remove my transdermal nitroglycerin patch at bedtime and reapply each morning."

   D. "Arising slowly and avoiding sudden position changes will keep me from getting dizzy and possibly falling."

4. The nurse is reinforcing health teaching for a patient who has stable angina. Which statement by the patient indicates a correct understanding of the teaching?

   A. "I will stay indoors during heat advisories, using fans to keep cool."

   B. "I will use a small, lightweight shovel for removing snow from my drive."

   C. "I am able to have sex if I can climb a flight of steps without chest pain."

   D. "I will rest for 30 minutes after eating any large, heavy meals."

5. An IV infusion of nitroglycerin is prescribed for a patient with unstable angina (UA), but after reviewing current medications taken within the last 24 hours, the nurse should withhold this order because of which drug?

   A. Vardenafil (Levitra)

   B. Enoxaparin (Lovenox)

   C. Eptifibatide (Integrilin)

   D. Clofibrate (Atromid-S)

6. Post MI, a patient in cardiogenic shock is complaining of chest pain rated 10 on a pain scale of 1 to 19. Of the following prn medications, which is the priority for this patient?

   A. Morphine titrated intravenously (IV)

   B. Oxygen by nasal cannula

   C. Nitroglycerin sublingual (SL)

   D. Aspirin (ASA)

7. Post cardiac catheterization, the patient complains of severe pain in the leg below the femoral artery access site. No pulses can be palpated and the leg is pale, cool, and dry while the unaffected leg is warm, moist, and pink. In addition to notifying the physician, which next action by the nurse is the priority?

   A. Quickly pack the affected leg in ice.

   B. Gently elevate the affected leg on two pillows.

   C. Administer prescribed injectable prn analgesia.

   D. Position the cold leg over the warm one, covering both with a blanket.

8. Following an acute MI, the patient is in cardiogenic shock. Which of the following parameters will provide the best indicator for evaluating the adequacy of left ventricular function?

   A. Measure hourly urine output using a urometer.

   B. Monitor continuous blood pressures via an arterial line.

   C. Perform anterior/posterior chest auscultation hourly.

   D. Monitor skin for color, temperature, and the presence of moisture.

9. A patient with heart failure awakens during the night with a "pounding heart" and sudden severe shortness of breath. After raising the head of the bed and applying oxygen, which next action by the nurse is the priority?

   A. Auscultate the chest.

   B. Observe for jugular venous distention (JVD).

C. Administer prn morphine sulfate.

D. Administer prn Lasix.

10. Which of the following signs and symptoms would a patient with cardiac valve disease develop first?

A. Shortness of breath

B. Pale, ashen skin color

C. Substernal chest pain

D. Cyanosis of the lips and nail beds

References

1. Gary R. Self-care practices in women with diastolic heart failure. *Heart Lung 35*(1):9–19, 2009.

2. Sauerbeck LR. Primary stroke prevention. *Am J Nurs 106*(11):40–49, 2006.

3. Tune JD. Withdrawal of vasoconstrictor influences in local metabolic coronary vasodilation. *Am J Physiol Heart Circ Physiol* 291:H2044–H2046, 2006.

4. Kumar R, Gandhi SK, Little WC. Acute heart failure with preserved systolic function. *Crit Care Med 36*(1):S52–S56, 2008.

5. Trujillo TC, Dobesh PP. Traditional management of chronic stable angina. *Pharmacotherapy 27*(12):1677–1692, 2007.

6. The Diabetes Control and Complications Trial/Epidemiology of Diabetes Interventions and Complications (DCCT/EDIC). Intensive diabetes treatment and cardiovascular disease in patients with type 1 diabetes. *NEJM* 353:2643–2653, 2005.

7. DeVon HA, Ryan CJ, Ochs AL, Shapiro M. Symptoms across the continuum of acute coronary syndromes: Differences between women and men. *Am J Crit Care 17*(1):14–24, 2008.

8. Molinaro RJ. Metabolic syndrome: An update on prevalence, criteria and laboratory testing. *Medical Laboratory Observer,* www.mlo-online.com, 2007.

9. Hong Y, Jin X, Mo J, et al. Metabolic syndrome, its preeminent clusters, incident coronary heart disease and all-cause mortality: Results of prospective analysis for the Atherosclerosis Risk in Communities study. *J Int Med* 262:113–123, 2007.

10. Dietrich T, Jimenez M, Krall Kaye EA, et al. Age dependent associations between chronic periodontitis/edentulism and risk for coronary heart disease. *Circulation 117*(13):1668–1674, 2008.

11. Berg AH, Scherer PE. Adipose tissue, inflammation and cardiovascular disease. *Circ Res* May 13, 2005. Downloaded from circres.ahajournals.org at UNIVARKANSAS MED SCI LI: B on September 8, 2008.

12. DeVon HA, Ryan CJ. Chest pain and associated symptoms of acute coronary syndromes. *J Cardiovasc Nurs 20*(4):232–238, 2005.

13. Beers MH, ed. *The Merck Manual of Medical Information.* White Station, NJ: Merck Research Laboratories; 2003.

15. Berg AH, Scherer PE. Adipose tissue, inflammation and cardiovascular disease. *Circ Res* May 13, 2005. Downloaded from circres.ahajournals.org at UNIVARKANSAS MED SCI LI:B on September 8, 2008.

16. Boyd S. Cardiovascular system. In: Hurst M, ed. *Hurst Reviews: Pathophysiology Review.* New York: McGraw-Hill; 2008.

17. Metules T, Bauer J. Unstable angina: Is your care up to snuff. *RN* 68(2):22–27, 2005.

18. Porth CM. *Pathophysiology: Concepts of Altered Health States.* 6th ed. Philadelphia: Lippincott Williams & Wilkins; 2002.

19. DeVon HA, Penckofer SM, Zerwic JJ. Symptoms of unstable angina in patients with and without diabetes. *Res Nurs Health* 28:136–143, 2005.

20. Ferguson HW. Lippincott Manual of Nursing Practice. 8th ed. New York: Lippincott Williams & Wilkins; 2006.

21. McSweeney J, Cody M, O'Sullivan P, et al. Women's early warning symptoms of acute myocardial infarction. *Circulation* 108:2619–2623, 2003.

22. Kunadian B, Vijayalakshmi K, Dunning J, et al. Should patients in cardiogenic shock undergo rescue angioplasty after failed fibrinolysis? Comparison of primary versus rescue. *J Invas Cardiol* 19(5):217–223, 2007.

23. Chojnowski D. Managing systolic heart failure. *Nursing 2006* 37–42, 2006.

24. Ehrat KS. *The Art of EKG Interpretation: A Self-Instructional Text.* Dubuque, IA: Kendall/Hunt; 2002.

25. Wennberg P, Eliasson M, Johansson L, et al. The risk of myocardial infarction and sudden cardiac death amongst snuff users with or without a previous history of smoking. *J Int Med* 262:360–367, 2007.

26. Shiga T, Hagiwara N, Ogawa H, et al. Sudden cardiac death and left ventricular ejection fraction during long term follow-up after acute myocardial infarction in the primary percutaneous coronary intervention era. Results from the HIJAMI-II Registry. *Heart* published online September 5, 2008. Downloaded from heart.bmj.com on September 9, 2008.

27. Peterson ED, Bynum DZ, Roe MT. Association of evidence-based care processes and outcomes among patients with acute coronary syndromes. *J Cardiovasc Nurs* 23(1):50–55, 2008.

28. ACC/AHA 2007 Guideline Revision. (2007) Guidelines for the management of patients with unstable angina/non-ST-elevation myocardial infarction: Executive summary. *J Am Coll Cardiol* 50(7):652-726. Downloaded September 15, 2008 from http://content.onlinejacc.org/cgi/content/full/50/7/652.

29. Rush P, Unger B, Endelstein K, et al. Therapeutic hypothermia feasibility in a critical, ST-elevation myocardial infarction, postcardiac arrest population. National Teaching Institute Research Abstracts. *Am J Crit Care* 16(3):315, 2007.

30. Wennberg P, Eliasson M, Johansson L, et al. The risk of myocardial infarction and sudden cardiac death amongst snuff users with or without a previous history of smoking. *J Int Med* 262:360–367, 2007.

31. Shiga T, Hagiwara N, Ogawa H, et al. Sudden cardiac death and left ventricular ejection fraction during long term follow-up after acute myocardial infarction in the primary percutaneous coronary intervention era. Results from the HIJAMI-II Registry. *Heart* published online September 5, 2008. Downloaded from heart.bmj.com on September 9, 2008.

32. Dressler DK, Dressler KK. Caring for patients with femoral sheaths. *AJN* 106(5):64A–64H, 2006.

33. Hurst M. *Hurst Review's NCLEX-RN Review*. New York: McGraw-Hill; 2008.

34. Koreny M, Riedmüller E, Nikfardjam M, et al. Arterial puncture closing devices compared with standard manual compression after cardiac catheterization: Systematic review and meta-analysis. *JAMA* 291(3):350–357, 2004.

35. Applegate RJ, Sacrinty MT, Kutcher MA, et al. Propensity score analysis of vascular complications after diagnostic cardiac catheterization and percutaneous coronary intervention 1998–2003. *Cathet Cardiovasc Intervent* 67:556–562, 2006.

36. Hamner JB, Dubois EJ, Rice TP. Predictors of complications associated with closure devices after transfemoral percutaneous coronary procedures. *Crit Care Nurs* 25(5):30–37, 2005.

37. Galli A, Palatnik AM. Ask the experts. *Crit Care Nurse* 23(2):88–94, 2005.

38. Tremper RS. Home study program: Intra-aortic balloon pump therapy: A primer for perioperative nurses. *AORN J* 84(1):33–48, 2006.

39. Weil KM. On guard for intra-aortic balloon pump problems. *Nursing 2007* 37(7):28, 2007.

40. Hamlin SK, Villars PS, Kanusky JT, Shaw ALD. Role of diastole in left ventricular function. II: Diagnosis and treatment. *Am J Crit Care* 13(6):453–468, 2004.

41. Doyle BJ, Ting HH, Bell MR, et al. Major femoral bleeding complications after percutaneous coronary intervention. *J Am Coll Cardiol Cardiovasc Intervent* 1:202–209, 2008.

42. Olson D, Lynn M, Thoyre S, et al. Factors associated with percutaneous coronary intervention (PCI) access complications. In: 2007 National Teaching Institute Research Abstracts. *Am J Crit Care* 16(3):302–315, 2007.

43. Pagana KD, Pagana TJ. *Mosby's Diagnostic and Laboratory Test Reference*. 6th ed. St. Louis: Mosby; 2003.

44. Ho PM, Eng MH, Rumsfeld JS, et al. The influence of age on health status outcomes after acute myocardial infarction. *Am Heart J* 155(5):855–861, 2008.

45. Chojnowski D. Managing systolic heart failure. *Nursing 2006* 37–42, 2006.

46. Smeltzer SC, Bare BG, Hinkle JL, Cheever KH. *Brunner and Suddarth's Textbook of Medical-Surgical Nursing.* 11th ed. St. Louis: Lippincott Williams & Wilkins; 2008.

47. Smeltzer SC, Bare BG, Hinkle JL, Cheever KH. *Brunner and Suddarth's Textbook of Medical-Surgical Nursing.* 11th ed. St. Louis: Lippincott Williams & Wilkins; 2008.

48. Hunt SA, Abraham WT, Chin MH, et al. ACC/AHA 2005 Guideline update for the diagnosis and management of chronic heart failure in the adult. Summary article: A report of the American College of Cardiology/American Heart Association Task Force on practice guidelines to update 2001 guidelines. *JACC 46*(6):1116–1143, 2005.

49. Bluemke DA, Achenbach S, Budoff M, et al. Magnetic resonance angiography and multidetector computed tomography angiography: A scientific statement from the American Heart Association Committee on Cardiovascular Imaging and Intervention of the Council on Cardiovascular Radiology and Intervention, and the Councils on Clinical Cardiology and Cardiovascular Disease in the young. *Circulation* 118:586–606, 2008.

50. Daleiden-Burns A, Stiles P. Proactive monitoring: Implications of implantable devices for future heart failure management. *Crit Care Nurse Q 30*(4):320–328, 2007.

51. Carbucicchio C, Santamaria M, Trevisi N, et al. Catheter ablation for the treatment of electrical storm in patents with implantable cardioverter-defibrillators. *Circulation* 117:462–469, 2008.

52. Simmons-Holcomb S. Recognizing and managing different types of carditis. *Nursing: Apr 2006 36P*:4–9, 2006.

53. Apte M, McGwin G Jr, Vila LM, et al. Associated factors and impact of myocarditis in patients with SLE from LUMINA: A multiethnic US cohort. *Rheumatology (Oxford) 47*(3):362–367, 2008.

54. Sengupta PP, Krishnamoorthy VK, Abhayaratna WP, et al. Comparison of usefulness of tissue Doppler imaging versus brain natriuretic peptide for differentiation of constrictive pericardial disease from restrictive cardiomyopathy. *Am J Cardiol 102*(3):357–362, 2008.

55. Imazio M, Brucato A, Cumetti D, et al. Corticosteroids for recurrent pericarditis: High versus low doses: A nonrandomized observation. *Circulation 118*(6):612–613, 2008.

56. Nishimura RA, Carabello BA, Faxon DP, et al. ACC/AHA 2008 guideline update on valvular heart disease: Focused update on infective endocarditis: A Report of the American College of Cardiology/American Heart Association Task Force on Practice Guidelines. *Circulation* 118:887–896, 2008.

57. Gold MM, Spindola-Franco H, Jain VR, et al. Coronary sinus compression: An early computed tomographic sign of cardiac tamponade. *Comp Assist Tomogr 32*(1):72–77, 2008.

58. King OF. Shock. In: Hurst M, ed. *Hurst Reviews: Pathophysiology Review*. New York: McGraw-Hill; 2008.

59. Paraskevas KI. Treatment of choice for Buerger's disease (thromboangiitis obliterans): Still an unresolved issue. *Clin Rheumatol* 27:547, 2008.

60. Paraskevas KI, Liapis CD, Briana DD, Mikhailidis DP. Thromboangiitis obliterans (Buerger's disease): Searching for a therapeutic strategy. *Angiology 58*(1):75–84, 2007.

61. Puechal X, Fiessinger J-N. Thromboangiitis obliterans or Buerger's disease: Challenges for the rheumatologist. *Rheumatology 46*:192–199, 2007.

62. National institute of Arthritis and Musculoskeletal and Skin Diseases. Questions and answers about Raynaud's phenomenon. NIH publication no. 06-4911, also available at www.niams.nih.gov, 2006.

63. Lazarides MK, Georgiadis GS, Papas TT, Nikolopoulos ES. Diagnostic criteria and treatment of Buerger's disease: A review. *Lower Extremity Wounds 5*(2):89–95, 2006.

64. Pagana KD, Pagana TJ. *Mosby's Manual of Diagnostic and Laboratory Tests*. St. Louis: Mosby Elsevier; 2006.

65. DeVon HA, Ryan CJ. Chest pain and associated symptoms of acute coronary syndromes. *J Cardiovasc Nurs 20*(4):232–238, 2005.

66. Beers MH, ed. *The Merck Manual of Medical Information*. White Station, NJ: Merck Research Laboratories; 2003.

67. Dietrich T, Jimenez M, Krall Kaye EA, et al. Age dependent associations between chronic periodontitis/edentulism and risk for coronary heart disease. *Circulation 117*(13):1668–1674, 2008.

68. Giovannucci E, Liu Y, Hollis BW, Rimm EB. 25-Hydroxyvitamin D and risk of myocardial infarction in men: A prospective study. *Arch Intern Med 168*(11):1174–1180, 2008.

69. Pagana KD, Pagana TJ. *Mosby's Manual of Diagnostic and Laboratory Tests*. St. Louis: Mosby Elsevier; 2006.

70. Peterson ED, Bynum DZ, Roe MT. Association of evidence-based care processes and outcomes among patients with acute coronary syndromes. *J Cardiovasc Nurs 23*(1):50–55, 2008.

71. Giovannucci E, Liu Y, Hollis BW, Rimm EB. 25-Hydroxyvitamin D and risk of myocardial infarction in men: A prospective study. *Arch Intern Med 168*(11):1174–1180, 2008.

5 Shock and Multisystem Failure

OBJECTIVES

In this chapter you will review:

- Various forms of shock and the underlying pathophysiology of each.
- Similarities and differences in circulatory shock, distributive shock, and obstructive shock.
- Nursing priorities and medical management indicated with various forms of shock.
- Stages and progression of shock from compensatory to irreversible multisystem failure.
- Multisystem organ dysfunction syndrome and its implications for the patient and the family/significant others.

✚ SHOCK STATES
Let's get the normal stuff straight first!

Our bodies are optimized to maintain circulating volume and perfusion to vital organs at all times, so a backup system is available in the event that volume within the vascular space or the blood pressure drops. The vascular space is the network that enables blood to be moved throughout the body. The vascular space includes all of the blood vessels in the body (veins, arteries, capillaries). Does the vascular space also include the heart? Yes, it does! The heart is continuous with the vascular space, and is a partner in circulation. The heart serves as the pump to support circulation, keeping the blood in the vascular space moving forward (Fig. 5-1).

▶ Figure 5-1. The Vascular System. The heart pumps blood through the vascular system, perfusing the tissues with oxygen.

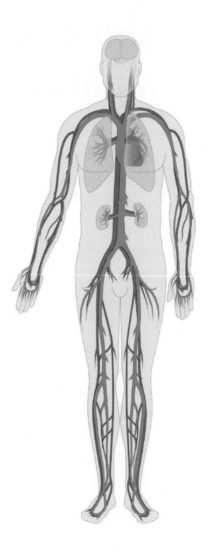

The blood vessels have a muscular layer (the tunica media) capable of vasoconstriction or vasodilation and the size of the blood vessels has a direct relationship with the blood pressure:

• When vessels become larger (vasodilated), the pressure within the vessels decreases.

• When vessels become smaller (vasoconstricted), blood pressure increases (Fig. 5-2).

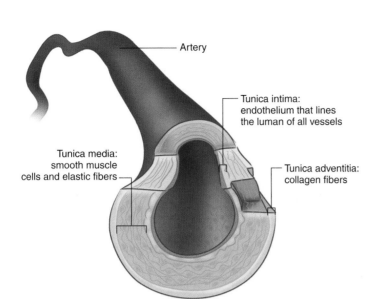

◀ Figure 5-2. Musculature of the Blood Vessels. The tunica media can dilate or contract vessels to increase or decrease blood pressure.

The systolic blood pressure is directly related to the cardiac output:

- When the cardiac output drops, the systolic pressure drops.
- When the cardiac output goes up, the systolic pressure goes up.

Any time the cardiac output drops (for any reason), compensatory mechanisms kick in to raise the blood pressure and the circulating volume:

- Aldosterone (the primary mineralocorticoid from the adrenal cortex) causes the body to retain sodium and water, increasing blood volume.
- ADH (antidiuretic hormone from the pituitary gland) causes the body to retain water, also increasing blood volume (Fig. 5-3).

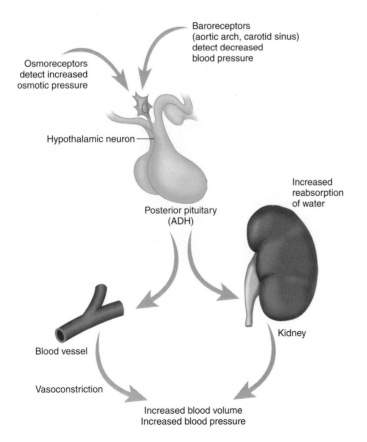

◀ Figure 5-3. Antidiuretic Hormone. Antidiuretic hormone increases blood volume by causing the body to retain sodium and water, resulting in increased blood pressure.

- Catecholamines (epinephrine and norepinephrine) secreted by the adrenal medulla cause the vessels to constrict to raise the blood pressure and shunt blood to vital organs (heart, brain, lungs, and kidneys). Catecholamines also cause the heart to beat faster, moving the little available volume around faster.

What is it?

Shock is a deadly "end of the road" syndrome characterized by circulatory failure and decreased perfusion. Shock by definition is not really a disease, but an adverse effect of many different disease conditions. When shock states occur, the body's compensatory mechanisms are immediately activated. If the underlying cause of shock is not promptly remedied, shock progresses, compensatory mechanisms will begin to fail (decompensate), and the circulatory system will no longer be able to supply peripheral tissues and body organs with needed oxygen.

The three stages of shock are defined as:

- *Early shock* is also called compensatory or nonprogressive shock. Adaptive mechanisms are compensating and managing to maintain circulation to all vital organs.

- *Advancing shock* is progressive. Decompensation is beginning, which results in a falling cardiac output, and dysfunction of vital organs is caused by hypoperfusion.[1]

- *Late shock* is irreversible depending on the degree of failed compensatory mechanisms (Figs. 5-4 to 5-6).

▶ Figure 5-4. Early Shock (Compensatory/Nonprogressive).

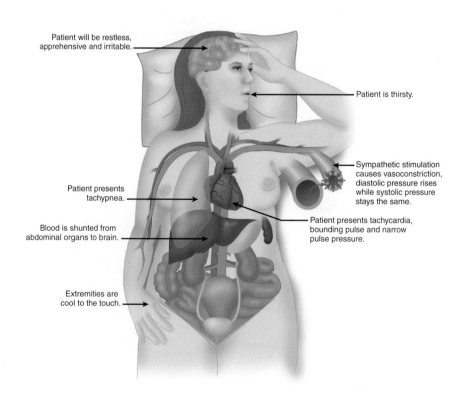

Patient will be restless, apprehensive and irritable.

Patient is thirsty.

Sympathetic stimulation causes vasoconstriction, diastolic pressure rises while systolic pressure stays the same.

Patient presents tachypnea.

Patient presents tachycardia, bounding pulse and narrow pulse pressure.

Blood is shunted from abdominal organs to brain.

Extremities are cool to the touch.

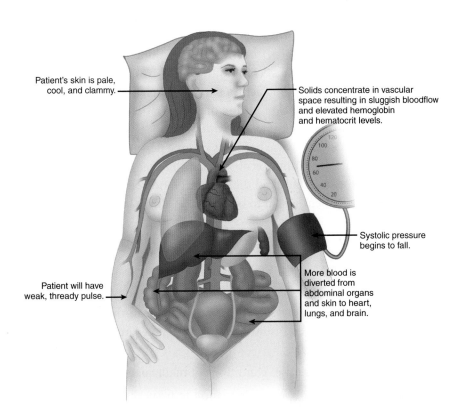

Patient's skin is pale, cool, and clammy.

Solids concentrate in vascular space resulting in sluggish bloodflow and elevated hemoglobin and hematocrit levels.

Systolic pressure begins to fall.

Patient will have weak, thready pulse.

More blood is diverted from abdominal organs and skin to heart, lungs, and brain.

◀ Figure 5-5. Advancing Shock (Progressive).

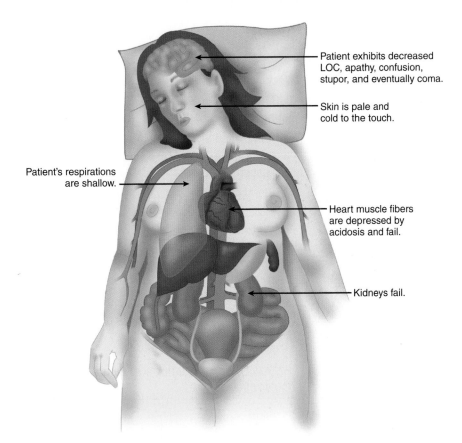

Patient exhibits decreased LOC, apathy, confusion, stupor, and eventually coma.

Skin is pale and cold to the touch.

Patient's respirations are shallow.

Heart muscle fibers are depressed by acidosis and fail.

Kidneys fail.

◀ Figure 5-6. Late Shock (Irreversible/ Fatal).

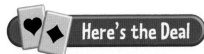

Here's the Deal

Early shock is called "nonprogressive" because the compensatory mechanisms are working! The systolic blood pressure in early shock may be unaffected because the responsive tachycardia (an adaptive mechanism) is maintaining the cardiac output. (Remember the formula? Stroke Volume × Heart Rate = Cardiac Output)

Causes and why?

All shock states happen either because of heart failure or circulatory failure! When the heart fails, most commonly caused by myocardial infarction, a resulting weak pumping action prevents the heart from moving blood forward and adequately meeting the oxygenation needs of the body. This type of shock is known as *cardiogenic shock*. Failed circulation occurs when the vascular space becomes volume depleted, too vasodilated, for the available volume, or obstructed (blocked). When this happens, the cardiac output falls and the systolic blood pressure decreases critically, and the patient is said to be in shock. This is known as *circulatory shock*.

CIRCULATORY SHOCK

The three types of circulatory shock are named to give you a hint as to the underlying problem that is interrupting adequate circulation to body tissues:

1. *Hypovolemic shock* describes conditions of inadequate blood volume.

2. *Obstructive shock* occurs when circulation to tissues is obstructed (blocked).

3. *Distributive shock* describes loss of vascular tone that inhibits blood from being distributed to tissues (Table 5-1).

Table 5-1 Types of circulatory shock, causes, and examples

Type of shock	Cause of shock	Examples of conditions leading to shock
Hypovolemic shock	Hemorrhagic/loss of whole blood from the vascular space.	• Massive trauma • DIC • Aortic aneurysm • Surgical procedures involving ligation of arteries Obstetric causes: • Placental abruption • Placenta previa • Postpartum uterine atony
	Intravascular dehydration owing to fluid loss.	• Polyuria • Diarrhea • HHNK • Diabetes insipidus • Addisonian crisis Removal of fluid accumulation: paracentesis or thoracentesis
	Massive fluid shifts and third spacing of fluid, leaving the vascular space dry.	• Burns • Ascites • Pleural effusion

(Continued)

Table 5-1 Types of circulatory shock, causes, and examples

Type of shock	Cause of shock	Examples of conditions leading to shock
Obstructive Shock	In obstructive shock, the normal heart is unable to pump because it is impaired by outside forces. The healthy heart either cannot fill or cannot contract.	• Cardiac tamponade • Pulmonary embolus • Thoracic tumors • Tension pneumothorax • Diaphragmatic hernia
Distributive shock	Loss of vasomotor tone to the vessel walls produces *neurogenic* shock.	• Spinal cord injury • Dissection of the spinal cord • Severe acute pain • Brain injury that alters the vasomotor center in the brain stem or sympathetic outflow to vessels • Hypoxemia • Insulin reaction • CNS depressants • Adverse effects of anesthetic agents
	The trigger for *anaphylactic* shock is release of substances in the blood that cause vessels all over the body to dilate.	Severe allergic reactions to: • Chemicals (sulfobromophthalein sodium, sodium dehydrocholate, radiographic contrast media) • Foods (legumes, nuts, berries, seafood, egg albumin) • Drugs (penicillin, antibiotics, sulfonamides, local anesthetics) • Enzymes • Hormones • Insect venom • Vaccinations • Allergen extracts • Serums (horse serum) • Sulfite-containing food additives
	In *septic shock* it is the presence of systemic inflammatory mediators that activate generalized systemic vasodilation.	Most frequent cause: gram-negative bacteremia although other organisms are implicated such as gram-positive bacilli and fungi.[2] Urosepsis is a common systemic infection of the elderly,[3] especially when an indwelling catheter is in place.

✚ Hypovolemic Shock

What is it?

Circulating blood volume must be adequate to maintain cardiac output. The amount of blood in the vascular space for the typical adult male is about 5 liters.[4] When volume within the vascular space drops, stroke volume drops, and the cardiac output drops as evidenced by a fall in systolic blood pressure.

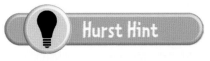

Hurst Hint

Less Volume = Less Pressure

The body has a wonderful set of biological and chemical mechanisms (backup systems) to compensate for fluid volume losses. Blood stored in the liver and pooled blood in the venous system (called *venous capacitance*) provides a readily available supply when the body is in crisis.

- This stored fluid can be mobilized and delivered to central circulation very quickly if there is any sudden threat to the critical level of intravascular blood volume.

- Hopefully, this mechanism, coupled with sympathetic stimulation (tachycardia and vasopressor effects), and hormonal regulation (aldosterone and ADH) will initiate compensation to restore volume and blood pressure to halt the progression of shock.

Our body cannot tell the difference among the various clinical shock syndromes; therefore, only one set of mechanisms is available to attempt in restoring or maintaining circulating volume. These compensatory mechanisms help the person in *hypovolemic shock* because more volume is what this patient really needs! Hypovolemic shock refers to a particular set of symptoms that represent the body's failed attempt to compensate for the acute loss of circulating blood volume.

There are degrees of shock:

- *Mild* shock occurs when <20% of blood volume is lost.

- *Moderate* shock occurs when 20% to 40% of blood volume is lost.

- *Severe* shock occurs when >40% of blood volume is lost.

What causes it and why?

See Table 5-1.

Loss of vascular volume can occur because of a number of reasons:

- Whole blood (plasma and solids) is lost from circulation during internal or external hemorrhage.

- The liquid portion of the blood (plasma) can be lost as a result of anything that increases capillary permeability, such as vessel injury resulting from a burn wound.

- Any disease associated with polyuria: diabetic ketoacidosis (DKA), diabetes insipidus (DI), Addison's disease, or particle-induced diuresis (PID).

- Excessive fluid loss through vomiting or continuous excessive gastric suction, diarrhea, diaphoresis, or hyperventilation.

- Third-space fluid shifts are when fluid is still present within the body, but is lost to circulation. Third spacing can be caused by fluid secreting tumors, organ failure, hypoalbuminemia, or any condition causing fluid to collect within a cavity, creating a need for evacuation (thoracentesis or paracentesis).

Signs and symptoms and why?

At the onset of early shock the body is compensating; therefore, the patient may be virtually asymptomatic. As shock progresses the patient begins to decompensate, and the following signs and symptoms are produced as a result of decreased cardiac output (Table 5-2).

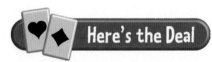

Here's the Deal

Shock symptoms occur because of rapid loss of circulating fluid volume. Did I say loss of TOTAL volume? No! A person can have fluid volume that is not within the vascular space, and is therefore not available for circulatory transport of oxygen and nutrients to the tissues or removal of metabolic waste products. When the vascular space is depleted, vital organs no longer receive the essential oxygen and nutrients necessary to sustain life.

Table 5-2 Characteristics of circulatory chock: hypovolemic presentation

Signs and symptoms	Cause and underlying pathophysiology
EARLY shock	
Restlessness	Activation of sympathetic nervous system stimulation causes the release of epinephrine and norepinephrine (also called catecholamines, or stress hormones for fight or flight).
Apprehension, irritability	Cerebral hypoxia owing to decrease in cardiac output and the sense of impending doom, that something is very wrong.
Tachypnea	Beta receptors respond to cellular hypoxia to initiate brochodilation.[5]
Bounding pulse (the heart is pumping harder to get what blood is left out to the vital organs)	Sympathetic stimulation has a direct effect on the myocardial cells to increase the force of contraction causing adaptive efforts to combat early shock.[5]
Thirst	A very basic compensatory mechanism for any condition of hemoconcentration to replace fluid volume. As vascular volume decreases, serum osmolarity increases and the thirst center in the hypothalamus is activated. The kidneys release angiotensin II, which has a direct effect on the hypothalamus as an added trigger to thirst.[12]
Reduced urinary output	Kidneys sense low circulating volume and begin to reabsorb water, decreasing the amount of urine excreted to offset existing hypovolemia.
Tachycardia	Sympathetic stimulation has a direct action on the pacemaker of the heart to speed up the heart rate and increase the force of contraction.
Narrowed pulse pressure	Sympathetic stimulation causes vasoconstriction, which causes the diastolic pressure to rise, but the systolic pressure stays the same.
ADVANCED shock	
Pulse quality: weak, thready	Progressive fluid volume deficit results in a small vascular space, and coupled with the vasoconstriction from continued sympathetic stimulation, the pulse feels like a very small threadlike string of a vessel when palpated and the low volume is reflected in the low pulse pressure exerted on the wall of the vessel.
Skin changes: cool, pale, clammy	Fat, bone, and skin can better survive ischemia than organs with high oxygen consumption. Blood flow is therefore diverted away from the skin as well as the GI tract and the liver in an effort to direct more blood flow to the heart, brain, and lungs.

(Continued)

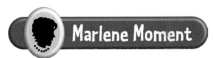

Marlene Moment

Hurst definition of third spacing: Fluid is in a place that does you no good; in other words, anywhere other than the vascular space.

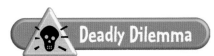

Deadly Dilemma

Once you see signs of shock, don't wait on the body to compensate, because compensatory mechanisms have *already* failed!

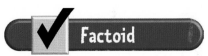

Factoid

A *rapid* drop in blood pressure is poorly tolerated by the body. A slow, gradual decline allows the body needed time for compensatory mechanisms to restore balance.

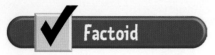

If whole blood is lost, the fluid volume (plasma) *plus* solids (RBCs, WBCs, platelets, etc.) are reduced; therefore, the HCT and Hgb will be low rather than high.

Table 5-2 Characteristics of circulatory chock: hypovolemic presentation (*Continued*)

Signs and symptoms	Cause and underlying pathophysiology
Oliguria	As blood pressure drops in shock, renal perfusion decreases, therefore reducing kidney function of filtration and excretion.
Hemoconcentration: elevated HCT, Hgb	Progressive fluid volume loss through intravascular dehydration leaves a concentration of solids within the vascular space, which in turn causes sluggish blood flow and can lead to tissue damage, which may trigger another potentially lethal complication of DIC.
Hypotension	The hallmark of failed compensatory mechanisms is reflected in a decreased systolic blood pressure. The cause of the shock has not been corrected, the backup system can no longer hold the cardiac output steady, and the cardiac output decreases, as reflected by the progressive decline in the systolic blood pressure.
LATE shock	
Decreasing LOC: apathy, confusion, stupor, finally coma	When the cardiac output falls below a critical level, the brain does not receive adequate blood flow. Brain cells, which require high levels of oxygen and glucose, cannot continue normal functions of orientation, comprehension, responsiveness, and wakefulness.
Shallow respirations	With progressive brain dysfunction because of critically insufficient oxygen supply, the medulla oblongata (which normally regulates respirations) ceases to relay the lifesaving message for the lungs to take in more oxygen.
Oliguria Anuria	With continued lack of perfusion secondary to failed compensatory mechanisms and a drastic reduction in cardiac output, the kidneys can no longer function. Kidneys shut down secondary to continued loss of circulating volume and sluggish blood flow, triggering the onset of anaerobic metabolism, which produces acidosis that depresses heart muscle fibers.

Testing, testing, testing

Although shock is usually diagnosed by the clinical picture, hypovolemia resulting from hemorrhage or third spacing can be identified with the following diagnostic tests:

Test	Clinical significance
Complete blood count (CBC) Hemoglobin, hematocrit, red blood cell count	Decreased: hemorrhagic shock. Increased: loss of volume resulting from third spacing which leaves the vascular space concentrated.
Clotting studies: Prothrombin time (PT) and partial thromboplastin time (PTT)	May be prolonged if coagulopathy is present.
Arterial blood gases (ABGs)	Will reflect decreased oxygen saturation and hypoxemia as tissue perfusion decreases. A base deficit occurs with tissue acidosis and is an index of the severity of shock.[7]
Serum lactate	This will be elevated because hypoperfusion causes anaerobic metabolism and resultant lactic acidosis.
Potassium	**Decreased:** early shock because increased aldosterone secretion causes renal excretion of potassium. **Increased:** when cellular death leaks potassium into the blood stream and in the presence of acidosis.
Blood urea nitrogen (BUN)	**Increases** with loss of plasma volume resulting in hemoconcentration.
Imaging Studies: CT, MRI	May be indicated to locate the source of internal bleeding.

Interventions and why?

Shock must be treated promptly and aggressively, restoring oxygen and nutrients to the tissues to prevent irreversible damage to vital organs. Permanent brain damage can develop in a matter of minutes if adequate oxygenated blood is not available to the brain cells. So first things first:

- A = Ensure a stable airway, with oral and nasopharyngeal airway as needed.
- B = Ensure adequate ventilation, with intubation and mechanical ventilation if needed.
- C = Restore circulation! Locate and terminate the source of volume loss.

As we said earlier, shock is an adverse effect of an underlying cause, so let's treat the cause(s).

If hypovolemic shock is caused by hemorrhage, the priority is to stop the bleeding:

- Frequently surgery may be required (ruptured spleen or lacerated liver resulting from trauma).
- Pneumatic antishock garments may be used to control internal or external hemorrhage by direct pressure.
- Military antishock trousers (MAST) may be in place to raise blood pressure.

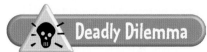
Deadly Dilemma

When late shock is well established, critical injury can occur to vital organs. Blood pressure and perfusion must be restored promptly before multiple system organ failure occurs.

If hypovolemic shock is caused by intravascular dehydration resulting from fluid loss (diarrhea, vomiting, polyuria, DI), then treatment may include the following:

- Antidiarrheal agents are prescribed for diarrhea.
- Antiemetic agents are prescribed for vomiting.
- Desmopressin (DDAVP) is administered for diabetes insipidus (DI).

The general nursing intervention during shock resuscitation is to:

- Administer supplemental oxygen to combat tissue hypoxia, hopefully to produce the following indicators of adequate tissue perfusion: PaO_2 > 80 mm Hg, SaO_2 > 92%, MAP > 65 mm Hg.
- Obtain venous access (two antecubital sites with a large-gauge IV catheter) to accommodate simultaneous infusion of crystalloids, colloids, and transfusion of blood and blood components.
- Administer isotonic crystalloid (electrolyte solutions) IV for fluid resuscitation: normal saline, lactated Ringer's, correct hypotension, and improve tissue oxygenation.[8] Hypertonic saline 3% may be ordered to pull fluid from the intracellular space into the extracellular space to achieve fluid balance, reducing the volume of required IV fluid.
- Administer colloids (plasma proteins/albumin) as prescribed if fluid is in a third space (ascites, burns, etc).
- Administer whole blood, packed red blood cells, platelets, clotting factors, and/or other blood components as prescribed, following protocols and safeguards.
- Position the patient to increase central circulation: modified Trendelenburg with lower extremities elevated, trunk horizontal and knees extended, and head slightly elevated.
- Monitor hemodynamic parameters: CVP, mean arterial pressure (MAP), and blood pressure (preferably continuously by arterial line) and SaO_2.
- Be alert to signs of FVE during rapid fluid resuscitation (see Chapter 2): The CVP should be monitored closely.
- Provide factual reassurance and reduce fear and anxiety with your physical presence and explanations of procedures and the treatment plan.

The patient needs ongoing assessment and frequent monitoring of the following parameters to detect progression of shock, and to evaluate the client's response to resuscitation (above):

- Monitor LOC and vital signs (BP, pulse pressure, pulse, respirations, SaO_2).
- Auscultate the lungs (posterior and bilaterally) to detect fluid before excessive accumulation can occur.
- Monitor skin color, temperature, and presence or absence of mottling.
- Assess the quality of peripheral pulses.
- Monitor urine output hourly.

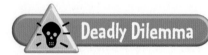

Deadly Dilemma

A patient in shock receiving large volumes of fluid may develop hypothermia and coagulopathy. Crystalloid and colloid solutions are often warmed to prevent hypothermia. Coagulopathy can result if the client is receiving large volumes of packed red blood cells because they don't have clotting factors.

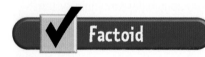

Factoid

The optimal CVP level for a client is 5 to 10 cm H_2O or 2 to 8 mm Hg depending on the monitoring system. Don't confuse these two systems of measure.

If the patient has persistent hypotension after adequate fluid administration, vasoactive medications (Levophed [norepinephrine bitartrate], phenylephrine (Neo-Synephrine, dopamine [Intropin, Revimine], and vasopressin [Pitressin]) may be prescribed. During administration of vasoactive medications, the nurse closely monitors the patient response and uses the following precautions:

- Flow rate control pump to ensure safe, accurate delivery of dosage.
- Documentation of vital signs: BP, pulse, and MAP a minimum of every 15 minutes and more often if unstable.
- Titrating vasopressors: tapering down as blood pressure rises, gradually weaning from medication, never abruptly discontinuing.

After the acute episode is resolved, the nurse always reinforces the importance of follow-up appointments and continuing medical care for any patient recovering from a shock state.

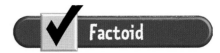

Titrating is a method for administering a medication or fluid to obtain a desired effect: bumping up a flow rate for hypotension, or bumping down the flow rate if blood pressure rises above the desired perimeter.

PATIENT TEACHING: DISCHARGE PLANNING   Patient teaching will be directly related to the underlying cause of the shock.

All postoperative patients going home with incisions and drains are taught to:

- Refrain from lifting and resume driving per doctor instruction to avoid danger from sudden jerky movements (slamming on breaks) or an increase in intra-abdominal pressure (straining, lifting, climbing stairs), which can cause bleeding.
- Monitor drainage and immediately report change in color from pink to bright red, or increasing amounts of drainage, as this can represent new bleeding.
- Increase dietary sources of protein and iron for anemia secondary to blood loss.

Patients with Addison's disease (loss of sodium and water) are taught to:

- Weigh daily and adjust Florinef accordingly (weight gain >2–3 lb hold or reduce the dosage; weight loss <2–3 lb increase the dosage.
- Increase intake of sodium and water during times of increased losses, and use sports drinks during strenuous activity.

Patients having GI losses are taught to:

- Seek treatment for the underlying cause before the onset of dehydration.
- Recognize the early signs of hypovolemia (thirst, dry mouth, fast heart rate) and seek medical attention promptly.

✚ Obstructive shock

What is it?

Obstructive shock is a type of circulatory shock that occurs when blood flow (into or out of) the heart is blocked because of mechanical factors. This blockage will lead to decreased ventricular filling and ejection capacity, resulting in decreased cardiac output and impaired circulation.

The blood in the vascular space is not effectively moved forward; therefore, the body responds to poor perfusion with the shock syndrome.

What causes it and why?

See Table 5-1. Any condition that causes the heart to be compressed (squeezed) or displaced from the center of the mediastinum will result in decreased ventricular filling, decreased ejection capacity, and a drop in the cardiac output. Now the patient is experiencing hypotension (systolic), poor perfusion of vital organs, and obstructive shock. The following conditions can produce obstructive shock. Specifically:

- Pulmonary embolism interferes with right ventricular emptying.
- Cardiac myxoma (a tumor) obstructing inflow and outflow of the heart.
- Cardiac tamponade owing to seepage of fluid into the sack surrounding the heart, squeezing the heart from the outside so blood can't enter the chambers.
- Mediastinal shift secondary to tension pneumothorax pushing the heart to the opposite side and kinking off the great vessels.
- Diaphragmatic hernia or diaphragmatic rupture crowding the heart with stomach and abdominal contents.

Signs and symptoms and why?

My patient will display many of the same signs as those previously described with hypovolemic shock, the prototype of circulatory shock (see Table 5-2). Obstructive shock has some unique differences related to the specific cause of circulatory obstruction (Table 5-3).

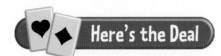

Here's the Deal

A diaphragmatic hernia can cause obstructive shock because there is no room in the thorax for the heart and lungs PLUS abdominal organs. When the stomach moves up into the chest cavity with the heart and lungs, there is not enough room for everybody. So, the heart is compressed by the extra pressure and ventricular filling is compromised. The resultant stroke volume is inadequate to produce an effective cardiac output.

Table 5-3 Differences in obstructive shock presentation

Signs and symptoms	Cause and underlying pathophysiology
Respiratory problems: dyspnea, tachypnea	Occurs when blood flow through the lungs is compromised by crowding of abdominal organs in the thoracic cavity (diaphragmatic hernia), or blood can't get into the lungs to be oxygenated.
Distended neck veins	Related to elevated right heart pressure, which elevates central venous pressure and causes blood to backflow, which engorges jugular veins.
Systolic hypotension with decreased stroke volume and falling cardiac output	Occurs because the heart is displaced or compressed: the chambers cannot properly fill; therefore, cardiac output and systolic pressure decrease.
Displaced trachea	Air or blood in the pleural space collapses the lung, and pushes mediastinal structures (heart, esophagus, trachea, etc.) toward the opposite side.

(Continued)

Table 5-3 Differences in obstructive shock presentation (*Continued*)

Signs and symptoms	Cause and underlying pathophysiology
Pulsus paradoxus	As the heart is being compressed, the cardiac output falls. With inspiration, the lungs inflate and draw blood into the right heart, pushing the intraventricular septum to the left, increasing compression to the already compressed left chamber and the cardiac output falls further. (Think of this as a "double squeeze.") With inspiration, the systolic pressure falls at least 10 mm Hg and rises 10 mm Hg with expiration, reflecting a little better cardiac output with reduced internal pressure on the heart during expiration.
Muffled heart sounds	Heart sounds are muffled when auscultated through a mass (tumor) in the cardiac muscle or a volume of blood or exudates in the pericardial sack.
Narrowing of pulse pressure	Occurs because the obstructive pathology hinders the movement of blood in or out of the heart chambers and systolic pressure (cardiac output) falls to meet the rising diastolic pressure.

Testing, Testing, Testing

The clinical picture gives indication of obstructive shock, which may be confirmed with the following:

- Chest X-ray, which demonstrates widening of the cardiac silhouette indicating cardiac tamponade, a collapsed lung, or a mass

- Echocardiogram, which demonstrates obstruction of great vessels and chambers of the heart and poor ejection fraction of the left ventricle

- VQ (ventilation/perfusion) scan, which demonstrates blood flow through the lungs

Interventions and why?

Here we go with the A-B-Cs again!

- Monitoring cardiac output and vital signs
- Chest auscultation for bilateral breath sounds
- Maintain patent airway and prepare for intubation and mechanical ventilation
- Supplemental oxygen to enhance oxygenation
  Fix the problem:
- Chest tubes with water seal and suction to promote re-expansion of collapsed lung
  - Care of chest tubes, monitoring drainage, maintaining water seal and one-way flow out of the lung, monitoring ABGs and oxygenation status
- Surgery to repair the diaphragmatic abnormalities or injuries
  - Postoperative care: turn, cough, deep breathe, incentive spirometry, assisting with ambulation, pain control, and surgical wound care following repair of the diaphragm

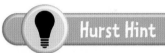

Beck's triad (three signs of tamponade) includes:
- Hypotension
- Jugular venous distention
- Muffled heart sounds

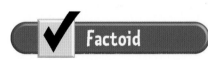

The falling cardiac output coupled with increasing myocardial ischemia may induce pulseless electrical activity (PEA). This is a fatal arrhythmia because conduction continues with an identifiable rhythm on the monitor, but no actual mechanical contraction of the heart occurs.

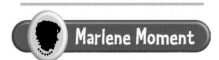

Don't forget who you are taking care of ... the PATIENT! Treat the patient not the MONITOR!

- Restore circulation with pericardiocentesis: needle aspiration to remove excess blood, fluid, or exudates (whatever) compressing the heart
  - Close monitoring of the patient after pericardiocentesis: fluid or blood could recur following aspiration. Watch for a decline in cardiac output and Beck's triad!

PATIENT TEACHING: DISCHARGE PLANNING

- Report any chest discomfort or palpitations immediately. The underlying cause may be returning.
- Report difficult breathing, fever, or change in the color of sputum immediately.
- Refrain from vigorous or strenuous activities or driving until released by your physician.
- The outcome is good if prompt diagnosis and treatment can be instituted to relieve the cause. The bad news is that the problem may recur: important.

✚ Distributive shock

Distributive shock occurs in the presence of normal blood volume, but because of vasodilation, there is insufficient blood pressure to support circulation.

What is it?

Distributive shock is the type of shock that differs from all other forms of circulatory shock or cardiogenic shock. Normally when a person is in shock, a compensatory response of systemic vasoconstriction occurs to raise the blood pressure, but not in distributive shock. This patient's entire vascular system is vasodilated.

- All forms of distributive shock are normovolemic, but the blood volume does not fill up the vascular space, which has become too large because of generalized vasodilation.
- Systemic vasodilation decreases blood return to the heart, which reduces the ventricular filling, ejected stroke volume, and cardiac output, causing a rapid drop in systolic blood pressure.
- Low cardiac output coupled with low systolic blood pressure results in a reduced delivery of oxygen to the vital organs.
- Distributive shock is classified as neurogenic, anaphylactic, or septic in origin.

✚ Neurogenic shock
What is it?

- *Neurogenic* shock, also called *vasogenic* shock, is characterized by a disruption in the sympathetic nervous system, which normally keeps the muscle layer of vessels partially contracted. A number of factors can override this normal action of the sympathetic system to cause gross vasodilation over the entire vascular system. As a result, blood pools in the venous system, blood returned to the right side of the heart is decreased, cardiac output drops, and the patient becomes hypotensive.

Causes and why?

See Table 5-1.

Pathways resulting in vasodilation:

* This can be a brief self-limiting condition as occurs with syncope/fainting or can be a prolonged course when related to a spinal cord injury.

* Neurogenic shock can be precipitated by spinal anesthesia when patients are improperly positioned and the anesthetic agent travels higher up in the cerebrospinal fluid, causing higher nerve blockade. Also general anesthesia can alter the sympathetic system and cause dilation of vessels.

Neurogenic shock is caused by an impaired baroreceptor response or altered autonomic spinal cord injury and spinal shock (reflex depression of cord function below the level of the injury). The higher the spinal cord injury, the more severe the neurogenic shock.

* Horror and severe pain overriding autonomic controls (eg, severe burns)

* Hypoglycemia/insulin shock disrupting brain metabolism/function caused by glucose deficit

Signs and symptoms	Why
Bradycardia	The sympathetic nervous system is not responding properly so symptoms are signs of parasympathetic stimulation. The skin is warm and dry instead of cool and moist and bradycardia instead of tachycardia
Dry, warm skin	Vasodilation causes the skin to be warm.
Orthostatic hypotension	Vasodilation makes the vessels feel like they do not have enough volume (even though no volume has been lost). Less volume, less pressure.
Fainting	When cardiac output decreases, not as much blood makes it to the brain.
No sweating below the level of the injury	Sympathetic activity is blocked.
Flaccid paralysis below level of injury	Blood vessel tone is lost below level of injury causing general dilation of vessels.

Source: Hurst M. *Hurst Reviews: Pathophysiology Review* New York: McGraw-Hill; 2008.

Testing, testing, testing

Imaging studies: CT or MRI may be indicated with neurogenic shock to identify spinal cord injury.

Interventions

We always use A-B-Cs in "shocky" emergencies requiring resuscitation:

- Provide airway and ventilator support in patients with high spinal cord injury (above T6).
- Prevent hypotension associated with spinal anesthesia with prescribed pre-bolus of LR or NS.
- After spinal anesthesia, elevate the head of the bed to keep the anesthetic agent from ascending up to the spinal cord.
- Prepare the trauma patient for surgery to stabilize the spinal cord injury.
- For insulin shock: Administer 50% glucose as prescribed.
- Continuous cardiac monitoring.
- ACLS protocols for significant bradycardia.
- Continuous blood pressure monitoring.
- Administration of vasopressors as prescribed.

✚ Anaphylactic shock

What is it?

- *Anaphylactic* shock is a type of distributive shock that involves the immune system. The immune system responds to foreign substances by activating an antigen–antibody response. This life-threatening antigen–antibody reaction occurs in a sensitized individual that produces a systemic response, which spirals rapidly downward without immediate intervention. This allergic response, or hypersensitivity, occurs as a result of previous contact with the foreign substance. Oddly enough, this dramatic antigen–antibody response does not occur after the first exposure to the antigen but to the second exposure (Fig. 5-7).

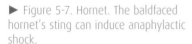

► Figure 5-7. Hornet. The baldfaced hornet's sting can induce anaphylactic shock.

Graciously provided by the Centers for Disease Control and Prevention, Harvard University and Dr. Gary Alpert (2006).

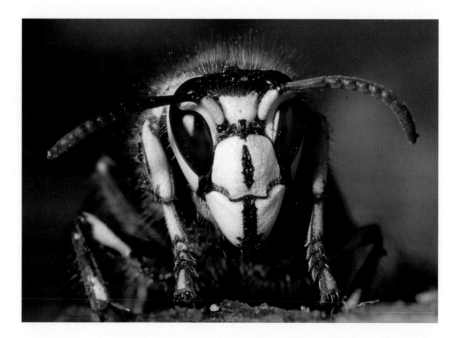

Causes and why?

See Table 5-1. Systemic exposure to sensitizing agents (Fig. 5-8):

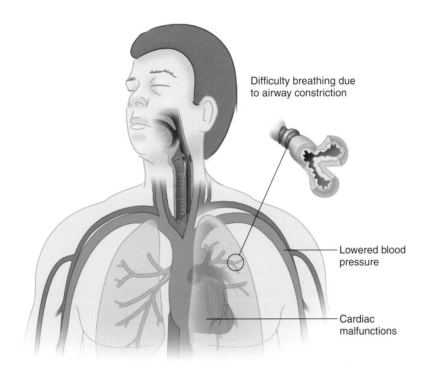

Difficulty breathing due to airway constriction

Lowered blood pressure

Cardiac malfunctions

◀ Figure 5-8. Effects of Anaphylactic Shock. Anaphylactic shock results in bronchospasm and laryngeal edema obstructing oxygen intake and fluid shift from the vascular space to the tissues, which causes a drop in blood pressure.

Signs and symptoms	Why
Sudden nasal congestion	Histamine and other biochemicals cause mucosal swelling and excess mucous production.
Flushed, moist skin	Blood vessels dilate bringing increased blood flow to the surface[11]
Nervousness, anxiety, feeling of doom	Decreased cerebral blood flow secondary to a decrease in cardiac output.
Red, itchy wheals (urticaria and pruritus)	Reaction to allergens.
Tachypnea and crowing (stridor)	Bronchospasm and laryngeal edema obstruct the intake of oxygen on inspiration. Oxygen lack triggers more rapid breathing.
Generalized edema	Leakage of fluid into extracellular tissues because of increased capillary permeability.
Hypotension	Fluid shifting from the vascular space into the tissues results in a fluid volume deficit in the vascular space and a drop in blood pressure.

Source: Hurst M. *Hurst Reviews: Pathophysiology Review* New York: McGraw-Hill; 2008.

Testing, testing, testing

Skin testing: develops a specific antigen.

Interventions and why?

Anaphylactic shock occurs suddenly and can be lethal. If the cause of distributive shock is an anaphylactic reaction, remove the antigen responsible for the response, administer medications to restore vascular tone, and provide required emergency life support.

- Discontinue antigen source if possible such as an IV antibiotic.
- Epinephrine is given first and early.[8]
  Oxygen therapy:
- IV fluid administration
- Antihistamines: H1 and H2 histamine receptor antagonists
- Corticosteroids[9]
- Bronchodilators

  After initial anaphylaxis resuscitation, continued monitoring and evaluation of effectiveness of treatment:

- Monitor for wheeze, stridor, or difficult breathing.
- Monitor vital signs being alert to fever, tachypnea, or tachycardia.
- Monitor effectiveness of respiratory therapy if indicated.
- Monitor pulse oximetry, ABGs, and parameters of tissue oxygenation.
- Administer decreasing doses of corticosteroids.
- Investigate the presence of previous allergies to medications, foods, latex, etc. Be alert to strawberry- and kiwi-sensitive patients, because they may also be allergic to latex, although as-yet unknown.
- Monitoring patients for 30 minutes before discharge after they have injections in the ED or outpatient settings.
- Educate patients with a history of anaphylaxis about their condition.
- Advise such patients to keep an epinephrine autoinjector kit available at all times.
- Refill prescription for autoinjector epinephrine kit well before the expiration date.
- Teach correct use of the Epi-Pen (autoinjector kit) using a simulator for self-injection.
- Advise that the patient procure a medic alert bracelet or medallion and list sensitivities, wearing it at all times.

✚ Septic shock

What is it?

Septic shock is the most common cause of circulatory shock, and this form of shock occurs in patients who have a widespread or overwhelming infection. Septic shock is caused by systemic infection wherein bacterial toxins act on blood vessels, producing vasodilation and pooling of blood.

What causes it and why?

See Table 5-1. Sepsis can be caused by any pathogenic organism that invades the body. Patients who have a compromised immune system are at a high risk for this type of shock. Cytokines, substances released by the immune system to fight infection, and toxins produced by the pathogenic organism cause blood vessels to dilate. This vasodilation decreases venous return to the heart causing cardiac output to drop. This drop in cardiac output results in decreased perfusions of all vital organs.

Signs and symptoms and why?

See Table 5-4.

Table 5-4 Signs and symptoms of septic shock

Signs and symptoms	Why?
Alteration in temperature: hyperthermia or hypothermia	Fever and a high white count may accompany the bacteremia in early shock, but hypothermia owing to a decreasing basal metabolic rate in late shock[3] and low white count may be present in the immune suppressed patient or those whose bone marrow is unable to continue production of mature WBC.
Warm, flushed skin	Febrile conditions coupled with bacterial toxins in the blood cause excessive vasodilation.[10]
Hypotension	Excessive systemic vasodilation reduces the pressure within the vascular space.
Confusion, behavioral changes	Decreased perfusion to brain tissues and toxins alters cerebral function.
Hyperventilation (early shock) and hypoventilation (late shock)	Fast breathing occurs in response to cellular hypoxia and can result in respiratory alkalosis.[9] Lactic acidosis may result from hypoventilation when the respiratory center becomes depressed.

Source: Hurst M. *Hurst Reviews: Pathophysiology Review* New York: McGraw-Hill; 2008.

Testing, testing, testing

Complete blood count (CBC): White blood cells (total count and differential) are significant because these blood cells fight infection and react against foreign bodies:

- WBC >10,000 usually means infection, inflammation, or tissue necrosis.
- WBC <4000 occurs with overwhelming infections.
- Neutrophils, which kill and digest bacteria, increase with bacterial infections.[1]
- Basophils and eosinophils are involved with allergic reactions and are capable of phagocytosis of antigen–antibody complexes.

Other tests give evidence of the severity of oxygen debt (deficit):

- Arterial blood gases (ABGs) reflect falling oxygen saturation/hypoxemia and base deficit as tissue perfusion decreases.[11]
- Serum lactate is elevated: Lactate is elevated because of anaerobic metabolism (increased lactic acid).
- Blood urea nitrogen (BUN) and creatinine increase when kidneys are damaged and filtering has been impaired.

Interventions and why?

The speed and appropriateness of therapy has a direct influence on outcomes:

- Administer prescribed crystalloid or colloid fluid resuscitation.
- Obtain blood cultures before antibiotics.
- Administer broad-spectrum antibiotic therapy until cultures return.
- Maintain mean arterial pressure with prescribed vasopressors (norepinephrine, dopamine).
- Continuously monitor all hemodynamic parameters available: CVP, PWP, and tissue oxygenation indicators.
- Notify the physician of fever, tachycardia, tachypnea, or decreasing O$_2$ saturation.
- Monitor ABGs and report promptly.
- Monitor hourly urine output, being alert to decreasing volume.

High-risk patients are taught health maintenance and preventive strategies to avoid infection and prevent recurrence:

- Adhere to meticulous personal hygiene.
- Maintain balanced, nutritious diet (increase protein and vitamin C for healing).
- Obtain pneumonia (pneumococcal) vaccine with a 5-year booster.
- Maintain seasonal influenza prophylaxis.
- Utilize diapers for incontinence rather than indwelling catheters (home bound patients).

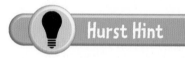

Hurst Hint

When you see cardiogenic shock, there will always be something wrong with the heart.

✚ Cardiogenic shock

What is it?

Cardiogenic shock is failure of the heart to pump blood to supply itself—and other vital organs and peripheral tissues—with a sufficient amount of oxygen to support and maintain cellular metabolism.

- When the heart is so damaged that it can no longer perfuse itself, the cardiac output falls quickly and dramatically and the patient becomes "shocky."
- The hypoxic, failing heart cannot keep blood moving forward; therefore, blood backs up into the lungs, causing pulmonary edema.
- With prolonged reduction of blood flow to vital organs, tissue hypoxia and multisystem organ failure occur.

- Oxygen is not being delivered to the vital organs and eventually without oxygen the cells go into the no-oxygen mode (anaerobic) of metabolism.

- Anaerobic metabolism leaves behind acid by-products that depress the muscle cells of the heart, causing cardiac arrhythmias and cardiac arrest.

Causes and why?

Cardiogenic shock occurs as a result of some kind of damage, insult, or injury to the heart that hinders its ability to effectively contract and pump the blood forward. In cardiogenic shock, the heart is too damaged to effectively perfuse itself or any other vital organ. When this happens, the heart cannot eject blood forward because the ischemic heart muscle can't pump effectively. In the presence of sustained ischemia, the heart beats erratically and cardiac output falls drastically.

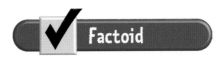

Factoid

When your patient develops cardiogenic shock, compensatory mechanisms have already failed, and the mortality rate has just increased significantly (Table 5-5)!

Table 5-5 Cardiogenic shock: understanding the why

Cause	Why
Myocardial infarction	Damaged heart cannot eject blood and cardiac output drops suddenly. The systolic pressure falls as compensatory mechanisms fail. The heart will do the best it can at any given moment under the existing circumstances, until finally the pump can no longer perfuse itself.
Lethal ventricular arrhythmias	The patient in sustained ventricular tachycardia will rapidly become unstable. Systolic blood pressure and cardiac output decrease because rapid heart rates reduce ventricular filling time. Ventricular tachycardia and ventricular fibrillation may occur because of myocardial ischemia after an acute MI.[12]
End-stage heart failure	Scarring of the myocardium from previous heart attacks, ventricular dilatation, and chronic myocardial ischemia damages the heart muscle, and wall motion becomes uncoordinated. (The ventricular chambers are not pumping together in synchrony.)

Signs and symptoms and why?

The patient will begin to display symptoms of shock secondary to a pump that can no longer move blood forward! Compensatory mechanisms common to hypovolemia are immediately activated, but sadly, these mechanisms only add to the workload of the already failing heart (Table 5-6).

Table 5-6 Signs and symptoms of cardiogenic shock

Signs and symptoms	Why
Tachycardia	The heart beats faster because of sympathetic stimulation, which is attempting to improve cardiac output. Unfortunately, this increases the workload on the heart and increases oxygen consumption resulting in myocardial hypoxia.
Cool, ashen skin	Vasoconstriction secondary to sympathetic stimulation brings less blood flow (warmth and color) to the skin.

(Continued)

Table 5-6 Signs and symptoms of cardiogenic shock (*Continued*)

Signs and symptoms	Why
Diaphoresis	Sympathetic stimulation activates the sweat glands.
Cyanosis of lips and nail beds	Stagnation of blood in the capillary bed after available oxygen has been extracted.
Increased central venous pressure (CVP) and pulmonary capillary wedge pressures (PCWP)	The failing pump cannot eject blood, yet more blood keeps coming into the heart, adding to blood that is already there, which increases the preload.

Interventions and why?

- Administer oxygen.
- Administer PRN morphine to relieve pain, anxiety and vasodilating properties to reduce preload and afterload.
- Administer prescribed IV diuretics to reduce circulating volume.
- Hemodynamic support: An intra-aortic balloon pump (IABP) is indicated to take over the workload of the left ventricle.
- Dobutamine is used to increase the cardiac output and systolic blood pressure, increasing perfusion of vital organs.
- Maintain bed rest in a low Fowler's position to promote oxygenation of the brain.
- First identify patients who are at risk and assess them very closely for early cardiac decompensation.
- Monitor vital signs, including LOC, and notify the doctor when you note early signs of falling cardiac output.
- Perform a focused cardiac assessment at frequent intervals (see Chapter 4).
- Monitor CVP and PWP (see Chapter 4) and notify the physician immediately for increasing pressure.
- Monitor hourly intake and output, being alert to any decrease in urinary output that could signal acute renal failure.
- In absolute physical and emotional arrest, the patient cannot tolerate any increase in workload to the heart. The patient will probably be sedated.
- Limit visitors to a minimum and avoid any lengthy or controversial conversations with the patient.

  The following measures can be put in place to support the failing heart and avoid volume excess:
- Diuretics (Lasix, Bumex)
- Vasodilators (Primacor, Nipride, Tridil)
- CRRT (continuous renal replacement therapy)
- Oxygen as indicated per pulse oximetry or ABGs

- Vasopressors to raise BP and increase CO
- Antiarrhythmics to correct major dysrhythmias
- Rescue percutaneous angioplasty if indicated

For a complete list of cardiac patient teaching, refer to Chapter 4. Teaching topics include self-care, monitoring, and medications to risk reduction and cardiac rehab.

✚ Multiple organ dysfunction syndrome

What is it?

Multiple organ dysfunction syndrome (MODS) is the progressive failure of two or more organs that results from an acute, severe illnesses or injury (sepsis, trauma, burns) requiring medical intervention to achieve homeostasis. Once organs begin to fail, there is a sharp increase in the mortality rate.

What causes it and why?

Any form of shock (which produces systemic inflammatory mediators) or systemic inflammatory response syndrome (SIRS) can activate the deadly cascade that ends in MODS. MODS results from SIRS. SIRS is a systemic inflammatory response that is triggered by many different processes, such as sepsis, burns, crushing injuries, pancreatitis, myocardial infarction, shock states, and post-resuscitation. Prevention of the progression from SIRS to MODS is the key to improving mortality rates.

Interventions

- Prevention is priority since mortality rate is 80% to 100% once multiple organs have failed. Patients at high risk for hypoperfusion must be identified and monitored intensely to recognize early warning signs of shock/tissue hypoxia (see hypovolemic shock).
- Refer to resuscitation guidelines for septic shock.

Frequently, the patient may experience more than one type of shock simultaneously. A patient in hypovolemic shock may develop septic shock as well, and low perfusion to organs will trigger MODS. Therefore, patient needs are the same as for hypovolemic and septic shock. (Refer to previous teaching outlined.)

For those unfortunate circumstances in which my patient has failure of three or more organs and reaches the end point of resuscitation, family members are advised that there is no coming back. Those awaiting the inevitable are taught:

- Realistic expectations and end of life physical signs (eg, mottling, first distally in feet/hands, gradually, creeping up the extremities with them becoming cold) as comfort measures are implemented.
- Customary protocols and usual care of the terminal patient to hopefully relieve some of the uncertainty and (possibly) avert anger toward health care providers for designating an end point to resuscitation.

PATIENT TEACHING Because MODS can occur later, after the acute symptomatic stage of shock from which the patient has seemingly recovered, the patient/significant other/family members should be taught to:

- Be on guard for subtle changes that could signal organ dysfunction, and access the health care delivery system immediately.
- Avoid overstressing the body with added oxygen demand during the recovery period following serious illness, injury, or shock.
- Closely monitor urinary output, and change in volume or color of urine.
- Report even subtle changes forewarning of organ dysfunction, especially mental changes (brain) and shortness of breath (lungs) or fatigue (heart).

SUMMARY

Shock is a life threatening condition that can result as a response to a variety of diseases. Regardless of the cause of shock, the central concern is inadequate tissue perfusion that can result in cell death in vital organs. Nursing care should be focused on prevention of shock progression through skilled assessment and prompt interventions.

PRACTICE QUESTIONS

1. Which of the following patients would the nurse monitor most closely for the development of *hypovolemic* shock?

    A. An adult man who has acute myocardial infarction

    B. A middle-aged patient in acute Addisonian crisis

    C. An elderly woman following insertion of a central line

    D. A young adult man who has a pulmonary embolism

2. Which of the following interventions would the nurse predict to be of *least* benefit for hypotension when the patient is in cardiogenic shock following acute myocardial infarction?

    A. Prompt, aggressive thrombolysis

    B. Vasopressor agents (catecholamines)

    C. Vasodilating agents (eg, nitrates)

    D. Plasma volume replacement therapy

3. When assessing shock states, which type of shock would the nurse recognize as being different from all other classic presentations of shock?

    A. Burn shock

    B. Septic shock

    C. Hemorrhagic shock

    D. Cardiogenic shock

4. Following spinal anesthesia, a hypotensive mother and unborn baby are at risk for the effects of distributive shock resulting from loss of sympathetic vasomotor tone. Which nursing intervention is the priority upon recognition of this shock state?

   A. Place the woman in a Trendelenburg position.

   B. Administer an IVF bolus of isotonic solution.

   C. Rotate tourniquets on both lower extremities.

   D. Lower the head of the bed and apply oxygen at 2 L/min.

5. A patient has severe respiratory distress following a bee sting. The nurse will anticipate the need to administer which first-line drug?

   A. Oxygen

   B. Albuterol

   C. Epinephrine

   D. Hydrocortisone

6. Which nursing implementation is the priority when the patient is in septic shock?

   A. Obtain cultures.

   B. Administer steroids.

   C. Administer vasopressors.

   D. Notify the next of kin.

7. Post insertion of a central line, the nurse notes that the patient's CVP is elevated, yet the systolic blood pressure is steadily decreasing. Which first intervention is indicated?

   A. Notify the physician.

   B. Lower the head of the bed.

   C. Apply oxygen per nasal cannula.

   D. Hang the patient's legs dependent.

8. A post-MI patient shows signs and symptoms of early cardiogenic shock. Which nursing intervention is the priority?

   A. Administer oxygen per nasal cannula.

   B. Change the patient's gown and linens.

   C. Administer prescribed sedation for restlessness.

   D. Set up an intra-aortic balloon pump (IABP) for immediate usage.

9. An unresponsive patient arrives in the ED wearing a medic-alert bracelet stating severe peanut allergy. Respiratory arrest and collapse occurred after ingestion of a chocolate candy topped ice cream dessert. Which intervention is the priority?

A. Prepare to assist with endotracheal intubation.

B. Administer 100% oxygen per nonrebreather face mask.

C. Administer epinephrine and antihistamines as prescribed.

D. Initiate an additional IV access for a hypotonic IV fluid bolus.

10. An infant is delivered, and with the birth cry develops cyanosis and marked dyspnea. Which nursing assessment would confirm obstructive shock?

A. Concave abdomen

B. Mottled, splotchy extremities

C. High systolic blood pressure

D. High-pitched crowing sounds with respirations

References

1. George-Gay B, Chernecky CC. *Clinical Medical Surgical Nursing: A Decision Making Reference.* Philadelphia: Saunders; 2002.

2. Porth CM. *Pathophysiology: Concepts of Altered Health States.* 7th ed. Philadelphia: Lippincott Williams & Wilkins; 2007.

3. Russel JA. Current treatment of septic shock. *Minerva Med* 99(5):433–458, 2008.

4. Lee LN. *The Physics Factbook.* http://hypertextbook.com/facts/1998/LanNaLee.shtml. Accessed January 15, 2009.

5. Hogan MA, Hill K. *Pathophysiology: Reviews and Rationales.* Upper Saddle River, NJ: Pearson Education; 2004.

6. Kelly DM. Hypovolemic shock: An overview. *Crit Care Nurs* 28(1):2–19, 2005.

7. Ghafari MH, Moosavizadeh SA, Moharari RS, Khashayer P. Hypertonic saline 5% vs lactated ringer for resuscitating patients in hemorrhagic shock. *Middle East J Anesthesiol* 19(6):1337–1347, 2008.

8. Johnson RF, Peebles R Jr. Anaphylactic shock: pathophysiology, recognition and treatment. *Semin Respir Crit Care Med.* Accessed January 31, 2009.

9. Yong PFK, Birns J, Ibrahim MAA. Anaphylactic shock: The great mimic. *So Med J.* Posted on Medscape April 12, 2007; Accessed February 21, 2009

10. Pagana KD, Pagana TJ. *Mosby's Diagnostic and Laboratory Test Reference.* 6th ed. St. Louis: Mosby; 2003.

11. Husein FA, Martin MJ, Mullinex PS, et al. Serum lactate and base deficit as predictors of mortality and morbidity. *Am J Surg* 185(5):484–491, 2003.

12. Corwin EJ. *Handbook of Pathophysiology.* 2nd ed. Philadelphia: Lippincott Williams & Wilkins; 2000:406–407.

6 Respiratory Disorders

OBJECTIVES

In this chapter you will review:

- The pathophysiology associated with common respiratory disorders.
- The key concepts and priorities associated with respiratory nursing care.
- The technologic advances that improve the quality of life and reduce threat to life when the respiratory system fails or is compromised.
- Risk reduction to promote respiratory health and optimal pulmonary function.
- The body's compensatory response to respiratory dysfunction.
- Treatment modalities and nursing care to promote restoration of highest level respiratory function.
- The impact of lifestyle choices, genetics, chemicals/pollutants, and comorbidities that alter pulmonary ventilation, perfusion of blood through the lungs, and diffusion of oxygen.
- Components of a teaching plan to enhance self-care monitoring for the patient recovering from an acute exacerbation of a chronic respiratory condition.

OBSTRUCTIVE PULMONARY DISORDERS

A number of acute and chronic disorders can result in pulmonary obstruction.

✚ Asthma

See Figure 6-1.

▶ Figure 6-1. Respiratory System/ Upper and Lower Airways. The respiratory system is comprised of the upper and lower airways and is responsible for gas exchange within the body.

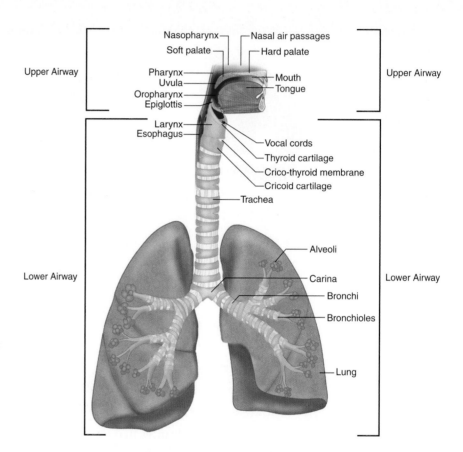

Let's get the normal stuff straight!

The function of the respiratory system is to exchange oxygen and carbon dioxide. This gas exchange is dependent upon three factors: ventilation, perfusion of blood through the lungs, and diffusion. Parasympathetic stimulation (vagus nerve and cholinergic receptors) produce bronchial constriction, and sympathetic stimulation (B_2-adrenergic receptors) produces bronchodilation. During exercise when a person needs more oxygen, the sympathetic nervous system is stimulated, causing bronchodilation and increased air intake.

What is it?

Asthma is a disease that is caused by an overreaction of the airways to irritants or other stimuli. In normal lungs, irritants may have no effect. Asthma is considered both chronic and inflammatory and a type of chronic obstructive pulmonary disease (COPD). As a result, the client with asthma experiences bronchial constriction, spasm, increased mucus secretions, mucosal edema, and air hunger. The episodes of asthma are usually recurring and attacks may be caused by exposure to irritants, fatigue, and/or emotional situations. It often occurs in childhood, but can occur at any age. The disease can be intrinsic or extrinsic, and many patients experience a combination of both (Fig. 6-2; Table 6-1).

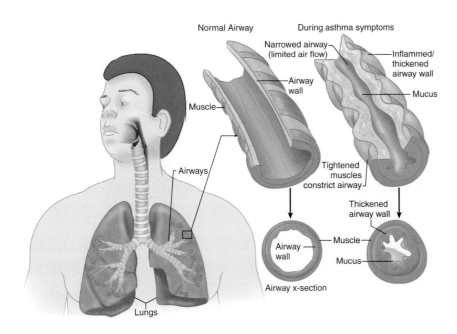

◀ Figure 6-2. Bronchial Spasm and Asthmatic Bronchiole. During asthma attacks mucous production is increased and is difficult to dislodge, and the airway becomes narrow because of the spasm of smooth muscle of the airway and edema that results from increased vascular permeability.

Table 6-1 Intrinsic and extrinsic asthma

Intrinsic (nonatopic)	Extrinsic (atopic)
Caused by anything except an allergy	Associated with allergens such as pollen, pet dander, and dust mites.
Can be caused by chemicals such as cigarette smoke or cleaning agents, taking aspirin, a chest infection, stress, laughter, exercise, cold air, or food preservatives	Starts in childhood/teenage years.
May be caused by irritation of nerves or muscles of the airway	Familial predisposition: One-third of clients have at least one family member with a diagnosis of asthma.
Most episodes occur after an infection of the respiratory tract	Usually have other allergy problems such as hay fever, hives, allergic rhinitis, or eczema.

Causes and why?

Airway inflammation related to asthma occurs because of cells that cause inflammation—mainly lymphocytes, eosinophils, and mast cells. The inflamed airway becomes damaged and narrowed, which increases the work of breathing.

These attacks may be brought on by exposure to irritants, fatigue, and/or emotional situations that would ordinarily have no effect on normal lungs (Table 6-2).

Table 6-2 Asthma: causes and why

Causes	Why
Environmental irritants: pet dander, dust and dust mites, cockroaches, fungi, mold, pollen, feathers, smoke, foods, cold air, food additives	Allergens cause histamine release, smooth muscles swell, airway narrows, poor gas exchange results.
Stress	Hormones can influence gas exchange.
Exercise	Increases work of breathing, making air exchange more difficult.

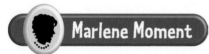

I always knew that I was allergic to exercise; now I realize this is a legitimate excuse!

Once the offending agent/ condition triggers an acute episode of asthma, the following pathophysiology develops quickly, usually within 10 to 20 minutes.

- Mast cells to the rescue! The IgE-coating of the uppermost mucosal mast cells release chemical mediators to do their dirty work: histamines, bradykinins, prostaglandins, and leukotrienes.
- Chemical mediators open the door to the underlying more abundant submucosal mast cells, moving the antigen/irritant into deeper tissue.
- Edema occurs because of increased vascular permeability. Resultant swelling of the mucosal surface lining the airways reduces the size of already tiny bronchioles.
- Bronchospasm caused by direct parasympathetic stimulation produces constriction of smooth muscles criss-crossing the airways, even further reducing the diameter of airways.
- Goblet cells go wild and start producing mucus like crazy! Mucus in bronchial airways reduces size of conducting airways, and can even plug off smaller bronchioles.

Fibrotic changes and remodeling of the airways can occur over time as a result of chronic inflammation:

- Enlarged mucus glands produce thick mucus.
- Leaky (permeable) vessels attract white blood cells (WBCs) to the area, causing even more sludging in the airways.
- Hypertrophy (enlargement) of bronchial muscles.
- Fibrosis develops in the sub-basement membranes to permanently change the size and shape of bronchioles.

Signs and symptoms and why?

The episodes of respiratory distress associated with asthma involve the following common signs and symptoms:

- Coughing: This is often worse at night or early morning, making it hard to sleep.
- Mucus production: Thick, sticky, tenacious mucus is hard to raise, making the cough productive only infrequently.
- Wheezing: Noisy respirations, a whistling or squeaky sound on inspiration.
- Chest tightness: Like something is squeezing or there's a weight on the chest.

- Shortness of breath: Not being able to catch the breath or feeling out of breath, or not able to get air out of the lungs.

Sometimes the symptoms go away spontaneously or with minimal treatment, and sometimes they get progressively worse until a trip to the emergency department is necessary because of ineffective airway clearance. During an acute episode, the patient may become very frightened and anxious.

Testing, testing, testing

Test	Clinical significance	Nursing care	Common interfering factors
Allergy testing	Identifies a trigger or triggers to avoid	Obtain a patient history of recent exposure to new or different items.	
Sputum specimen	Reveals elevated eosinophils	Provide mouth care prior to obtaining the specimen (rinse mouth with water only). Obtain the specimen in the morning upon wakening if possible.	
WBC (blood test)	May reveal elevated eosinophils		
ABGs (arterial blood gases) Pulmonary function tests	Reveals hypoxemia and hypocapnia with respiratory alkalosis initially (because of fast breathing)		

Pulmonary function tests are a group of tests that measure lung function (Table 6-3).

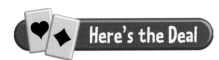

If the episodes of asthma are seasonal, the physician will suspect pollens, but if the attacks are recurrent, then other environmental agents, such as new clothing, fabrics/starches, soaps/detergents, etc may be the offending agent.

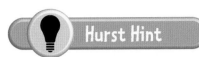

Sputum specimens are sterile, even though the mouth is not! Have the patient rinse his or her mouth first to reduce the bacterial count, and expectorate into a sterile sputum cup, not allowing the lips to touch (contaminate) the container.

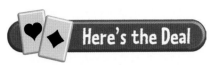

During episodes of fast breathing, respiratory alkalosis and hypocapnia may be present (because of the loss of CO_2, which is acid), but this changes as the patient begins to tire and hypoxia worsens.

Table 6-3 Diagnostic tests to measure pulmonary function

Test	Clinical significance	Nursing care	Common interfering factors
SPIROMETRY A common test to monitor air volume and flow rates, and graphs on the screen show volume/time curves and flow volume loop graphs.	*Forced vital capacity* (FCV) is the maximum amount of air that can be inhaled and exhaled. *Forced expiratory volume (FVE-1).* The maximum amount of air that can be exhaled in 1 second.	Provide patient teaching regarding procedure. The patient wears a nose clip and breathes into a mouthpiece with tubing connected to the spirometer.	
Methacholine challenge test.	Used in conjunction with spirometry, the agent (methacholine) is inhaled as an aerosol mist in increasing amounts to simulate inhaled allergens. The test is positive if lung function drops by at least 20%.	A bronchodilator is given on completion of the test to reverse the effects of the methacholine. Assess respiratory status before, during, and after the procedure. Ensure emergency equipment is available in the event of respiratory distress.	

 Hurst Hint

Prior to pulmonary function tests, instruct the patient to avoid stimulants (caffeine/chocolate), exposure to cold air, exercise, or smoking on the day of the test. Also advise the patient not to eat a heavy meal before the test.

Interventions and why?

Administer the following classifications of antiasthmatic medications as prescribed:

- Short-acting bronchodilators for quick relief
- Systemic and/or inhaled corticosteroids
- Short-acting beta$_2$ adrenergic agonist (SABA)
- Long-acting inhaled beta$_2$ agonist (LABA)
- Leukotriene receptor antagonist blocker (LTRA)
- Leukotriene modifier (LTM)
- Xanthine bronchodilator
- Mast cell stabilizer

If symptoms are poorly controlled, the patient is evaluated for how well he or she is adhering to the prescribed treatment plan, whether self-administration techniques for medication administration are effective, and environmental exposure to triggers is under control (Table 6-4).

Table 6-4 Medications used to treat asthma

Recommended	Indications	Example: trade name/generic name
Short-acting beta$_2$ adrenergic agonist (sympathomimetic) (SABA)	Rescue inhaler: fast acting bronchodilator; U, used for acute or intermittent asthma and chronic asthma. Inhibits histamine release by the mast cells. Also used for prevention of exercise-induced asthma.	Proventil, Ventolin, Salbutamol (albuterol)
Inhaled corticosteroid (ICS)	Can be used alone (step 1) to reduce the inflammatory response or combined with LABA (step 2) bronchodilator.	Beclovent (beclomethasone dipropionate) Pulmicort Turbuhaler (budesonide) AeroBid (flunisolide)
Long-acting inhaled beta$_2$ agonist (LABA)	Produces rapid relief of bronchoconstriction: Also used for prevention of exercise-induced asthma (EIB).	Serevent (salmeterol xinafoate) Formoterol
Leukotriene receptor antagonist blocker (LTRA)	Bronchodilator, respiratory smooth muscle relaxant. Inhibits the enzyme necessary to convert arachidonic acid to leukotrienes.	Singulair (montelukast) Accolate (zafirlukast)
Leukotriene modifier (LTM)	Inhibits the leukotriene pathway to inflammation.	Luteol, Zyflo (zileuton)
Xanthine bronchodilator	Respiratory smooth muscle relaxant, respiratory and cerebral stimulant.	Elixophyllin, Slo-Bid, Theo-Dur, Bronkodyl (theophylline)
Mast cell stabilizer	Antiasthmatic, anti-inflammatory agent. Inhibits release of inflammatory mediators histamine and prostaglandin D$_2$.	Tilade (cromolyn, nedocromil sodium)

Source: Berger W. (2007) New approaches to managing asthma: a US perspective. *Therapeutics and Clinical Management.* 4(2):363-379.

PATIENT TEACHING: DISCHARGE PLANNING   The priority teaching focus for the patient with asthma is self-management behaviors. My patient needs to understand how to manage his or her asthma so that acute severe attacks are kept to a minimum to minimize complications and permanent damage from chronic inflammation that results in remodeling of the airways.

Teaching should always begin with the most basic healthy behaviors:

- Drink adequate water (64 oz daily) to liquefy secretions so they can be easily raised.

- Practice relaxation techniques to reduce the reaction to stress and stressors.

- Hand hygiene (washing frequently) to reduce contact with cold germs (rhinovirus in particular)[1] that can live on inanimate objects for weeks, being transferred from hand to face to nose!

- Daily exercise with warm-up and pretreatment medications for EIB (see specific guidelines for exercise induced bronchospasm [EIB]).[2]

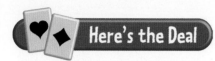

Here's the Deal

If patients don't use aerosol inhaler devices correctly, they will not receive maximum benefit of the medication. If the patient has special needs (has poor coordination or limited dexterity), the nurse can collaborate with the physician regarding the type of device prescribed. Supervised practice should be available well before hospital discharge.

Hurst Hint

Focus discharge teaching on common errors that asthma patients tend to make:

- Breathing in too fast: Teach slow deliberate breaths.
- Getting teeth and tongue in the way of the medication spray: Have the patient open the mouth wide, then close lips around the mouthpiece.
- Avoid complications of inhaled steroids (candidiasis and dysphonia) by remembering to either use a spacer or rinse the mouth after use.[3]

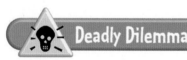

Deadly Dilemma

Treatment of hypoxia resulting from an acute asthma attack is always the top priority!

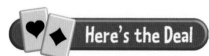

Here's the Deal

Two to four puffs of a short-acting bronchodilator, usually an inhaled beta$_2$-agonist, can be used and repeated up to three times after intervals of 20 minutes.

The revised guidelines set forth by the NAEPP and the Global Initiative for Asthma (GINA) recommends the following target areas for patient teaching:

- Monitor peak expiratory flow (PEF).
- Avoid or remove known triggers.
- Adhere to the prescribed medication regimen.
- Prevent the development of osteoporosis associated with use of corticosteroids: adequate calcium and vitamin D intake.
- Treat symptoms as soon as possible to prevent a severe exacerbation (flare-up).
- Continue to take controller medicine, even when there are no symptoms—the disease is still there, and can flare up at any time.

What can harm my patient and why?

- Bronchial constriction and spasm can severely reduce air flow during acute attacks.
- Chronic inflammation from repeated episodes causes thickening of the epithelial layer of the airways and remodeling of the bronchioles.
- Poorly controlled asthma interferes with a person's life, and the quality of life suffers.
- Repeated sick days because of incapacitating symptoms may cause missed work or school, and strained relationships.
- Even without a current acute flare-up, the patient may be chronically fatigued from lost sleep because of night time mucus secretions and coughing.
- If episodes are frequent, and trips to the emergency department are often, the person does not have the physical or psychic energy to focus on any other aspect of life. When a person can't breathe, then nothing else really matters.
- Depending on the severity of the attack, with status asthmaticus being the most severe, the patient could die from airway obstruction and hypoxia.
- The mortality rate at the last official census was >4000 deaths during a two-year period.[4]
- Intravenous epinephrine for emergency use will produce immediate bronchodilation.
- Based on ABGs, oxygen administration may be indicated before and/or after emergency nebulizer treatment.
- Because the inflammatory response (with edema of the airways) is a usual cause of exacerbation, intravenous corticosteroids may be administered.
- The patient with diagnosed asthma has quick relief medications for opening up airways during acute exacerbations.

✚ Chronic obstructive pulmonary disease (COPD)

Let's get the normal stuff straight!

Respiration involves the exchange oxygen and carbon dioxide. This gas exchange (ventilation, perfusion of blood through the lungs, and diffusion) takes place throughout the upper and lower airways. Working like billows, the lungs move air in and out of the lungs effortlessly and quietly with equal bilateral excursion. The tiny, spongelike alveolar sacs are normally elastic and contain surfactant-secreting cells. The surfactant stabilizes the alveolus and allows them to collapse on end respiration, thereby decreasing the work of breathing.

What is it?

Chronic obstructive lung disease is the name given to a condition in which two pulmonary diseases exist at the same time: chronic bronchitis and emphysema. Also chronic asthma in combination with emphysema or bronchitis may cause COPD.

COPD is a condition that is characterized by obstructed air passageways that limit airflow, restricting ventilation. Bronchitis occurs when the bronchi are chronically inflamed and irritated. Swelling and production of thick mucus produces obstruction of large and small air passageways. Emphysema causes the lungs to lose their elasticity, becoming stiff and noncompliant with trapping of air and chronically distended alveoli.

Destruction of alveolar tissue reduces surface area for gas exchange. This results in a ventilation-perfusion mismatch and impaired gas exchange. The loss of elastic fibers reduces expiratory airflow resulting in trapped air, carbon dioxide retention, and collapse of airways.

Causes and why?

Cigarette smoking (active or passive) is the most important risk factor, and leading cause of chronic bronchitis and emphysema. Smoking causes irritation and inflammation, which over time causes remodeling (structural changes) of the alveoli.

A less common cause of emphysema (approximately 1% of cases) results from an inherited deficiency of a lung protective enzyme (antiprotease). When this enzyme is lacking, protease digests proteins, which leads to the decreased elasticity of alveolar walls. If emphysema occurs prior to age 40, the antiprotease enzyme is most probably deficient.

Signs and symptoms and why?

COPD has two presentations: the "pink puffer," the patient with emphysema, and the "blue bloater," the patient with chronic bronchitis. Refer to Table 6-5 for characteristic signs and symptoms of Type A (pink puffer) and Type B (blue bloater), keeping in mind the fact that longstanding illness will produce a combined form of COPD characteristics (Fig. 6-3).

Table 6-5   Signs and symptoms of bronchitis and emphysema

Pink puffer: pulmonary emphysema	Blue bloater: chronic bronchitis
Dyspnea, tachypnea, use of accessory muscles because of increased work of breathing and decreased alveolar ventilation	Excessive mucus production: may be gray, white, or yellow
Barrel-shaped chest with increased AP diameter because of hyperinflated lungs and trapped air	Edema, ascites because of right heart failure causing blood/fluid backing up into systemic circulation
Grunting and prolonged expirations in an effort to keep the airways open	Dyspnea and poor exercise tolerance because of air-flow obstruction
Clubbing of fingers and toes because of chronic hypoxia causing tissues changes	Dusky, cyanotic nail beds and lips because of hypoxia
Inspiratory wheezes, crackles because of the collapse of bronchioles	Expiratory wheezes, rhonchi, crackles
Productive morning cough as secretions pool over night while sleeping	Chronic cough in effort to expel excess mucus
Weight loss because of excessive energy expenditure with work of breathing and decreased caloric intake because of dyspnea	Weight gain because of fluid retention secondary to cor pulmonale (right heart failure) caused by pulmonary hypertension
Sits upright and uses pursed lip "puffer" breathing, exerting pressure to keep alveoli open (positive airway pressure)	Dyspnea, tachypnea, and use of accessory muscles because of hypoxia
Decreased chest expansion because of trapped air and stiff lungs	Polycythemia because of chronic hypoxemia, which triggers release of erythropoietin

Source: Hurst M. *Hurst Reviews: Pathophysiology Review.* New York: McGraw-Hill; 2008.

▶ Figure 6-3. Clubbing of the Fingers. One sign of patients with COPD is the clubbing of the fingers and toes. The chronic hypoxia causes tissue changes that alter the angle of the nail beds.

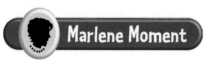
Marlene Moment

If you can't breathe, forget trying to eat. It won't happen!

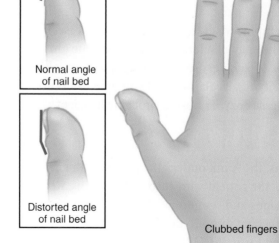

Normal angle of nail bed

Distorted angle of nail bed

Clubbed fingers

Testing, testing, testing

Refer to diagnostic tests for asthma (earlier in this chapter) for a more detailed description of the following:

- Pulmonary function tests
- Pulse oximetry
- Chest X-ray
- ABGs (See Chapter 3 for detailed explanation of respiratory acidosis and respiratory alkalosis.)

Interventions and why?

- Monitor ABGs and relay reports to physician.
- Monitor oxygen saturation (pulse oximetry) frequently (to determine adequate oxygenation).

    Monitor for early signs of respiratory acidosis (eg, headache, lethargy, confusion).

    Administer prescribed medications and monitor effectiveness:
- Bronchodilators
- Mucolytics
- Anticholinergics
- Steroids
- Leukotriene antagonists
- Anxiolytics
- Diuretics (indicated with right-sided heart failure)

    Because of real, potential, or high risk for infection:
- Administer prescribed antibiotics, prophylactic antibiotics.
- Provide meticulous mouth care several times per day.
- Monitor effectiveness of respiratory therapy and pulmonary rehabilitation.
- Monitor sputum for change in color (which may indicate infection).

    Because of debilitation and low energy level:
- Position patient high Fowler's or orthopneic, with support to elbows.
- Assist with personal hygiene, spacing activities to avoid fatigue.
- Place personal items within easy reach, and check on patient often.

PATIENT TEACHING   Give factual information about the benefits and availability of smoking cessation programs. However, smoking cessation requires that the patient desire quitting because of excessive mucus production, the patient needs to be taught how to clear airways:

- Vibration or clapping to loosen thick secretions.
- Hydration to liquefy viscous secretions.
- Postural drainage allows gravity to clear lobules of the lung.

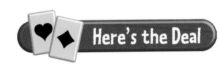

Here's the Deal

It is always better to assess your patient closely and notify the rapid response team in advance of calling a "code" when respiratory arrest is in progress.

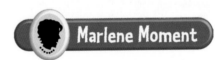

Marlene Moment

Yellow certainly means caution/danger, but green does not mean go when it comes to sputum color. It means INFECTION!

Because of weight loss and malnutrition the patient is taught to:

- Eat small, nutrient dense foods (three meals and three snacks).
- Foods should not require much chewing (interferes with breathing).

Because of the high risk of infection, the patient is taught to:

- Stay away from people who are sick.
- Keep immunizations current: influenza and pneumococcal pneumonia.
- Monitor sputum for change in color: Notify health care provider for yellow, green, or rusty sputum.

What can harm my patient and why?

Patients with COPD are totally consumed with the work of breathing, and this permeates their life. Psychosocial issues are related to withdrawal, decreased ability to communicate (because it requires air), and decreased enjoyment of life. Like any disease state, there are degrees of COPD, but when the condition is advanced, the patient can become totally disabled and debilitated, which places him or her at risk for:

- Infection
- Injury from falls
- Respiratory failure

A-B-Cs are always first! If the patient has respiratory arrest, immediate resuscitation is required:

- Ventilatory assistance (manual Ambu-bag breathe)
- Endotracheal intubation and ventilator with positive end expiratory pressure to hold airways open (PEEP).
- Monitor ABGs and administer oxygen accordingly as prescribed.
- Administer bronchodilators and steroids as prescribed.

Cutting edge

The COPD diet calls for fruits, vegetables, and fish with a minimum of other meats if your patient wants to have fewer respiratory symptoms and avoid a decline in lung function.[5] Fruits and vegetables and fish are packed with antioxidants, omega-3 fatty acids, and are alkaline rich[6] to help counteract retained acid (CO_2) from poor expiratory function. Cured meats are particularly harmful to lung tissue because the nitrite preservatives cause structural damage to lungs similar to the damage seen with COPD.[7] Two major eating patterns have been the focus of a long-range study (12 years) and their effects compared in relation to development of nitrogenous damage to lung tissue:

- The Western way of death: Cured and red meats, french fries, desserts, and sweets
- The prudent diet: Whole grains, fruits, vegetables, and fish

As the Western diet scores increased in adult men, so did the incidence of newly diagnosed COPD. An additional advantage of the prudent diet

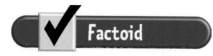

Factoid

If your patient has COPD, administering oxygen >2 to 3 L/min can lead to respiratory failure.

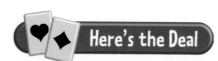

Here's the Deal

The normal stimulus to breathe is high levels of CO_2, but because the patient with COPD has chronically high levels of CO_2, chemoreceptors become insensitive to carbon dioxide; therefore, the lack of oxygen becomes the stimulus to breathe. As long as your COPD patient is hypoxic, he or she will continue to breathe. However, if this patient is given too much oxygen, breathing will stop.

was noted when cough with phlegm disappeared as nonstarch polysaccharides were added to the diet. Dietary fiber (fruits, vegetables, whole grains) are loaded with these beneficial nonstarch polysaccharides!

✛ Pulmonary embolus

Let's get the normal stuff straight!

The function of lung tissue is respiration, which enables gas exchange, producing the oxygenation of the blood and the removal of carbon dioxide. This normal respiratory exchange cannot take place unless the lungs are adequately perfused with oxygenated blood. Let's review circulation to the lungs:

- The lungs have two sources of blood flow: pulmonary circulation and bronchial circulation.
- Bronchial arteries branch off the thoracic aorta and enter the lungs with the right and left bronchi.
- Bronchial circulation supplies oxygen to the structures and supporting tissue of all the air passageways.
- Larger bronchial veins drain back into the vena cava.
- Pulmonary circulation is responsible for gas exchange.
- The pulmonary artery leaves the right heart and carries deoxygenated blood to the lungs to pick up oxygen and leave behind CO_2.
- The four pulmonary veins drain blood from the lungs, returning oxygenated blood to the left heart.
- Bronchial blood vessels have the unique capability of being able to form new vessels (angiogenesis) to produce collateral circulation in the event of obstructed pulmonary circulation (as with pulmonary embolism).
- Collateral bronchial blood flow is a back-up mechanism to help keep lung tissue alive while pulmonary circulation is being restored.

What is it?

Pulmonary embolus is a life-threatening condition that happens when a thrombus travels with the direction of blood flow toward the heart, and from the right ventricle goes via the pulmonary artery to the lungs (Fig. 6-4).

▶ Figure 6-4. Pulmonary Embolism from Lower Extremity. A pulmonary embolism is a life-threatening condition that occurs when a thrombus travels with the direction of blood flow until it arrives in the lungs via the pulmonary artery.

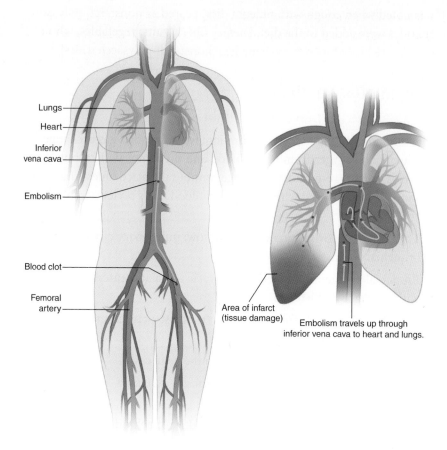

Lungs
Heart
Inferior vena cava
Embolism
Blood clot
Femoral artery
Area of infarct (tissue damage)
Embolism travels up through inferior vena cava to heart and lungs.

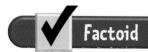

Factoid

One out of four patients hospitalized for acute exacerbation of COPD may have a pulmonary embolus![10]

Causes and why?

In order to have an embolus, the patient must first have a thrombus. Some patients are at greater risk of thrombus formation because of disease states such as diabetes, heart failure, and obstructive lung disease. Pregnancy, advanced age, and obesity also increase risk for development of a thrombus.[9]

Thromboembolism is directly related to venostasis and/or trauma to the vessel wall, which could occur in any of the following situations:

• Prolonged bed rest in excess of 1 week: Because the skeletal muscle pump is inactive when the patient is nonambulatory, reducing venous return to the heart, leading to venostasis. Also, bed rest induces diuresis because of improved renal perfusion, which also contributes to sluggish venous blood flow.

• Chronic lung disease with bed rest in excess of 3 days: Low oxygen levels lead to polycythemia and increased blood viscosity. Added to bed rest and inactivity, this even further reduces venous blood return.

• Vessel trauma, because endothelial injury at the site of trauma leads to local inflammation and influx of WBCs, platelets, and fibrin.

• Major surgery within four weeks, because surgical stress increases blood clotting factors.

- Use of oral contraceptives leading to increased coagulability, especially when coupled with nicotine, which is a powerful vasoconstrictor.
- Any diagnosis of cancer, with or without chemotherapy.[15]
- Conditions that increase blood viscosity, such as obesity or polycythemia (increased red blood cells sludging up blood flow).
- Venostasis from any reason: dehydration, prolonged sitting or standing, burns during the plasma to interstitial fluid shift, diuresis from alcohol abuse, or FVD caused by ulcerative colitis or ileostomy[11]

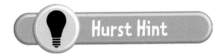

Hurst Hint

Be on the lookout for patients at high risk for PE! They will all have venostasis and increased coagulability!

Signs and symptoms and why?

When a thrombus has traveled to the lung and obstructed perfusion of blood into the lung, alveolar ventilation is halted; therefore, the patient has an oxygenation problem!

The symptoms associated with a small area of obstructed pulmonary vasculature may be subtle and easily overlooked or they could be confused with other respiratory problems. If the embolus occludes one branch of the pulmonary artery, or >50% of the pulmonary vasculature, death may be the first indication of a PE.[10]

A small clot obstructing a small vessel will hopefully remain a small, manageable problem, but a large clot obstructing a large vessel is a massive problem! The patient will have the following signs and symptoms:

- Chest pain (classic three "S" type), sudden, sharp, and stabbing! Or the discomfort could be referred to the back, shoulder, or abdomen.
- Shortness of breath with wheezing or rales on auscultation.
- Productive cough with hemoptysis (coughing up bloody sputum).
- Low and/or declining oxygen saturation.
- Tachycardia, possibly arrhythmias if oxygen deprived.
- An area of atelectasis over the affected lung field on auscultation.
- Hypotension, which accompanies decreased cardiac output.
- EKG changes, which demonstrate hypoxia and right ventricular strain:
  - Tachycardia
  - S wave in lead I
  - Q wave in lead III[10]
  - Right bundle branch block[15]
  - Inverted T wave in lead III
- Jugular venous distention (JVD)[10]

Testing, testing, testing

See Table 6-6.

Table 6-6   Tests for pulmonary embolus

Test	Clinical significance	Nursing care	Common interfering factors
D-dimer	This blood assay detects fragments of blood clots that are produced by the body's mechanism for breaking up clots. D-dimer in excess of 500 mg/mL (in a nonsurgical patient) may indicate a pulmonary embolus.		
Pulmonary arteriography (angiography): X-ray dye is injected into the pulmonary vessels through a central line in the right heart.	Vascular filling defects or an abrupt disruption of blood flow can be visualized.		
Lung scan (ventilation-perfusion scan or VQ scan) Radiopaque dye is injected peripherally and outlines lung tissue.	This test helps provide a diagnosis of PE because areas of actual pulmonary ventilation and pulmonary perfusion can be directly visualized.		
Computed tomography (CT of the lung: spiral CT or CT angiography)	Provides visualization of a blood clot in the lung or in the leg.[15]		

Interventions and why?

The patient having respiratory distress that occurs suddenly and without warning will be anxious and apprehensive, especially if he or she is struggling to breathe. Hypoxia can begin to affect vital organs quickly. If PE is suspected because of identified risk factors and patient symptoms, here's what to do first:

- Stay with the patient and call for help, equipment, and supplies (ie, IV start kit, oxygen flow meter, pulse oximeter, etc) (Table 6-7).
- Notify the physician of respiratory distress.
- Obtain a quick bleeding history (recent surgery, dental extractions, peptic ulcer disease, etc) to determine candidacy for thrombolysis.
- Call for stat ABGs and relay results to physician immediately.
- Elevate the head of the bed and apply oxygen as indicated to maintain SpO_2 >90%.

Table 6-7   Delivery of oxygen to acutely breathless adults

Simple face mask with open side port	Side port allows room air to enter mask, diluting oxygen; can deliver 40%–60% oxygen with flow rates of 10–12 L/min.
Partial rebreather face mask with one-way discs over side ports and reservoir	Side ports covered with rubber disc lets two-thirds exhaled air escape and utilizes the other one-third exhaled air in the reservoir bag containing carbon dioxide to be rebreathed as a respiratory stimulant. Can deliver 70%–90% oxygen at flow rates of 6–15 L/min.

(Continued)

Table 6-7 Delivery of oxygen to acutely breathless adults (*Continued*)

Nonrebreather mask with one-way valves in side ports and reservoir	Exhaled air leaves via the one way valves, and oxygen enters the reservoir through a one-way valve, letting higher concentrations of oxygen to accumulate in the reservoir for the patient to inhale. Can deliver 90%–100% oxygen at a flow rate of 15 L/min.
Venturi mask with interchangeable color coded valves: • Blue (24% on 2 L/min) • White (28% on 4 L/min) • Yellow (35% on 6 L/min) • Red (40% on 8 L/min) • Green (60% on 12 L/min)	The Venturi valve allows different amounts of room air to be sucked into the mask to dilute the oxygen concentration to deliver varying amounts of oxygen, ranging from 24% up to a maximum of 60% oxygen.

Source: Reference 12.

- Calmly explain to the patient or family member what is being done to relieve the difficult breathing.[13]
- If the patient is to be transferred to an intensive care setting, call for portable oxygen and a nonrebreather mask (and stay with him or her until the "hand off" to the ICU nurse).
- Obtain venous access (two reliable antecubital sites).
- Monitor pulse oximetry: Select and apply appropriate sensor (finger, nasal, ear, or forehead), check sensor for proper position and set alarms (Table 6-8).[14]

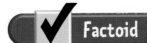

Never leave an unstable patient!

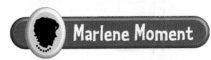

Don't you DARE send your patient to the intensive care unit with a transporter! These are not medical people! You accompany your patient personally and don't leave until you have given report to his or her new nurse! And, unless you want to be giving mouth-to-mouth ventilation to a stranger (who may have any number of bad bugs), you had better take the Ambu-bag during transport, just in case.

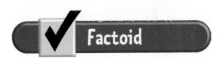

Not giving enough oxygen kills more patients than giving too much oxygen.[1]

Table 6-8 Tips for accurate pulse oximetry measurements

Finger or toe sensor	• Remove nail polish (if any). • Apply detector on finger pad. • Apply the emitter over fingernail. • Make sure it's not wrapped too tightly!* • Patient must have good peripheral circulation.
Nasal sensor	• Clean nose with acetone pad (remove skin oils). • Apply sensor over bridge of nose. • Provides more accurate reading when patient has poor peripheral circulation. • Patient must weigh >110 lb.[1] • Appropriate for long-term monitoring.
Ear clip sensor	• Can't be used at site of ear lobe piercing. • Appropriate for continuous monitoring.

(Continued)

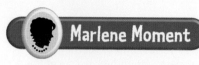

Marlene Moment

If your patient is acutely breathless, you can just forget oxygen by nasal cannula. Here's my rule: "If the patient is blue, don't even ASK ... go for the MASK!"

Table 6-8 Tips for accurate pulse oximetry measurements (*Continued*)

Forehead sensor	• Held in place with Velcro band for patients who have diaphoresis and tape won't stick.
	• Used for patients with poor peripheral circulation.
	• May not be appropriate with mechanical ventilation or lying supine if indicated by manufacturer guidelines.
All types sensors	• Check sensor placement and intactness of skin every 8 hours.
	• Move location of sensor at intervals to avoid skin breakdown.
	• Recognize limitations of pulse oximetry: false readings can be related to low (or high) hemoglobin, irregular heart rate, cold extremities, or vasoconstriction.

*Forget getting accurate SpO_2 if you cut off circulation!
Source: Reference 13.

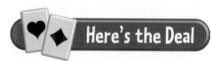

Here's the Deal

The more hypoxemic the patient, the greater concentration of oxygen is required to raise his or her oxygen saturation. The oxygen cannot be picked up in the affected lung tissue because that area is not being perfused: the emboli has lodged and is obstructing blood flow into the lung. When there is a ventilation-perfusion mismatch, such as with PE, higher concentrations of oxygen are required to treat hypoxemia.[15]

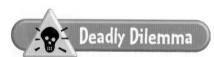

Deadly Dilemma

Oxygen toxicity can occur when high concentrations (>50%) are given in excess of 48 hours: Minimize duration and reduce concentration as soon as possible!

- Monitor ECG with continuous cardiac monitor, watching for arrhythmias and conduction defects.
- Administer thrombolytic medication as ordered.
- Administration of dopamine (Intropin) or dobutamine (Dobutrex) IV to improve cardiac output and raise the blood pressure if cardiogenic shock is present.[15]

The hypoxemic patient requires close monitoring. General nursing care priorities are to:

- Administer oxygen by Vento-mask or nasal cannula for documented hypoxemia (PO_2 <90% on room air).
- Administer non-narcotic analgesia as prescribed for pain to avoid depressing the respiratory center.

Differing methods of oxygen delivery provide the following concentrations:

- Nasal cannula can provide 24% to 40% with flow rates 2 to 6 L/min.
- Various types of oxygen masks deliver 35% to 60% with flow rates 5 to 10 L/min.[15]
- 100% oxygen can be delivered by tight-fitting nonrebreathing face mask or endotracheal intubation with mechanical ventilation.

Prompt and timely medical management is dependent upon nurse identification and close monitoring of patients at risk for venous thrombus. Early recognition of signs and symptoms and immediate collaboration with the physician is essential to initiate correct diagnosis and thrombolysis when indicated.

- If the patient is not a candidate for thrombolysis and/or anticoagulation, other medical options involve risk, but may be lifesaving.

- The nonpharmacologic approach may include surgical or mechanical (catheter) embolectomy when thrombolysis and anticoagulation are absolutely contraindicated.

- Patients who have repeated thrombus may be candidates for a vena caval shunt, a procedure in which the inferior vena cava is partitioned into small channels with clips allowing blood flow, but keeping large clots out of the right ventricle.

- An umbrella filter, which can be placed in the inferior vena cava, is another option to catch large clots, while allowing blood to pass through (Fig. 6-5).

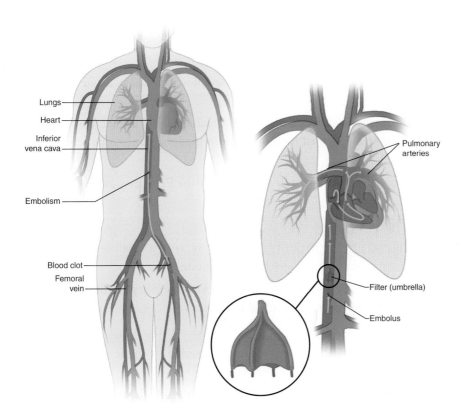

◀ Figure 6-5. Vena Cava Umbrella. In persons who have deep vein thrombosis, part of a blood clot in an affected leg vein may break off and travel through the blood stream and may become an embolus. After traveling through veins and the heart, the embolus can become lodged in one of the arteries that carry blood to the lungs (pulmonary arteries). It may block blood flow and may cause pulmonary embolism. To prevent pulmonary embolism, the physician may recommend that a filter, called an umbrella, be permanently placed in the vein that carries blood from the legs to the heart (inferior vena cava). The filter traps emboli before they reach the heart but allows blood to flow through freely.

PATIENT TEACHING   The underlying pathophysiology and cause of PE is venous thrombosis related to venostasis, hypercoagulability, and trauma, so prevention is always best! Teach patients how to avoid a repeat performance:

- Maintain adequate hydration.

- Utilize the "muscle" pump to increase venous return to the heart.

- Avoid prolonged sitting or standing, and long distance travel.

- Elevate legs periodically to increase venous return.

- Use of prescribed compression hose compresses superficial veins and forces circulation to deeper veins.

- Avoid known agents associated with thrombus formation such as oral contraceptives, smoking.

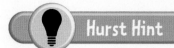

Teach active exercises for the non-ambulatory patient: ankle rolling, plantar flexing/dorsiflexing (point toes and pull back to squeeze calf muscle).

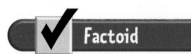

More volume (coming in to the lung blocked by a clot) means more pressure!

- Limit vitamin K foods while taking oral anticoagulant Coumadin and observe bleeding precautions (outlined in Chapter 2).
- Immediately report any calf pain, especially if associated with local warmth, redness, and heat.

What can harm my patients and why?

Sudden death can occur with pulmonary embolus without warning. If my patient survives the initial respiratory insult, the following resultant life-threatening problems may occur:

- Hypoxia, leading to fast breathing (tachypnea)
- Respiratory alkalosis caused by increased respiratory rate, blowing off too much CO_2
- Pulmonary hypertension caused by blood backing up behind the clot obstructing the pulmonary vessel
- Dilation of cardiac chambers, myocardial ischemia, tricuspid regurgitation
- Right heart failure (cor pulmonale) resulting from the increased work load, pumping against high pressure in the lung (pulmonary hypertension)
- Cardiogenic shock[16] can occur quickly if the PE is massive

✚ Lung trauma

The lungs occupy the majority of the thorax, with a small center space called the mediastinum where the heart resides.

- The thorax is a closed cavity with the diaphragm separating the thoracic cavity from the abdominal cavity.
- The rigid, bony rib cage supports and protects the lungs.
- Expansion of the chest cavity is made possible by the intercostal muscles and the diaphragm as air is pulled in.
- Arteries and veins supply each intercostal muscle that separates each rib.
- Pressure in the thorax fluctuates with respirations.
- Fluctuating pressures (negative and positive) in the alveoli are responsible for air entering and leaving the lungs.

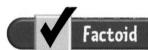

Negative pressure = below atmospheric pressure
Positive pressure = above atmospheric pressure

RESTRICTIVE PULMONARY DISORDERS

Restrictive lung disease has many forms that can occur across the life span. Other respiratory conditions (ie, asthma, COPD) cause the patient to have trouble EXHALING, but the patient with a restrictive lung disease cannot INHALE.

✦ ARDS

Let's get the normal stuff straight!

The cells that line the alveolar walls make surfactant that reduces surface tension of pulmonary fluid. Surfactant is necessary to maintain stability of the alveolus, prevent alveolar collapse, reduce the work of breathing, and keep the alveoli from going underwater!

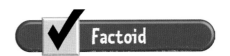

Dry is good when we're talking about the alveoli: Oxygen cannot diffuse through lung fluid!

What is it?

Acute respiratory distress syndrome (previously known as adult respiratory distress syndrome) is associated with a wide range of conditions that can cause direct or indirect lung injury.

ARDS is a clinical condition characterized by sudden (noncardiac) development of pulmonary edema in previously healthy lungs. Onset is rapid, within 12 to 18 hours of the initiating injury. The mortality rate is as high as 60%, and survivors may be left with stiff, scarred lungs.

What causes it and why?

ARDS is caused by direct or indirect injury to the pulmonary epithelium, which results in:[17]

- Accumulation of activated neutrophils in the alveoli and release of inflammatory mediators
- Reduction in the utilization of existing surfactant
- Decreased production of surfactant
- Alveolar flooding
- Development of a fibrous matrix inside the alveoli
- Remodeling of the alveoli

The pulmonary epithelium is the primary site of direct injury caused by:

- Aspiration of caustic fluid (gastric acid)
- Inhalation injury (smoke, corrosive chemical fumes, or high concentrations of oxygen)
- Lung infections (bacteria, fungi, viruses)
- Fat or air embolism

A site away from the lungs (extrapulmonary) may sustain injury and transmit effects to the lungs. Examples of these extrapulmonary etiologies of ARDS include:

- Urosepsis
- Pancreatitis (circulating enzymes injure the pulmonary capillary bed)
- Uremia (circulating toxins cause injury to the pulmonary vessels)
- All forms of shock that reduce pulmonary perfusion
- Massive trauma and DIC, causing hypotension and decreased pulmonary perfusion

Signs and symptoms

The patient initially complains of fatigue and mild shortness of breath with a dry cough at the onset of ARDS. Symptoms very quickly become increasingly severe:

- Dyspnea, nonproductive cough (initially) and increased respiratory rate.
- ABGs drawn during early onset will reflect respiratory alkalosis caused by tachypnea.
- As the ventilation-perfusion mismatch continues and the patient tires, ABGs will reveal hypoxemia and respiratory acidosis.
- Mottled skin and cyanosis of lips and nail beds.
- Restlessness, anxiety, agitation, and confusion caused by hypoxia.
- Decreasing LOC, lethargy, and stupor as hypoxia worsens.
- Hypoxemia causes cells to switch to the anaerobic mode of operation and the by-product lactic acid is released.

Testing, testing, testing

Depending on the causative factor, additional tests may be performed, but diagnosis is based on bilateral consolidation of lung tissue visible on chest X-ray. ABGs reflect hypoxemia and the severe ventilation-perfusion mismatch. Blood moves through the lungs but the nonfunctional alveoli are unable to diffuse oxygen through damaged membranes. Additional studies will document:

- Elevated plasma neutrophil elastase levels (>220 ng/mL)[18]
- P/F ratio <200 mm Hg (this is the difference between amount of oxygen administered [FIO_2 = inspired oxygen] and the amount of oxygen in the patient's blood (PaO_2)[18]
- Decreased functional residual lung capacity
- Pulmonary wedge pressure (PWP) <18 mm Hg[19]

Interventions and why?

Identify patients at risk and be alert to early signs to facilitate earliest possible respiratory support. High-risk patients include those with:

- Endotracheal intubation
- Mechanical ventilation with PEEP

Treatment will be implemented according to the initiating event. The "5 Ps":[18]

- Perfusion: administer crystalloids, colloids, and blood transfusions with close monitoring of hemodynamic parameters to avoid circulatory overload. Administer prescribed inotropes such as dobutamine (Dobutrex) and milrinone lactate (Primacor) to increase blood pressure, cardiac output, and pulmonary perfusion.
- Positioning: alternate three therapies (kinetic, lateral positioning, and prone) to improve ventilation. The greatest amount of time (18 hours per 24-hour period) is to be spent in the prone position.

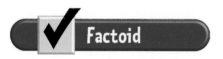

Factoid

Primacor dilates the pulmonary bed to get more blood flow into the lung.

- Protective lung ventilation: limit pressure (<30 cm H_2O) and maintain PEEP. Keep oxygen levels as low as the patient can tolerate (50%–60%) without compromising oxygenation.
- Protocol weaning: "sedation vacations" and spontaneous breathing trials to help wean patients off the ventilator as soon as possible.
- Prevent complications: DVTs (refer to prevention of PE later in this chapter), poor nutrition, pressure ulcers, and ventilator-associated pneumonia (discussed later in this chapter).

PATIENT TEACHING: DISCHARGE PLANNING The patient who has recovered from ARDS may be left with stiff lungs and remodeled alveoli, making him or her more susceptible to infections because of decreased ability to clear airways (loss of recoil). It is important to take very good care of these lungs!

- Do not smoke and avoid being around others who smoke.
- Get immunizations against pneumonia and influenza.
- Avoid sick people and crowds during the flu and cold season.
- Use antiseptic wipes for grocery baskets and door knobs to kill germs. (You don't want to pick up the rhinovirus!)
- See a health care provider at the first sign of a respiratory illness.
- Eat healthy! (Refer to COPD diet guidelines.) A prudent diet full of antioxidants and nonstarch polysaccharides: fruits, veggies, whole grain breads, and fish! No cured meats containing nitrites!

What can harm my patient and why?

Blood comes into the capillary bed surrounding the alveoli, but no oxygen is received there (ventilation-perfusion mismatch), and the patient will rapidly become severely hypoxic. Even with the best care the patient may not survive, and survivors may be left with stiff, noncompliant lungs. Prognosis is not good. The deadly chain of events consists of:

- Pulmonary edema as plasma fluid pours into the alveoli
- Hypoxemia resulting from ventilation perfusion mismatch
- Respiratory acidosis as lactic acid builds up because of anaerobic metabolism
- Severe hypotension and hypovolemia because of third spacing of fluid
- Decreased cardiac output caused by PEEP (right heart pumping against high pressure in the pulmonary system)
- Respiratory failure caused by inability of the lungs to diffuse O_2 into the blood and remove CO_2
- Multisystem organ failure caused by lack of oxygen and cellular energy (ATP) to support organ function
- Death occurs because vital organs shut down caused by sustained perfusion deficit

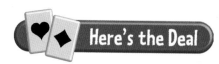

Here's the Deal

The patient on mechanical ventilation will require parenteral nutrition plus fat solutions periodically, and small enteral feeds are also indicated, not necessarily for nutrition, but to maintain health of intestinal mucosal surfaces.

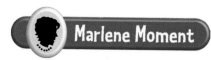

Marlene Moment

I don't think we have to worry about pressure ulcers when our ARDS patient has to be repositioned so frequently! We don't do the prone position for many patients, but for the ARDS patient, a big part of every day is "bottoms" side up!

Cutting edge

The controversy of sterile isotonic saline instillation into an endotracheal tube versus no isotonic saline prior to suction is still raging. Some studies say yes. This practice decreases the incidence of ventilator-associated pneumonia (VAP),[20] whereas others recommend avoiding instilling sterile normal saline into the tube when suctioning.[18] It is easy to understand the risk and the benefits of either practice. If thick infected stuff won't come up without thinning, the patient is in trouble. On the other hand, contamination can occur if the nurse isn't careful and organisms just got introduced directly into the tube.

✚ Sleep apnea

Sleep apnea with loud snoring makes nighttime miserable for bed partners, but the person with obstructive sleep apnea-hypopnea syndrome is also miserable during the daytime!

Let's get the normal stuff straight!

Bony nasal passageways and the hard palate provide structure and support for the upper airway. Other upper airway structures are composed of soft tissue and muscles that assist with speech, mastication, and maintenance of the airway:

- The soft palate and uvula at the back of the oropharynx
- The tongue
- Muscles of the pharynx

During sleep, the normal pattern of respirations is characteristically slower, rhythmic, gentle, and quiet.

What is it?

Obstructive sleep apnea-hypopnea syndrome (OSAHS) is a widespread disorder affecting almost 18 million individuals in the United States.[21] A diagnosis of OSAHS is confirmed when five or more episodes of apnea or hypopnea occur per hour of sleep. The apneic or hypopneic periods are of 10 or more seconds' duration and occur repeatedly throughout sleep.[22] Noisy breathing disturbances during sleep interfere with rest and leave patients (and bed partners) grumpy and tired during the day. Fatigue interferes with work and leisure, but related public safety issues of untreated patients can pose health hazards.

Causes and why?

- Decreased muscle tone, weak muscles of the upper airway
- The tongue drops backward against the soft palate
- Air moving through nasal passages over the soft palate cause vibrating motions of the tongue against the soft palate, uvula, and pharynx
- Loud snoring signals partial oropharyngeal obstruction
- Sedatives, muscle relaxants, alcohol ingestion add to the problem of insufficient muscle tone and can contribute to airway collapse[21]

Testing, testing, testing

Sleep clinics are well equipped to perform the following diagnostic tests:

- Polysomnogram based on stages of sleep, as evidenced by brain wave-forms
- Electroencephalography, which measures brain waves
- Electromyography, which records movements of the lower facial muscles by an electrode placed on the chin
- Electrocardiogram (EKG), which records electrical activity of the heart
- Chest wall motion and nasal airflow measures respiratory activity
- Limb leads on lower legs monitor limb movement (restless leg syndrome)
- Body position is recorded by a video camera mounted on the wall facing the bed
- A sound meter records snoring
- The apnea-hypopnea index (AHI) is determined from the monitor of respiratory activity. The number of times the patient experienced apnea or shallow ineffective breathing (hypopnea) per hour of sleep is calculated. An AHI of five or more episodes per hour of sleep plus video recording of sleep disturbances and daytime sleepiness/fatigue confirms the diagnosis of OSAHS.

Signs and symptoms

Number one complaint: The patient can't get a good night's sleep! He or she may report:

- Feeling progressively more fatigued and irritable during the day
- Yawning and dosing off anytime during the day when sitting or just being still
- Difficulty concentrating and memory loss for things that are ordinarily remembered
- Awakening frequently during the night with loud snoring and getting up to urinate
- Awakening with a headache every morning and just feeling bad with no energy
- Medical history of hypertension poorly controlled with two antihypertensive agents
- Gastroesophageal reflux (GERD), heartburn, and frequent belching
- Loud snoring with periods of not breathing, but respiratory movement and gasping continuing till awakened, especially when lying supine

    Physical assessment and history may reveal one or more risk factors:

- Large abdomen with BMI = 28 kg/m^2
- Enlarged neck circumference
- Craniofacial findings: A narrow high hard palate is visualized with a large tongue, big tonsils, and adenoids.

- Frequent nasal congestion and stuffiness
- History of smoking
- Regular alcohol use

Interventions and why?

The patient with OSAHS has to first recognize that he or she actually has a problem! Many times it is the nurse who performs a physical exam and recognizes patients at risk followed by inquiry regarding symptoms. Risk factors include:

- Age
- Male gender
- Obesity
- Family history
- Menopause[23]

Diagnosis is the first order of business! Collaboration with the patient's health care provider will get a referral to a sleep clinic for a comprehensive sleep study and evaluation. Once OSAHS is verified, a treatment plan can be established.

- Dosage reduction (or discontinuation) when sleep dysfunction is remedied

The patient needs something to keep his or her airways open during sleep. Continuous positive airway pressure (CPAP) is just what the doctor ordered (literally)!

- A face mask is worn during sleep with tubing connected to the CPAP machine, which uses room air with pressure (5–20 cm H_2O) as prescribed.
- The continuous pressure prevents airway collapse and eliminates snoring and other symptoms.

Many patients do not like the CPAP because the mask is tight and it leaves a slight indention around nose and mouth (briefly) when taking it off after a good night's sleep.

- Encourage patient compliance by informing the patient how much better and more alert he or she will feel.
- Cite the positive benefits and avoidance of health consequences.
- Encourage the patient to join an OSAHS support group.

PATIENT TEACHING   Because compliance with CPAP is less than optimal (50%–80%)[21] patient teaching should include behavioral strategies to compliment CPAP to improve outcomes. These strategies may effectively relieve symptoms in mild cases of OSAHS and reduce health hazards:

- Lose weight. Even a little weight loss has a big effect on the apnea-hypoxia index (AHI). Portion control is effective and is the least drastic dietary intervention, but elimination of sweets and fatty foods will achieve results.
- Get physical. Walking daily will compliment any weight loss plan.

- Avoid smoking and all agents having a sedative effect (alcohol, and prescribed and OTC sleep aids).

- Investigate FDA-approved dental devices (oral mouthpiece) that hold jaw/tongue in a forward position.

- Avoid sleeping supine. Use oversized, elongated pillows to help maintain a side-lying position during sleep.

- Have blood pressure monitored periodically, as antihypertensive medications may be required.

What can harm my patient and why?

In addition to being tired all day and not being able to concentrate or think clearly, there are serious health consequences associated with OSAHS:

- Hypotension: Blood pressure drops dramatically during episodes of apnea.

- Reduced myocardial oxygen supply: Apnea up to 90 seconds can drop oxygen saturation to 40%.

- Arrhythmias may occur during periods of myocardial ischemia and hypoxia.

- Intermittent hypoxia impairs myocardial contractility and cardiac output drops.

- Impaired mood and alertness result.

  Denial can harm my patient. Most people with OSAHS remain undiagnosed[21] until the disorder is well advanced and cardiovascular and neurobehavioral signs are severe.

Cutting edge

Advances are being made in sleep medicine as the public is becoming more knowledgeable about health hazards associated with OSAHS. More nonpharmacologic options are becoming available (eg, pupillometry, which documents daytime sleepiness),[21] but pharmacology is lagging behind because OSAHS research is hindered by many variables.

- To date there is no standard widely accepted pharmacologic option, but there are promising strategies for treating metabolic syndrome and obesity.

- Modafinil, a drug used for narcolepsy, is shown to decrease daytime sleepiness, improving quality of life and maximizing safety when used in conjunction with CPAP.

✛ Lung infections/inflammation

What is it?

Pneumonia is an acute lower respiratory tract infection of the lung tissue usually caused by bacteria, but can be caused by a virus (ie, influenza). Lung tissue is colonized by an invading organism and an intense inflammatory reaction occurs, which results in consolidation of lung tissue

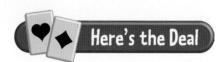

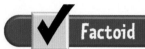

(tissue becomes more solid and less elastic, increased lung density) and production of increased amounts of exudates (mucous, secretions). In addition, bacteria can release toxins that damage lung tissue and surfactant-producing cells. Consolidation, exudates, and decreased surfactant all result in increased work of breathing and decreased gas exchange.

Some various types of pneumonia are as follows:

- Community-acquired pneumonia/infection: Infections acquired at home or in the community. A client is either **admitted with or develops s/s within 24 to 48 hours** after admission. The one- to two-day time frame suggests that the client has been exposed to the pathogen and was incubating the disease **prior to admission.**

- Hospital-acquired pneumonia/infection: Pneumonia occurring 48 to 72 hours **after** the client is admitted to the health care facility and shows **no evidence of incubation on admission (cultures negative upon admission).** Ventilator-assisted pneumonia is an example of hospital-acquired pneumonia.

- Aspiration pneumonia: Pneumonia resulting from aspiration of a substance containing gastric acid contents.

- Opportunistic pneumonia: Pneumonia caused by an organism that is usually nonpathogenic in a healthy individual. If the immune system (resistance) is decreased, nonpathogenic organisms may cause infection.

One of the major causes of VAP is unsterile equipment used in suctioning, poor/infrequent mouth care, and contaminated water solutions used in mouth care (the bottle of water by the bed). Thirty-one percent of the infections in medical-surgical units are pneumonia.

Mechanically ventilated patients are especially prone to nosocomial pneumonia (ventilator-associated pneumonia).

Causes and why?

Pneumonia is generally acquired when a person's immune system is unable to resist or defend itself against an invading organism. Pneumonia is the fifth leading cause of death, with the highest incidence among older adults, nursing home residents (or people in other crowded living situations), hospitalized clients, clients with chronic illnesses, and those being mechanically ventilated. Community-acquired pneumonia (CAP) is more common than nosocomial and is seen commonly in late fall and winter as a complication of influenza. Common gram-negative pathogens associated with CAP include *Streptococcus pneumoniae, Haemophilus influenzae, Legionella pneumophila, Pseudomonas,* and *aeruginosa.* Hospital-acquired pneumonia (HAP) or nosocomial pneumonia has a mortality rate of 20% to 50%. This high mortality rate is caused in part by the virulence of organism, the resistance of the organism to antibiotics, and the patient's underlying disease process. Common pathogens associated with HAP include *Enterobacter* spp., *Escherichia coli, H. influenzae, Klebsiella* spp., and methicillin-resistant *Staphylococcus aureus* (MRSA). These organisms can invade from many common places in a person's environment such as bedside tables, hospital equipment, visitors, and staff (Table 6-9).

Table 6-9   Risk factors associated with pneumonia

Causes	Why
Bacterial or viral infection	Decreased cough impedes lungs from expelling mucous.
Aspiration	Bacteria that cause pneumonia reside in the oropharynx and nasopharynx, migrate to the lungs by aspiration, and cause lung inflammation.
Antibiotic use	Alters normal flora of lungs allowing bacteria to grow rapidly.
Smoking	Tobacco smoke decreases cilia, which impedes lungs from expelling mucous.
Client illness: diabetes, chronic lung disease	Alters normal flora of lungs, allowing bacteria to grow rapidly.
Near drowning	Aspiration of bacteria-laden water; clean water may also cause severe lung inflammation.
Inhaling noxious gases	Lung inflammation; impaired gas exchange.
Steroid therapy, malnutrition, alcoholism, very old, very young, AIDS	Suppressed or impaired immune system.
Clients who are NPO	If proper mouth care is not provided bacteria will migrate from the mouth to the lungs.
Clients who've undergone abdominal or thorax surgery	Postop pain impedes deep breathing, which allows fluid to accumulate in the lungs.
Clients who have artificial airways (endotracheal tube or tracheostomy)	The presence of tube allows direct portal of entry for pathogens to the lower respiratory tract.
Clients who have not received influenza or pneumococcal immunizations	Pneumonia may occur as a complication of influenza. Pneumococcal vaccine may reduce or eliminate the risk of pneumonia.

Who is at risk for aspiration pneumonia?

- Geriatric patients
- Patients with decreased level of consciousness (LOC)
- Postop patients
- Patients with a poor gag reflex
- Patients who are weak
- Patients receiving tube feedings
- Patients who are intoxicated

Testing, testing, testing

CBC with differential (differential will help determine if infection is bacterial or viral). The WBC count will be high with bacterial infection (>15,000 with the presence of bands, which are immature neutrophils). This will be normal/low in viral infection.

Chest X-ray (infiltrates may be through lung fields or patchy; consolidation (filling of air spaces with exudate); possibly pleural effusion.

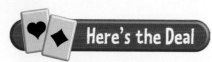

Here's the Deal

How do I know I am infected with TB? The little red wheal 48 hours after my TB skin test tells me that I have been exposed. Does it mean I have active disease? Not necessarily, the body can keep it walled off until such time as the body's defense mechanisms are suppressed (as with corticosteroid therapy or malnutrition).[24] If the organism breaks out of its surrounding waxy protective shell and replicates more bacilli, active symptomatic infection will occur.

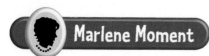

Marlene Moment

I have the same problem that macrophages have when they come into contact with *Mycobacterium tuberculosis hominis*! My body does this with D. (dark) mint chocolinis! I engulf it and digest. After I eat it, the scales reveal the ugly truth: It stays with me in another form, very similar to the way the TB nuclei stay in our body, infecting the macrophages that transfer antigens to the T lymphocytes, who become sensitized and produce the very enzymes that destroy the lung.

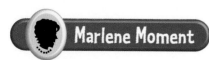

Marlene Moment

TB or no TB, that is the question. My answer is, "No, thank you!" I'd rather not Tah-B infected with *Tuberculosis mycobacterium*, even though almost half the world is, and WHO predicts that 10% of the latent infections will become active at some point in life.[24]

Sputum cultures and sensitivity (to determine specific bacteria and effective antibiotic).

✚ Tuberculosis

Let's get the normal stuff straight!

Healthy people (no cancer, leukemia, diabetes, chronic renal failure, or HIV) have a red alert system that is activated when foreign substances (and microorganisms) enter the body:

* Macrophages are on the scene immediately, seeking to destroy the tubercle bacillus by ingestion. This works with other organisms, but the waxy coating on the tubercle bacillus provides protection against total eradication.
* Natural killer cells and T lymphocytes are attracted to the area where macrophages congregate to help muster a defense.
* When the immune system has surrounded the tubercle bacillus it can no longer multiply, but the few remaining bacteria in tissues will produce a positive reaction to a TB skin test.
* This cell-mediated response (sensitization of T lymphocytes, which make lytic enzymes to finish off the job started by the macrophages) is usually effective, but not so with *M. tuberculosis hominis* (human)!

The World Health Organization (WHO) reports that one-third of the world population is infected with the *Tuberculosis mycobacterium* and has either latent or active disease.[25]

What is it?

Pulmonary tuberculosis is the number one infectious killer in developing countries, and worldwide is the leading cause of AIDS deaths.

Causes and why?

The only known cause of tuberculosis is infection with the tuberculosis mycobacterium, and this occurs by either inhaling an airborne droplet containing the nuclei of the organism or inhaling the dried nuclei moved about through air currents. This can happen in the grocery isle when a host walks past you and coughs or sneezes. Talking, laughing, or singing can spew infected droplets into the air. Not everyone will get TB, because the nuclei must make its way deeper through the airways to lodge in the alveoli where it will multiply.

Signs and symptoms and why?

Signs and symptoms of active pulmonary tuberculosis are easy to spot when coupled with the two distinctive symptoms that accompany typical respiratory symptoms: cough lasting longer than 3 weeks, fatigue, and pleuritic chest pain. Two red flags that are highly suspicious of TB are:

* Night sweats
* Weight loss

Once the lesion is well advanced in the lung tissue and caseation is in progress, the patient will know that something is wrong and may become alarmed when sputum becomes blood streaked (hemoptysis).

Testing, testing, testing

There are two skin testing methods for determining a person's exposure to TB:

- The Mantoux TB skin test uses tuberculin purified protein derivative (PPD) injected intradermally and will produce a local inflammatory reaction at the site within 48 to 72 hours.[24]
- The newer QuantiFERON-TB Gold test (QFT-G) is a blood test that provides results in 24 hours, and unlike the TB skin test using PPD, false-positives don't occur with repeat testing.[24]
- Chest X-ray can reveal craters, cavities, pulmonary effusion, and associated lung damage, but does not diagnose latent or primary TB.
- Sputum specimen for culture and sensitivity.
- Acid-fast smear: The waxy outer capsule of the tubercle bacillus will absorb the red dye when the acid-fast stain is applied to the slide.
- Thoracentesis to obtain pleural fluid for cytology will reveal heat sensitive, nonmotile, aerobic acid-fast bacillus.
- Bronchoscopy will reveal inflammation and pathologic changes in lung tissue. Sputum for cytology can be collected via the bronchoscope if the patient is unable to produce an adequate specimen.

Interventions and why?

Recognition of symptoms is paramount! The nurse conducting the admission interview will ask questions about weight loss, night sweats, exposure to communicable illness, and conduct a survey of conditions known to increase risk for TB infection. If the patient is admitted to the hospital with known or suspected tuberculosis, the nurse will immediately implement airborne isolation precautions:

- Isolation room with negative air flow with at least six air exchanges per hour.
- Ultraviolet lights mounted on the wall kill evaporated nuclei settling on flat surfaces.
- High particulate air filters boost room efficiency in containing the bacillus.
- Use of N-95 fit tested particulate filter masks by any health care provider entering room.
- If the patient leaves the room for diagnostics, the patient must wear a snug fitting particulate filter.

Because the patient is infected with a difficult to eradicate bacillus and is already malnourished, pharmacologic therapy and nutritional support are essential:

- Administer prescribed TB medications, being alert to possible drug interactions with other patient medications.

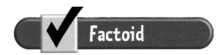

Factoid

After TB skin test, the size of the inflammatory reaction (wheal) determines whether the test is positive or negative. A reaction measuring 10 mm induration is the usual criterion for a positive reaction in the normal population, but in immunocompromised populations (steroids, HIV, organ transplants) 5 mm induration is significant. A reaction of 4 mm or less is a negative skin test.

- Collaborate with physician or pharmacist for dosage adjustments.
- Monitor for side effects and toxicity to anti-TB medications: GI disturbances, elevated liver enzymes, and creatinine.
- Obtain sputum specimens as ordered: In the early morning, rinse mouth first and don't let the lips touch the lip of sterile specimen container.
- Monitor effectiveness of prescribed anti-TB medications: reduction in fever, cough and improved sense of well-being.
- Enhance appetite by removing evidence of expectorated secretions and providing mouth care before meals.
- Weigh patient daily and monitor intake and output.
- Collaborate with dietician for juice at the bedside and nutritious between-meal snacks.
- Serve high calorie nutritious diet and monitor daily calorie count.

PATIENT TEACHING   Airborne isolation and continuous dosing with effective anti-TB medication is a priority.

- The patient with active TB will require isolation for a period of 2 to 3 weeks of continuous antibiotic therapy, but given the correct antibiotics, the person is less likely to spread the disease after only a few days.
- Respiratory hygiene, hand washing, proper containment, and disposal of contaminated tissues are emphasized.
- Compliance is necessary to safeguard their health, avoid later disability, and prevent infecting others.
- Caution patients against missing doses or stopping medications because they can develop resistance to the medication.

Compliance with medications and follow-up testing is essential:

- To reduce uncomfortable side effects with INH, caution patients to avoid tyramine- and histamine-containing foods such as tuna, aged cheese, red wine, soy sauce, and yeast extracts.
- Advise patients to take INH on an empty stomach for better absorption, even though this causes GI upset.
- Return to the health department or clinic for sputum cultures to evaluate the effectiveness of the treatment.
- Report to the hospital or clinic laboratory for periodic testing to detect liver or renal toxicity. BUN, creatinine, and liver enzymes are monitored.
- Report a fever or change in respiratory status immediately, as this may indicate worsening of TB and possible drug resistance.

Nutritional considerations are an important component of a teaching plan to promote health maintenance:

- Nutritious meals and high calorie nutritional supplements are needed.
- Small, frequent, nutrient-dense meals and snacks are better tolerated in the presence of fatigue, excessive mucus, and chronic cough.

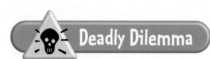

Deadly Dilemma

Nurses with latent TB who refuse prophylactic treatment can unknowingly develop active TB, and many patients can become infected! One such nurse working on the neonatal/maternal unit of a large hospital exposed 1500 new mothers, babies, and coworkers.[23]

- Community facilities (Meals on Wheels, shelters, food stamps, soup kitchens) are recommended when resources are lacking.

What can harm my patient and why?

TB can turn lungs into cheesecake! Not really, but same consistency: the Ghon focus (the tubercle lesion) forms in the mid-lung region (upper part of lower lobes, or the lower portion of upper lobes):

- The granulomatous lesion becomes soft and cheeselike in the necrotic center.
- The cheesy necrotic center is full of the tubercle bacillus and infected macrophages and other immune cells.
- When the necrotic tissue is coughed up, a cavity is left behind.
- Functional lung tissue is lost, as is surface area for oxygen diffusion.
- Pleural effusions (fluid in the pleural space) can collapse the lung (pneumothorax).
- *Mycobacterium tuberculosis* can mutate and can become resistant to antibiotics.
- Pulmonary TB can spread by "seeding" and lymph to other parts of the body.
- Common sites of extrapulmonary TB are pleura, bones, brain and meninges, peritoneum, genitourinary tract, and reproductive organs.
- Sneaky hidden (occult) TB that has spread to the kidney may cause progressive renal damage before being diagnosed.[26]

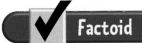

Factoid

When caseation (kay-see-A-shun) on X-ray, it usually means TB. Nothing else looks quite like the soft, crumbly, or liquefied cheese (necrotic lung tissue) that caves in and loses its normal shape.

Cutting edge

The BCG (Bacille Calmette-Guérin) vaccination (not routinely given in the United States) has been implemented worldwide since 1921. BCG is effective in preventing severe TB infections in children but doesn't provide protection against adult infection because it only lasts 10 to 15 years. A promising new bivalent intranasal vaccine that will boost and prolong immunity in previously vaccinated people is ready for human testing.[27]

The three Rs: recovery, risk reduction, rehab

After diagnosis of active long-term disease, pharmacologic interventions are initiated. The following first-line drugs may be prescribed according to various regimes' options and combinations:

- Isoniazid (INH)
- Rifampin
- Pyrazinamide
- Ethambutol

If the patient fails to respond to the above standard first-line drugs or multidrug resistance occurs, second-line drugs are employed:

- Capreomycin
- Ethionamide

- Para-aminosalicylate sodium
- Cycloserine

If resistance to second-line drugs occurs (extensively drug resistant TB), the patient becomes essentially untreatable.[28]

+ Pleuritis

The only nice thing about pleuritis is that diagnosis is easy because the symptoms are so distinctive!

Let's get the normal stuff straight!

A thin, transparent two-layered membrane lines the chest wall on the outermost side, and covers the lungs on the innermost side. A thin layer of pleural fluid is contained within the two layers to provide lubrication for ease of ventilation as the lungs move rhythmically with inhalation and exhalation.

What is it?

Pleuritis is inflammation of the pleura, and this condition is commonly called pleurisy, which can be fibrinous (dry) or wet (accumulation of fluid in the pleural space).

Causes and why?

Pleuritis is caused by an injury (trauma or mechanical, such as thoracotomy) to the chest wall, or an inhaled irritant (eg, asbestos) that produces inflammation. Pleuritis may also be associated with other disease conditions such as:

- Systemic lupus erythematosus (SLE)
- Rheumatoid arthritis (RA)
- Pneumonia
- Metastasis of cancer
- Lung infarction (PE)
- Pancreatitis
- Tuberculosis

When pleurisy occurs, fluid can seep across capillary walls as a result of local inflammation.

Signs and symptoms and why?

In addition to a squeaky pleural friction rub, chest pain is the characteristic sign of pleuritis:

- Sudden onset of sharp, stabbing pain that worsens with chest wall motion associated with deep breathing, coughing, or sneezing.
- Pain is relieved by breath holding.
- Pain can be referred to the upper abdomen, neck, or shoulder.
- Pain decreases as fluid accumulates because pleural layers are no longer rubbing.

Testing, testing, testing

Depending on the clinical picture and the presence of comorbidities placing the patient at risk for pleuritis, the following diagnostic tests may be performed:

- Chest X-ray will reveal accumulation of fluid in the pleural space.
- Employ sputum examinations and acid-fast staining if TB is suspected.
- Obtain pleural fluid for cytology via thoracentesis.

Interventions and why?

Diagnosis of the underlying cause and ensuring adequate oxygenation is the priority. Chest pain is scary for the patient, and control of pain also relieves accompanying anxiety.

What does my patient need?

Pain control is accomplished through the use of:

- Administration of prescribed analgesics and NSAIDs
- Teaching the patient to splint the chest to decrease chest wall motion, especially with coughing
- Application of heat to relax tense intercostal and back muscles
- Application of cold to numb cutaneous nerve endings

Anxiety is reduced by physical presence and explanations of why pleuritis occurs. Factual reassurance can relieve fear of the unknown as well as fear related to preconceived notions and dread of serious illness.

PATIENT TEACHING   Teach the patient about prescribed medications and alternate therapies for pain control:

- Do not exceed the prescribed amount of NSAIDs in a 24-hour period.
- Use caution with heating pads and use insulation to avoid burns.
- Call the health care provider if fever occurs or symptoms worsen.

What can harm my patient and why?

A number of complications can occur because of the underlying cause of pleuritis, but complications specifically related to pleural inflammation are:

- Pleural effusion can develop and cause pneumothorax.
- Fibrosis and adhesions can result from the inflammatory response and cause pleural layers to stick together.

Cutting edge

When chest X-rays are negative, real-time ultrasound can identify pleuritis. In patients with pleuritic pain of unknown cause, real-time b-mode lung ultrasound (LUS) enables the diagnosis of radio-occult lung and pleural lesions.[29]

✚ Trauma

Let's get the normal stuff straight!

The lungs occupy the majority of the thorax, with a small center space called the *mediastinum* where the heart resides.

- The thorax is a closed cavity with the diaphragm separating the thoracic cavity from the abdominal cavity.
- The rigid, bony rib cage supports and protects the lungs.
- Expansion of the chest cavity is made possible by the intercostal muscles and the diaphragm as air is pulled in.
- Arteries and veins supply each intercostal muscle that separates each rib.
- Pressure in the thorax fluctuates with respirations.
- Fluctuating pressures (negative and positive) in the alveoli are responsible for air entering and leaving the lungs.

What is it?

Injuries to the thorax can cause a wide range of injuries to airway structures, lung tissues, and the pleural space and/or the diaphragm, all of which can compromise respirations:

- Contusion of lung tissue (the most common injury)[30]
- Rib and sternum fractures, causing an unstable segment in the rib cage that sinks in with inspiration and billows out with expirations (flail chest)
- Hemothorax/pneumothorax
- Sucking chest wounds/flail chest
- Tension pneumothorax

Causes and why?

Lung trauma can occur as a result of an accident (vehicular, falls, job related) or as a result of violence (guns, knives, blunt force). A common cause of lung contusion is steering wheel injury, many times involving deployment of airbags.

Signs and symptoms and why?

Depending on the type and severity of chest trauma, the patient can have a number of clinical problems. See Table 6-10 for patient complaints and signs and symptoms of various types of chest trauma (Fig. 6-6).

✔ **Factoid**

Negative Pressure = Below Atmospheric Pressure
Positive Pressure = Above Atmospheric Pressure

Table 6-10 Signs and symptoms of chest trauma

Description of chest injury	Patient complaints and signs and symptoms
Pulmonary contusion: • Bruising of the lung tissue. • Tissue can rupture because of the force of the injury. • Greater injury is sustained when the chest wall has less muscle and fat tissue to protect lungs. • Edema and leakage of blood into the area caused by permeable vessels that are injured.	• Chest pain • Abrasions on back or chest • Respiratory distress, dyspnea • Ineffective cough • Hemoptysis
Rib/Sternum fractures: • Commonly seen in motor vehicle crashes with blunt force to chest • Most commonly fractured ribs are 5–9	• Anterior chest pain worsening with coughing or deep breathing • Ecchymosis • Crepitus • Swelling • Chest deformity • Muscle spasm over the area
Flail chest: • Involves multiple (two or more) rib fractures, usually of anterior chest, which has less muscular protection. • Free-floating, unstable segments of broken ribs create an unstable, moveable chest wall.	• Chest pain • Dyspnea with increased work of breathing • Paradoxical respirations visible as the chest wall sucks in during inspiration and puffs out on expiration • Crepitus around the unstable area as rib segments rub each other • Decreased tidal volume as the patient fatigues
Hemothorax/pneumothorax: • Accumulation of blood in the pleural space. • Caused by lacerated lung tissue or intercostal blood vessels. • Small bleeds will self-seal, but large bleeds can lead to shock. • Increased intrathoracic pressure can lead to a mediastinal shift.	Depending on the amount of blood in the pleural space the patient may exhibit: • Hypotension • Tachypnea • Decreased venous return • Flat neck veins If mediastinal shift occurs the patient will display symptoms (below) of tension pneumothorax.
Sucking chest wound/Flail chest: • Penetrating injury creates an opening through the chest wall. • The lung on the affected side collapses. • Sucking wound pulls atmospheric air into the cavity. • Increased intrathoracic pressure causes a mediastinal shift.	Depending on the size of the sucking chest wound, the patient will experience: • Restlessness • Tachypnea, dyspnea • Decreased breath sounds on the injured side • Asymmetric chest expansion • Hypoxia and cyanosis • Respiratory distress
Tension pneumothorax: • Accumulating air or blood in the pleural space is trapped, with no way to get out. • Increasing pressure in the thorax pushes everything to the opposite side (mediastinal shift). • Once the heart is displaced, the great vessels are kinked and blood can't get into (or out of) the heart.	The patient has profound respiratory distress because the heart and lungs are compressed. • Distended neck veins • Asymmetric chest wall motion • Trachea deviated from the midline • Cyanosis caused by hypoxia • Hypotension because of decreased cardiac output • Shock

▶ Figure 6-6. Hemothorax. A hemothorax consists of blood accumulating in the pleural space and can cause a mediastinal shift.

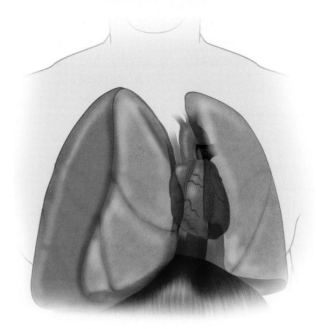

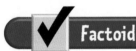

If the patient has an endotracheal tube in place when a mediastinal shift occurs, the trachea will NOT be deviated from the midline because the ET tube acts like a splint, holding the trachea in the midline.

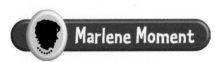

When your patient's trachea is lined up with his left ear lobe, there is a big problem! Sometimes all it takes to fix the problem is to release one side of a dressing to relieve pressure in the chest cavity.[29]

Testing, testing, testing

Test	Clinical significance	Nursing care	Common interfering factors
Chest X-ray	Identifies infiltrates at the area of lung contusion, pneumonia, or pleural effusion. Reveals multiple broken and displaced ribs associated with flail chest. Reveals pneumothorax or hemothorax following trauma wounds that penetrate into the chest cavity.		
Computed tomography and ultrasound	Useful for identifying trauma, especially when bleeding is suspected.		
ABGs	Evaluates: • Effectiveness of ventilation. • Hypoxemia and hypercapnia • Acid–base imbalance.		

Interventions and why?

For pulmonary contusion:

• Monitor ventilatory effort and effectiveness of gas exchange.

• Administer non-narcotic analgesics to avoid depressing respirations.

- Monitor oxygen saturation (pulse oximetry) and ABGs.
- Administer oxygen PRN or as ordered.
  For flail chest:
- Splint the injured area with gloved hands while awaiting help.
- Use a bag of IV fluid as a splint over the injured area, or a sand bag, and on inhalation (when the chest sucks inward) cover the concave area and tape the splint to the chest.
- Give support, encouragement, and factual information to the patient who is facing endotracheal intubation and mechanical ventilation.
- Explain that the ventilator with positive end expiratory pressure (PEEP) will keep the lungs inflated (even on exhalation) to realign the broken ribs and stabilize the chest wall so the ribs can begin healing.
- Assist with intubation and implement safety precautions for the patient with an artificial airway and mechanical ventilation.
  For pneumothorax or hemothorax:
- First things first: Have the patient exhale and cover the sucking chest wound with a sterile gloved hand.
- Chest tubes will be inserted for aspiration/drainage of air and/or fluid.
- When there is a large amount of fluid or air in the pleural space, another option is to connect chest tubes to water seal drainage and/or suction for evacuation of whatever has collapsed the lung (Fig. 6-7).

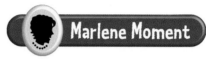

Marlene Moment

You can't have an "inney" and an "outey" at the same time! It's one way OR the other with the lungs, and you know nobody can hold their breath long enough to heal! The ribs have to be still if they are ever going to knit back together.

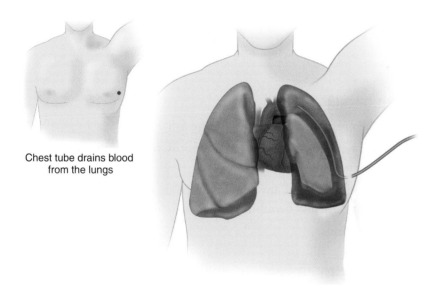

Chest tube drains blood
from the lungs

◀ Figure 6-7. Using Chest Tube to Drain Blood. A chest tube can be inserted into the pleural space to drain the accumulated blood and allow the collapsed lung to reinflate

For tension pneumothorax or hemothorax: A Heimlich (one-way) valve with needle is used to aspirate fluid or air that can cause a mediastinal shift.

- A-B-Cs are always the priority, especially after trauma.
- If the airway is collapsed or obstructed with blood, patent airway is accomplished by a mechanical airway (nasotracheal, oropharyngeal, or tracheal tube) with suction to remove blood and secretions.

- Breathing is supported mechanically, first with a bag/mask device, and later with a ventilator if respiratory effort is ineffective.
- Circulation requires normotension, and hemorrhage/shock may necessitate volume replacement using isotonic and electrolyte solutions, plasma products, and blood transfusion.

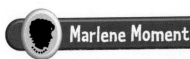

Marlene Moment

When my patient is on a ventilator with a rate setting, I know that at least one of us can breathe easier (Uh … that would be ME) after I have given morphine as prescribed for pain. And here is why: I don't have to worry about depressing my patient's respirations because the ventilator controls breathing for my patient.

Effective Ventilation is the Patient Priority

- Position patients in Semi-Fowler's and occasionally use high Fowler's to help the patient take deeper breaths. This position favors increased lung capacity.[311]
- Monitor ABGs, respiratory rate, depth, and character.
- Monitor oxygen saturation and administer oxygen as prescribed.
- Assist patients to turn, cough, and deep breathe, manually splinting the chest at the site of chest tubes.
- Administer non-narcotic analgesics as prescribed to avoid depressing the respiratory center.
- Administer morphine cautiously and monitor respirations closely.
- Monitor chest drainage, color, and amount. Notify the physician if pink drainage becomes bright red (fresh bleeding) or increases in volume.

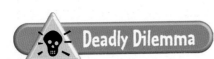

Deadly Dilemma

Notify the doctor for chest drainage >100 mL/h or for change in color from pink to red. This means excessive or fresh (new) bleeding.

Chest Trauma Is Never Nice, Tidy, and Clean. Traumatic Wounds Are Always Contaminated and Prone to Infection.

- Administer prescribed prophylactic antibiotics.
- Monitor wounds, drainage for signs of infection.
- Monitor temperature QID, administering antipyretics for oral temperature >101°F.
- Reinforce damp dressings or reapply sterile dressings when soiled.

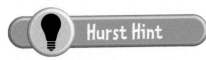

Hurst Hint

Postoperative hypoventilation is common after thoracic surgery because of pain and ineffective coughing!

PATIENT TEACHING

- Take the prescribed antibiotics for the full 10 days.
- Monitor temperature every day and notify your health care provider of any fever or listlessness.
- Notify your doctor of any cough, chest pain or tightness, shortness of breath, or difficulty breathing.
- Care for drains.

What can harm my patient and why?

Depending on the type and extent of injury to structures of the respiratory tract, a number of complications may develop:

- Bloody secretions can accumulate in the airways if the patient cannot clear secretions with effective coughing.
- Respiratory failure can develop either immediately or over time.
- Blood or air can accumulate in the pleural space, collapsing a lung and/or creating tension, which could lead to a mediastinal shift and death resulting from obstructive shock.

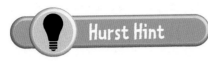

Hurst Hint

Removing chest tubes is really scary for the patient! Prepare the patient by telling him or her what to expect and be sure to mention your plan to administer an analgesic in advance of the tube removal.

Auscultate and document findings, noting any tachypnea or use of accessory muscles. Report any diminished or absent breath sounds, and patient reports of restlessness, anxiety, or chest discomfort immediately.

PRACTICE QUESTIONS

1. The nurse is teaching an asthma patient who has exercise-induced bronchospasm (EIB) how to best prevent an exacerbation. Which statement by the patient is most appropriate?

   A. "I will premedicate with Singular (montelukast sodium)."

   B. "I only have to warm up before exercise when it is cold outside."

   C. "I will take an extra dose of prescribed long-acting inhaled beta$_2$-agonists (LABA) just before exercising."

   D. "I will keep my corticosteroid inhaler on my person during exercise."

2. An obese, postoperative patient experiencing sudden sharp stabbing chest pain is breathless and highly anxious. Which nursing intervention is of most immediate priority?

   A. Stay with the patient and try to calm him or her.

   B. Apply oxygen by nonrebreathing face mask.

   C. Obtain a rapid bleeding history for possible thrombolysis.

   D. Position the patient upright with arms supported on overbed table.

3. The teaching plan for a patient with COPD should include which food facts?

   A. A diet high in fruits, vegetables, and fish promotes lung health.

   B. Red meat stimulates erythropoiesis and improves oxygen-combining capacity.

   C. Meats such as chicken and turkey reduce the buildup of carbon dioxide, a by-product of metabolism.

   D. Limit liquids with meals to have an improved appetite and greater stomach capacity for food.

4. Which of the following patients would be at *greatest* risk for the development of a pulmonary embolus?

   A. A young adult patient who is two days postop emergency appendectomy

   B. A frail elderly patient receiving fluid resuscitation following a severe burn wound

   C. A 45-year-old male patient on bed rest because of a suspected myocardial infarction

   D. A light smoker who is planning elective tubal ligation and discontinuation of birth control pills

   E. A four-day postoperative patient who has sequential compression device (SCD) and refuses to walk because of pain

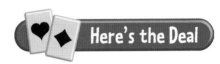

Here's the Deal

Be ready with a sterile occlusive dressing (a strip of petroleum gauze and dry dressing material) when your patient's chest tube is being removed. He or she should have already have practiced the Valsalva maneuver (bearing down, forced air against a closed glottis) and is instructed to do this during removal to prevent atmospheric air from being sucked into the pleural space. As the tube is coming out, be ready to immediately cover the opening and tape down three sides, leaving one side open to act as a flutter valve, just in case there is any little air bubble still in there that wants out!

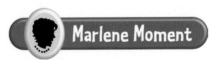

Marlene Moment

Don't be a mean nurse! If your patient is having chest tubes removed, don't make him or her "bite the bullet." Be generous with physical/emotional support and premedication!

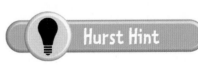

Hurst Hint

A chest X-ray is done prior to removal of chest tubes to make sure the lung has re-expanded. Another postprocedural chest X-ray is done to verify that the lung is still expanded.

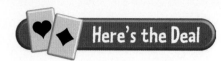

5. Which method for oxygen delivery would the nurse select for the post-operative patient whose acute breathlessness was just preceded by a sudden, sharp pain in the chest?

   A. Vento-mask with 40% oxygen

   B. Nasal cannula with 4 to 6 L oxygen flow rate

   C. Nonrebreather face mask with a reservoir and 15 L/min flow rate

   D. Any low pressure (2 L/min) is indicated because of the high pressure in the lung

6. Which of the following breakfast choices would be most beneficial for the patient with chronic obstructive lung disease?

   A. Whole wheat toast, eggs with cheese, grilled steak strips, and yogurt

   B. Low-fat milk, scrambled eggs, sausage, and toast with sausage gravy

   C. Orange juice, cereal with whole milk, fruit cup, and hash brown potatoes

   D. Oatmeal with butter and brown sugar, bacon and fried eggs, toast, and coffee

7. An unrestrained driver has several broken and displaced ribs. Respiratory effort is increasing and blood pressure is decreasing. Which assessment would most definitely lead the nurse to suspect that a collapsed lung has produced a mediastinal shift?

   A. Distant muffled heart sounds

   B. Expectoration of bloody sputum

   C. Absent breath sounds on the unaffected side

   D. Trachea deviated toward the unaffected side

8. Your COPD patient is experiencing respiratory distress and ABGs reveal PaO_2 is 50 mm Hg and the $PaCO_2$ is 60 mm Hg. Which next intervention is indicated?

   A. Elevate the head of the bed.

   B. Administer 40% oxygen by Venturi mask.

   C. Call respiratory therapy to administer a PRN updraft.

   D. Prepare to assist with intubation and mechanical ventilation.

9. The 40-year-old adult with cystic fibrosis already has extensive bronchiectasis and the current lung infection has deteriorated into respiratory failure. Considering the fact that this patient does not have an advanced directive, which option is the priority for this patient at this time?

   A. Support the patient in a peaceful, comfortable death.

   B. Ask the patient if he or she has thought about end of life care.

   C. Encourage the patient to sign a do not resuscitate (DNR) directive.

   D. Advise the patient that lung transplant organs come available suddenly and unexpectedly.

10. Which of the following positions would be most helpful for the patient with acute respiratory distress syndrome (ARDS)?

A. Prone

B. Supine

C. Semi-Fowler's

D. Trendelenburg

References

1. Tousman S, Zeitz H, Taylor LD, Bristol C. Development, implementation and evaluation of a new adult asthma self-management program. *J Commun Health Nurs 24* (4):237–251, 2007.

2. Holcomb SS. New asthma guidelines encourage more activity and a better night's sleep. *Nurs Pract 33*(3):9–11, 2008.

3. Leyshon J. Correct technique for using aerosol inhaler devices. *Nurs Standard 21*(52):38–40, 2007.

4. Collins A. Asthma: Implications and nursing interventions. *Kansas Nurse 82*(10):6–8, 2007.

5. Hirayama F, Lee AH, Binns CW. Dietary factors for COPD: Epidemiological evidence. *Sum Expert Rev Med 2*(4):645–653, 2008.

6. Vormann J, Remer T. Dietary, metabolic, physiologic and disease-related aspects of acid-base balance. *J Nutr* 138:413S–414S, 2008.

7. Jiang R, Paik D, Hankinson JL, Barr RG. Cured meat consumption, lung function and chronic obstructive pulmonary disease among United States adults. *Am J Respir Crit Care Med* (175):798–804, 2007.

8. Smeltzer SC, Bare BG, Hinkle JL, Cheever KH. *Brunner & Suddarth's Textbook of Medical-Surgical Nursing*. 11th ed. Philadelphia: Lippincott Williams & Wilkins; 2008.

9. Rizkallah J, Man SFP, Sin DD. Prevalence of pulmonary embolism in acute exacerbations of COPD: A systematic review and metaanalysis. Available at: http://www.chestjournal.org/content/early/2008/09/23/chest.08-1516. Abstract. Accessed March 24, 2009.

10. Sims JM. An overview of pulmonary embolism. *Dimen Crit Care Nurs 26*(4):182–186, 2007.

11. Henderson Y. Delivering oxygen therapy to acutely breathless adults. *Nurs Standard 22*(35):46–48, 2008.

12. Beattie S. Respiratory distress: Second in a four-part series. *RN 70*(7):34–38, 2007.

13. Editors. *Nursing 2008*. Monitoring your adult patient with bedside pulse oximetry. *Nursing 38*:42–44, 2008.

14. Slessarev M, Somogyi R, Preiss D, et al. Efficiency of oxygen administration: Sequential gas delivery versus "flow into a cone" methods. *Crit Care Med 34*(3):829–834, 2006.

15. Masotti L. Diagnosis and treatment of acute pulmonary throboembolism in the elderly: Clinical practice and implication for nurses. *J Emerg Nurs 34*(4):330–339, 2008.

16. Rocco PRM, Pelosi P. Pulmonary and extrapulmonary acute respiratory distress syndrome: myth or reality? *Curr Opin Crit Care* 14(1):50–55, 2008.

17. Kodama T, Yukioka H, Kato T, et al. Neutrophil elastase as a predicting factor for development of acute lung injury. *Int Med* 46(11):699–704, 2007.

18. Powers J. The 5 P's spell positive outcomes for ARDS patients. *Am Nurse Today* 2(3):34–39, 2008.

19. Caruso P, Denari S, Ruiz SAL, et al. Saline instillation before tracheal suctioning decreases the incidence of ventilator-associated pneumonia. *Crit Care Med* 37(1):32–38, 2009.

20. Willard RM, Dreher HM. Wake-up call for sleep. *Nursing2005* 35(3):46–49, 2005.

21. Merritt SL, Berger BE. Obstructive sleep apnea-hypopnea syndrome. *AJN* 104(7):49–52, 2004.

22. Punjabi NM. The epidemiology of adult obstructive sleep apnea. *Proc Am Thorac Soc* (5):136–143, 2008. Available at: http://pats.atsjournals.org/cgi/content/abstract/5/2/136. Accessed March 24, 2009.

23. Todd B. The quantiFERON-TB gold test. *AJN* 106(6):33–37, 2006.

24. Rockwood R. Extrapulmonary TB: What you need to know. *Nurs Pract* 32(8):44–49, 2007.

25. Langemeier J. Tuberculosis of the genitourinary system. *Urol Nurs* 27(4):279–284, 2007.

26. Mu J, Jeyanathan M, Shaler CR, et al. Immunization with a bivalent adenovirus-vectored tuberculosis vaccine provides markedly improved protection over its monovalent counterpart against pulmonary tuberculosis. *Mol Ther* (Epub ahead of print) Available at: http://www.ncbi.nlm.nih.gov/pubmed/19319120?ordinalpos=4&itool=EntrezSystem2.PEntrez.Pubmed.Pubmed_ResultsPanel.Pubmed_DefaultReportPanel.Pubmed_RVDocSum. Accessed March 28, 2009.

27. World Health Organization. TB fact sheet. Available at: http://www.who.int/tb/publications/2008/factsheet_april08.pdf. Accessed March 28, 2009.

28. Volpicelli G, Caramello V, Cardinale L, Cravino M. Diagnosis of radio-occult pulmonary conditions by real-time chest ultrasonography in patients with pleuritic pain. *Ultrasound Med Biol Med* (11):717–723, 2008.

29. Yamamoto L, Schroeder C, Believeau C. Thoracic trauma, the deadly dozen. *Crit Care Nurs Quart* 28(1):22–40, 2005.

30. Pruitt B. Hospital nursing: Help your patient combat postoperative atelectasis. *Nursing2006* 36(5):641–646, 2006.

31. Hurst M. *Hurst Reviews: Pathophysiology Review*. New York: McGraw Hill; 2008.

7 Neurologic Dysfunction

OBJECTIVES

In this chapter you will review:

- The underlying pathophysiology associated with manifestations of common neurologic disorders.
- The key concepts and priorities associated with management of care for patients having acute, chronic, autoimmune, and degenerative neurologic conditions.
- The effects of neurologic dysfunction related to priority needs of oxygenation, circulation, and physical safety.
- Treatment modalities and nursing care to promote restoration of maximum neurologic function.
- The technologic advances that improve the quality of life and reduce threat to life when the neurologic system is compromised by trauma, infection, or autoimmune or degenerative conditions.
- The impact of age, nutritional status, lifestyle choices, genetics, and comorbidities that alter neurologic health.
- Components of a teaching plan to enhance self-care and monitoring when the patient has a neurologic disorder.

NEUROLOGIC DISORDERS

Disorders affecting the brain and spinal cord have the potential to affect patient safety, functional ability, and quality of life.

✚ Headaches

Almost everybody has experienced a headache at some time during their life. However, for some headaches are more frequent and severe, requiring clinical investigation and medical management.

Let's get the normal stuff straight first!

The thalamus relays pain signals to cortical pathways (somatosensory cortex, parietal cortex, and limbic cortex) for discrimination of pain characteristics and interpretation of the pain sensation.

- Pain perception has both a physical and a psychic component, which are under neurohormonal control (serotonin and norepinephrine).
- Endogenous (naturally produced) analgesia in the form of endorphins, dynorphins, and opioid peptides have sites of synthesis throughout the central nervous system (CNS).

People respond to pain according to their individual pain threshold, pain tolerance, and sensitivity to pain:

- Pain threshold is the point at which a stimulus is perceived to be painful. It is the lowest intensity at which pain is perceived.
- Pain tolerance is the maximum pain intensity level a person will tolerate before seeking relief.
- Trigger points are points at which pain can follow a stimulus and are capable of giving rise to the perception of intense pain.[1]
- Trigger points to the sensation of pain are abundant in the muscles around the eyes, the back of the head and neck, and the upper and lower back (Fig. 7-1).[2]

▶ Figure 7-1. Trigger points for headache.

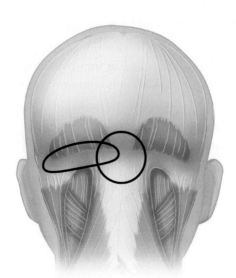

What is it?

Cephalgia (pain in the head), commonly called headache, can be a primary or secondary disorder.

- Primary headaches are not related to organic causes.
- Secondary headaches have an underlying organic cause such as injury, infection, or tumors.
- Clinical investigation and diagnosis are required for all secondary headaches because medical management is directed toward the underlying cause.

Headaches are classified based on diagnostic criteria from the International Headache Society (IHS). The primary classification of headaches includes migraine, cluster, and tension-type headaches.

- Migraine headaches comprise of pulsating, throbbing, and disabling severe pain that can occur with or without an aura (neurosensory involvement) and are often accompanied by nausea and vomiting.
- Cluster headaches follow the trigeminal nerve pathway, producing bouts of severe unilateral pain with periods of exacerbation and remission.
- Tension-type headaches are a band of mild to moderate pain around the entire head.

Causes and why?

Table 7-1 shows the causes of headache and why these causes occur.

Table 7-1 The causes of headache and why

Causes	Why
Tension	Muscle tension from fatigue, emotional stress, or body position. Characteristics include mild to moderate pain that may be constant OR bandlike pressure.
Migraine	Constriction and then dilation of arteries to the brain. The pain is usually severe and throbbing in nature. They are commonly unilateral, but can occur on both sides. They can be brought on by emotional upset, fatigue, nitrite- or tyramine-containing foods, or menstruation. They may be related to the neurotransmitter serotonin.
Cluster	Vasodilation that may be triggered by alcohol and tobacco. They are most common in men, especially those who drink alcohol. A very common feature of the cluster headache is tearing of one eye. Pain is unilateral and is often described as a stabbing pain through one eye (knifelike or icepick). These headaches can be extremely severe and have been known to cause suicide.
Symptom of serious illness	Underlying abnormality, such as arteritis, vascular abnormalities, subarachnoid hemorrhage, a brain lesion, bleeding, and disorders of the eyes, ears, sinus, or teeth.
	Headaches caused by intracranial masses or lesions usually present as dull and constant. Don't think that it's not a big deal just because it's not severe. Approximately one-third of clients with brain tumor present with headache as their primary symptom.
	Ocular or periocular pain usually accompanies a headache that has an ophthalmologic origin.
	Sinus headaches usually have an accompanying tenderness overlying the skin and bone. This is known as maxillary or frontal sinus tenderness and is elicited by gentle percussion over these areas.

(Continued)

Table 7-1   The causes of headache and why (*Continued*)

Causes	Why
Depression	Aches and pains are a common symptom of depression because of an abnormality of serotonin in the brain. Certain neurotransmitters in the brain play a part in the interpretation of pain.
Temporomandibular joint dysfunction (TMJ)	The TMJ joint is misaligned, which triggers headache that is usually precipitated by chewing.
Hypertension	Increased pressure can precipitate headache.

Source: Created by the author from Reference 2.

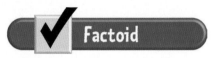

About 23 million Americans suffer from a migraine each year.

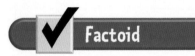

Genetics are implicated,[3] with an inherited tendency for the development of headaches.

The etiology of migraines is thought to be vascular, biochemical, and/or the result of muscular tension.

Testing, testing, testing

Diagnosis of the headache does not usually involve testing unless the neurologic exam suggests a problem. If indications from the history or physical indicate that headaches are secondary (rather than primary), the physician may request the following:

- CT of the head to rule out tumors, masses, or abnormalities
- MRI of the head to rule out pathology, dilated ventricles, or pituitary involvement
- Cerebral angiography (looking for aneurysm)
- Electroencephalogram (EEG) to record brain waveforms and patterns, which could be consistent with electrical pathology
- Electromyography to evaluate head, neck, and myofascial muscle tonus[4]
- Labs: CBC with differential, erythrocyte sedimentation rate (ESR) for possible infectious secondary causes of headache; electrolytes, glucose, and thyroid for possible neurohormonal disturbances

Signs and symptoms and why?

The signs and symptoms and rationales associated with headache are listed in Tables 7-2 and 7-3.

Table 7-2   Signs and symptoms and rationales associated with headache

Signs and symptoms	Why
Pressure, pain, or a tight feeling in the temporal areas of the brain	Tight muscle fibers prevent or reduce blood flow to that area.
Pain	Nervous system dysfunction or injury may trigger an inflammatory response.
Nausea	Nervous system response or nervous system dysfunction.
Headache pain with sensitivity to light (photophobia) and nausea	A response in the brain stem causes a reaction in the trigeminal nerve, an important pain pathway.

Source: Created by the author from Reference 1.

Table 7-3 Migraine headaches: signs and symptoms

Signs and symptoms	Why
• Mood change (depression, irritability) • Behavioral changes (activity level) • Changes in patterns of elimination • Neck pain, back pain, flulike aches • Photophobia	Premonitory symptoms for nonaura migraine headaches may begin one to two days before onset of a headache. The behavioral signs that accompany pain differ according to the severity of the pain and individual coping patterns. Some patients can't be still, whereas others curl into a ball and hold or rub their head.
Aura: • Dizzy feeling • Seeing flashes of light or spots • Numbness or tingling of face or hands • Feeling unusually sleepy at an abnormal time • A heavy or weak-feeling extremity[4]	The patients who experience an aura usually describe sensory or neurologic symptoms that are related to decreased cerebral blood flow with resultant loss of normal regulatory mechanisms

The typical signs and symptoms vary according to the type of headache. Refer to Table 7-4 for characteristics and patterns of pain.

Table 7-4 Characteristic pain and patterns of primary headaches

Location of primary headache and accompanying symptoms	Pain intensity and characteristics	Pain onset/pattern	Attack duration
Migraine Pain is accompanied by at least one of the following: • Nausea/vomiting • Photophobia (sensitive to light) • Phonophobia (sensitive to sound without any change in normal quality of ambient stimuli)	• Throbbing • Worse with movement • Moderate to severe pain At least two of the above defining characteristics are present.	The aura, which serves as a warning sign, may precede the headache by up to one hour, which gives the patient time to self-medicate to reduce the intensity of the attack.[4]	Duration: 4–72 hours[3]
Cluster • Unilateral pain • Ipsilateral autonomic symptoms: tearing, red eye, edematous lid, nasal stuffiness, ptosis, miosis[5] • Located behind or around eyes and crown of head to neck	• Boring • Stabbing • Burning • Squeezing • Severe (never mild)	Periods of remission between cycles of daily headaches. Some cycles are long (up to 1 year) and some remissions are short (1 month).	Duration can be 15–180 minutes[5,6,7] with average headache lasting 1 hour
Tension-type headache Some (not all) patients report: • Photophobia • Unilateral headache • Nausea • Anorexia[8]	• Pulsating quality • Aggravated by routine physical activity	Pain is preceded by a steady constant frontal or temporal pressure and builds to a band of pain around the head with tension in the back of the neck.	Usually relieved within two hours

What can harm my patient and why?

In addition to physical suffering and misery, painful primary headaches that occur with frequency can disrupt lives, wreck relationships, and cause sufferers to change plans and goals. Because they are unpredictable, school attendance or job performance is sporadic. Some sufferers are reported to have contemplated suicide during a severe attack.[7]

Interventions and why?

Abortive treatment (to stop the pain) without delay is the priority when an attack is in progress! Refer to Table 7-5 for commonly prescribed medications and interventions.

Table 7-5   Abortive therapy for headaches

Type of headache	First-line abortive intervention(s)	Alternate abortive intervention(s)
Migraine headache	• An ergotamine preparation plus caffeine (Cafergot) taken at the onset may abort the attack. • Imitrex (sumatriptan) is widely used, but can aggravate ischemic heart disease and cannot be taken concurrently with an ergotamine preparation.	Other triptans may be used: • Amerge (naratriptan) • Maxalt (rizatriptan) • Zomig (zolmitriptan) • Almotriptan
Cluster headache	• Sumatriptan injection or nasal spray (>90% effective) • 100% oxygen administered by means of a face mask at 8–15 L/min (70% effective) Since duration is short, the goal of abortive therapy is to stop the pain within 20 minutes.	• Dihydroergotamine (IM, IV, SQ) • Ergotamine (PO or rectal) • Zolmitriptan (nasal spray or PO) • Intranasal lidocaine (<33% effective) • Greater occipital nerve (GON) blockade[7]
Chronic tension headache	• Ibuprofen (800 mg) • Naproxen sodium (825 mg) A low number of patients in clinical trials have been pain free after two hours.	• Addition of caffeine 130 or 200 mg is a boost to the NSAIDs[8]

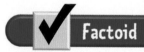

Long-term indomethacin use is associated with peptic ulcer disease.

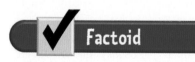

Some patients get immediate relief from cluster headaches with 100% oxygen; others get relief during oxygen administration, but the headache recurs when oxygen is discontinued.[7]

Nursing care during an acute episode to compliment prescribed abortive medication may include any or all of the following supportive and comfort measures:

- Provide a quiet dark environment (pull shades, close curtains, close door, notify switchboard to hold incoming calls).
- Elevate the head of bed to 30 degrees and assist the patient to a position of comfort.
- Make provisions for uninterrupted rest/sleep. (Put a sign on the patient's door directing visitors to the nursing unit to leave a message.)
- Administer prescribed PRN medications such as antiemetics, antidepressants, or muscle relaxants.

Once relief is obtained, the patient will need a thorough medical evaluation and a prescriptive plan for prophylactic medications to reduce the frequency and duration of attacks. Prophylactic therapy is aimed at preventing attacks from occurring and reducing the incidence of migraines. Prophylactic therapy is useful for patients who experience frequent (two to three per month) or severe attacks.[9]

Commonly used drugs for migraine prophylaxis are:[10]
Amitriptyline
Propranolol/timolol
Divalproex sodium
Topiramate

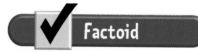

More than two migraines per month is an indication for prescribing prophylactic medicine.

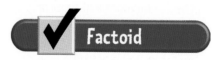

Because of its effect on the heart, verapamil necessitates an EKG after each dosage change and serial EKGs every 3 to 6 months with stable dosing.

Prophylactic medications effective for preventing cluster headaches include:

- Verapamil
- Lithium carbonate
- Divalproex sodium, extended release
- Topiramate
- Melatonin

Polypharmacy actually enhances control with the cluster headache, rather than stopping a medication that gives partial relief; additional drugs are often added for cluster headache prophylaxis.[5]

Acupressure is evolving as an effective alternative approach to migraine and tension-type headaches.[9,11]

A thorough nursing history can provide clues for the physician when prescribing therapy, and should include:

- Medication history: Some diuretics, antihypertensives, and anti-inflammatory drugs can aggravate headaches, as do monoamine oxidase (MAO) inhibitors.
- Stress history: personal, family, job-related stress, emotional problems
- Previous exposure to toxic substances or chemicals and relationship to headache
- Detailed pain history: location, quality, frequency, patterns, precipitating factors, aura, nighttime awakenings with pain
- Family history of headaches

PATIENT TEACHING General teaching includes topics such as stress management, exercise, meditation, lifestyle changes, regular sleep, regular meals, and relaxation. Preventing attacks by avoiding known triggers and using prophylactic medications is an important part of any headache management plan.

Teach patients to avoid migraine food triggers:

- Chocolates
- Coffee

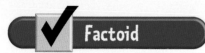

Factoid

Alcohol is the only dietary trigger for cluster headaches.

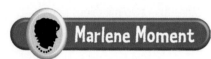

Marlene Moment

When teaching the cluster "head-acher," remember that most of them are smokers![7] If they are using oxygen in the home, they don't want to be buying a new roof, do they?

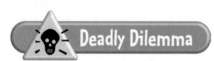

Deadly Dilemma

The terrible trio: early morning headache, vomiting, and papilledema is not a simple primary headache! Think intracranial pressure (ICP) when you see these three!

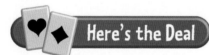

Here's the Deal

When a person lays supine all night, cerebral vessels don't drain as freely, and the ICP increases to cause early morning awakening with a terrible headache that triggers the vomiting reflex. After arising and being up a while (erect position draining cerebral vessels) the headache subsides, but the retinal exam will reveal edematous retinal vessels. This is not a primary headache! This is increased intracranial pressure, which must be evaluated immediately by a physician (preferably a neurologist).[12]

- Dairy products
- Foods containing tyramine
- Alcohol

More specific patient teaching is directed toward underlying pathophysiology, for example:

- The patient who is prone to sinus headaches that have been thoroughly evaluated can be taught to take an NSAID at bedtime (with milk) and use warm moist heat over the face an hour prior to bedtime for help getting to sleep.
- The patient who is prone to cluster headaches and chooses to drink alcohol can benefit from teaching to hydrate, hydrate, hydrate: alternating water with fruit juice.
- If high flow oxygen is prescribed, the patient needs to be taught oxygen safety if tank and mask are available to abort attacks at home.
- Teach the patient never to discontinue prescribed prophylactic medications without first consulting the doctor.
- Teach the patient to take indomethacin with food or milk to reduce gastrointestinal (GI) side effects.
- Teach the patient taking indomethacin to report stomach pain or black stools immediately.

Cutting edge

Positron emission tomography (PET) scans during nitroglycerin-induced cluster headaches have pinpointed a pathway in the brain that modulates the cluster headache. This new surgical intervention (stimulator surgery) involves placing an electrode into the posterior inferior hypothalamus. A high percentage of chronic cluster headache patients who are unresponsive to conventional therapy report a reduction in their frequency of headaches and some have become pain free.[7]

Each type of headache is very selective in its response to treatment, so correct diagnosis is very important. A thorough evaluation should match the patient symptoms to the classification criteria set forth by the International Headache Committee. Careful management is indicated because of the tendency of migraine and cluster headaches to develop medication overuse syndrome. When headaches are recurring or are found to follow circadian rhythms, prophylactic medications are considered.

✚ Seizure disorder

Like headaches, seizures can be related to many secondary causes and a treatment plan hinges on the underlying cause.

Let's get the normal stuff straight!

Thought processes, sensory sensations, speech, and voluntary movement, as well as control of bowel and bladder are made possible by electrical communication between the brain and the spinal cord and electrical communication within the brain. Different lobes of the brain are responsible for different functions. The cerebellum is responsible for smooth coordinated voluntary skeletal muscle movements made possible by electrical impulses within the brain, these impulses are transmitted to the spinal cord, nerves, and muscles.

What is it?

Seizures are a temporary dysfunction of the brain that cause changes in mentation, sensation, and motor activity. Seizures can be partial, and begin in a single part of the brain, or generalized, characterized by abnormal electrical charges over the entire brain. Seizures can occur with or without convulsions, and they may or may not cause unconsciousness depending on the extent of the brain cells involved.

Causes and why?

Seizures are a result of abnormal electrical activity in the brain owing to known and unknown causes. Genetics is implicated in the neuronal changes that result in increased excitatory transmission or reduced inhibitory transmission, and enhanced connectivity between neurons.[13]

Epilepsy is a common cause of seizures; however, many other disease states and physiologic alterations may be implicated:

- High fever
- Hypoglycemia
- Traumatic brain injury,[14] stroke, or brain tumors
- Electrolyte imbalances (sodium, calcium, magnesium)
- Drug or alcohol withdrawal

Testing, testing, testing

- Lab tests will be prescribed to rule out electrolyte imbalance or abnormal blood glucose.
- An EEG will record the electrical activity of the brain.
- Computed tomography (CT) scan of the head.
- Magnetic resonance imaging (MRI) of the head.

Signs and symptoms and why?

Seizures come in many different forms, all having characteristic signs and symptoms. Refer to Table 7-6 for various manifestations of involuntary activity associated with seizures.

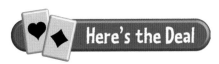

Here's the Deal

Prophylactic medications are taken so you don't get a headache. Don't stop taking prescribed medications because your headaches have stopped! The medication is why you have relief! If side effects are bothersome, consultation with the health care provider can result in an alternative medication which may be better tolerated.

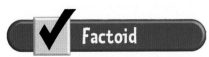

Factoid

A circadian pattern headache is one occurring during the night or early morning.[12]

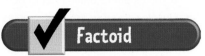

Factoid

A negative EEG does not necessarily mean that the patient is free of epilepsy and/or primary seizure pathology.

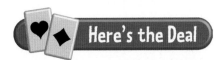

Here's the Deal

When a single EEG is negative, yet the patient is experiencing seizure disorder, the epilepsy specialist may prescribe special EEGs. The video EEG records all motor activity over a period of time as the EEG is in progress to correlate motor activity with brain wave patterns. Another more sensitive EEG is the sleep-deprived version, which may pick up abnormalities when regular EEGs are normal.

Table 7-6 Various manifestations of involuntary activity associated with seizures

Seizures: classification, defining characteristics, examples, and seizure activity	
Simple partial seizures: • No loss of awareness • Can be focal (localized) or generalized • Involve sensory experiences • Motor manifestations • Autonomic phenomena • Can begin as simple partial and spread over the brain to become complex partial seizure	• Duration 5–30 seconds. • Posturing or repetitive movements of one hand (depending on area of onset). • Unpleasant smells or tingling may be reported. • Fearful or déjà vu experience can accompany a sense of being out of touch with surroundings.[15]
Complex partial seizures: • Involves a larger area of the brain • Impaired awareness • Automatic motor movements • Motor manifestations • Can begin as complex partial seizure and spread over the brain to culminate in a generalized tonic-clonic seizure[15]	• Duration 15 seconds to 3 minutes • Hand/mouth movements consist of picking, fumbling, smacking, chewing motions • Limp posturing of hands opposite side from where seizure started (contralateral) • Short period of confusion at end of seizure
Generalized seizures: • Involves entire brain so both hemispheres react. • Onset without warning or progression from localized manifestations. • Loss of awareness or loss of consciousness (with exception of clonic seizure which can occur with or without loss of awareness). • Followed by deep sleep with confusion upon awakening and no memory of the seizure. • Urinary incontinence common and occasional fecal incontinence. • Aura uncommon, but patients usually have a premonition that a seizure is coming.[15]	• Duration 50–120 seconds (except for brief absence seizure of 5–10 seconds). • Absence seizures (petit mal): sudden cessation of activity with staring or blinking eyes (Fig. 7-4). • Tonic-clonic: All muscles contract in a rigid, tight hold for a period before the onset of clonus. • Tonic: sustained bilateral rigid posturing. • Clonic: involuntary muscle contraction alternates with muscle relaxation to produce jerking movements. • Atonic: sudden loss of all muscle tone, causing the patient to drop into a fall.
Unclassified seizures: • Seizure pattern fits neither partial nor generalized characteristics • Insufficient defining characteristics for diagnosis	• Variable duration • Overlapping and variable characteristics • May or may not experience loss of awareness or loss of consciousness

What can harm my patient and why?

Any loss of voluntary control and protective reflexes can place the patient at risk for injury:

• Falls

• Head injury

• Tongue chewing

• Broken, damaged teeth or bones

- Aspiration of secretions or vomitus
- Back strain and muscle injury

In addition to potential for physical injury, the seizure patient is at risk for decreased quality in all aspects of life; psychological, vocational, and social. This can be exhibited in many ways, including:

- Depression
- Limited independence
- Social embarrassment[15]

Interventions and why?

The A-B-Cs are always the priority when the patient has an altered state of consciousness and/or is prone to aspiration:

- Take note of the duration of the seizure and the affected body parts.
- When the seizure ends, open the airway with the head tilt/chin lift maneuver.
- Suction the oropharynx first and then the nose.
- Check breathing and begin rescue breathing if necessary.
- Insert an oral or nasal airway if necessary.
- Place the patient in a side-lying position (Fig. 7-2).

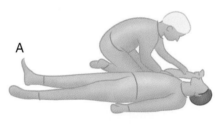
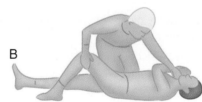
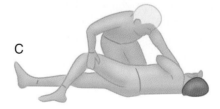
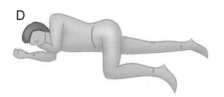

◀ Figure 7-2. Recovery position after seizure.

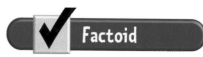

Factoid

It would seem that the frequency of seizures would be the primary determinant of decreased quality of life, but patients with epilepsy resistant to pharmacologic control report adverse drug effects as the primary interference with quality living.[16]

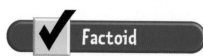

Factoid

Status epilepticus (repeated succession of seizure activity or prolonged seizure duration) is an emergency because hypoxic brain damage may occur.[17]

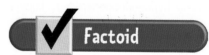

Factoid

Ictus or ictal refers to the seizure. *Preictus* is the time before the seizure. *Interictal* is what's going on in your brain when the seizure is in progress. *Postictus* or *postictal* is the time after the seizure.

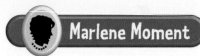

Marlene Moment

Don't get ictus confused with icterus, or you will be having a "yellow" seizure. (Icterus or icteric refers to jaundice, totally different word, so don't get messed up.) Learning a new (medical) language is hard, but it gets better over time as you use these words.

The treatment plan is totally dependent upon proper diagnosis.

● When seizures are unprovoked and the EEG confirms interictal discharges and laterality of a seizure focus, a diagnosis of epilepsy is established.

● If seizures are secondary to other problems, they are expected to subside when the underlying condition is remedied.

● The selection of an antiepileptic medication is based on the type of epilepsy and individual issues, for example, pregnancy or coexisting multiple medical problems).

Refer to Table 7-7 for the "old" (much cheaper) medications used to treat epilepsy and seizure disorder, and the newer (more expensive) antiepileptic drugs (AEDs) approved by the Food and Drug Administration (FDA) since 1993.[15]

Table 7-7 Pharmacologic therapy for seizure disorder and epilepsy: advantages and disadvantages

Disadvantages of drugs used for seizure disorder prior to 1993	Advantages of antiepileptic drugs approved since 1993
Five older seizure control agents: ● Phenytoin (Dilantin) ● Carbamazepine (Tegretol, Carbatrol) ● Phenobarbital (Luminal, Barbita) ● Valproate (Depakene, Depakote) ● Primidone (Mysoline, Apo-Primidone)[15]	FDA-approved AEDs: ● Felbamate (Felbatol) ● Gabapentin (Neurontin) ● Levetiracetam (Keppra) ● Lamotrigine (Lamictal) ● Oxcarbazepine (Trileptal) ● Pregabalin (Lyrica) ● Tiagabine (Gabitril) ● Topiramate (Topamax) ● Zonisamide (Zonegran)[15]

Disadvantages of older anticonvulsants:
● High incidence of adverse and toxic effects:
  ● Phenytoin: arrhythmias, cardiovascular collapse, gingival hyperplasia, aplastic anemia, agranulocytosis, toxic epidermal necrosis
  ● Carbamazepine: respiratory depression, heart block, aplastic anemia, agranulocytosis, hepatitis and jaundice, leukopenia, leukocytosis, and aplastic anemia
  ● Phenobarbital: bronchospasm, laryngospasm, circulatory collapse liver damage, agranulocytosis. Overdose leads to CNS depression, coma, and death
  ● Valproate, valproic acid: hepatic failure, prolonged bleeding time, hypofibrinogenemia, leukopenia, bone marrow depression, anemia
  ● Primidone: leucopenia, thrombocytopenia, eosinophilia, rare megaloblastic anemia, osteomalacia
	Advantages of newer AEDs:
	● Better tolerated by patients
	● Fewer drug interactions
	● Reduced side effects and adverse effects
	● Do not require routine serum monitoring

A pharmacologic option effective for epilepsy with partial seizures is phenytoin, carbamazepine, or any of the newer AEDs. When epilepsy is refractory to medications (uncontrolled), there are two options for seizure control:

- Surgery, which is curative and consists of resection of the area that is generating the seizures, for example, a temporal lobe resection).
- Vagal nerve stimulator which is palliative to relieve seizures when medications have failed.

Patients are referred to a neurologist or neurosurgeon when seizures cannot be controlled with medications, when patients cannot tolerate the side effects of medications, or when epilepsy is complicated with pregnancy or comorbidities.

PATIENT TEACHING   Safety issues are priority, so the patient must be taught to:

- Recognize and heed the aura or other premonitory symptoms as a warning sign to stop all activity and lie down in a safe place immediately.
- Have someone immediately available when engaging in activities (swimming or tub bathing, climbing a ladder) that could be hazardous in the event of seizure.[18]

To reduce the frequency of seizures, caution the patient against:

- Prolonged exposure to flashing lights (computer or electronic games or casino gaming), which could trigger a seizure
- Abruptly stopping antiseizure medications by refilling before vacations or trips
- Ingestion of alcoholic beverages
- Losing sleep or excessive stress/tension[18]

Family members/significant others should be taught what to do (or not do) when a seizure is in progress and afterward:

- Added injury can occur (broken bones) if attempts are made to hold a patient down during a seizure.
- Never put anything into the patient's mouth, or try to open a clenched jaw.
- Loosen anything constricting (eg, a necktie or necklace) to facilitate breathing.
- Turn the patient to the side in a recovery position (bend the uppermost leg) to promote drainage of any oral secretions.
- Call 911 if the seizure lasts longer than 5 minutes or another seizure starts soon after the initial one.

Cutting edge

An implantable device to stimulate the vagal nerve sends weak signals to the brain to prevent seizures! The patient is provided with a magnet, which turns on the device during the aura to stop a seizure! Patients with intractable epilepsy report improved quality of life. How cool is that?[18]

✚ Traumatic brain injury (TBI)

Traumatic brain injury (TBI) presents a challenge to nursing because TBI impacts all aspects of the patient's life.

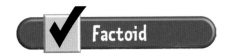

Factoid

Not all patients are candidates for surgical cure of epilepsy.

Let's get the normal stuff straight!

The brain has two hemispheres with a connecting isthmus and resides within the cranium (Fig. 7-3).

▶ Figure 7-3. Lobes of the brain.

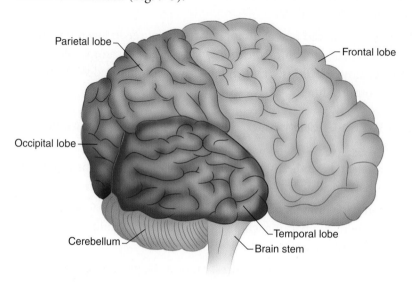

The cranium is the hard bony portion of the skull that encases and protects the brain. The brain has four lobes (frontal, parietal, temporal, and occipital) and five parts (cerebrum, cerebellum, pons, medulla oblongata, and the spinal cord). Membranes (called meninges) cover the brain and the cord, and between each membrane there is a potential space. There are three layers of meninges (Fig. 7-4):

- Dura mater (tough fibrous external covering)
- Arachnoid (middle weblike delicate layer)
- Pia mater (internal layer)

▶ Figure 7-4. Layers of covering over the brain.

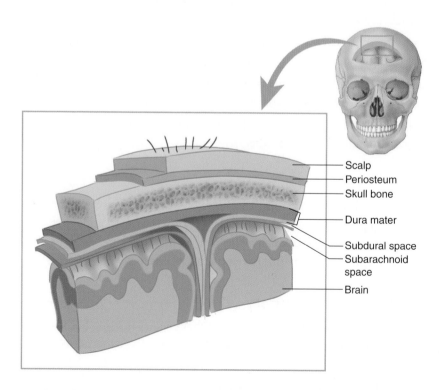

The cavities of the brain (called ventricles) are filled with cerebrospinal fluid (CSF), which is formed by the choroid plexus in the walls and the roof of the ventricles.[19] CSF also circulates around the brain, floats in the cerebral hemispheres, and fills the spinal column. Its watery cushion serves a triple function: to bathe, nourish, and protect the brain and spinal cord from shock.[19]

What is it?

Traumatic brain injury (TBI) consists of primary and secondary damage. The first occurs on impact, causing surface lacerations and contusions to brain tissue and vessels. Secondary damage is visible later as edema appears, which increases intracranial pressure and leads to hypoxia. Infection may ensue later[14] as a result of contaminating organisms from penetrating injuries or from internal injury with organisms ascending from the nasal cavity or mouth. TBI is classified as being either open or closed. Open wounds actually penetrate the skull, but the skull is intact with a closed head injury. Specific types of injuries occurring with TBI include:

- Skull fractures: Simple, comminuted, depressed, or basilar fracture.
- Coup-contrecoup injury: The brain accelerates to hit the inner cranial vault, and then slams backward in the opposite direction, producing injury on both sites, bruising the brain, and tearing blood vessels.
- Concussion: Transient neurologic dysfunction without structural or residual brain damage.
- Contusion: Bruising to brain tissue in single or multiple places where the brain comes in contact with the interior of the hard bony skull.
- Hematoma: Epidural, subdural, or intracerebral bleeding into an enclosed space.
- Diffuse axonal injury: Nerve cells are stretched and torn within the white matter of the brain.

Causes and why?

Obviously *trauma* causes traumatic brain injury. Common causes of such injury are:

- Motor vehicle accidents (including automobiles, motorcycles,[20] and all-terrain vehicles)
- Acceleration/deceleration forces to the head, as in sports (football) injury or shaken baby syndrome[21]
- Any direct blow to the head, which could be an accidental sports injury or an act of violence
- Blast injuries or gunshot wounds, such as those affecting the military during acts of war[14]

Testing, testing, testing

Upon arrival to the emergency department, while still on a spine board, initial testing will consist of X-rays of the neck and skull to rule out fractures and assess spine stability. Secondary imaging studies include the following::

Test	Clinical significance	Nursing care
CT (can be with or without contrast)	CT or CAT scanning is the primary neuroimaging technique in the initial evaluation of the acute head trauma patient. CT imaging uses a computer to digitally construct an image based upon the measurement of the absorption of X-rays through the brain.	• Ask about allergies because the contrast dye used is iodine based. • Have the patient sign a consent form prior to the test. • Instruct the patient that the head (which will be in a holder) must remain still, and no talking!
MRI (magnetic resonance imaging)	MRI is the most sensitive of the structural tests. MRI, as its name indicates, utilizes magnetic fields to image the brain's tissue, as opposed to the X-ray radiation of the CT scan.	Picks up on pathology earlier than CT • Because a magnet is used: no jewelry, no credit cards, no pacemakers (ever)! • Screen for old tattoos that may contain lead based paint. • Instruct the patient that a thumping sound will be heard (which is normal). • Claustrophobia is not usually a problem with the newer open MRIs (no tight tube).[22]
EEG (electroencephalogram): • Damaged areas of the brain will produce decreased electrical activity.[22]	Monitors brain wave patterns produced by electrical activity.	• Electrodes are applied to the scalp with water-based glue. • Hold sedatives and caffeine prior to the test. • The patient is NOT NPO, because this would drop blood sugar and alter normal brain wave patterns.
Cerebral angiography	X-ray of cerebral circulation • A catheter is inserted via the femoral artery and advanced to an artery in the neck. • Dye (iodine based) is injected into the artery to outline cerebral blood vessels. • Gives more detailed images than the magnetic resonance angiography (MRA). MRA is non-invasive and is used with MRI.	• Ask about allergies to iodine and shellfish.
Positron emission tomography (PET) scan	Shows metabolically active areas of the brain (in color) picking up oxygen and sugar labeled with a tracer. • Less metabolically active areas obviously pick up less of the tracer radionuclide. • Different levels of activity show up in different colors.	

Signs and symptoms and why?

Depending upon the type and degree of damage within the brain after traumatic injury, the patients, score on the Glasgow coma scale (GCS) varies according to his or her ability to arouse, process information, and follow a command. The GCS is a standardized tool used to quickly measure, record, and communicate the severity of brain trauma to other members of the health care team.[24] The GCS assigns a number from 3 to 15 based on three categories of observed patient behaviors:

- Eye opening = ranges from 1 (no response) to 4 (spontaneous)
- Motor = ranges from 1 (no response) to 6 (obeys command)
- Verbal = ranges from 1 (no response) to 5 (appropriate, oriented conversation)

The sum of each category is totaled to provide the GCS score.[25] When evaluating the patient's Glasgow coma score, think: If less than 8, intubate, as these patients generally require ventilation because of the severity of their TBI.

The patient will display varying signs and symptoms based on the severity of brain trauma. Refer to Table 7-8 for signs and symptoms of mild, moderate, and severe TBI.

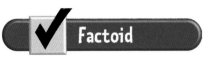

Factoid

The earlier after injury that the initial CT is done and the larger the initial size of the hematoma, the greater the likelihood of the hematoma expanding on the next CT.[23]

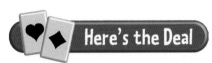

Here's the Deal

Hemorrhages within the brain can expand over time and naturally will increase the most while the injury is still "fresh." Especially when there is a large area of brain damage, you should expect it to bleed more.

Table 7-8 Manifestations of mild, moderate, and severe TBI

Mild TBI	Moderate TBI	Severe TBI
Clinical examination reveals concussion with normal Glasgow coma scale (GCS) score (14–15) and minimal to absent brain damage	Clinical examination may reveal Coup-contrecoup injuries: contusion with possible extra-axial hematoma formation (epidural, subdural) Glasgow coma scale score (9–13), but may deteriorate later because of secondary injury[21]	Clinical examination may reveal skull fracture, any intracranial contusion, hematoma, or brain tear is considered severe.[21] Diffuse axonal injury may be present. Glasgow coma scale score 8 or less.
The patient signs and symptoms include: - Possible brief loss of consciousness at time of injury - No evidence of direct external trauma - Awake and aware - Headache The postconcussive syndrome symptoms are: - Longer reaction time - Increased distractibility - Decreased attention span - Decreased concentration - Impaired balance and coordination - Decreased memory - Dizziness - Tinnitus - Sensory sensitivity[24] - Sleep disturbances[21]	The patient signs and symptoms include: - Possible brief loss of consciousness - Possible brief post-traumatic seizure - Worsening headache - Facial trauma usually present - Focal neurologic deficits - Nausea and vomiting - Restless - Agitated - Irritable - Confusion - Memory loss	The patient signs and symptoms reveal: - Pattern of loss of consciousness, waking up for an interval of clear thought pattern, followed by deterioration of consciousness again[22] - Paralysis or weakness on opposite side of injury (contralateral) - Pupil dilation on same side as injury (ipsilateral) (Fig. 7-12) - Breathing difficulties Cushing's reflex (also called Cushing's phenomenon), which consists of three clinical signs (triad): - Hypertension - Bradycardia - Decreased or irregular respirations Cushing's phenomenon means dangerously high intracranial pressure (ICP) and may forewarn of impending herniation syndrome.[21]

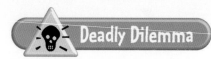

If there are changes in the LOC (no matter how subtle), don't wait for the next scheduled CT to prove what you already suspect. Call the doctor STAT!

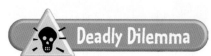

The patient with moderate TBI who has a Glasgow Coma Scale score of 9 or above and deteriorates to a score of 8 is in trouble! This patient is predicted to have a worse outcome than the patient with severe TBI who was admitted with a Glasgow Coma Scale score of 8!

What can harm my patient and why?

Mild brain injury causes a change in behavior, thought patterns, sensory perception, mood, and emotions related to ultrastructural damage not detected with conventional MRI.[26] Because an injured brain causes symptoms that encompass all aspects of living, the patient may experience:

- Depression[27]
- Suicidal ideation[14]
- Seizures
- Persistent cognitive impairment[28]
- Alterations in gait and mobility[29]
- Sleep deprivation

  Moderate brain injury:
- All of the above (mild brain injury) possible outcomes
- Progressive deterioration to severe brain injury
- Secondary injury can lead to transtentorial herniation[30]

  Severe brain injury:
- Infections of the brain (encephalitis) from penetrating injury or invasive pressure monitoring catheters
- Vegetative state caused by diffuse axonal injury
- Increased intracranial pressure leading to neural compression, hypoxia, and death
- Brain stem herniation syndrome and death

Interventions and why?

Because even mild traumatic brain injury can deteriorate, CT scanning is a safer (but more expensive) option for patients who have loss of consciousness or memory loss of the trauma.

- Repeat CT scanning is performed at 12 and 24 hours to monitor for slow bleeds.
- Longer periods of observation in the emergency department with serial observations can help physicians make discharge decisions after a minor head injury.
- In-hospital observation for 24 hours provides quick access to surgical intervention if the need arises.
- Moderate head injuries (risk for subdural, epidural hematomas) can deteriorate quickly and must be closely observed and re-evaluated for early neurosurgical intervention.
- Brief hyperventilation and osmotic therapy can reduce ICP to buy time for transfer to a trauma center (availability of neurosurgery) for more definitive measures to relieve pressure.
- Immediate surgical intervention (drilling burr holes, evacuation of hematomas) is indicated for increased intracranial pressure with signs of herniation syndrome.[21]

Traumatic brain injury results in persistent neurologic deficits and an entire team of professionals and specialists is required:

- Neurologist
- Psychiatrist
- Nurses
- Social worker/case manager
- Occupational therapist
- Speech therapist
- Psychologist
- Rehab specialist

The problem of postconcussion syndrome following mild brain trauma, although not life threatening, is distressing and in some instances debilitating. Donepezil (cholinesterase inhibitor used with dementia and head injury) has been used with success in the treatment of post-TBI cognitive impairment and memory deficits,[31] and further clinical studies are currently in progress.

Always take time to assess first. Even in emergencies when you want to act fast, this initial step is even more important! Determine the Glasgow coma scale baseline score for comparison with later scores and neurologic checks.

Priorities for the patient with severe TBI are A-B-Cs using the stepwise approach and include the following:

- Secure the airway with rapid-sequence intubation and ventilation, especially in the presence of agitation and combative behavior.[21]
- Maintain systolic BP >90 mm Hg with fluids and blood products because the trauma patient will likely have other injuries.[20]
- Administer prescribed agents (eg, mannitol or hypertonic saline) to reduce brain swelling and ICP.
- Administer seizure prophylaxis (rapid-acting benzodiazepines such as lorazepam or diazepam)[21] as prescribed.

Mild to moderate traumatic brain injury requires close observation to detect deterioration that can occur with secondary injury.

- Assessment is always the first phase of the nursing process, and the priority "neuro" assessment will always be LOC!
- Perform neurologic checks frequently (usually every two hours): pupils, reflexes, vital signs, and LOC.
- Calculate and record the Glasgow coma scale score with each neurological check.
- In addition to the usual "oriented × 3" you will be watching for any behavioral change or change in cognition.
- Attention span, concentration, and memory can be monitored with a five-minute conversation while you are getting vital signs.
- Ask questions that can evaluate the patient's speech and language for changes.

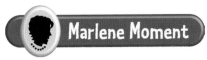

Marlene Moment

Once the patient is intubated, it's going to be pretty hard to elicit a best "verbal response," and if both eyes are swollen shut, you can also forget the "eye opening" part of the Glasgow coma scale! Better at least get a good baseline to identify "starting point" patient status. It can be beneficial to break the Glasgow down to an EVM score, and report a separate score for eye, verbal, and motor response. This helps to better evaluate the patient who is intubated or whose eye is swollen shut.

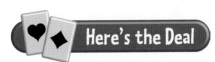

Here's the Deal

Intracranial pressure monitoring is recommended for severe TBI with low Glasgow coma scale scores (3–8), abnormal admission CT scans (hematomas, contusions, edema, and compression of basal cisterns) or normal CT if any two additional criteria are present: neurologic posturing, hypotension <90 systolic, or age >40 years.[32]

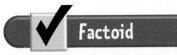

Factoid

Intracranial pressure monitoring is not without risk because of the invasive catheter required. It is often worth the risk because it enables the nurse to detect worsening pressure, trends well in advance of discovering deadly signs of impending herniation syndrome.

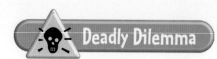

Hypotension resulting from a head injury is a sign of herniation, and if clinical evidence doesn't lead you there, you had better be looking for other injuries causing the blood pressure to drop!

Hypertonic agents pull fluid from cerebral tissues into the vascular space, thereby lowering the intracranial pressure.[33-35]

Don't worry about depressing respirations with "benzos," the ventilator has a built in "tolerance" to these drugs: it will keep right on breathing for my patient!

Post-traumatic seizures increase secondary brain injury by causing more brain hypoxia owing to increased metabolism of brain tissue and ICP.

In the absence of ICP monitoring (not recommended for mild to moderate TBI),[32] be alert to any subtle change that can mean huge things happening inside your patient's brain-injured head. Even with a normal admission CT, edema or slow bleeding could be increasing the ICP.

• Affect, mood, and behavior should be noted at each scheduled "neuro" check.

My patient needs close monitoring for early detection of worsening trends, so all of the above "first things first" neurologic checks and Glasgow coma scale scoring will continue.

• Severe TBI will require intracranial pressure monitoring in an intensive care setting.
• Risk for infection with ICP monitoring (ventricular catheters or subarachnoid screws) requires dry dressings and tight connections at all times.
• Cerebral perfusion pressure (CPP) is calculated by subtracting the ICP from the mean arterial pressure (MAP).
• Any drainage from ears, nose, or dressings about the head is checked for glucose to identify the presence of CSF.

Nursing care to meet basic and special needs of the patient with traumatic brain injury is summarized in Table 7-9.

Table 7-9 Nursing care for the patient with traumatic brain injury

Nursing care of the patient with traumatic brain injury	Rationales for interventions
Maintain temperature neutrality: • Monitor temperature frequently. • Utilize cooling blanket with rectal probe to maintain constant temperature. • Use thin sheeting for cover. • Remove blankets or bedspread. • Administer prescribed antipyretics for temperature >100.4°F. • Tepid sponge bath PRN.	Hyperpyrexia may result from brain injury or as a result of infection secondary to invasive lines and ICP monitoring devices. Thermal control pads cool or warm as indicated to achieve set temperature as monitored by the rectal probe. Hypothalamus may be dysfunctional because of brain trauma. Fever increases cerebral metabolism, which increases ICP. Antipyretics reduce fever by internal mechanisms, and sponge bathing reduces fever by evaporation, which may be less desired because of increased tactile stimulation, which could trigger a seizure.

(Continued)

Table 7-9 Nursing care for the patient with traumatic brain injury *(Continued)*

Nursing care of the patient with traumatic brain injury	Rationales for interventions
Structure surroundings to provide quiet, nonstimulating, safe environment: Use indirect light source. Pull curtains, close blinds. Block incoming calls. Monitor activity of visitors. Keep bed in low position with padded side rails. Insure availability of suction and oxygen at the head of the bed.	Bright lights, a streak of sunlight across the patient's face, ringing of telephone, loud noises, and sudden touch may startle the patient and initiate a seizure. Low bed with padded rails is a safety issue in the event of seizure activity. Nausea and vomiting or excessive secretions may necessitate suction. PRN oxygen is indicated after tonic seizure activity, during which time the patient may not be breathing.
Support nutrition compatible with patient needs and physical capabilities: • Monitor total parenteral nutrition TPN infusion as prescribed via central or peripherally inserted central (PIC) line. • Administer fat emulsions (lipids) as prescribed. • Administer nasogastric (NG) tube feedings as prescribed, being cautious to test (commercial glucose strips touched to drainage will produce color change if glucose is present) any nasal drainage for CSF. • High caloric, nutrient-dense diet PO as prescribed. • Collaborate with speech therapy when swallowing evaluation is indicated. • Assist with oral feedings and thicken thin liquids with tasteless commercial products to facilitate swallowing as indicated. • Feed patients in an upright position with head tilted forward and chin down to swallow. • Monitor labs: total protein or serum albumin, and urine for ketones as indicators of nutritional status.	Parenteral nutrition bypasses the GI tract and is used when patients cannot eat or when extra calories are needed. Fats supply added calories and enable utilization of fat-soluble vitamins. Head-injured patients have increased caloric needs to meet added metabolic demands of fever, seizure activity, and neurologic posturing that places muscles in a constant tight hold. Steroids (given to reduce inflammation and ICP) cause increased breakdown of fats and proteins, increasing nutritional needs. CSF rhinorrhea is an absolute contraindication for NG tube feedings. Oral insertion or G-tube insertion are alternate routes for enteral feed in the presence of CSF leakage. Thickened liquids are better tolerated with less risk of aspiration when the brain-injured patient has swallowing difficulties. The trachea is positioned to the front with the esophagus posterior, tilting head forward and directing chin downward helps direct food/liquids toward the esophagus. Total protein and serum albumin are laboratory indicators of nutritional adequacy. Absence of urinary ketones is indicative of positive nitrogen balance because fats are not being utilized to maintain metabolic processes.

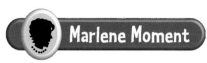

Here you are turning on the lights and doing "neuro" checks at 2 a.m., and I haven't slept for 24 hours! Forget mood and affect! I don't think I'm going to be a happy camper! I will however be less grumpy if you remind me that I am staying in the hospital for observation, so you can wake me up every two hours to make sure that I am okay!

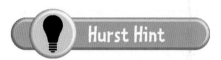

These "neuro" checks are giving me a headache. Listen, instead of fully awakening me to talk, can't you just check my mood ring?

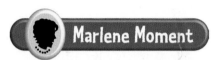

Notify the doctor/neurologist/neurosurgeon at the first indication of increasing ICP, because patients can deteriorate rapidly, in just minutes.

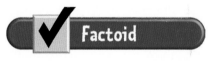

The TBI patient may become a little slower to respond (not affecting GCS score) when mental status declines, and within minutes may lose the ability to follow commands. ICP can happen very rapidly! Be alert to subtle changes!

(Continued)

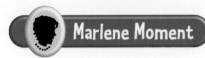

Marlene Moment

Please do NOT wait until my pupils are fixed and dilated before you call the doctor! You know better than that! I need help while it can actually still *help!*

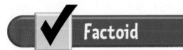

Factoid

Normal ICP is 10 to 20 mm Hg.

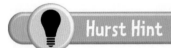

Here's the Deal

Cerebral perfusion pressure (CPP) is the amount of pressure required to adequately perfuse cerebral tissues with oxygen (normally between 70 and 80 mm Hg).[4]

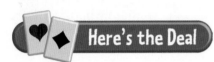

Hurst Hint

CSF is easy to spot because it makes halos on dressings and linens.

Table 7-9 Nursing care for the patient with traumatic brain injury *(Continued)*

Nursing care of the patient with traumatic brain injury	Rationales for interventions
Provide protective positioning to reduce ICP and promote safety: • Keep HOB elevated 30 degrees at all times. • Use pillows to support side-lying position keeping hips and legs aligned with torso. • Keep head and neck straight (no flexed) and in perfect alignment at all times. • Observe patient 5–10 minutes after each position change to evaluate patient response. • Monitor vital signs and ICP after each position change: Return to baseline readings should occur within 15 minutes.	Elevating the head of the bed (HOB) reduces ICP by promoting gravity drainage. Elevating the HOB reduces potential for aspiration when NG tube feedings are in progress. Side-lying position facilitates drainage of oral secretions. Neutral position and proper alignment promotes venous drainage by reducing obstruction (kinking) of jugular veins. Staying physically present is necessary to determine whether the patient is tolerating a position. ICP that remains up, blood pressure fluctuation, increased heart rate, or change in breathing pattern are all indicators for immediate repositioning.
Make provisions for hygienic and oral care: • Provide total hygienic care for the unconscious patient: bed bath, perineal care, and oral care. • Evaluate patient tolerance to full bed bath and terminate activity if poorly tolerated: bathe instead face, axilla, and groin (the triangle). • Provide meticulous mouth care with sponge swab and hydrogen peroxide–based cleanser, using Yanker suction to retrieve solution when patient is unable to expectorate. • For intubated patients, collaborate with respiratory therapy to assist and stabilize the ET when bite block is removed for mouth care (above).	A full bath does not justify any increase in ICP or excessive stimulation that could initiate seizure activity or neurologic posturing. Bacteria from the mouth can accumulate around the ET tube and be forced into the lung around the tube when the patient coughs or breathes against the ventilator. Frequent meticulous mouth care reduces bacterial count in the mouth to help prevent lung infection. Manual stabilization of the ET tube during oral care when everything is out of the mouth is necessary to prevent accidental extubation.
Provide protective eye care: • Instill sterile liquid tears or methylcellulose as a wetting solution when the blink reflex is lost. • Close eyes and apply eye pads with thin strips of hypoallergenic paper tape when indicated. • Apply Steri-Strips. Suture-alternate thin skin adhesive strips from lid to cheek may also be used to keep eyes closed.	Corneal abrasion can occur when the blink reflex is lost. Lubrication prevents dry eye and risk for abrasion. Eye pads keeps the lids closed, and provide protection against a lid being open and in contact with the pillow cover. Skin adhesive strips (suture alternative) are easily removed for pupil checks, leaving no residue behind.

(Continued)

Table 7-9 Nursing care for the patient with traumatic brain injury (*Continued*)

Nursing care of the patient with traumatic brain injury	Rationales for interventions
Maintain fluid balance and monitor for electrolyte imbalance: • Monitor and record 24-hour intake and output and daily weights. • Monitor IV flow rates being alert to all fluids, flushes for central lines and IV medications, restricting total fluids to 1200–1500 mL/d. • Monitor serum sodium and correlate with urinary output and blood pressure. • Monitor serum glucose and administer insulin per sliding or weight based scale as prescribed.	Fluid balance is reflected by 24 hour intake and output. Rapid fluid gain or loss is reflected in daily weight. Multiple infusions plus diluent for IVPB plus flush solutions for each invasive line can dramatically increase the 24-hour fluid total and predispose to added water in brain tissue. Head injury can produce syndrome of inappropriate antidiuretic hormone secretion (SIADH), which dilutes serum sodium causing fluid volume excess and increased BP. Post-traumatic diabetes insipidus (DI) can occur, leading to fluid volume deficit, hypotension, and shock. Stress, steroids, and TPN increase the blood sugar, which can cause polyuria.
Maintain bladder and bowel function: • Exercise caution when inserting Foley catheter when the TBI patient has additional trauma: inspect urinary meatus for evidence of blood prior to insertion. • Secure the catheter to leg with tension loop using Velcro or paper tape fastener. • If external sheath is used (males), check for constriction and monitor skin care. • Monitor bowel movements and record. • Perform digital rectal exam if impaction is suspected. • Collaborate with physician for stool softener and/or addition of fiber to diet or tube feedings.	When the head injury occurs in conjunction with a motorcycle accident, bladder trauma is common.[20] Stability of indwelling catheter prevents additional mechanical trauma. Immobility decreases intestinal peristalsis. Voluntary muscle tone may be lost with brain injury. Velcro strap for external sheath can reduce circulation, causing tissue ischemia or decrease venous return causing edema. Constant moisture/urine can irritate and macerate tissue. Stool softeners increase the water content of the stool to reduce constipation and straining. Fiber stimulates peristalsis.

(*Continued*)

Table 7-9 Nursing care for the patient with traumatic brain injury (*Continued*)

Nursing care of the patient with traumatic brain injury	Rationales for interventions
Implement measures to decrease ICP: • Space nursing interventions to allow for uninterrupted periods of rest. • Avoid use of restraints. • Keep frequency and duration of suction to an absolute minimum. • Caution coherent patients against coughing, nose blowing, straining, or tensing muscles and hanging head down. • Administer corticosteroids (dexamethasone) as prescribed. • Administer furosemide as prescribed.	ICP increases with each intervention, position change, or physical contact, especially when noxious (eg, veni-punctures). Struggling against restraints, suction, coughing, nose blowing, straining, isometrics, bending at the waist, leaning head down (and any other noxious stimuli) are all activities that increase ICP. Corticosteroids reduce the inflammatory response in the brain to decrease cerebral edema. Furosemide promotes diuresis of excess fluid.
Monitor and report signs/symptoms of increased ICP and worsening neurologic status: • Decreasing LOC • Changes in pupils (asymmetry, fixed, and dilated) • Slurred speech • Patterned respirations: Cheyne stokes, ataxic • Lethargy, drowsiness • Mood changes (labile, agitated) • Behavioral changes (quiet to restless) • Diminished to absent reflexes • Flaccid extremities • Projectile vomiting • Neurologic posturing • Paralysis (facial or hemiplegia)	The brain is contained within the rigid skull which accommodates brain tissue, CSF, and blood flow. Full capacity of the bony cranium is exceeded when cerebral edema and increased intracranial pressure occurs. ICP compresses neural tissue to cause physiologic changes in vital signs, awareness/consciousness, and voluntary muscle control. Projectile vomiting occurs when the vomiting center in the brain is stimulated. Neurologic posturing that is rigid and involuntary is classified as: Decorticate: Arms flexed inwardly, legs extended with plantar flexion Decerebrate: Arched spine, plantar flexion indicates greatest neurologic involvement
Implement measures to prevent complications of bed rest: • DVTs use antiembolism stockings and sequential pneumatic compression devices. • Pneumonia: Position for optimal chest expansion, alternate position side to side, instruct in deep breathing.	External compression forces circulation deep to improve blood flow. Alternating pressure simulates the muscle pump that is activated with ambulation. Upright position with arms/elbows supported maximizes chest expansion with less effort.

(Continued)

Table 7-9 Nursing care for the patient with traumatic brain injury *(Continued)*

Nursing care of the patient with traumatic brain injury	Rationales for interventions
Decubitus ulcers: • Turn frequently, pad pressure points, maintain adequate nutrition and hydration (Refer to Chapter 1 for specific interventions.)	Turning and repositioning reduces pressure on local tissues to improve blood flow and reduce ischemia. Hydration and nutrition promote cellular health and well-being.
Reorientation for the confused patient: • Large calendars, clocks. • Family photos visible. • Reiterate date, time, and place with each neurologic check. • Give frequent reminders and hints to facilitate recall. For the patient awakening from coma: • Reorient frequently to help dispel fears. • If combative give assurance that he or she is safe and maintain distance to avoid appearance of threat. • Provide for physical needs, explaining each intervention with rationales and expectations.	Constant visual reminders of day and time assist with orientation. Familiar photos reinforce previous relationships and serve as memory "joggers." Repetition, repetition, repetition hastens re-learning. Persons awakening from a coma are frightened, being in a strange place with unfamiliar surroundings and people. Combativeness is a primitive self-protection mechanism. Distance is less threatening because the person's space is not being invaded. Explanations are fundamental to understanding.
Assist patient and family members to integrate the experience and make realistic plans: • Provide emotional support by listening and empathizing with fears and concerns. • Provide updates and meaning of signs (ie, posturing, Glasgow scores) • Inform patient/family members of available resources/options • Encourage patient and family members by giving optimistic (but factual) information.	Patients and family members are frightened because of known and uncertain outcomes. Factual information is essential for decisions that must be made by next of kin or designated power of attorney. Family members may interpret involuntary neurologic movement (posturing) as signs of improvement because the patient is "moving." Knowledge of resources is helpful for advance planning. Accepting reality is best accomplished in small increments with hopeful anticipation.

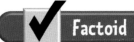

Fever increases metabolic demands and can lead to cerebral hypoxia with resultant deterioration of brain function!

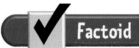

Extraneous stimuli can trigger seizures.

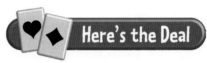

Exercise caution when inserting a Foley catheter on a trauma patient! Always check for blood around the urinary meatus first, especially if the TBI patient was riding a motorcycle! Bladder trauma is common.[20]

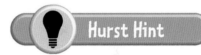

Rhinorrhea that tests positive for CSF is an absolute contraindication against NG tube feedings.

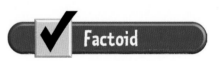

Detecting CSF on bloody dressings is easy: Just look for the halo!

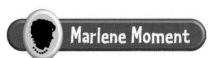

Obviously you can't give a tube feeding if your patient has CSF running out the nose! You don't want to get Ensure into the brain, do you?

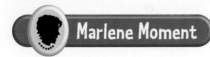

If you're not a patient person, don't sit with somebody who needs re-orienting. You will be pulling out your hair (and theirs too)!

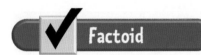

Second-impact syndrome (SIS) can occur with a minimal repeat impact following the initial concussion. SIS produces serious brain injury and possibly death.

PATIENT TEACHING   Patient teaching following mild to moderate traumatic head injury will include signs of postconcussive syndrome (see Table 7-5) and implications of further injury:

- Athletes are cautioned against return to play after a concussion for at least one week (even if symptom free) because of possible serious reinjury.[21]

- Patients released after minor head injury are advised to have telephone access and a competent adult available to monitor (4–6 hours) for delayed signs and symptoms.

- Watch for early signs of increasing ICP (pressure inside the head), the earliest being a change in level of consciousness. Slowed speech pattern and delayed responsiveness are other early indicators to return to the emergency department.

- Call 911 for vomiting, slurred speech, behavioral changes, lethargy, and difficult arousal, which are signs that intracranial pressure is already high and is compressing neural tissue.

- Consultations and referrals are recommended for postconcussion syndrome.

Cutting edge

In the past, postconcussion syndrome was thought to be psychosomatic, and one recent study of post-traumatic concussion syndrome has supported that assumption. Certain individuals were found more likely to develop the syndrome than others: those having higher intelligence scores, previous affective/anxiety disorders, and women (one-third more likely than men).[36] The conclusion showed a correlation between pain and development of postconcussion syndrome, but NOT mild traumatic brain injury. Other experts believe that shearing of white matter connections and neural fiber tracts necessary for memory, attention, and goal-oriented behaviors[37] are responsible for postconcussion syndrome. With the advent of more refined imaging (analysis of diffusion tensor MRI),[26,28] white matter ultrastructural damage has been well documented months to years after mild traumatic brain injury.

✚ Spinal cord injury (SCI)

The Spinal Cord Injury Network reports that 2008 data revealed 12,000 new cases of spinal cord injury (SCI) per year, not counting victims who did not survive the injury.[38]

Let's get the normal stuff straight!

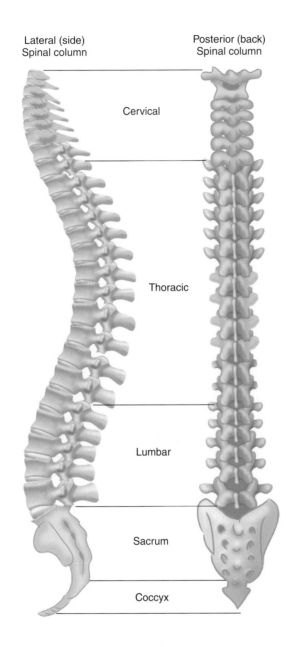

Lateral (side)
Spinal column

Posterior (back)
Spinal column

◀ Figure 7-5. Sections of spinal column.

Cervical

Thoracic

Lumbar

Sacrum

Coccyx

The spinal column is filled with glucose-rich cerebrospinal fluid, which bathes the brain and spinal cord (Fig. 7-5). The spinal column (and brain) is encased in a triple-layered covering (pia mater, arachnoid, and dura mater) and is surrounded by bony vertebral bodies to protect the cord and the column of fluid. The spinal cord descends from the brain and spinal nerves branch outward. The vertebral bodies are listed as:

- Cervical: C1 through C7 are relatively smaller vertebrae whose function is to provide support to the skull and allow for forward, backward, right, and left lateral movement of the neck.[39]

- Thoracic: T1 through T12 are joined with the ribs to provide protection for internal organs.

• Lumbar: L1 through L5, and some people have an L6! These vertebrae are larger and thicker because they have to support the weight of the body.

The spinal cord is a downward progression of the brain, which has three segments (Fig. 7-6):

▶ Figure 7-6. Spinal cord.

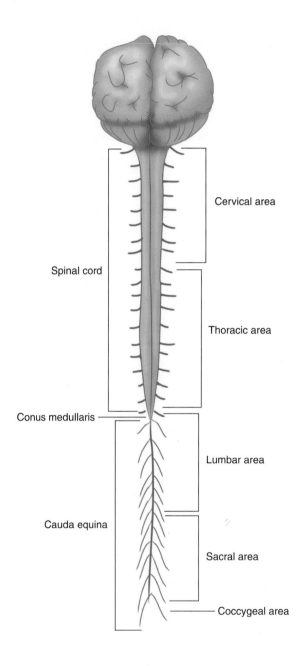

Cervical area

Spinal cord

Thoracic area

Conus medullaris

Lumbar area

Cauda equina

Sacral area

Coccygeal area

• A tiny central cavity
• Inner gray matter surrounding the central cavity
• Outer superficial layer of white matter

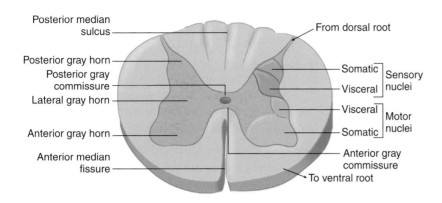

Posterior median sulcus

From dorsal root

Posterior gray horn

Posterior gray commissure

Lateral gray horn

Somatic ⎤ Sensory
Visceral ⎦ nuclei

Visceral ⎤ Motor
Somatic ⎦ nuclei

Anterior gray horn

Anterior median fissure

Anterior gray commissure

To ventral root

◄ Figure 7-7. Cross-section of spinal cord.

Bilateral pairs of dorsal root and ventral root branch from the inner gray matter of the cord (Fig. 7-7).

- The dorsal half, called the dorsal "horn," contains sensory afferent neurons.
- The ventral half, called the ventral "horn," contains motor efferent neurons.

The reflex arc in the spinal cord makes automatic responses possible without waiting on the brain to send the appropriate message. For example, the hand will have already dropped a hot skillet before the brain even knows there is a problem!

What is it?

Injury to the spinal cord can be complete or incomplete and can occur at different spinal cord levels. Complete spinal cord injury (SCI) is characterized by total loss of function (motor and sensory) below the level of the injury. Incomplete SCI implies that there is some motor or some sensory function remaining.

Spinal cord injury (SCI) is classified according to the type and extent of motor and sensory loss:

- Tetraplegia (previously called quadriplegia): Loss of muscle strength and movement in all four extremities
- Paraplegia: Lower level SCI occurs in thoracic, lumbar, or sacral segments (cauda equina and conus medullaris), resulting in loss of muscle strength and movement in the lower extremities.

Causes and why?

Bones in the spinal column can be injured by twisting, pulling, compression, or fractures and when the vertebra is damaged, all or portions of the cord can also suffer damage. The cervical spine is most vulnerable to injury because the cervical vertebrae are smaller and capable of a greater range of movement. Thoracic vertebrae are the most stable, being attached to the ribs.

Trauma to the spinal cord results from various causes, some of which could be preventable by wearing seat belts, safety harnesses, checking depth of water before diving, and sobriety while operating motorized recreational all-terrain vehicles (ATVs):

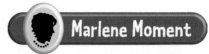

Marlene Moment

The inner gray matter of the cord looks like a butterfly to me! The cross-section of the cord shows the gray butterfly with ventral and dorsal horns making a "swallow tail." The dorsal (input) horn contains sensory afferent fibers (A = arriving) and the ventral (output) horn contains motor efferent fibers (E = exiting).

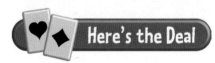

Here's the Deal

Ipsilateral refers to same side. *Contralateral* refers to the opposite side.

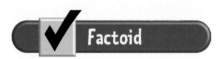

Factoid

The higher up the level of SCI, the greater the severity of symptoms.

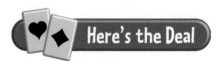

Here's the Deal

A higher level of SCI will affect the patient's ability to breathe, but a lower level of injury will affect the bladder, bowel, and legs.

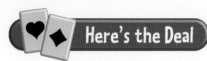

Hemi-section means "half-cut," which is what happens with Brown-Séquard syndrome. Half of the cord is cut, so the patient has movement (motor function intact) on one side, but no sensation; and the other half of the body can feel sensation but is unable to move.

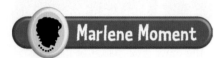

Marlene Moment

If I had Brown-Séquard syndrome, I know which arm I'm going stick out for my shot! You betcha! Can you guess which one? Yup! The only one that I can move is the one the student nurse will get to practice on!

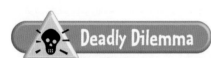

Deadly Dilemma

When a lumbar puncture is performed to measure and reduce CSF there is a danger that the opening into the spinal column gives high ICP an outlet for escape. The brain can be sucked downward, herniating through the tentorium and the foramen magnum.[22]

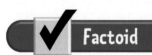

Factoid

Lumbar puncture is performed by inserting a long thin spinal needle into the lumbar subarachnoid space between L-3 and L-4 to prevent accidental puncture of the cord, which normally stops at the level of L-1.

- Vehicular accidents (most common)
- Falls (from high places: roofs, ladders, tree deer stands)
- Acts of violence (knives, bullets)
- Sports and recreational activities[38]

Complete SCI is caused by complete transverse disruption of the cord. The cord is either totally severed with the initial injury from direct compression by the fractured vertebral body, stretching or tearing arteries that supply that portion of the cord; or are destroyed by a secondary injury related to hemorrhage, expanding hematoma, or edema at the site of injury.[40] Incomplete SCI is caused by damage to a portion of the cord.

Depending on the site of the injury, the patient can lose motor function and/or sensory function. When incomplete injury occurs, the patient can lose motor and retain sensory or vice versa. Brown-Séquard syndrome (hemi-section) is a combination of loss of sensory on one side and loss of motor on the other.

Upper motor neuron damage will result in spastic paralysis and reflexes. Lower motor neuron damage will result in flaccid paralysis and areflexia.

Testing, testing, testing

Initial tests will include a CBC and electrolytes for any trauma patient, and the following specific tests to evaluate spinal cord–related injury:

- ABGs: Arterial blood gases are correlated with shock and tissue hypoxia as a guide to ventilator management and oxygen delivery.
- X-ray can reveal fracture and/or displacement of vertebral bodies.
- CT reveals fractures with displacement of vertebral bodies as well as hematomas.
- MRI: Magnetic resonance imaging can detect primary as well as secondary spinal cord injury related to edema and hemorrhage.[41]

A myelogram may be indicated if there are progressive neurologic deficits. This test is an X-ray of the spinal subarachnoid space that uses radiopaque dye (water base or oil base). The patient is NPO for this test and a permit is signed. Associated nursing implications are to:

- Warn the patient that the table will tilt around to disperse the dye.
- Administer a light pre-procedural sedative as prescribed.
- Position the patient in a side-lying position with knees drawn up to arch the back and separate the intervertebral disks for lumbar puncture, which is performed for injection of the dye into the CSF.
- Force fluids after the procedure to replenish CSF volume and prevent spinal headache.
- Observe the site for leaking of CSF (usually just a Band-Aid dressing is applied).
- Continuous leaking of CSF is an indication for an epidural blood patch to seal the site. (A small amount of blood is drawn from the patient and injected into the lumbar site to clot and seal the leak.)

● Monitor for signs/symptoms of infection: chills, spike in temperature, vomiting, stiff neck, and abnormal posturing (Kernig's sign and Brudzinski's sign).

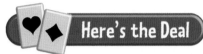
◄ Figure 7-8. Kernig's sign.

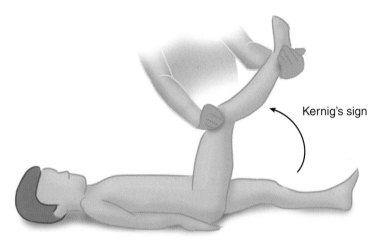

Kernig's sign

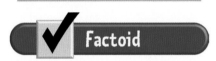
Here's the Deal

Oil-based dye does not mix with CSF and must be aspirated back out, but water-based dye does mix with CSF, and therefore cannot be aspirated for removal.

Factoid

The dye used for a myelogram is irritating to the meninges and should be removed (oil base can be aspirated back out) or excreted in a timely manner, hastened by forcing fluids.

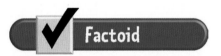
◄ Figure 7-9. Brudzinski neck sign.

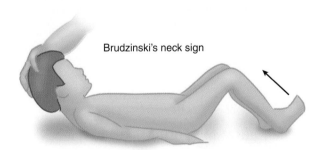

Brudzinski's neck sign

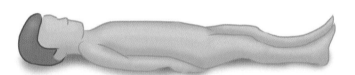
Factoid

Kernig's sign is elicited with the patient lying flat: One leg is flexed at the hip and knee and then straightened at the knee. Pain and inability to extend (straighten) at the knee = positive sign (Fig. 7-8)!

Signs and symptoms and why?

Spinal cord injury produces loss of innervation to muscles below the level of the injury. Refer to Table 7-10 for signs and symptoms of spinal cord lesions.

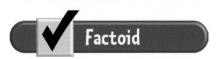
Factoid

Brudzinski's sign is elicited with the patient lying flat: Flex the neck and if the hip and knee involuntarily flex = positive sign (Fig. 7-9)![22]

Table 7-10 Signs and symptoms of spinal cord lesions

Level of SCI (Fig. 7-10)	Patient signs/symptoms of functional, motor, and/or sensory loss
C1-2	Tetraplegia and respiratory paralysis requires mechanical ventilation. No control of head and neck. Mobility is limited to sip and puff electric wheelchair.
C3-4	Tetraplegia with a weak diaphragm and loss of intercostal muscle function; has some neck control. Can be off mechanical control for short periods of time. Can use electric wheelchair with voice-, mouth-, head-, chin-, or shoulder-activated controls.
C5-6	Tetraplegia with good head and neck control as well as some shoulder movement. No fine motor ability, but gross arm and shoulder movement is preserved. Can operate electric wheelchair but requires transfer assistance. Diaphragm could be initially involved, but resolves after the initial injury.
C6-7	Tetraplegia with functional ability of bicep and deltoid muscles. Loss of triceps. Fully innervated shoulders plus extend and dorsiflex wrists. Can be independent with minimal assistance.
C7	Tetraplegia with functional triceps muscles has full elbow extension and can flex wrists. Has some finger control. Can independently use manual wheelchair.
T1-5	Diaphragmatic breathing is possible and arm muscles are intact and functional with full hand and finger control. Has sensation down to nipple line. Paraplegia is present with bladder and bowel involvement. Independently uses manual wheelchair.
T6-10	Paraplegia with loss of abdominal reflexes at T12. Has partial to good balance with trunk muscles. Spastic paralysis of lower extremities, feels sensation down to groin level.
T11-L5	Can flex and abduct hip, flex and extend knees (L1-L3). Can flex knees and dorsiflex ankles (L2-L4). Can ambulate short distances with assistance.
Below T12: conus medullaris	Dysfunction of bowel and bladder. Weakness of lower extremities; loss of sensation to areas in sacral dermatome and back pain.
Below T12: cauda equina	Lower motor neuron dysfunction results in areflexic paralysis with muscle atrophy, sphincter dysfunction, and loss of outer aspect of legs, ankles, and posterior lower extremities.
S1-5	Loss of bladder, bowel and sexual dysfunction at S-1. No paralysis of legs below S3; loss of sensation in the saddle area: perineum, scrotum, penis, anus, and upper back of thighs.

Sources: References 2 and 94.

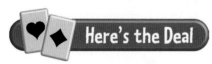

Here's the Deal

Don't take any patient off the spine board or remove the cervical collar until the radiologist has "cleared" the C-spine!

What can harm my patient and why?

- Spinal shock occurs because of transient loss of reflexes below the level of the injury. Flaccid paralysis of the muscle layer around vessels results in immediate vasodilation and hypotension.

- Neurogenic shock consists of a triad of symptoms: hypotension, bradycardia, and hypothermia.

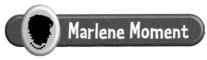

Figure 7-10. Levels of spinal cord injury.

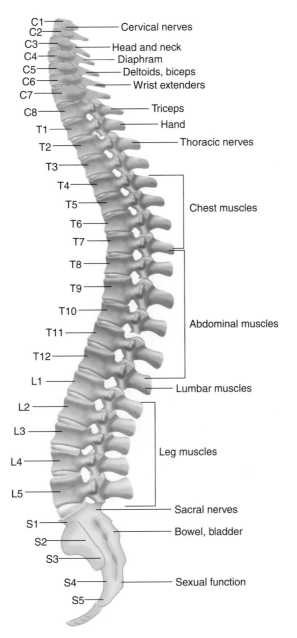

C1 — Cervical nerves
C2
C3 — Head and neck
C4 — Diaphram
C5 — Deltoids, biceps
C6 — Wrist extenders
C7
C8 — Triceps
T1 — Hand
T2 — Thoracic nerves
T3
T4
T5 — Chest muscles
T6
T7
T8
T9
T10 — Abdominal muscles
T11
T12
L1 — Lumbar muscles
L2
L3
L4 — Leg muscles
L5
— Sacral nerves
S1
S2 — Bowel, bladder
S3
S4 — Sexual function
S5

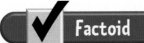

Marlene Moment

And don't be checking for a Brudzinski's sign if cervical spine injury is suspected: You might cause one!

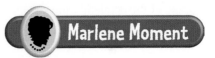

Factoid

Cauda equina literally means a *horse's* tail, because this bundle of nerves extending from the bottom of the spinal cord looks like a horse's tail. The cauda equina syndrome produces erectile dysfunction and incontinence.[17]

Marlene Moment

Just because you know medical terms and your non-nursing friends don't, it would not be nice for you to use big words on them! Example: "You are acting just like a cauda equina!"

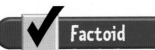

Factoid

Motorcycle crashes are common causes of spinal cord injury as well as other trauma, which could cause massive hemorrhage (ie, traumatic amputation of a leg).[20] Neurogenic shock or spinal shock that occurs simultaneously with hemorrhagic (hypovolemic) shock is a "double whammy!"

- Alterations in thermoregulation: Poikilothermy (pronounced POY-key-low-thermia), which occurs with high level SCI is characterized by body temperature the same as that of the environment.

- Postural hypotension at the T4-T6 level.

- Neurogenic bladder with frequent urinary tract infections owing to incomplete emptying and contamination from multiple catheterizations.

- Autonomic hyperreflexia (also called dysreflexia): Greatest risk when spinal cord lesion is at the level of T6 or higher. Noxious stimuli can trigger a potentially life-threatening sympathetic response.[39]

- Death at the scene of the accident because of respiratory failure when the spinal cord is severed at the C1-C2 level.

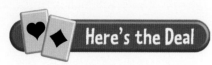

Here's the Deal

The CNS response to hemorrhage is immediate sympathetic stimulation to produce vasoconstriction and thereby raise the blood pressure. If hypovolemic shock occurs simultaneously with neurogenic shock or spinal shock, the sympathetic outflow is blocked (neurogenic shock) and the blood vessels are paralyzed (spinal shock) and unable to respond. Obviously this is a deadly "double whammy," because the body's primary defenses mechanism against shock is ineffective in maintaining cardiac output to support perfusion of vital organs.

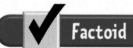

Factoid

Spine immobilization and respiratory support must begin at the scene of the accident if the patient is to arrive alive!

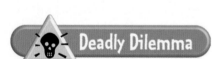

Deadly Dilemma

Do not (I repeat, do NOT) open the airway using the head tilt, chin lift maneuver when a cervical spine injury is suspected or possible. The jaw thrust chin lift will effectively pull the tongue forward without flexing the neck.

Interventions and why?

A-B-Cs mandate immediate respiratory support at the scene for high cervical spine injuries.

- Initial airway management and bag/mask breathing.
- Endotracheal intubation and mechanical ventilation.
- Cardiac support for vasovagal response and severe bradycardia.[2]
- Treatment of neurogenic shock because of autonomic nervous dysfunction below the level of the SCI causing vasodilation: Trendelenburg position, inotropes such as dopamine and fluid resuscitation; epinephrine or atropine to speed up the heart rate (see Chapter 5).
- Methylprednisone or dexamethasone to reduce local inflammatory reaction.

Once stabilized, my patient needs implementation of a treatment plan to guard against additional spinal cord injury and a comprehensive plan aimed toward preventing complications. Refer to Table 7-11 for a summary of nursing care for the spinal cord–injured patient.

Table 7-11   Nursing care of the spinal cord–injured patient

Possible complications following spinal cord injury	Nursing care to safeguard the spinal cord–injured patient against potential harm
Autonomic dysreflexia, which occurs when the CNS responds to noxious stimuli (usually bladder or bowel distention) with the following symptoms: - Hypertension - Bradycardia - Severe headache - Nasal congestion - "Goosebumps" (piloerection) - Profuse perspiration above the level of spinal cord injury - Cold dry skin below the level of spinal cord injury	If autonomic dysreflexia is recognized as being in progress: - Immediately elevate the head of the bed to a sitting position to drop the pressure quickly before a blood vessel in the brain ruptures! - Stay with the patient and call for supplies to perform an immediate bladder catheterization and empty the bladder. - Perform a digital rectal exam to check for fecal impaction. Manual removal of the fecal mass is required to remove the source of visceral stimulation causing the autonomic dysreflexia. - Examine the skin surface for any source of irritation that could have precipitated the attack (broken skin, pressure area, a needle cap, or thermometer cover inadvertently left in the bed). Remove any such objects and relieve pressure points. - Administer PRN hydralazine (Apresoline) if the source of noxious stimuli cannot be quickly found. Prevention: Keep bladder decompressed, stools soft, and bowels moving regularly. (See measures to promote elimination.)

(Continued)

Table 7-11   Nursing care of the spinal cord–injured patient (*Continued*)

Possible complications following spinal cord injury	Nursing care to safeguard the spinal cord–injured patient against potential harm
High risk for DVT resulting from venostasis with risk for possible pulmonary embolus: • Related trauma and head injury as well as other systemic bleeding injuries activate the stress response to increase clotting mechanisms. • Bedrest and paralysis renders the muscle pump ineffective for promoting venous return to the heart. • Disruption of innervation to vessels below the level of SCI promotes lifetime risk because of venous pooling when the patient has tetraplegia or paraplegia. Other SCI risk duration may extend up to several months after the initial injury.	Prevent DVT formation: • Apply compression stockings (TED hose). • Utilize sequential compression devices (SCDs) to improve venous return. • Administer prescribed heparin or low molecular weight heparin (Lovenox) as prescribed after head injury or other sources of bleeding are ruled out. • Implement passive range of motion every two hours. • Ensure adequate hydration and monitor fluid intake. For early detection of a possible DVT: • Check calf of legs for local warmth or redness every shift. • Measure and record calf circumference daily. Alert the physician of any hint of DVT, chest pain, or dyspnea immediately.
	Prevent decubitus ulcers: • Utilize alternating pressure mattress. • Alternate positions every two hours. • Pad pressure points: hips, knees, ankles, shoulders. • Maintain adequate nutrition and hydration.
Alteration in bladder and bowel function owing to loss of muscle tone below the level of the SCI: • Urinary retention resulting from atonic bladder. • Risk for urinary tract infections resulting from urinary stasis and frequent catheterizations.	Measures to promote elimination: • Perform intermittent catheterizations as needed, taking the opportunity to teach the patient and family members by show and tell. • Monitor for bladder distention between catheterizations. • Monitor the site of the suprapubic catheter (if present) for redness or leakage. • Monitor urine for odor and color, and note sediment or cloudiness. • Obtain specimen for urine C&S if indicated. • Force fluids and monitor hydration status.

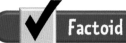

Factoid

Neurogenic shock occurs more commonly in injuries above T6 because sympathetic outflow from T1-L2 ceases when the cord is injured and there is nothing to oppose and balance all the vagal tone, resulting in generalized vaso-dilatation and hypotension.

(Continued)

Table 7-11 Nursing care of the spinal cord–injured patient *(Continued)*

Possible complications following spinal cord injury	Nursing care to safeguard the spinal cord–injured patient against potential harm
• Risk for pyelonephritis and urosepsis resulting from low bladder wall compliance creating stasis along the entire (upper and lower) urinary tract.[39] • Risk for nephrolithiasis (kidney stones) resulting from demineralization of bones secondary to bed rest and lack of weight-bearing on long bones. • Risk for paralytic ileus resulting from disruption of visceral innervation below the level of SCI during the first week after injury. • Risk for fecal impaction related constipation and to loss of abdominal muscle tone and ability to bear down to evacuate the bowel.	• Monitor 24-hour intake and output. • Auscultate for bowel sounds and monitor for abdominal distention frequently. • Insert NG tube as ordered to intermittent suction for relief of abdominal distention and to prevent nausea and vomiting. • Monitor stools and pattern of fecal elimination. • Perform digital rectal exam to check for fecal impaction if no bowel movement (BM). • Administer daily stool softener. • Provide a high-fiber diet after the return of bowel activity as evidenced by active bowel sounds and passage of stool.
Risk for orthostatic hypotension resulting from disruption of the spinal reflex arc that produces vasoconstriction when upright. • Greater risk for SCI above T-7. • Increased venous capacitance resulting from venous pooling in lower extremities and abdomen can drastically reduce systolic blood pressure and cardiac output. • Patients with tetraplegia may react drastically to minor upright positional changes.	Improve capability for mobilization to wheel chair by reducing positional blood pressure fluctuations: • Apply knee high compression stockings (open toe preferred for assessment) to apply external pressure to vessel walls, improving venous return. • Monitor three-step blood pressure readings: lying supine, 30–45 degrees and 90 degrees. Change positions slowly, monitoring and recording as you go! If there is a 20 mm Hg decrease in systolic blood pressure, lower to the previous position, wait 15 minutes, and try again. • Apply elastic abdominal binder as ordered to apply pressure to encourage venous return and support to the diaphragm. • Collaborate with the physician for the feasibility of a tilt table or special beds with conversion capability to arm chair.

(Continued)

Table 7-11 Nursing care of the spinal cord–injured patient *(Continued)*

Possible complications following spinal cord injury	Nursing care to safeguard the spinal cord–injured patient against potential harm
High risk for disuse syndrome and muscle atrophy resulting from immobility.	
High risk for decubitus ulcer resulting from pressure leading to tissue ischemia.	Promote skin integrity by relieving pressure: • Use an alternating pressure mattress if available. • Turn the patient every two hours, log rolling if indicated. • Inspect under and around any appliances or fixation devices (eg, C-collar). • Inspect back, buttocks, and heels where the patient is strapped to a spine board for transfer and diagnostic imaging. • Keep the skin clean and dry at all times. • Maintain adequate hydration and nutrition to promote cellular health of tissues. • Procure a gel flotation cushion for wheelchairs of patients with paraplegia and tetraplegia. Teaching patients to lean; the cushion will do the rest of the work to relieve the pressure on buttocks and scrotum when seated.

Get them real help by investigating all complaints and being an advocate! Methylprednisolone or dexamethasone is administered as soon after the injury as possible to reduce secondary SCI related to local edema and ischemia; thereafter, damage control and rehab are the priorities.

• High spinal cord lesions can lead to respiratory and cardiovascular dysfunction, which must be treated as they arise.

• Stabilization of cervical spine injuries may be accomplished through cervical traction to reduce the fracture or application of a halo vest for cervical stabilization.

• For most patients who receive external stabilization, adequate bony healing occurs within 12 weeks of halo immobilization.

• Surgical stabilization is required for severe comminuted fractures of the vertebral body.[40]

• Physical rehab is consulted for an activity/exercise program to prevent disuse syndrome. Bladder and bowel retraining programs (begun as early as neurologically possible) are a vital part of rehab.

• The enterostomal therapy (ET) nurse has an integral part of these bladder/bowel retraining programs, as well as patient motivation.

• Psychology and psychiatry consults are scheduled as soon after the injury as feasible, and occupational rehab is added as the patient becomes more stable.

Maximizing physical capabilities is essential to rehabilitation, as is the involvement and support of family and significant others.

PATIENT TEACHING When teaching the spinal cord–injured patient, the significant other, responsible family member, or caregiver should be included in teaching sessions in the event that assistance is required. (Refer to Table 7-7 for functional abilities and possible areas of dependency.)

- Patients with SCI above T6 (and caregivers) are cautioned about the risk for development of autonomic dysreflexia, signs and symptoms, and preventive measures (see Table 7-8).
- Teach site care when screws, wires, or pins are used to maintain skeletal traction.
- Teach the patient with halo traction to change the liner periodically and monitor the skin underneath the shoulder harness for redness and irritation. Powder is to be avoided.
- If a screw or pin appears loose or falls out of the halo head band, stabilize it in a neutral position (using two hands) and have someone else notify the neurosurgeon immediately.
- After the return of bowel peristalsis (usually one week after injury), dietary teaching should focus on increasing fiber with fruits, vegetables, and whole grain breads and cereals.
- Reinforce the bladder and bowel retraining instructions given by physical therapy/rehab team.

The show and tell method plus skills practice is helpful for teaching skills such as:

- Safe application of external catheter (for males)
- Catheter insertion technique for intermittent catheterization
- Manual checking for and removal of fecal impaction
- Transfer techniques bed to chair, chair to vehicle, etc.

Cutting edge

The Christopher and Dana Reeve Paralysis Act was signed into law by President Obama on March 30, 2009. This is a landmark for all spinal cord–injured Americans that promotes collaborative research, rehabilitation, and quality of life initiatives.[41]

✚ Herniated nucleus pulposus (HNP)

Degenerative disk disease with incapacitating back pain can certainly make life miserable!

Let's get the normal stuff straight!

An intervertebral disk separates each of the bony vertebrae to absorb shock. The disk and the vertebral column are surrounded by ligaments that provide added support and protection. The disk has a soft gelatinous center that changes shape with movement but is surrounded with a tough protective fibrous ring of cartilage called the *annulus*. The annulus takes a lot of wear and tear over the years, and with aging, the center gelatin (nucleus pulposus) naturally dries out and loses elasticity.[2]

What is it?

When the nucleus pulposus slips out of place or herniates through a tiny fracture in the annulus, the disk becomes dysfunctional and creates pressure on one or more spinal nerves.

- This condition is commonly called a slipped disk or a herniated disk, which usually takes place in the lower lumbar spine (L5-L5-S1) where the bulk of body weight is carried and the greatest twisting and bending motions occur.
- Another vulnerable area prone to injury and dysfunction are the disks in the cervical spine between C6-C7 and between C5-C6.
- When the nucleus starts to bulge outward, it usually occurs at the weakest point of the structural support around the vertebral bodies posteriorly where the nucleus and the supportive ligament are the thinnest.[2]

Causes and why?

Herniated nucleus pulposus (HNP) is usually caused by years of wear and tear with little cracks in the annulus that weaken the supportive cartilaginous ring. Then one day the person sneezes and suddenly herniation occurs.

- Another scenario can occur over time as the nucleus pulposus protrudes through a weak place in the annulus to apply pressure to spinal nerves before it finally herniates.
- Acute trauma from a fall or a blow to the back or neck can also cause sudden herniation.
- Following an initiating event that injures the annulus, symptoms can abate only to reappear months or years later with herniation at the site of old injury that weakened the supportive ring.
- Because HNP tends to occur in families, the annulus fibrosus is believed to be congenitally weak, which is why it herniates with any increase in intradiscal pressures.[42]

Testing, testing, testing

Based on the neurologic examination and patient subjective symptoms, several tests can be used to diagnose degenerative disk disease and rule out other causes of symptoms:

- MRI is the gold standard for diagnosis of disk disease because even small herniations are readily visible.
- CT scan or myelogram may be indicated if MRI findings are not consistent with the clinical picture.
- Use of lumbar discography to visualize the nucleus pulposus (using contrast dye and pressure manometry) when considering surgery after

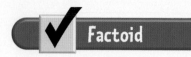

failed conservative therapy has been associated with vascular uptake of the dye (even after verification of needle placement).[43]

Electromyography can determine the presence of muscle disorders and other causes of neuropathy when the MRI or CT scan is not diagnostic.

- Needle electrodes are inserted into skeletal muscles.
- Amplitude of electrical waveforms are visible (and auditory) on a screen.
- Changes in electrical potential of muscles and the nerves to the muscle are measured.

Signs and symptoms and why?

The patient may give a history of back or neck injury (recent or remote) and will have the following characteristic complaints. Development of these complaints is dependent upon how quickly damage developed (acute or chronic) and which spinal nerves are being compressed by the bulging or herniated nucleus pulposus:

- Pain at the local site (lumbar or cervical)
- Muscle weakness and atrophy (both)
- Referred pain to the sacroiliac joint, thigh, or down either leg (lumbar)
- Sciatica when the disk is impinging on a nerve root in the low back (lumbar)
- Tingling, numbness, or burning sensations in the arms and hands (cervical)
- Pain that is aggravated by sitting, bending, twisting, or lifting (lumbar)
- A preference to walk, stand, or lie down rather than sit (lumbar)
- Alterations in bladder or bowel control when spinal nerves are irritated or compressed (lumbar)

What can harm my patient and why?

- Loss of mobility, strength, and endurance for ADLs, work, and play occurs.
- Work loss because of chronic back pain contributes to poor work history and unemployment.
- Loss of bladder and bowel sphincter is embarrassing and may restrict social interactions and recreational activities.

Interventions and why?

Pain relief is paramount:

- Administer prescribed NSAIDS, analgesia, muscle relaxants, and anti-anxiety agents.
- Create a calm, quiet, restful environment to compliment prescribed medications.
- Assist with turning and maintaining good alignment while on bed rest.
- Evaluate the effects of prescribed physical therapy.
- Provide interest and age-appropriate distraction if indicated and desired.

The patient needs some relief! Because of the nature of disk disease, conservative treatments will help for a while, then pain reoccurs, and the patient is likely to become discouraged. The patient may be fearful of surgical options because of having heard horror stories about worst case scenarios. Therefore:

- Provide factual information regarding surgical and nonsurgical options and alternatives.
- Actively listen to fears, complaints, and concerns with empathy, allowing the patient to vent.
- Encourage the patient with optimism, sharing cases of positive outcomes from surgical and nonsurgical options.
- Support individual research into the pros and cons of available options and alternatives.

Conservative (nonsurgical management) is attempted for low back pain unless worsening neurologic deficits are present and verified by MRI.[44]

- Short term (one- to two-day) bed rest to take pressure off the disk
- Physical therapy
- Massage therapy
- Nonsteroidal anti-inflammatory drugs: NSAIDs
- Analgesics such as Tylox (oxycodone) and Vicodin (hydrocodone) for acute pain
- Nerve root injection with lidocaine and dexamethasone after locating the affected nerve root with radiculography with contrast medium has effectively relieved pain[45]

Surgical intervention may be varied depending on the nature of the patient's problem, age, and disability:

- Removal of the herniated disk and bridging the space using a bone graft (discectomy with fusion)
- Subtotal (partial rather than total) discectomy decreases reherniation after lumbar discectomy [46]
- Foraminotomy: opening up the space within the foramen to make more room for the bulging or herniated disk to reduce compression and relieve pain
- Laminectomy or hemi-laminectomy: excision of all or half of the posterior arch of the vertebra to relieve pressure
- Solid fusion, with or without laminectomy, which limits mobility of the spine
- Total discectomy and replacement with bone graft
- Total disk replacement with prosthetic devices, which has complications related to the particular device (migration, polyethylene inlay pushes out, device wear, degeneration, and ossification around the device, particle disease)[47]

PATIENT TEACHING   Because of the nature of nursing, many patients with low back pain and degenerative disk disease may be nurses or individuals whose occupation requires manual lifting and stress/strain to the lumbar or cervical spine.

- Muscle-strengthening exercises and good body mechanics are a vital part of injury prevention programs.
- Use lumbar support wraps when lifting and pulling patients.
- Get help rather than trying to move or lift heavy objects.
- Do not exceed the prescribed dosage of NSAIDs and take medication with food to reduce GI upset.

Cutting edge

- An FDA-regulated Investigational Device Exemption clinical trial following up on 688 patients in 14 centers across the United States compared conventional surgery with total disk replacement using the CHARITE artificial disk in phase 1. The results revealed that removal of the original device and replacement revisions with the newer motion-preserving device, or the original alternate procedure of pedicle screw arthrodesis are viable options.[48,49]
- An international study using an American made product (ProDisk II prostheses by Spine Solutions, New York City) did 21 implants and followed patients for more than three years. Nearly all reported less intensity of pain, and the disability index improved dramatically.[50]
- Stem cell research is in progress in the United States and abroad using rats[51] and pigs[52] implanting human mesenchymal stems cells (MSCs) into intervertebral disks and monitoring differentiation and survival of MSCs in the disk following xenotransplantation. An important finding is that there is an acidic microenvironment surrounding a damaged human disk. This acidic microenvironment negatively impacted the survival and replication of rodent MSCs when subjected to a similar low pH environment. The implication is that if and when humans become recipients, regeneration of the disk must begin in earlier rather than later stages of disease.

INFECTIOUS DISORDERS

The brain and spinal cord are the most common sites of central nervous system (CNS) infections.

✚ Meningitis and encephalitis

Infectious diseases are bad anywhere in the body, but when infectious agents attack the brain and spinal cord, they are horrible!

Let's get the normal stuff straight!

Capillaries in the brain are different from capillaries anywhere else in the body:

- Their endothelial cells are tightly bound together and they are completely surrounded by a basement membrane, which forms the blood-brain barrier.

- The blood-brain barrier is very selective and allows only essential substances to enter the brain, while unwanted substances are excluded.
- Highly water-soluble drugs are in the excluded category, but highly lipid-soluble drugs such as chloramphenicol can pass through the blood-brain barrier with ease.

The triple-layered meninges form the covering of the brain and spinal cord (Fig. 7-11).

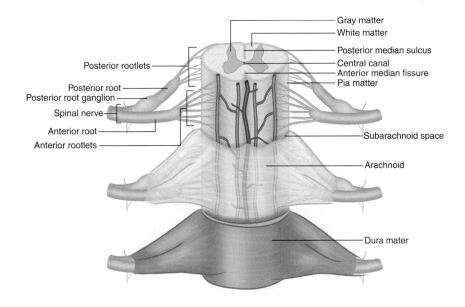

◀ Figure 7-11. Layers of the meninges.

- The outermost layer (called the *dura mater*) is tough and fibrous for protection.
- The middle weblike, delicate layer (called the *arachnoid layer*) has a subarachnoid layer that contains the CSF.
- The *pia mater* is the innermost delicate connective tissue sheath that covers the brain and spinal cord.
  Infectious agents cannot cause illness until they gain access to the body:
- A portal of entry is required via penetration, inhalation, direct contact, or ingestion.
- Once inside, the agent incubates and the patient experiences prodromal signs.
- The maximum impact of the infectious process is called the *acute phase* of an illness.
  When the patient is acutely ill, the body has already mobilized the immune response with lymphocytes to the rescue: T lymphocytes, B lymphocytes, the natural killer lymphocytes, as well as all available immunoglobins.[2]

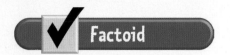

Anytime CSF is leaking OUT, infection can creep IN.

What is it?

Meningitis (inflammation of the meninges) is inflammation with infection affecting the spinal cord, whereas encephalitis is an inflammation with infection of actual tissue within the brain.

Causes and why?

Both diseases (meningitis and encephalitis) can be caused by bacterial or viral infections, but can also follow traumatic brain injury when the skull has been fractured and CSF is leaking out. Additional causes include the use of invasive procedures to monitor or reduce ICP.

ICP such as intracranial pressure monitoring devices or drilling burr holes in the skull as an outlet for pressure.

- Meningitis can be a complication of other infections such as otitis, sinusitis, or herpes simplex infections; sepsis; or pneumonia.
- Encephalitis can occur from infection with arboviruses transmitted by mosquitoes and ticks (West Nile encephalitis, St. Louis encephalitis, La Crosse encephalitis, and rarely Equine encephalitis).[53]

Testing, testing, testing

The cause (bacterial versus viral) of meningitis or encephalitis must be determined for selection of effective anti-infective therapy:

- A lumbar puncture may be performed to evaluate pressure and obtain a CSF specimen.
- Evaluation of CSF for protein, glucose, WBC
- Culture and sensitivity of spinal fluid
- CBC and blood cultures
- WBC and differential
- CT or MRI to check for sinus infection
- EEG to evaluate the patient for seizure disorder
- Solid-phase antibody-binding assays: ELISA (enzyme-linked immunosorbent assay)
- Rapid serologic assay: IgM capture ELISA (MAC-ELISA) and IgG ELISA (IgM reacts early and IgG antibody reacts later)[54]
- Monoclonal antibodies (MAbs) for identification of viruses

Signs and symptoms and why?

The signs and symptoms of both meningitis and encephalitis may be preceded by a prodromal flulike syndrome before fever spikes and prostration occurs. The patient with meningitis will display a stiff neck (nuchal rigidity), a positive Kernig's sign, and a positive Brudzinski's sign (see Figs. 7-8 and 7-9). Other symptoms of both include:

- Headache
- Diaphoresis

- Nausea and vomiting
- Seizure activity
- Increased sensitivity to light and noise (evokes pain)

What can harm my patient and why?

Because bacterial and viral infection attacks the central nervous system and causes inflammation, as many as 30% of survivors will have persistent neurologic damage, such as:[53]

- Deafness
- Seizures
- Learning disabilities
- Severe brain damage
- Death (5%–20% mortality rate)[55]

Interventions and why?

Protecting oneself and others from communicable disease, while initiating supportive and restorative interventions is the priority:
- Place the patient in isolation according to CDC guidelines.
- Assist with lumbar puncture for obtaining CSF fluid for analysis, culture, and sensitivity. (See guidelines with testing for spinal cord injury: myelogram.)
- Collect specimens for culture and sensitivity before initiating IV antibiotic therapy.
- Access multiple peripheral IV lines for administration of IV fluids and IVPB antibiotics.
- Administer prescribed antibiotic therapy for bacterial infection: vancomycin or ampicillin.
- Administer prescribed antiviral therapy for viral infection: acyclovir or ganciclovir.

My patient will require close monitoring to detect increasing ICP and worsening of neurologic status.

- Monitor LOC, speech, and mood behavior to detect early signs of ICP.
- Monitor the ability to swallow/clear airway and maintain airway patency.
- Monitor temperature and administer antipyretics PRN.
- Maintain a quiet darkened environment with the bed in a low position and padded rails up.
- Position to support ventilation and promote drainage of oral/nasal secretions, suctioning as needed.

Make provisions for elimination, nutrition, skin care, and comfort (refer to plan for brain injury, Table 7-6).

Supportive therapy for both meningitis and encephalitis involves therapy to maintain fluid and electrolytes in the presence of nausea, vomiting, and/or diaphoresis. The treatment plan may include:

- Antipyretics (acetaminophen) for stiff neck, headache, and fever
- Antiepileptics for seizure activity (see Table 7-4)
- Measures to reduce meningeal edema and ICP (see Table 7-6)

If residual neurologic damage is suspected, consider physical therapy, speech therapy, otology screening, and cognitive testing. Home and community health may also be required to provide long-term home recovery and surveillance.

PATIENT TEACHING The patient recovering from meningitis or encephalitis should be taught to boost the immune system by:

- Eating a nutritious diet with ample fruits and vegetables
- Getting adequate sleep and rest
- Avoiding undue stressors
- Avoiding tobacco, alcohol, and drugs

Once acute illness subsides, physical, speech, and occupational therapy may be necessary for residual CNS damage:

- Teach patients to expect slow but significant progress with speech and physical therapy.
- Teach patients to be open to change and expanding capabilities, new interests, and stimulating challenges if occupational therapy is required.

Teaching to prevent encephalitis and meningitis involves:

- Home and community mosquito control, removing all standing water-breeding grounds
- Wearing protective clothing and using insect repellent when outdoors, especially wooded areas where ticks are common
- Pneumonia and *Haemophilus influenza* type B (Hib) vaccines for susceptible patients
- Information regarding postexposure prophylactic antibiotics for exposure to meningococcal meningitis (This is not required for Hib meningitis for fully immunized adults.)
- Pneumococcal polysaccharide vaccine for all adults over age 65 who have decreased immunity because of chronic diseases
- MCV4 vaccine for those traveling to countries in which meningitis is common, or for susceptible individuals during a community outbreak

Cutting edge

The CDC has appointed a branch of the vector-borne infectious division (Arbovirus Diseases Branch) to identify dangerous mosquito viruses and develop rapid diagnostics and response to reduce the spread of disease from infected mosquitoes. The polymerase chain reaction (PCR) can provide speedy identification of viruses in the field to shorten public health response time, although PCRs have not yet been validated for routine clinical use.[54]

CRANIAL NERVE DISORDERS

A trio of neuralgia, palsy, and neuropathy can be distressing for the patient and decrease quality of life.

✚ Trigeminal neuralgia

Let's get the normal stuff straight!

Communication between the brain and peripheral nerve pathways is essential for normal motor, sensory, and autonomic functions. The 12 cranial nerves each have their own unique function and anatomical location that they serve.

What is it?

Trigeminal neuralgia (also known as tic douloureux) is an acquired condition that involves painful episodic dysfunction of the fifth cranial (trigeminal) nerve.

Causes and why?

Vascular compression of the fifth and seventh cranial nerves are documented by 3T magnetic resonance (MR) imaging and MR angiography[56,57] and may also be associated with age-related changes in the brain, because it is more likely to occur later in life (50s and 60s) and with structural damage such as scarring and plaque formation with multiple sclerosis.

Testing, testing, testing

Radiographic imaging (3T MRI, angiography, and echo) can identify indentions and distortion of the trigeminal nerve.[56]

Signs and symptoms and why?

The patient with trigeminal neuralgia can initiate a painful attack with ordinary activities such as brushing teeth, combing hair, or shaving. Any stimulation, a cold wind on the face or slight touch over a trigger point can set off an attack. During the attack the patient will:

- Grimace, moan, or cry in pain
- Pace or fidget and hold the affected side of the head
- Experience involuntary one-sided facial twitching

   Between attacks, the patient is fearfully anticipating the next episode, and reluctant to make any commitments or appointments, especially if the paroxysms are increasingly frequent.

What can harm my patient and why?

Never knowing when an attack will occur is unsettling; therefore, dread permeates all activities of living, causing decreased social commitments, early retirement, reclusive living, and anhedonia (no fun).

Interventions and why?

Pain relief and avoidance of light, sound, and any stimulation to the trigger point is the priority during an attack (refer to supportive nursing care for headaches). Pharmacologic therapy is aimed toward dampening abnormal electrical signals:

- Preventive therapy may include Tegretol (carbamazepine) taken daily to reduce neural transmission at selected terminals.
- Neurontin (gabapentin) and Lioresal (baclofen) are accepted medications for pain control.
- Dilantin (phenytoin) is another older alternate drug with many side effects (see Table 7-4).

If the attacks are frequent and disabling, surgical intervention may be the best option for uncontrolled trigeminal neuralgia. After pain subsides:

- Evaluate patient consistency in self-administration of preventive medications.
- Discuss preferences for and knowledge of invasive surgical therapies.
- Provide information regarding advantages and disadvantages of treatment options.

When patients are poorly responsive to the standard medications, 3T MR imaging can identify those patients who will benefit from microvascular nerve decompression, which releases pressure on the nerve without causing facial paralysis. Other less preferred options that cause facial muscle and eyelid weakness as well as recurrent pain after the expected three to five years of relief include:

- Radiofrequency thermal coagulation, which can also affect the corneal reflex
- Percutaneous balloon microcompression, which has a significant recurrence percentage and associated facial muscle weakness
- Gamma knife therapy, an emerging option especially for the elderly with other chronic illnesses who are not relieved with medications or other surgical options[58]

Because of the debilitating, recurring nature of trigeminal neuralgia, psychological consultation is indicated as a component of long-term care.

PATIENT TEACHING   For the patient who chooses to postpone surgical options, teach strategies for reducing the frequency of attacks:

- Chew on the unaffected side.
- Try mouthwash and careful flossing or tepid water pic rather than brushing. Avoid touching gums on the affected side.
- Avoid hot and cold everything: face cloths, foods, and drinks.
- Avoid direct currents of air: fans, open auto windows, air conditioning vents.

Teach patients to take prophylactic medication even when pain free, and to comply with lab tests to monitor for adverse effects (see Table 7-4).

Cutting edge

Surgeons performing microvascular decompression for relief of trigeminal neuralgia found that 10 of 98 patients had no visible sign of compression of the trigeminal nerve once it was exposed, so "nerve combing" with a fine microneedle was performed instead. Immediately postoperatively all 10 patients whose trigeminal nerve had been "combed" (scratched with a needle in a linear fashion) reported decreased sensation to sharp pain (a prick) on the affected side. After three years, 7 of the 10 patients who presented for microvascular decompression and got "combed" instead were still pain free. Of the remaining three, one had significantly less pain, one had recurrence after 18 months, and one experienced permanent neurologic deficits. It is theorized that surgical manipulation dampens the nerve's abnormal activity. Nerve "combing" is getting attention even though the sample size is small.

✛ Bell's palsy

Let's get the normal stuff straight!

The seventh cranial nerve is also called the facial nerve because the two branches innervate the entire face (upper and lower). The facial nerve is unique in that in order to reach the facial muscles, it must travel most of the way through the fallopian canal, a small bony passageway in the skull, beneath the ear.

The facial nerve is fairly resilient, being insulated with a fatty myelin sheath, and enclosed in an outer connective tissue sheath. The facial nerve supplies the following muscles and tissues:

- External auditory meatus: Awareness of sensation
- Nasopharynx: Awareness of gag reflex sensation
- Taste buds of anterior two-thirds of the tongue
- Lacrimal, sublingual, and submandibular glands
- Facial muscles controlling all facial expressions
- Stapedius muscle of the middle ear, which protects from loud sounds[2]

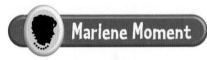

Marlene Moment

No, this is not a typo! I said the fallopian canal, not the fallopian tube! (Duh ... wrong end.) You know that can't be right, because men get Bell's palsy too.

What is it?

Bell's palsy is primarily a unilateral cranial neuropathy that causes inflammation and edema of the seventh cranial nerve (facial nerve). Bell's palsy is the most common cranial nerve dysfunction,[59] affecting 40,000 Americans yearly.[60]

Causes and why?

The cause is listed as *idiopathic,*[59] which means that Bell's palsy occurs without a clear cause. It is theorized that the pressure from inflammation and edema on the facial nerve within the bony fallopian canal causes ischemic damage to the myelin sheath or causes infarction of the nerve.[60] Additionally there are some theories of precipitating factors:

- Viral infection: herpes simplex (fever blister), herpes zoster (shingles), meningitis

- Higher incidence during third trimester pregnancy compared with early pregnancy[61]
- Upper respiratory infection (influenza or colds)[60]
- Chronic middle ear infection
- Other infections: sarcoidosis or Lyme disease

Testing, testing, testing

Generally, diagnosis is made based on the history and the clinical appearance of the patient, but the following tests may be prescribed if there is any conflicting clinical presentation:

- Skull films can rule out tumors or masses.
- EMG (electromyelogram) can confirm the absence and extent of innervation loss.
- Imaging: CT or MRI can rule out other causes of pressure on the nerve as a source of paralysis.

There is no specific test for Bell's palsy, but blood may be drawn to test for Lyme disease or sarcoidosis if suspected.[17]

Signs and symptoms and why?

Prodromal pain behind the ear begins several hours or possibly several days before unilateral facial paralysis occurs.[17] The onset of symptoms is sudden and usually peaks in intensity within 48 hours. The frightened patient appears in the emergency department holding the affected side with one hand and wiping drool and tears with the other.

- Facial features are distorted because of unilateral paralysis: The weak side pulls toward the midline when speaking.
- Unilateral upper and lower facial weakness.
- Abnormal sensitivity to sound may prompt the patient to cover the affected ear.
- Impaired sense of taste: The anterior two-thirds of the tongue are affected.[2]
- Lacrimation in one eye, with tears running down the cheek because of incomplete lid closure.
- Salivation and drooling from one side of the mouth.
- Impaired speech and slurring of words.
- Mild pain and twitching of facial muscles.

My patient needs an immediate "steroid boost" to reduce nerve injury and recovery time and improve outcomes:[59,62]

- Administer prescribed prednisolone as soon as possible after the onset of symptoms.
- Protect the affected eye from injury because the blink reflex is paralyzed!
- Lubricate the affected eye with liquid tears and methylcellulose drops.

- Close the eye at night and apply an eye pad with paper tape to prevent sleep trauma.

The patient is scared. Give factual information, assuring him or her that a stroke is not in progress.

- Recovery is gradual. Usually symptoms begin to abate within two weeks.

- Most patients regain normal neurologic function within three to six months, with longer recovery time for some, depending upon the extent of injury.

- A very few patients have residual damage, and cosmetic or reconstructive surgery can be considered.

My patient needs me (the nurse) for encouragement and supportive care:

- Provide emesis basin and tissues for oral secretions.

- Provide eye pads and paper tape (to take home).

- Recommend foam ear plug for affected ear to protect against loud sounds.

- Mechanically soft diet requiring minimal chewing.

Urge careful chewing food on the opposite side of the mouth.

Research documents the benefit of steroids (prednisolone) given early for all patients with Bell's palsy, and antiviral agents (acyclovir or valacyclovir) as indicated.

- There has been no documented benefit (or harm) from physical therapy or facial massage in an effort to maintain muscle; however, even the psychosomatic benefit of "doing something" may be helpful.

- Acetaminophen, ibuprofen, or aspirin are recommended for pain if needed, unless contraindicated by other prescription medications.

- Warm moist heat may be applied to the face in conjunction with NSAIDs as needed.

Alternative medicine (acupressure)[63] has documented benefit in some cases and facial reconstructive surgery may rarely be required for eyelid closure.

PATIENT TEACHING   Patient teaching includes the following protective measures:

- Wear sunglasses outdoors to protect from wind-blown dust and trash.

- Avoid chewing gum, which increases salivation and increases tissue trauma from chewing.

- An ear plug can be worn for comfort and protection.

- Avoid cleaning the ear with a cotton-tipped applicator because depth sensation is impaired.

- Night-time closure of the eye: Use a small strip of paper tape from lid to cheek and cover with an eye pad for double protection.

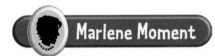

Marlene Moment

If you have Bell's palsy, don't be digging in your ear with a Q-tip or the neurosurgeon may have to remove it from your brain!

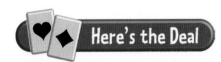

Here's the Deal

When *exogenous* steroids are taken, it causes the adrenal glands to halt *endogenous* production of corticosteroids. If steroids are abruptly discontinued, the adrenal glands do not have time to "wake up" and commence production of these essential hormones; therefore, hypotension and shock can quickly ensue.

- Take prescribed steroid medication exactly and taper down as instructed: Never abruptly stop taking a steroid!

What can harm my patient and why?

The small percentage of patients who have permanent residual damage will have a crooked smile and a drooping eyelid on the affected side. Until return of neurologic function, the patient is at risk for:

- A change in body image, decreased self-esteem, and social embarrassment
- Damage to the tongue and inner aspect of the cheek because of chewing and biting injury
- Drying and irritation of the affected eye because the lid does not fully close
- Corneal abrasion and blindness because the protective blink reflex is lost

Cutting edge

Skin-toned external eyelid weights (double-sided adhesive) are the newest development for an eyelid that will not fully close. The device, which works with gravity to assist blinking, is manufactured by MedDev Corp. (Sunnyvale, CA) and is available by prescription from an ophthalmologist.[66]

✚ Multiple sclerosis

The name *multiple sclerosis* literally means *many scars,* and for the patient who has the disease it means many problems.[64]

Let's get the normal stuff straight!

The brain, spinal cord, and 12 pairs of cranial nerves communicate with peripheral nerve pathways for normal motor, sensory, and autonomic functions. Cranial nerves each have their own unique function and anatomical location that they serve.

- Cranial nerve II (also called the optic nerve), located behind the globe of the eye, arises from the retina and therefore is not a peripheral nerve.
- Motor nerves stimulate movement and sensory nerves provide sensation.
- Every neuron has a cell body, lots of little nerve branches (dendrites) for receiving messages, and a long tail (the axon) for transmitting messages.
- Axons are covered with an outer sheath of connective tissue, and the innermost layer contains the Schwann cells that produce the myelin sheath surrounding peripheral nerves.
- The fatty (lipoproteins) membrane of the Schwann cell is tightly wrapped in layers around each segment of the axon like insulation on an electrical wire (Fig. 7-12).

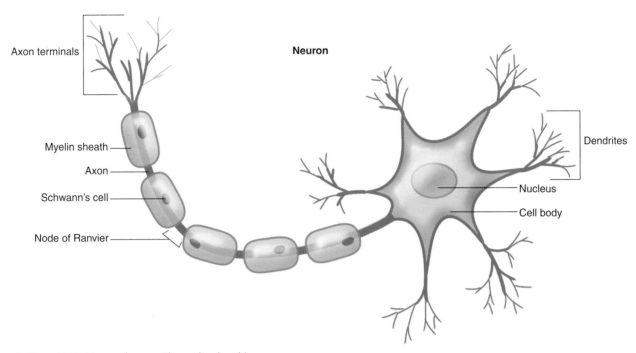

▲ Figure 7-12. Neuron (axon with myelin sheath).

- Each segment of the axon is connected by nodes (nodes of Ranvier) that are not myelinated and nerve impulses hop from one node to another down the length of an axon for really speedy transmission.
- Each Schwann cell provides myelin for one single segment of the axon.
- The next Schwann cell takes care of the next segment and so forth, so that myelination of nerve cells requires a long string of these specialized cells.

What is it?

Multiple sclerosis (MS) is a chronic incurable neurologic disease that causes patchy demyelination of the brain, spinal cord, and optic nerve (cranial nerve II). This disease affects more than twice as many women as men and occurs in young to middle-aged adults, often childbearing women and young mothers. It is an autoimmune, incurable disease that is characterized by exacerbations (acute relapses) and remissions (periods of time between attacks). Four characteristic patterns of presentation have been identified:

- Relapsing-remitting MS: The most common form has recurring attacks of worsening neurologic function followed by periods of remission with partial or complete recovery. During remission symptoms do not get any worse.
- Primary progressive MS: Once symptoms begin the disease gradually worsens with no clear relapses or remissions, but increasing, progressive disability.

- Secondary progressive MS: This starts with an initial pattern of relapsing-remitting, but then the disease worsens steadily, with or without relapses, remissions, or plateaus.
- Progressive-relapsing MS: The least common pattern begins just like primary progressive with symptoms gradually worsening from the start but distinct relapses also occurring without clear remissions.[7]

Causes and why?

MS is thought to be an autoimmune disease in which the body's own defense system attacks and destroys the myelin protective insulation layer over the nerves. Once myelin is gone, the nerves become damaged or destroyed. Genetic and geographic predispositions have been identified:

- The highest incidence is in Europe, New Zealand, southern Australia, northern United States, and southern Canada (colder climates). Exposure to these climates prior to age 15 carries increased risk, even following relocation to a warmer climate.
- MS in one identical twin predisposes the other twin with the exact same genetic makeup to have a 1 in 4 risk of developing MS; therefore, some additional factor must also be involved. Family history increases the risk to 1 in 40, significantly greater than the 1 in 750 incidence in the general population.[65]

Signs and symptoms and why?

The myelin pops off the neurons at multiple sites, causing a slowing of neurotransmission, with damage and deterioration of neurons. Multiple symptoms will be produced. Refer to Table 7-12 for site-specific symptoms. Frequently optic nerve involvement is a first symptom of MS.[66]

Table 7-12 Multiple sclerosis sites: specific signs and symptoms

Demyelination of the brain, cord, and optic nerve	Signs and symptoms related to dysfunctional impulse transmission at site of damage
Cerebrum: upper motor neurons (damage is within the cerebral cortex or through descending corticospinal structures from brain to spinal cord) • Cognitive dysfunction • Impaired sensory function • Dysfunction of upper motor neurons • Disorders of mood and temperament	• Decreased attention span • Impaired reasoning capabilities • Progressive dementia • Seizures • Spastic paralysis and hyperreflexia • Depression or euphoria
Cerebellum: • Balance and coordination • Gait patterns	• Postural and intention tremors • Limb incoordination • Gait ataxia • Spasm of limbs

(Continued)

Table 7-12   Multiple sclerosis sites: specific signs and symptoms   (*Continued*)

Demyelination of the brain, cord, and optic nerve	Signs and symptoms related to dysfunctional impulse transmission at site of damage
Brain stem (cranial nerves originating from medulla) • Cranial nerve XII: hypoglossal • Cranial nerve X: vagus • Cranial nerve IX: glossopharyngeal	• Severe dizziness • Nausea and vomiting • Difficulty swallowing • Slurred speech
Optic nerve: unilateral visual disturbances	• Painful optic neuritis • Blurring or gray vision • Nystagmus • Diplopia (double vision) • Impaired or vision loss in one eye
Spinal cord: lower motor neurons (damage is between the muscle and the spinal cord) • Upper cervical/spinal accessory nerve • Thoracic and upper lumbar segmental nerves (innervate all of viscera) • Lower sacral/upper sacral segmental nerves • Lower sacral segmental nerves	• Muscle weakness • Loss of muscle tone • Flaccid paralysis and areflexia • Sensory deficits in the face and neck area • Numbness or tingling of arm or hand • Bladder dysfunction • Sluggish bowel, constipation • Erectile dysfunction

Source: References 2, 64, and 66.

Testing, testing, testing

The patient history and clinical findings form a basis for diagnosis and testing to confirm suspicions:

- EEG will reveal abnormally slow electrical signals when compared with normal.
- CSF (if lumbar puncture is performed) will reveal oligoclonal bands.[64]
  MRI is prescribed to confirm the presence of:
- Plaques in more than one area of the CNS.
- Unexplained plaques in the white matter of the CNS that can only be attributed to MS. These plaque formations (sclerosed areas in the white matter) are what give MS its name: *multiple sclerosis.*[64]

What can harm my patient and why?

Chronic and progressive MS can lead to:

- Severe bladder and kidney infections, because stasis of urine from incomplete emptying of the bladder provides an environment for growth of microorganisms
- Osteoporosis owing to steroid use, lack of mobility, and weight-bearing

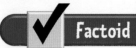

Factoid

Disease-modifying drugs mimic the basic properties of myelin to protect nerves and thereby decrease the formation of MS lesions, reducing the frequency and duration of attacks and slowing the onset of disability.[68]

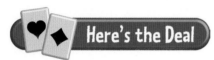

Here's the Deal

Disease-modifying therapies (all injections) only slow progression of MS; these drugs do not cure MS or make the patient feel any better. Adverse reactions and local reactions at the site may cause patients to have a negative attitude toward this therapy.

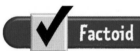

Factoid

Although immunosuppressant drugs are effective in the treatment of relapsing forms of MS, they increase the patient's susceptibility to infection.

- Aspiration pneumonia owing to loss of muscle tone, leading to dysphagia and reduction of the protective cough reflex
- Decubitus ulcers from prolonged wheelchair sitting or becoming bedridden
- Psychiatric and psychological problems
- Decreased quality in all areas of life: social, vocational, and personal[67]

Interventions and why?

The treatment plan focuses on return to function after attacks, reducing the frequency of attacks and preventing disability. The characteristic presentation pattern directs the course of treatment:

- Acute relapses may be treated with a short course of corticosteroid therapy to decrease inflammation and suppress the immune system gone awry.[68]
- Disease-modifying therapies are immune suppressants. Such drugs approved by the FDA are Copaxone (glatiramer) given SQ daily and Tysabri (natalizumab) given IV once weekly decrease exacerbations and reduce neuronal damage.
- Interferons approved by the FDA are beta interferon 1b (Betaseron) and beta interferon 1a (Avonex and Rebif). These are antiviral proteins that suppress the replication of virus cells.
- Tysabri (natalizumab) has been helpful for patients who don't respond to interferon drugs. It cannot be given until other drugs have cleared the system. A period of two weeks is required for interferon drugs or Copaxone, and a three-month "wash out" is needed following the use of Novantrone or other immunosuppressants.

The goal of rehabilitation is to preserve and improve function. This requires a full team of specialists in physical therapy, occupational therapy, speech therapy, and swallowing. Cognitive and vocational rehabilitation employs neuropsychologists and occupational therapists to assist patients to establish and attain realistic goals.

Early aggressive intervention at the initial onset of symptoms is essential for keeping early damage to the myelin from progressing to later disability.

- Intervene as an advocate for early interferon beta treatment at the first onset of symptoms.
- Administer prescribed beta interferon as prescribed to decrease early irreversible damage.
- Administer prescribed oral or IV methylprednisolone to reduce inflammatory response.[68]

The newly diagnosed patient needs information about the disease, the importance of not missing any doses of prescribed medication and self-help strategies (see Patient Teaching).

Disease-modifying medication therapies

Medication	Adverse effects/nursing care
Copaxone (glatiramer acetate)	Flushing, chest pain, palpitations, anxiety, dyspnea, hives
Tysabri (natalizumab)	Infusion reactions, hives, chest pain, headache, joint pain
Novantrone (mitoxantrone)	Nausea, vomiting, myelosuppression • Watch the site of infusion for red streaking (phlebitis) • Be alert to signs of extravasation and stop infusion promptly because necrosis can occur[68]

Administer medications prescribed for control of spasticity (and see Patient Teaching)

- Baclofen (GABA agonist)
- Dantrium (dantrolene)
- Valium (benzodiazepine)

Administer medications prescribed to combat disabling fatigue and lassitude (see also Patient Teaching)

- Symmetrel (amantadine)
- Cylert (pemoline)

Administer prescribed medications to treat ataxia:

- Inderal (beta-adrenergic blocker)
- Neurontin (antiseizure agent)
- Klonopin (benzodiazepine)

Nursing care and monitoring:

- Assist and monitor ambulation for weakness and balance problems.
- Provide juices at bedside (vitamin C to acidify urine) and monitor the bladder for distention.
- Provide a diet high in fiber and monitor bowel function.
- Assist with hygiene as needed because of weakness and fatigue.
- Assist with meals as needed (ie, cut meat or open cartons if the fingers are numb) and monitor for dysphagia.
- Monitor safe, effective use of assistive devices, canes, and walkers.
- Utilize therapeutic communication (see Chapter 1) and active listening to address expressed concerns and fears.

PATIENT TEACHING   In addition to urging compliance with prescribed medications to control symptoms, patients with MS can benefit from the following teaching.

Teaching regarding psychosocial issues and depression that many patients experience:

- Improve coping skills through family counseling and individual support services.
- Self-help patient groups may be a source of support and encouragement.
- Spiritual beliefs and practices can be a valuable source of strength (see Chapter 1).

Teaching strategies to improve compliance with prescribed injectable medications:

- Warm compresses prior to injecting certain medications (Copaxone, Betaseron, Avonex, Rebif) decreases local pain.[68,69]
- Use a 23-gauge needle for IM injections (beta interferon-1a), rotate sites, and give injections in the evening for more tolerable local reactions.[68]

Teach strategies to cope with physical problems resulting from dysfunction of nerve transmission.

For optic nerve involvement, advise the patient to:

- Rest the eyes periodically throughout the day.
- Consider talking books (a free service of the Library of Congress) and audio books.
- Avoid extended reading or prolonged computer work.
- Patch one eye to stop double vision during a short task.[66]

For lack of energy, fatigue, weakness, stiffness, or spasticity, instruct the patient to engage in:

- Moderate aerobic exercise, but avoid overheating (Don't overdo anything!)
- Timed rest periods throughout the day
- Stretching exercises or yoga to improve flexibility and mobility
- Manage stress by eliminating all nonessential activities and focus on activities that produce challenging interest and delight

For elimination problems:

- Advise a well-balanced low-fat, high-fiber diet to promote bowel function.
- Encourage bladder retraining exercises, such as drinking a measured amount of fluid and in the absence of bladder sensation, using a timer to provide the 30-minute signal to attempt voiding.[4]
- Teach self-catheterization and indications for bladder decompression (residual urine and retention).
- Teach application and care of male condom catheter to prevent tissue trauma and irritation.
- Advise the use of absorbent pads, which are a noninvasive alternative to urinary diversion procedures for female incontinence.

* Drink eight glasses of fluid daily (minimum), including cranberry juice and vitamin C to increase the acidity of the urine.

Cutting edge

Two recent studies add credibility to the link between the Epstein-Barr virus (EBV) and the development of multiple sclerosis. Epstein-Barr virus (EBV) is a herpesvirus that causes infectious mononucleosis and other disorders. One study suggests a link between EBV exposure and the loss of nerve tissue, whereas the other study explores interactions between a person's genes and EBV.[70]

PERIPHERAL NERVE DISORDERS

Peripheral neuropathy can occur as a singular dysfunction (mononeuropathy), such as carpal tunnel syndrome, in which a single nerve is compressed, or it can comprise multiple neurologic problems, as seen in diabetes (polyneuropathies), autoimmune diseases, and degenerative conditions that attack the peripheral nervous system.

✤ Guillain-Barré syndrome

Guillain-Barré syndrome is an example of polyneuropathy that can rapidly become a medical emergency.

Let's get the normal stuff straight!

Peripheral nerves include all nerves outside of the brain and spinal cord.

* The 12 cranial nerves and 31 pairs of spinal nerves that connect the spinal cord to the rest of the body comprise the peripheral nervous system.
* Motor nerves stimulate movement and sensory nerves provide sensation.
* Every neuron has a cell body, lots of little nerve branches (dendrites) for receiving messages, and a long tail (the axon) for transmitting messages.
* Axons are covered with a protective outer sheath of connective tissue, and an innermost layer containing Schwann cells, which produce the myelin sheath surrounding peripheral nerves.

What is it?

Guillain-Barré (pronounced *ghee-YAN bah-RAY*) syndrome (GBS) is an acute inflammatory demyelinating disorder that causes symmetric flaccid paralysis to move upward along segmental nerve tracts. The incidence is lowest in children and increases after age 50, with the highest rates of GBS reported in the elderly, especially those beyond age 75. GBS occurs more frequently in males than females. With the eradication of polio in the United States, GBS has become the most common cause of flaccid

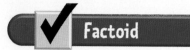

When GBS follows a head injury or surgery, the cause is thought to result from decreased cell and humoral immunity with subsequent production of antimyelin antibodies.[72]

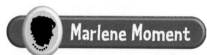

Marlene Moment

The autoimmune response is comparable with warfare situations in which our soldiers on foreign ground have opened fire on other US battalions there to help them. The myelin is there to insulate and protect, but in the confusion of battle, our own body attacks itself! This autoimmune response results in:

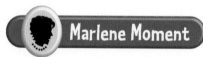

Marlene Moment

These little myelin secreting cells are NOT singing the Schwann song! Even though the myelin is peeled away exposing the axon, the Schwann cells will continue to make myelin to wrap and rewrap the nerve fiber, re-establishing communication between the brain and the muscles. No "Schwann song" for this baby (unless of course the axon was hit hard and damaged early on in the course of the disease or sustained secondary damage). Otherwise, full recovery is possible with no residual deficits.

paralysis in the United States. Fortunately, the incidence of GBS is low, occurring at a rate of 1.1 to 1.8 in 100,000.[71]

Causes and why?

The exact cause of the autoimmune attack is unknown, but most experts concur that the problem originates from an infectious organism containing an amino acid that imitates a protein in the peripheral nerve myelin to cause inflammation.[4] The syndrome usually (75% of cases) develops after a flulike respiratory or gastrointestinal illness with the onset of symptoms two to four weeks after the antecedent event. Others contracting GBS may not report an antecedent infection but antibodies against nerve gangliosides that react with *Campylobacter jejuni* are detected in their system. In addition to *C. jejuni*, there are other infections that commonly trigger the autoimmune response to go awry:

- Epstein-Barr virus
- *Mycoplasma pneumoniae*
- Cytomegalovirus
- Possibly *Haemophilus influenzae*[73]

Other less common triggers for Guillain-Barré include:

- Surgery or head injury
- Influenza immunization
- Human immunodeficiency virus
- Mononucleosis

Guillain-Barré syndrome is caused when the body's own immune system attacks the peripheral nervous system:

- Local inflammation results because of the cell-mediated response causing T cells (activated lymphocytes), B cells, and killer lymphocytes and other immune agents to rush to the area for "clean up" of what they perceive as foreign protein.
- The demyelination of sensory, motor nerves, cranial and autonomic nerves[73]
- Once the myelin has peeled away from the axon, secondary axonal damage may occur and produce residual dysfunction after GBS has subsided.
- Schwann cells are uninjured and can manufacture more myelin to initiate the recovery phase of the illness.

Testing, testing, testing

Many neurologic diseases can mimic GBS; however, a number of nonspecific tests can rule out other causes, such as a drug screen for exposure to toxic substances or serum electrolyte studies for possible hyponatremia. Specific tests for GBS include:

- Nerve conduction studies to evaluate waveform amplitude, velocity, conduction blocks, and latency. The presence of axonal waves on tibial nerve study and abnormal blink reflex (response of supraorbital nerve) are early indicators of GBS.[72]

- CSF obtained by lumbar puncture will show a higher concentration of protein with normal mononuclear cell counts.
- Stool culture and serology for *C. jejuni*.
- Electromyography (EMG) can determine the degree of axonal loss (usually performed later in the disease process).[72]

Signs and symptoms and why?

The initial symptoms of Guillain-Barré syndrome are weakness, tingling, or loss of sensation in the feet and legs that spreads upward to the trunk and arms. Progressive muscle weakness may rapidly become bilateral flaccid paralysis. Other signs and symptoms may include:

- Weak, sluggish, or delayed eye and facial movement
- Difficulty articulating words, and halting, slurred speech
- Chewing or swallowing problems, dysphagia
- Severe pain in the lower back
- Bladder control and dysfunction
- Bradycardia
- Hypotension
- Difficulty breathing because of a weak diaphragm
- Decreased respiratory excursion

What can harm my patient and why?

Life-threatening complications of GBS may occur early in the course of the illness, or may happen as a result of prolonged physical immobility or autonomic dysfunction and can include:

- Respiratory failure
- Cardiac arrhythmias
- Deep vein thrombosis and resultant pulmonary embolus
- Fear of outcomes and prognosis with possible residual damage
- Loss of control and independence because of paralysis
- Death because of rapidly progressing paralysis of the diaphragm before respiratory support can be initiated

Interventions and why?

A-B-Cs will always be the top priority with GBS because the paralysis that begins in the lower extremities can rapidly advance upward and cause paralysis of the diaphragm. Ventilator support is needed in 25% to 30% of cases[74] because of respiratory failure.

- Monitor bedside parameters for vital capacity and negative inspiratory force.
- Remain vigilant and alert to even minor reductions in respiratory capacity.

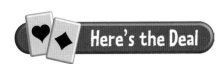

Here's the Deal

Mortality rate from GBS is 3% to 10%; an additional 20% still cannot walk after 6 months, but the good news is that about two-thirds of GBS patients will make a full recovery. If the axons aren't irreparably damaged the Schwann cells are unaffected and will make more myelin to restore a functional protective sheath.

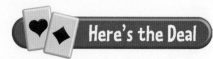

- Advocate for elective intubation in anticipation of emergency airway management and ventilation because of respiratory fatigue or paralysis.

- Suction as needed to maintain patency of the airway.

- Detect heart rate, rhythm, and electrical conduction abnormalities through continuous cardiac monitoring.

Intervene with prescribed pharmacologic and technologic maneuvers to decrease circulating antibody levels as quickly as possible to decrease the extent and severity of demyelination and length of recovery from GBS:

- Administer prescribed intravenous immune serum globulin (IVIG), which contains healthy antibodies extracted from donor plasma.

- Monitor the patient during plasmapheresis: vital signs, cardiac monitor, respiratory effort, tissue oxygen saturation

Cardiovascular supportive therapy is necessary because of autonomic hyperreflexia/dysreflexia:

- For tachycardia and hypertension, administer prescribed short-acting pharmacologic therapy such as alpha-adrenergic blockade.

- For decreased cardiac output and hypotension, implement orders for isotonic IVF and IVF bolus.

- Establish a communication system with the patient who is fully awake and aware cognitively, but unable to respond because of facial paralysis. Maximize use of any physical capability (eg, blink once for yes and twice for no).

- Give reassurance that even while being mechanically ventilated, the body is at work repairing itself.

- Reposition the immobile patient every 2 hours and maintain good body alignment.

- Apply compression stockings or sequential compression devices (SCDs) to improve venous return in the bedfast patient.

- Administer prescribed prophylactic anticoagulation for prevention of coagulopathies.

- Implement enteral or parenteral feedings as prescribed for the intubated patient.

- Monitor the patient receiving oral feedings for dysphagia and if noted, hold the patient NPO until a swallowing study can be obtained.

- Provide diversional activities and mental stimulation for the immobile, paralyzed patient: music, audio books, videos, etc.

- Encourage family members and visiting friends to interact with the patient.

PATIENT TEACHING Teach the patient self-care strategies and assisted care needs as the weakness and possible residual effects may persist for an extended period. As function gradually returns, reinforce teaching by other disciplines (physical therapy, speech and swallowing therapy, respiratory therapy, vocational or occupational therapy). Teach the patient:

- To use assistive devices and wheelchair for safety and conservation of energy.
- To balance activities with rest periods.
- To use thickening additives for liquids and mechanically soft diet as instructed for swallowing difficulties.
- That strict compliance with home or outpatient therapy will hasten return of strength and endurance, and prevent respiratory complications.
- To stay mentally active and emotionally involved in people, events, and activities outside of himself or herself.
- To continue all prescribed medications for the prescribed duration, even if he or she is feeling better.
- That GBS rarely occurs in the same individual, but just in case, to get to the nearest emergency department at the first sign of numbness or tingling of the feet.

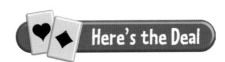

Here's the Deal

If intravenous immune serum globulin is administered, then plasmapheresis sucks off the plasma containing the IVIG, so what good have we done the patient? They aren't given together for this reason. Common sense dictates that either one or the other will be sufficient.

Cutting edge

Since Guillain-Barré syndrome commonly begins after viral or bacterial infection, scientists are focusing on correlating characteristics of these organisms that can trigger inappropriate activation of the immune system.[75]

✚ Myasthenia gravis

The name *myasthenia gravis* literally means a *grave (dead serious) muscle weakness.*

Let's get the normal stuff straight!

Voluntary movement depends on transmission of nerves to muscles at the myoneural junction.

- The motor neuron communicates with the innervated muscle cell at the end plate of the muscle membrane.
- The chemical acetylcholine normally attaches to receptor sites in the motor end plate to create the action potential causing muscle contraction.
- Acetylcholine is only active in the myoneural junction for a very brief time.
- The enzyme acetylcholinesterase inactivates any acetylcholine remaining after the synapse.
- Repeated muscle contractions or differing muscle force requires inactivation so another action potential can be generated in the innervated muscle cell.[2]

The thymus gland, located in the neck region above the heart, is an integral component of the immune system because it is responsible for mature, functional T lymphocytes, which are capable of detecting and reacting to foreign antigens (and not reacting to self-antigens).[2]

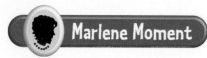

Marlene Moment

The myoneural junction is the place where "the rubber meets the road." Just like a car that's full of fuel with a dysfunctional fuel injection system, the car is still not going anyplace! It stops at the intersection! When acetylcholine receptor–binding sites are lacking at the myoneural junction, the electrical impulse isn't going anywhere. The acetylcholine binding sites are not available to enable transmission of the electrical stimulus across the intersection (myoneural junction) between the nerve and the muscle.

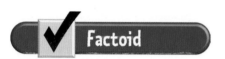

Factoid

As a rule, women are usually more prone to autoimmune diseases than men, and when women develop myasthenia gravis, they do so at an earlier age (20–40) as opposed to men, who do not develop symptoms until after age 60 or 70.

▶ Figure 7-13. Thymus gland.

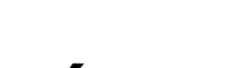

Factoid

A whopping 80% of patients with myasthenia gravis have hyperplasia or a tumor of the thymus (Fig. 7-13).[78]

What is it?

Myasthenia gravis (MG) is an autoimmune reaction that affects women earlier in life and with increased frequency compared with men.

- The characteristic muscle weakness that occurs in muscles all over the body is deemed "grave" because respiratory muscles can become too fatigued to support effective tissue oxygenation.
- MG causes a disruption in communication between the motor neuron and the muscle cell because of dysfunction at the myoneural junction,[2] the place where the nerve meets the muscle.
- Myasthenia gravis can be categorized into subtypes: ocular or generalized, with or without thymoma, early or late onset, or with or without antimuscle-specific tyrosine kinase antibodies.[76]

Causes and why?

The pathology of MG is within the myoneural junction, where antibodies attack the acetylcholine receptor sites within the motor end plate. The transmission of nerve impulses to the muscle does not take place because there is nowhere for the acetylcholine to attach.

- The majority of patients have autoantibodies directed against the postsynaptic nicotinic acetylcholine receptor (AChR).[77]
- The autoimmune damage at the receptor site keeps the nerve impulse from crossing over to the muscle.

Tumors or hyperplasia of the thymus gland are implicated in the autoimmune response and manufacture of antibodies at the acetylcholine receptor sites, possibly owing to abnormal T-lymphocyte function.[2]

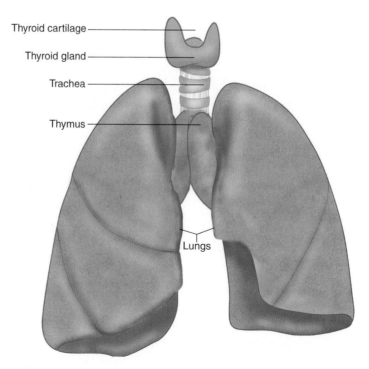

Testing, testing, testing

The acetylcholinesterase inhibitor test is also called the Tensilon or edrophonium test. Edrophonium chloride (Tensilon) given IV produces dramatic but short-lived improvement in muscle strength.

- A droopy eyelid that fully opens within 30 seconds after the injection is an example of a positive test.
- Because Tensilon is very short acting, the clinical improvement in muscle strength disappears in 5 minutes.
- If a total dose of 10 mg over three minutes is administered with no clinical improvement, the test is negative.[79]

    Other tests for the diagnosis of myasthenia gravis are:

- EMG electromyography reveals decreased amplitude reflecting delayed or absent neuromuscular transmission when muscles supplied by a selected nerve are stimulated.
- CT or MRI of the chest may reveal thymus enlargement or tumor.
- Immunoassay tests detect the presence of acetylcholine receptor antibodies in the serum.

Signs and symptoms and why?

Weakness of ocular muscles is the presenting sign of myasthenia gravis in 75% of cases, and all patients experience ocular muscle weakness at one time or another.[2,79]

What can harm my patient and why?

Generalized muscle weakness can cause a number of harmful events such as:

- Decreased quality of life
- Trauma caused by falls
- Aspiration pneumonia
- Corneal abrasion

The most life-threatening complication of myasthenia crisis or cholinergic crisis is characterized by severe generalized weakness and respiratory failure.

Interventions and why?

The stress of illness or surgery may cause exacerbation of myasthenia gravis, so monitoring of respiratory function can predict impending respiratory insufficiency (refer also to Guillain-Barré syndrome).

- Vital capacity
- Negative inspiratory force

    The priority need for the myasthenia gravis patient during an exacerbation or cholinergic crisis is oxygenation! As a result of extreme muscle

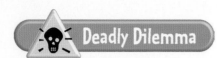

Deadly Dilemma

Atropine must be immediately available to reverse possible brady-cardia for cholinergic crisis caused by overdose or toxic levels of anti-cholinesterase drugs.

weakness, oxygen intake is compromised because the diaphragm and intercostal muscles are too weak to pull air into the lungs.

- Protect the airway with endotracheal intubation.
- Support respirations with mechanical ventilation.
- Monitor the patient who is receiving plasmapheresis (see guidelines with Guillain-Barré syndrome).
- Administer IV immunoglobulin therapy as prescribed.
- Administer corticosteroid drugs as prescribed.
- Administer prescribed anticholinesterase medications:
  - Neostigmine (Prostigmin)
  - Pyridostigmine (Mestinon)
  - Ambenonium (Mytelase)

Administer immunosuppressive therapy, which is prescribed when the desired effect is not obtained with anticholinesterase drugs or thymectomy:

- Prednisone (Apo-Prednisone, Deltasone)
- Azathioprine (Imuran)
- Cyclophosphamide (Cytoxan)

Postoperative thymectomy nursing care (usually a transsternal surgical procedure) involves:

- Preoperative plasmapheresis to decrease postoperative length of mechanical ventilation.[80]
- Postoperative monitoring in an intensive care setting with weaning from ventilator as indicated by respiratory function.

Once the exacerbation of acute, severe symptoms has subsided, the nursing plan will focus on the following basic needs:
Energy conservation:

- Incorporate rest periods before and after each activity of daily living.
- Develop energy conservation strategies to decrease fatigue and opti-mize activity.
- Schedule activities during times when energy level and strength are highest.
Nutrition:
- Consume a soft diet with viscous foods and thickened liquids.
- Position upright with head tilted slightly forward for meals. Instruct to eat slowly with small bites, chewing thoroughly and small sips of liquids.

To avoid the risk for injury because of muscle weakness and visual dis-turbance (falls), impaired swallowing (possible aspiration), and weak or delayed blink reflex and lid closure:

- Patch one eye to eliminate double vision and resultant dizziness.
- Employ frequent eye care with liquid tears (check expiration dates) and a protective shield to protect the eye during sleep.

- Assist the patient to the bathroom, and instruct him or her in the use of hand grips (for the toilet and shower).
- Collaborate with physical therapy for assistive devices as needed.
- Keep pathways in the room clear of obstruction with ample room for use of assistive devices.
- Instruct the patient not to attempt mobilization, but rather to use the emergency call bell in the event of increased weakness.
- Collaborate for swallowing study prior to oral intake with suspected high risk for aspiration.
- Defer meals during times of extreme weakness, eating at times of optimal strength.

Avoid medications that exacerbate myasthenia gravis or cause myasthenia crisis:
- Aminoglycoside antibiotics (amikacin sulfate, gentamycin sulfate, kanamycin, neomycin sulfate, tobramycin sulfate, streptomycin sulfate, paromomycin sulfate, netilmicin)
- Other antibiotics: polymyxins, tetracyclines
- Cardiac drugs: verapamil and beta blockers
- Drugs with CNS action: narcotics, hypnotics sedatives, barbiturates, phenothiazines, or tranquilizers

---

PATIENT TEACHING   To prevent excessive fatigue and worsening of symptoms:

- Take prescribed cholinesterase inhibitors on time to maintain blood levels and effectiveness.
- Take cholinesterase inhibitors 30 to 40 minutes before meals for maximum strength to chew and swallow.[78]
- Apply for a handicapped permit to reduce energy expenditure required walking distance to stores or offices.
- Patronize stores in which motorized shopping carts are available with carryout or curbside pick-up.
- Schedule timed rest periods throughout the day according to the pattern of fatigue or lowest ebb of energy.

Myasthenia crisis must be prevented, so the patient must be taught to avoid psychological or physiologic stressors that could lead to respiratory failure:

- Infection
- Pregnancy
- Emotional upset
- Alcohol ingestion
- Vigorous physical activity
- Exposure to cold or extreme heat
- Anticholinesterase drugs (too much or too little)

The patient with myasthenia gravis should be taught to wear a medic alert bracelet at all times, and if living alone, to invest in a life alert system (push button) necklace or bracelet to summon emergency responders from a community location.

Cutting edge

Data collected over a median time of 9.8 years following 172 patients who either had thymectomy or conservative treatment were evaluated to compare survival and quality of life. Thymectomy was found to have significantly better survival, remission, improvement, and quality of life scores than the conservative treatment group.[81]

DEGENERATIVE NERVOUS SYSTEM DISEASES

Slowly progressing incurable neurologic diseases eventually lead to disability.

✚ Parkinson's disease

The patient with Parkinson's disease will experience physical, social, and psychological challenges.

Let's get the normal stuff straight!

Nerve impulses travel to muscles along neural pathways with the help of chemical messengers called *neurotransmitters.*

- The basal ganglia consists of structures in the forebrain and part of the midbrain, the substantia nigra, and its axons that make up the nigrostriatal pathway.

▶ Figure 7-14. Substantia nigra.

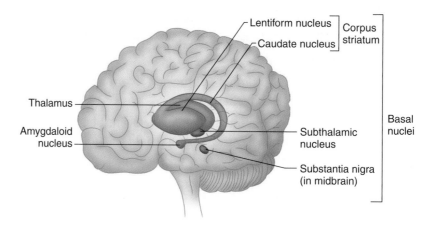

- Dopamine, the major neurotransmitter in the basal ganglia is produced and stored within the substantia nigra (Fig. 7-14).

- Dopamine, an inhibitory neurotransmitter and other neurotransmitters in the basal ganglia, make balance and smooth controlled voluntary movements possible.

- Looping circuits of the basal ganglia into the cortical areas add efficiency and graceful precision to motor movements.
- The basal ganglia (and the inhibitory action of dopamine) allow arms to swing naturally with running or walking and permits learned follow-through motions of throwing a ball or swinging a golf club to make contact with the ball.[2]

What is it?

Parkinson's disease is a slowly progressing degenerative disorder that affects the brain centers that control and regulate movement.

- The disease affects men more often than women.
- Onset is between 40 and 60 years of age. There is an increasing incidence with advancing age.

Causes and why?

Parkinson's disease can be idiopathic (cause unknown) or known/suspected based on genetics or head injury. Other suspected causes are atherosclerosis, excessive oxygen free radicals, toxic environmental exposure, and viral infections. The pathology involves the basal ganglia:

- Neurons in the substantia nigra and corpus striatum (where dopamine is produced) degenerate.
- Dopamine deficit upsets the balance between excitatory and inhibitory neurotransmitters.
- Dopamine lack results in overexcitability of the extrapyramidal pathways, causing tremors, rigidity, and abnormal, unstable gait.
- Heredity is implicated because having a close relative with Parkinson's disease (PD) increases the risk of developing PD three- to fourfold.[82]

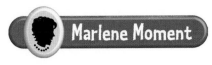

Marlene Moment

Don't even playfully call your Parkinson's patient a "Mover and a Shaker." That's not nice!

Testing, testing, testing

There is no current test to diagnose Parkinson's disease.[83,84] Diagnosis of Parkinson's disease is based on a thorough clinical examination and the presence of characteristic signs and symptoms.

- MRI can be used to rule out other non-Parkinson problems.
- Positron emission tomography (PET) scan and single photon emission computed tomography (SPECT) scans are being used to evaluate individuals at risk (see Cutting Edge).

Signs and symptoms and why?

Initial visible signs of Parkinson's disease are tremors that are worse at rest, and disappear with voluntary (intentional) movement. Eventually patients with Parkinson's disease develop the characteristic gait and the same "look" (Table 7-13).

Table 7-13   Parkinson's disease: signs and symptoms

Four cardinal signs	Secondary motor signs and symptoms	Nonmotor signs and symptoms
• Rest tremors • Bradykinesia • Rigidity • Loss of postural reflexes[85]	Characteristic gait: • Shuffling • Propulsive • Festination: gets faster and faster until the patient falls or runs into something to stop him or her Typical posture: • Head bent forward • Arms flexed • Thumbs turned into palms; "pill rolling" • Knees slightly bent Stiff muscles (dystonia) and joints (dysarthria): • Freezing • Cogwheel resistance to passive range of motion (ROM) • Lead pipe: stiff limbs remain where placed Facial/oral dystonia: • Dysphagia • Mask-like expression • Elevated eyebrows • Staring with decreased blinking • Slow measured speech • Soft muffled speech Loss of fine motor ability: • Inability to tie shoes • Difficulty with buttons • Slow, small handwriting	Autonomic dysfunction: • Insomnia • Oily skin • Diaphoresis • Excessive salivation (sialorrhea) • Heat intolerance • Orthostatic hypotension • Urinary retention • Constipation Cognitive neurobehavioral abnormalities: • Depression • Confusion • Personality change • Long- and short-term memory loss • Dementia (occurs late) Sensory abnormalities: • Absent sense of smell • Paresthesias with no physical cause for numbness, prickling, tingling, heat, or pain

Source: References 82, 83, and 85.

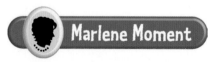

Sialorrhea (pronounced sigh-ah-lo-REE-ah) means excessive salivation, which is literally "a flow coming out" of the mouth. Now you have another new word to use on your non-nursing friends that sounds a lot nicer than "diarrhea of the mouth."

What can harm my patient and why?

The disease can cause premature disability and retirement, depression, declining physical and mental capabilities leading to loss of independence, social contacts, and quality of living. The greatest health hazard is related to:

• Aspiration pneumonia

• Injury from falls (fractured hip, subdural hematoma, etc)

• Neuroleptic malignant syndrome caused by long-term use of levodopa

Interventions and why?

If the patient is at high risk for aspiration, do not attempt feedings without a swallowing evaluation first. If the patient has aspirated during an attempted feeding:

• Immediately apply oropharyngeal and deep tracheal suction if needed.

• Position the patient upright and apply oxygen if effective breathing effort is present.

- Manually support respirations with bag-mask device and call a code from the room.
- Stay with the patient and notify the physician.

If the patient is at risk for neuroleptic malignant syndrome (NMS), signs must be recognized promptly because this is a potentially fatal complication:

- Hyperpyrexia
- Altered mental status
- Rigidity of muscles
- Irregular pulse, tachycardia
- Fluctuating BP
- Diaphoresis

Prepare to implement traditional treatment for NMS: bromocriptine, dantrolene, IVF, and supportive care.

My patient needs relief from symptoms that can be obtained through administration of prescribed medications. Refer to Table 7-14 for medications commonly used and nursing implications.

Table 7-14 Medications for control of Parkinson's symptoms

Pharmacologic therapy and nursing implications	Drug data, outcomes, and precautions	Side effects and adverse effects
Levodopa /carbidopa: (Sinemet/ Tagamet) (Sinemet-CR extended release) • Administer with food to minimize gastric irritation. • Teach patients to avoid B_6 supplements or excessive consumption of foods high in B_6. • Teach patients to arise slowly; monitor BP.	Converts to dopamine in the basal ganglia to produce symptomatic relief of tremors. Levodopa must be combined with carbidopa (enzyme inhibitor) because blood enzymes would break down most of the levodopa before it reached the brain. Controversy exits as to whether levodopa is toxic to neuronal cells or protective. There is no evidence that it worsens or slows the progression of Parkinson's disease.	Confusion, hallucinations, depression, and sleep disturbances Instruct patient to inform doctor if extrapyramidal symptoms occur, or if symptoms come and go ("off effect" and "on effect") Neuroleptic malignant syndrome can occur: Call 911 for severe rigidity, high fever, and stupor!
Trihexyphenidyl hydrochloride (Artane, Apo-Trihex) Benztropine mesylate (Cogentin) Biperiden hydrochloride (Akineton) Procyclidine (Kemadrin) • Have patient void before dosing. • Take after meals if dry mouth interferes with enjoyment • Take before meals if salivation is excessive to reduce saliva. • Monitor vital signs to determine response to drug.	Anticholinergic agents reduce tremors and rigidity. Used in combination with Levodopa to counteract action of acetylcholine. Contraindicated in narrow angle glaucoma. Effects of Artane potentiated by MAO inhibitors.	Blurred vision Dry mouth Rash Constipation Urinary retention Mental confusion Delirium Sedation Cardiovascular effects: • Tachycardia • Palpitations • Hypotension • Orthostatic hypotension

(Continued)

Table 7-14 Medications for control of Parkinson's symptoms (*Continued*)

Pharmacologic therapy and nursing implications	Drug data, outcomes, and precautions	Side effects and adverse effects
Amantadine hydrochloride (Symmetrel): • Administer with food or milk to reduce GI effects. • Schedule dose several hours before bedtime to reduce insomnia. • Monitor BP.	Developed as an antiviral agent, has anticholinergic (parasympatholytic) activity. May increase release of dopamine from neuronal storage sites. Reduces rigidity, salivation, dyskinesia, and postural changes. Little or no effect on tremors. NEVER abruptly stop the drug, as this can cause Parkinsonian crisis and neuroleptic malignant syndrome.	Orthostatic hypotension Sleep disturbances: insomnia, nightmares, agitation, and hallucinations May cause leg swelling as well as mottled skin, often on the legs. Causes difficulty concentrating and increased confusion in the elderly and those with cognitive deficits; therefore, rarely used for these patients.[83]
Bromocriptine mesylate (Parlodel) Pergolide (Permax) Pramipexole (Mirapex) Ropinirole (Requip) Apomorphine (Apokyn) Two additional drugs: cabergoline (Dostinex is not approved for use with Parkinson's) and lisuride (Dopergin) is not available in the United States. • Administer with food to reduce GI upset. • Monitor BP. • Monitor BUN and creatinine.	Dopamine agonists may be neuroprotective because of antioxidant effects, inhibiting free radical formation and scavenging free radicals. They may also slow the programmed cell death believed to be accelerated in Parkinson's disease.[93] Dopamine agonists have many side effects when beginning therapy, but resolve over several days. Dosages are reduced for creatinine clearance >60 mL/min. Not to be abruptly discontinued: must gradually be reduced and stopped over 1 week.	Nausea and vomiting Constipation Dysphagia Orthostatic hypotension Drowsiness Dry mouth Sleepiness, drowsiness, or sedation in some patients may pose safety hazard when driving. Report tardive dyskinesia (bizarre involuntary movements of the face, tongue, jaw, mouth).
Selegiline (Eldepryl, Atapryl, Carbex): • Monitor vital signs (especially during times of dosage change). • Monitor for behavior changes.	MAO inhibits the breakdown of dopamine; controls tremors by prolonging the action of dopamine in the brain. It also has a mild antidepressant effect. Used as adjunctive therapy with levodopa/carbidopa for patients who are responding poorly to therapy. Levodopa/carbidopa dose is reduced after 3 to 4 days of selegiline. NOT to be used in conjunction with tricyclic antidepressants (Elavil), as they can cause severe CNS toxicity.	Side effects may include sleep disturbances, agitation, heartburn, nausea, dry mouth, dizziness, confusion, nightmares, and hallucinations. Headache occurs less frequently and should be reported to the physician.
Entacapone (Comtan) Nitecapone Tolcapone (Tasmar) • Administer with food if GI upset occurs. • Monitor initial liver function studies, and teach patients about repeat studies. • Monitor BP and have patient arise slowly.	Catechol-*O*-methyltransferase inhibitors (COMT) extend the effect of levodopa or carbidopa, and reduce motor fluctuations in advanced disease. Must be gradually discontinued over time. Not to be combined with sedatives or alcohol. Hepatotoxic; therefore, only indicated for patients whose symptoms are poorly controlled with other drugs.	Diarrhea Dyskinesia Orthostatic hypotension Sleep disorders and excessive dreaming Adverse effect: Liver toxicity. Requires periodic liver function studies.

(*Continued*)

Table 7-14 Medications for control of Parkinson's symptoms (*Continued*)

Pharmacologic therapy and nursing implications	Drug data, outcomes, and precautions	Side effects and adverse effects
Diphenhydramine hydrochloride (Benadryl) Phenindamine hydrochloride (Neo-Synephrine) • Monitor BP (N-S) • Administer with food or milk (B)	Antihistamines: Mild sedative effects; Benadryl has antiemetic effect; Benadryl prolongs action of dopamine and may reduce tremors by central anticholinergic effects. Neo-Synephrine is NOT to be used within 21 days of MAO inhibitor. NOT to be combined with tricyclic antidepressants because of increased pressor effects!	Drowsiness (B) Tachycardia (B) Dry mouth (B) Elderly patients may experience dizziness, sedation, and hypotension (B) Tremors (N-S) Palpitations (N-S)
Amitriptyline (Elavil) Fluoxetine hydrochloride (Prozac) Bupropion hydrochloride (Wellbutrin) • Prozac (P): administer early morning. • Elavil (E): administer late afternoon or bedtime. • Wellbutrin (W): administer with meals to decrease nausea and vomiting.	Antidepressants: reduces depression. Elavil preferred because of anticholinergic and antidepressant effects, but interacts with levodopa and dosage must be reduced. Not to be combined with alcohol or sedatives. Prozac is NOT to be combined with selegiline! Can cause hypertensive crisis and death. Wellbutrin increases adverse effects of levodopa and MAO inhibitors.	Drowsiness (E) Orthostatic hypotension (E) Dry mouth (E) Dizzy (E) Sedation (E) Urinary retention (E) Headache (P) Nervousness (P) Anxiety (P), (W) Insomnia (P), (W) Nausea and vomiting (W)
Methylphenidate (Ritalin) • Administer 30–45 minutes before meals. • Monitor pulse and BP.	Amphetamine: stimulant that reduces the profound mental fatigue of PD that impacts quality of life.[86] Contraindicated in cardiac disease or psychiatric illness. NOT to be used with MAO inhibitors, as it will cause hypertensive crisis!	Nervous Insomnia Weight loss Rash Abrupt withdrawal can cause severe depression or psychotic behavior. Teach patients to take dose in the early morning and early afternoon to avoid insomnia.

Source: Reference 87.

PATIENT TEACHING My patient will need information for self-care and monitoring, which includes expected results of medications, and drug specific side effects/adverse effects.

• Keep a daily diary to record "on again/off again" symptoms and any side effects and effectiveness of treatments.

• Share your list of medications, side effects, and symptom relief or return of symptoms with your doctor.

Hurst Hint

If the PD drug ends in -capone, it's got to be a catechol-*O*-methyltransferase inhibitors (COMT)!

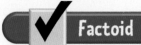

Factoid

Check for drug interactions with MAO inhibitors when new drugs are prescribed! Be alert to interactions between tricyclics and anti-depressants with anti-Parkinson medications.

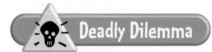

Deadly Dilemma

With all MAO inhibitors, caution the patient to avoid alcohol, fermented foods, and foods that contain tyramine. Teach patients how to recognize a hypertensive crisis, which can be a KILLER!

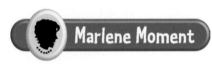

Marlene Moment

If you want life to be a bowl of cherries, you need to eat some!

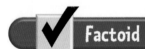

Factoid

Flat (no heel) shoes stimulate stronger eccentric contractions, stretching plantar flexors, which stimulates portions of the cerebellum to inhibit limbic structures and enhance neurogenesis.[89]

Teach nutrition tips from the *Official Journal of the National Parkinson's Foundation* for more healthy living:[90]

- Add cherries to the diet for antioxidant effects (PD is a very stressful disease that creates free radicals).
- Add blueberries to protect the brain against dementia.
- Add cranberries for antioxidative effect and to protect against urinary tract infections.
- Add strawberries, raspberries, and blackberries for protective phytonutrients.
- Add beans to the diet for fiber to prevent constipation and as an excellent source of B vitamins and magnesium, which are important to the nervous system.

Patient teaching to promote safety should include instructions to:

- Evaluate the home for safety hazards and remove throw rugs and obstacles from pathways.
- Ensure adequate lighting, leaving night lights on for visibility to the bathroom.
- Use assistive devices as prescribed with handrails around tub and elevated toilet seat.
- Prevent aspiration of food/fluids by eating/drinking in the upright position with head tilted forward, eating slowly.
- Mechanically soften and blenderize foods if dysphagia is present.

Instructions to maintain muscle tone include instructions to:

- Participate in a regularly scheduled exercise program. (Group programs are motivational and provide opportunities for interacting with others.)
- Keep going! Use motorized shopping carts, get handicapped parking permits to continue usual activities with modifications for fatigue. (See also teaching regarding energy conservation for multiple sclerosis.)
- Stay connected: Seek out support groups and activities to help you stay well.
- Dance classes are excellent exercise and provide stimulating social contacts.
- Walk daily, wearing flat-soled shoes to regenerate your brain as well as your muscles![89]

Cutting edge

Neurons are degenerating undetected for many years before the onset of physical signs of Parkinson's disease, such as slow movements and tremors. Characteristic symptoms do not appear until 80%[83] of the dopaminergic neurons have already been lost, and by that time the disease is well under way. Molecular markers based on gene expression in serum can identify patients (so a risk score can be assigned), thus opening the door to strategies to prevent or delay the onset of Parkinson's disease.[84]

Another promising development involves a large trial in progress (cosponsored by the NIH and the Parkinson study group) to further test the effects of coenzyme Q10. Brain cells need energy to survive and function, and this energy comes from the mitochondria. In Parkinson's disease, there seems to be mitochondrial dysfunction. Coenzyme Q10 seems to affect this energy-generating mechanism in cells, although the exact mechanism is unknown. A recent smaller study with 1200 mg/day of the coenzyme Q10 resulted in improvements in motor function.[87]

Once the diagnosis is made, anti-Parkinson medications are started as soon as possible. Refer to Table 7-11 for commonly prescribed medications.

- No current medication or treatment has been shown to stop the progression of PD.
- The focus is on controlling bothersome symptoms that impact quality of life.
- The treatment plan is highly individualized, so there is no standard or "best" treatment for Parkinson's disease.

Surgical options are reserved for select patients whose symptoms are poorly controlled by medications:

- Thalamectomy: Destruction of a portion of the thalamus with a stereotactic electrical stimulator to reduce tremors not controlled with conservative measures. Complications include hemiparesis and ataxia.
- Pallidus pallidotomy: Imaging is used to guide the electrode through a burr hole to a target area in the palladium to apply electrical stimulation to destroy the portion of brain causing rigidity. Only one side of the brain will be treated, followed by a second later procedure if rigidity or tremors are bilateral.
- Deep brain stimulation is being used for patients unresponsive to pharmacologic therapy. A pulse generator sends high-frequency electrical impulses via a lead anchored to the cranium into the thalamus to block nerve pathways and stop tremors. A magnetic wand over the site can turn the generator on or off.

Other treatment approaches, including general lifestyle modifications (rest and exercise), speech therapy, and physical therapy help to manage symptoms. Experimental therapies (transplantation of fetal cells or stem cells, growth factors, or gene therapy) are not available as treatment.[87]

✚ Alzheimer's disease

Alzheimer's disease accounts for almost three-fourths of all dementia, with the prevalence increasing after age 65 and doubling with every additional five years![2]

Let's get the normal stuff straight!

The hippocampus is the area in the cerebral cortex where memory (recent and remote) is stored and information is processed. Enzymatic activity (choline acetyltransferase) in the cortex and hippocampus supports synthesis of acetylcholine, the neurotransmitter associated with memory.

What is it?

Alzheimer's disease is a dementia that occurs in middle to later life that is characterized by progressive, irreversible atrophy of brain tissue and loss of mental function. Alzheimer's disease (AD) can be familial or sporadic (occurring early or late onset) (Fig. 7-15).

▶ Figure 7-15. Alzheimer's Brain. Cross-sections of normal brain and brain affected by Alzheimer's disease.

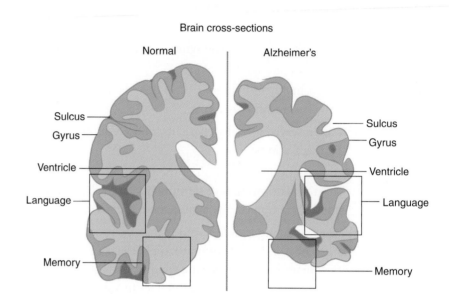

Brain cross-sections

Causes and why?

The brain pathology in AD is characterized by atrophy, plaques, and tangles of nonfunctioning neurons. Biochemically, the patient with AD has decreased levels of choline acetyltransferase and resultant decrease in acetylcholine available to the brain.[2] There is a link to heredity. If Alzheimer's is in the immediate family, chances of developing the disease are a little higher, but if you are a carrier of the AopE4 gene variant, there is a much higher chance of developing the disease. Other individuals who are at risk for developing Alzheimer's disease are:

* People with Down's syndrome who live into their fifties and sixties (linked to their chromosomal makeup).
* People who have had severe head or whiplash injuries also appear to be at increased risk.
* Boxers who receive continual blows to the head have an increased incidence.

Testing, testing, testing

There is no definitive test for diagnosis of Alzheimer's disease. The only positive confirmation is autopsy findings of plaque and neurotangles within the brain, but because dementia can be caused by other illnesses, lab tests and imaging can rule out everything else that could be causing symptoms:

- Thyroid profile (to rule out hypothyroidism)
- Drug screen (to determine alcohol or drug use)
- Serum levels of electrolytes and vitamins (looking for imbalance or deficiencies)
- CBC to make sure the patient is not anemic (decreased oxygen to the brain)
- CT or MRI imaging (to rule out brain tumor or other pathology)
- Electroencephalogram (EEG) to rule out other brain pathology

  Neuropsychological tests will be administered to gauge:
- Memory
- Attention
- Language skills
- Executive function
- Problem-solving ability

Signs and symptoms and why?

My patient will have gradual loss of memory, thinking, and language skills, and behavioral changes. Significant other or family members will report that the patient:

- Cannot remember recent information, new events, or placement of objects
- Is frequently disoriented to time and place
- Becomes lost in familiar places
- Struggles with ordinary, familiar activities such as hygiene, grooming, or dressing
- Has difficulty communicating; not being able to find the right words or complete sentences
- Has difficulty interpreting and processing directions and conversations
- Uses poor judgment when making decisions
- Has rapid mood swings with personality changes, disinterest in usually desired activities
- Demonstrates withdrawal behaviors with increased suspicion
- Cannot perform complex mental tasks such as balancing a checkbook[90]

What can harm my patient and why?

Anything can harm my patient, because the Alzheimer's patient cannot comprehend warning signs or danger. The patient is vulnerable to any physical threat because of the inability to interpret cues and get out of harm's way. Other threats to physical safety and well-being include:

- Risk for aspiration.
- Risk for physical injury related to wandering.

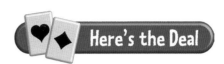

Here's the Deal

A shrinking brain (atrophy) leaves the ventricles larger as brain tissue recedes. This can be identified with imaging studies; however, confirming atrophy does not provide the diagnosis of Alzheimer's disease.

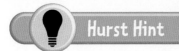

Always use persuasive talk and gentle urging first, UNLESS someone (staff member or another patient) is in danger;[91] then use nonviolent physical force to remove the patient to a safe, controlled environment.

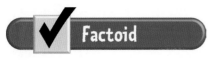

Restraints are avoided with the Alzheimer's patient (except in an emergency) because restraints increase agitation.

- Risk for violence related to paranoia and fear, causing others to retaliate.
- If the problem is combative behavior, back off and use verbal techniques, body language, personal space, and para-verbal communication to defuse actions of the patient.

Interventions and why?

In addition to personal care and assistance with activities of daily living allowing the patient to be as independent as possible (see Multiple sclerosis and Parkinson's disease), the patient needs pharmacologic therapy (cholinesterase inhibitors).

- Donepezil hydrochloride (Aricept)
- Rivastigmine tartrate (Exelon)
- Galantamine hydrobromide (Reminyl)

Refer to Table 7-15 for side effects and nursing implications associated with administration of cholinesterase inhibitors.

Table 7-15   Administration of cholinesterase inhibitors

Cholinesterase inhibitor and nursing implications	Side effects/adverse effects	Patient/family teaching
Donepezil hydrochloride (Aricept) • Administer at bedtime just prior to going to bed. • Begin with 5-mg tablet and increase to 10 mg after 4–6 weeks. • Monitor vital signs, watching for bradycardia because of the vagotonic effect of the drug.	The patient may experience: Headache Insomnia Nausea Diarrhea Vomiting Muscle cramps Anorexia GI bleeding	Patients/family members are taught to monitor for signs of GI bleeding: • Black, tarry stools • Coffee ground emesis • Epigastric pain
Rivastigmine tartrate (Exelon) Begin with 1.5 mg BID Increase to 3 mg/day every two weeks until the dosage reaches 6 mg BID in patch form, a 4.6 mg, 5-cm patch is worn once a day for 4 weeks. If well-tolerated, dosage is increased to a 9.5 mg patch daily.	The patient may experience: Nausea and vomiting Diarrhea Muscle weakness Anorexia and weight loss Dizziness, drowsiness, upset stomach	Instruct that Exelon may only postpone worsening of Alzheimer's disease for 6–12 months, but the effects are still worthwhile. Exercise caution when using NSAIDs because of the increased incidence of gastric ulceration. Exelon will not be available in generic form until Novartis' patent expires in 2014.

(Continued)

Table 7-15 Administration of cholinesterase inhibitors *(Continued)*

Cholinesterase inhibitor and nursing implications	Side effects/adverse effects	Patient/family teaching
Galantamine hydrobromide (Reminyl) Begin 4 mg BID In 4 weeks increase to 8 mg BID In another 4 weeks increase to 12 mg BID Administer morning and evening with food.	Watch for the following signs/symptoms: Headache Nausea and loss of appetite Mild diarrhea, especially when starting treatment. Changes in vision or balance Dizziness, fainting spells, or falls Severe diarrhea Skin rash or hives Slow heartbeat or palpitations Stomach pain Unusual bleeding or bruising, red or purple spots on the skin Vomiting Weight loss	Patients/family members are taught to monitor for signs of GI bleeding: ● Black, tarry stools ● Coffee ground emesis ● Epigastric pain

People who weigh less than 110 lb may experience more severe side effects and may need to stop taking Exelon.

A number of strategies are available for custodial care facilities to excite the imagination, shift mood, manage stress, stimulate positive interactions to combat depression, and facilitate motor movements and cognitive function:[83]

● Art therapy provides a channel of expression to allow patients who are unable to communicate through words to express delight, become more relaxed, and recover some fine motor skills.

● Music therapy: Music can stimulate or music can quiet. Make selections according to patient need (eg, falling asleep at mealtime may require stimulating music). Be alert to the patient's response to music. If the patient becomes agitated or restless, make another selection.

● Storytelling: Large colorful pictures can evoke memories or can encourage patients to make up stories (can be used in the home or in day care groups).

Strategies to reduce the incidence of sundowning:

● Keep patients active and busy during waking hours to discourage long daytime naps.

● During the afternoon make a shift to calm, restful, quieting activities.

● Turn the lights on before dusk, and keep the room well lighted until bedtime.

● Provide hydration and snacks.

● Make sure the room is neat and tidy with all clutter removed.

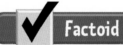

Cholinesterase inhibitors enhance uptake of acetylcholine in the brain to improve memory skills by slowing the degradation of acetylcholine released by the remaining intact neurons.

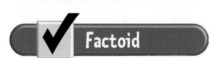

Depression (which is common in Alzheimer's disease) can worsen memory loss and cognitive impairment.

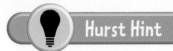

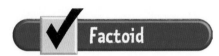

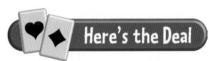

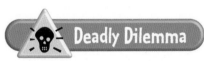

Strategies for dealing with wandering in the hospital include:

- Use weight-activated bed alarms.
- Use diversional and recreational strategies to reduce boredom (art, music, storytelling).
- Set a schedule for toileting, hydration, and snacks.
- Ask family members to bring familiar objects (photos, quilts, and a favorite pillow) to make it seem more like home.
- Put a strip of black duct tape on the floor across the doorway to define parameters, or a black rubber mat that will look like a black hole to make the patient turn around.

PATIENT TEACHING   The patient and/or caregiver (depending upon the progression of mental deterioration) is taught to:

- Wear a medic alert bracelet with personal information and phone number of contact person.
- Utilize home health aide and community resources for any available help.
- Place multiple locks on doors in hidden and high places.
- Mask exit doors with a curtain and alert a neighbor of the wandering pattern.
- Obtain a wristband transmitter to track a wanderer who has left the home.
- Turn on night lights to reduce the sundowning phenomenon and night time confusion.
- Never leave the patient alone or unsupervised.
- Utilize respite care or community resources for a day out to relieve caregiver strain.

Cutting edge

Clinical trials at sites across the United States are working to find something that will prevent, slow, or halt the progression of this relentless disease. One such trial, PREADVISE, is seeking to determine whether vitamin E and selenium can prevent memory loss and dementia such as that seen in Alzheimer's disease.[90]

There is currently no cure for Alzheimer's disease, but with optimal treatment the hope is to slow the progression of the disease and maintain quality of life for as long as possible. Medications (see Table 7-11) help for a while, and when dementia progresses, additives to prolong dopamine effects may extend effectiveness. Researchers are looking for new treatments to alter the course of the disease and improve quality of life. Family members are encouraged to utilize resources for respite care as needed.

PRACTICE QUESTIONS

1. A migraine-prone patient is experiencing an aura. Which medication is most appropriate for abortive therapy?

   A. Amitriptyline

   B. Verapamil

   C. Lithium

   D. Prednisone

2. A patient has received abortive medication for a headache in progress. What next nursing intervention is most appropriate?

   A. Make provisions for uninterrupted sleep.

   B. Awaken the patient to reassess in thirty minutes.

   C. Serve the scheduled meal tray and advise the patient to eat as much as possible.

   D. Provide supportive nursing care such as elevating the head of the bed and closing the curtains.

3. A trauma patient has a subdural hematoma and the next CT is scheduled in 12 hours. Which observation by the nurse would necessitate another stat CT to confirm expansion of the existing hematoma?

   A. The pupils are 2 mm and show a brisk reaction to light.

   B. The patient complains of a dull headache like a tight band around his head.

   C. The Glasgow coma scale score has dropped from 10 to 9 since the last check.

   D. The systolic blood pressure has dropped 10 mm Hg since administration of analgesia.

4. Which first action by the nurse is the priority when autonomic dysreflexia is in progress?

   A. Sit the patient upright.

   B. Find and remove the trigger source.

   C. Notify the physician from the bedside.

   D. Administer prescribed Apresoline IV slowly.

5. The patient with a herniated nucleus pulposus (who is sitting in the bedside chair) requests additional medication because analgesia given one hour ago has been ineffective in relieving low back pain. Because this analgesia has previously been highly effective, the nurse can correctly assume that:

   A. The patient may be developing drug dependency.

   B. The patient has developed a tolerance to the medication.

C. The patient is experiencing increased nerve compression.

D. Some added stressor has decreased the patient's pain threshold.

6. The patient with multiple sclerosis complains of injection site pain associated with self-administered (SQ) Betaseron (interferon beta-1b) every day. From which of the following instructions will the patient derive the most benefit?

A. Use a smaller-gauge needle.

B. Apply a warm compress at the injection site.

C. Administer concurrently prescribed NSAID medication.

D. Administer the medication very slowly using the push and pause method.

7. Which factor if identified in the nursing history could the nurse identify as having the greatest predisposition to the development of Guillain-Barré syndrome (GBS)?

A. Recent viral infection

B. First-degree relative has GBS

C. Poorly controlled diabetes

D. Enlargement of the thymus gland

8. Which will be *least effective* in reducing inflammation and resultant demyelination when the patient has Guillain-Barré syndrome?

A. Plasmapheresis treatments

B. Methylprednisolone (corticosteroid)

C. IV immune serum globulin

D. None. All are effective as monotherapy but not combined.

9. The Parkinson patient is hospitalized for monitoring during a change in the levodopa/carbidopa dosage since selegiline has been added to the medication regime. Which home medications must the nurse withhold pending collaboration with the physician?

A. Colace

B. Elavil

C. Benadryl

D. Ibuprofen

10. The patient with Alzheimer's disease experiences "sundowner syndrome" every afternoon at 5 p.m. Which initial nursing strategy will be most helpful to provide symptomatic relief of confusion and agitation?

A. Administer prescribed Ativan 0.5 mg IVP as needed for restlessness.

B. Turn on the TV and close the door to the room.

C. Increase the lighting in the room and provide a nutrient-dense snack.

D. Notify a family member that someone is needed to stay in constant attendance.

References

1. Penas CF, et al. Referred pain elicited by manual exploration of the lateral rectus muscle in chronic tension type headache. *Pain Med* 10(1):43–48, 2009.

2. Porth CM. *Pathophysiology: Concepts of Altered Health States.* 7th ed. Philadelphia: Lippincott Williams & Wilkins; 2007.

3. Goadsby PJ. Pathophysiology of migraine. *Neurol Clin* 27(2):335–360, 2009.

4. Smeltzer SC, Bare BG, Hinkle JL, Cheever KH. *Brunner and Suddarth's Textbook of Medical-Surgical Nursing.* 11th ed. Philadelphia: Lippincott Williams & Wilkins; 2008.

5. Leroux E, Ducros A. Cluster headache. *Orphanet Rare Dis* Available at http://www.ncbi.nlm.nih.gov/pubmed/18651939?ordinalpos=1anditool=EntrezSystem2.PEntrez.Pubmed.Pubmed_ResultsPanel.Pubmed_DiscoveryPanel.Pubmed_Discovery_RAandlinkpos=5andlog$=relatedreviewsandlogdbfrom=pubmed. Accessed March 30, 2009.

6. Bell's Palsy Information Site. Eye care. Available at http://www.bells-palsy.ws/eye.htm. Accessed April 15, 2009.

7. Rozen TD. Trigeminal autonomic cephalalgias. *Neurol Clin* 27(2):537–556, 2009.

8. Penas CF, Schoenen J. Chronic tension type headache: What is new? *Curr Opin Neurol* Available at http://www.ncbi.nlm.nih.gov/pubmed/19300250. Accessed March 31, 2009.

9. Jena S, Witt CM, Brinkhaus B, et al. Acupuncture in patients with headache. *Cephalalgia* 28:969–979, 2008.

10. Yaldo AZ, Wertz DA, Rupnow MFT, Quimbo RM. Persistence with migraine prophylactic treatment and acute migraine medication utilization in the managed care setting. *Clin Ther* 30(12):2452–2460, 2008.

11. Willich SN. Acupressure reduced intensity and pain frequency of primary migraine or tension-type headaches. *Evidence-Based Nursing.* Available at http://ebn.bmj.com.libproxy.uams.edu/cgi/content/full/12/2/47. Accessed March 30, 2009.

12. Larner AJ. Not all morning headaches are due to brain tumors. *Pract Neurol* 99(2):80–84, 2009.

13. Jacobs MP, Leblanc GG, Brooks-Kayal A, et al. Curing epilepsy: Progress and future directions. *Epilepsy Behav* 14(3):438–445, 2009.

14. Stevens J. Traumatic brain injury. *Kansas Nurse* 83(3):3–5, 2008.

15. McElroy-Cox C. Caring for patients with epilepsy. *Nurse Pract* 32(10):34–40, 2007.

16. Perucca P, Gilliam FG, Schmitz B. Epilepsy treatment as a pre-determinant of psychosocial ill health. *Epilepsy Behav* Available at http://www.ncbi.nlm.nih.gov/pubmed/19303947?ordinalpos=9andito ol=EntrezSystem2.PEntrez.Pubmed.Pubmed_ResultsPanel.Pubmed_ DefaultReportPanel.Pubmed_RVDocSum. Accessed April 06, 2009.

17. Beers MH, ed. Seizure disorders. *The Merck Manual of Medical Information.* Whitestation, NJ: Merck Research Laboratories; 2003.

18. Nursing 2008. Patient education series. *Nursing2008 38*(5):33, 2008.

19. Taber CW. Brain. Venes D, ed. *Taber's Clyclopedic Medical Dictionary.* 20th ed. Philadelphia: F.A. Davis; 2007.

20. Pirrung JM, Woods P. Motorcycle crashes. *Nursing2009 39*(2):29–33, 2009.

21. Heegaard W, Biros M. Traumatic brain injury. *Emerg Med Clin North Am 25*(3):655–678, 2007.

22. Hurst M. *Neurology On-line Review.* Brookhaven, MS: Hurst Review Services; 2008.

23. Naravan RK, Maas AI, Servadei F, et al. Progression of traumatic intracerebral hemorrhage: A prospective observational study. *J Neurotrauma 25*(6):629–639, 2008.

24. Ghajar J, Ivry RB. The predictive brain state: Timing deficiency in traumatic brain injury? *Neurorehab Neural Repair 22*(3):217–227, 2008.

25. McNett M. A review of the predictive ability of Glasgow Coma Scale scores in head injured patients. *J Neurosci Nurs 39*(2):68–75, 2007.

26. Lo C, Shifteh K, Gold T, et al. Traumatic brain injury. *J CAT 33*(2):293–297, 2009.

27. Homaifar BY, Brenner LA, Gutierrez PM, et al. Sensitivity and specificity of the Beck Depression Inventory-II in persons with traumatic brain injury. *Arch Phys Med Rehabil 90*(4):652–656, 2009.

28. Lipton ML, Gellella E, Lo C, et al. Multifocal white matter ultrastructural abnormalities in mild traumatic brain injury with cognitive disability: A voxel-wise analysis of diffusion tensor imaging. *J Neurotrauma 25*(11):1335–1342, 2008.

29. Williams G, Morris ME, Schache A, McCrory PR. Incidence of gait abnormalities after traumatic brain injury. *Arch Phys Med Rehabil 90*(4):587–593, 2009.

30. Rehman T, Rushna A, Tawil I, Yonas H. Rapid progression of traumatic bifrontal contusions to transtentorial herniation: A case report. Available at http://www.casesjournal.com/content/1/1/203. Accessed April 6, 2009.

31. Foster M, Spiegel D. Use of Donepezil in the treatment of cognitive impairments of moderate traumatic brain injury. *J Neuropsychiatry Clin Neurosci 20*(1):106, 2008.

32. Brain Trauma Foundation, American Association of Neurological Surgeons, Joint Section on Neurotrauma and Critical Care. *Guidelines for the Management of Severe Traumatic Brain Injury: Indications for*

Intracranial Pressure Monitoring. New York: Brain Trauma Foundation; 2003.

33. Bratton SL, Chestnut RM, Ghajar J, et al. Hyperosmolar therapy. *J Neurotrauma 24*(S14–S20), 2007.

34. Himmelseher S. Hypertonic saline solutions for treatment of intracranial hypertension. *Neuroanesthesia 20*(5):414–426, 2007.

35. Cajigal S. Hypertonic saline found to reverse transtentorial herniation. *Neurol Today 8*(11):1–9, 2008.

36. Meares S, Shores EA, Taylor AJ, et al. Mild traumatic brain injury does not predict acute postconcussion syndrome. *J Neurol Neurosurg Psychiatry* 79:300–306, 2008.

37. Ghajar J, Ivry RB. The predictive brain state: Timing deficiency in traumatic brain injury? *Neurorehab Neural Repair 22*(3):217–227, 2008.

38. Spinal Cord Injury Information Network. Facts and figures at a glance. Available at:http://www.spinalcord.uab.edu/show.asp?durki=1 16979andsite=4716andreturn=19775. Accessed April 6, 2009.

39. Fonte N. Urological care of the spinal cord-injured patient. *Wound, Ostomy Continence Nurs 35*(3):23–331, 2008.

40. Bailes JE, Petschauer M, Guskiewicz KM, Marano G. Management of cervical spine injuries in athletes. *J Athletic Training 42*(1):126–134, 2007.

41. The National Spinal Cord Injury Association. Christopher and Dana Reeve Paralysis Act. Available at http://www.spinalcord.org/news.php?dep=1andpage=0andlist=2237. Accessed April 12, 2009.

42. Choy DS. Familial incidence of intravertebral disc herniation: An hypothesis suggesting that laminectomy and discectomy may be counterproductive. *J Clin Laser Med Surg 18*(1):29–32, 2000.

43. Smuck M, Yoon T, Colwell M. Intravascular injection of contrast during lumbar discography: A previously unreported complication. *Pain Med 9*(8):1030–1034, 2008.

44. Madigan L, Vaccaro AR, Spector LR, Milam RA. Management of symptomatic lumbar degenerative disk disease. *J Amer Acad Orthop Surg 17*(2):102–111, 2009.

45. Harbayshi H, Takhashi J, Hashidate H, et al. Characteristics of L3 nerve root radiculopathy. *Surg Neurol* [Epub ahead of print]. Available at http://www.ncbi.nlm.nih.gov/pubmed/19150111?ordinalpos=4anditool=EntrezSystem2.PEntrez.Pubmed.Pubmed_ResultsPanel.Pubmed_DefaultReportPanel.Pubmed_RVDocSum. Accessed April 14, 2009.

46. Wera GD, Dean CL, Ahn UM, et al. Reherniation and failure after lumbar discectomy: A comparison of fragment excision alone versus subtotal discectomy. *J Spinal Disord Techniqes 21*(5):316–319, 2008.

47. Murtagh RD, Quencher RM, Cohen DS, et al. Normal and abnormal imaging findings in lumbar total disk replacement: Devices and complications. *Radiographics 29*(1):105–119, 2009.

48. Blumenthal S, McAfee PC, Guyer RD, et al. A prospective, randomized, multicenter Food and Drug Administration Investigational device exemptions study of lumbar total disc replacement with the

CHARITE artificial disc versus lumbar fusion. Part 1: Evaluation of clinical outcomes. *Spine 30*(14):1565–1575, 2005. Erratum in *Spine 30*(20):2356, 2005.

49. McAfee PC, Geisler FH, Saiedy SS, et al. Revisability of the CHARITE artificial disc replacement: Analysis of 688 patients enrolled in the U.S. IDE study of the CHARITE Artificial Disc. *Spine* 31(11):1217–1226, 2006.

50. Mirovsky Y, Shalmon E, Halpern Z, et al. Lumbar disk replacement with the ProDisc prosthesis. *Orthopedics 31*(2):133, 2008.

51. Wuertz K, Godburn K, Iatridis JC. MSC response to pH levels found in degenerating intervertebral discs. *Biochem Biophys Res Commun 379*(4):824–829, 2009.

52. Henriksson HB, Svanvik T, Jonsson M, et al. Transplantation of human mesenchymal stem cells into intervertebral discs in a xenogeneic porcine model. *Spine 34*(2):141–148, 2009.

53. Matthews C, Miller L, Mott M. Getting ahead of acute meningitis and encephalitis. *Nursing2007 37*(11):37–41, 2007.

54. National Multiple Sclerosis Society. What is multiple sclerosis? Available at http://www.nationalmssociety.org/about-multiple-sclerosis/what-is-ms/index.aspx. Accessed April 16, 2009.

55. Centers for Disease Control and Prevention Fact Sheet: Arborviral Encephalitis. Available at: http://www.cdc.gov/ncidod/dvbid/arbor/arbofact.htm. Accessed April 12, 2009.

56. Miller JP, Acar F, Hamilton BE, Burchiel KJ. Radiographic evaluation of trigeminal neurovascular compression in patients with and without trigeminal neuralgia. *J Neurosurg 110*(4):627–632, 2009.

57. Russell D, Baloh RW. Gabapentin responsive audiovestibular paroxysmia. *J Neurol Sci* April 3, 2009. [Epub ahead of print]. Available at http://www.ncbi.nlm.nih.gov/pubmed/19345961?ordinalpos=2andito ol=EntrezSystem2.PEntrez.Pubmed.Pubmed_ResultsPanel.Pubmed_ DefaultReportPanel.Pubmed_RVDocSum. Accessed April 14, 2009.

58. Prasad S, Galetta S. Trigeminal neuralgia: Historical notes and current concepts. *Neurologist 15*(2):87–94, 2009.

59. Gilchrist JM. Seventh cranial neuropathy. *Semin Neurol 29*(1):5–13, 2009.

60. National Institute of Neurological Disorders and Stroke. Bell's palsy fact sheet. Available at http://www.ninds.nih.gov/disorders/bells/detail_bells.htm. Accessed April 14, 2009.

61. Vrabec JT, Issacson B, Van Hook JW. Bell's palsy and pregnancy. *Otolaryngol Head Neck Surg 137*(6):858–861, 2007.

62. Tyler KL. Prednisolone-but not antiviral drugs-improves outcome in patients with Bell's palsy. *Nat Clin Pract Neurol 5*(2):74–75, 2009.

63. Wong CL, Wong VC. Effect of acupuncture in a patient with 7 year history of Bell's palsy. *J Alt Comp Med 14*(7):847–853, 2008.

64. Palmieri RL. Caring for a medical-surgical patient with MS. *Nursing2008 38*(10):34–40, 2008.

65. National Multiple Sclerosis Society. About MS. Available at http://www.nationalmssociety.org/about-multiple-sclerosis/who-gets-ms/index.aspx. Accessed April 16, 2009.

66. National Multiple Sclerosis Society. Visual symptoms. Available at http://www.nationalmssociety.org/about-multiple-sclerosis/symptoms/visualSymptoms/index.aspx. Accessed April 16, 2009.

67. Ross AP, Hackbarth N, Rohl C, Whitmyre K. Effective multiple sclerosis management through improved patient assessment. *J Neurosci Nurs* 40(3):150–157, 2008.

68. Blasier MG. Pharmacologic management of multiple sclerosis. *Urol Nurs* 28(3):217–219, 2008.

69. Jolly H, Simpson K, Bishop B, et al. Impact of warm compresses on local injection-site reactions with self-administered glatiramer acetate. *J Neurosci Nurs* 40(4):232–239, 2008.

70. National Multiple Sclerosis Society. Research news. Available at http://www.nationalmssociety.org/research/research-news/news-detail/index.aspx?nid=999. Accessed April 17, 2009.

71. McGrogan A, Madle GC, Seaman HE, deVries CS. The epidemiology of Guillain-Barré syndrome worldwide. *Neuroepidemiology* 32(2):150–163, 2009.

72. Vucic S, Kiernan MC, Cornblath DR. Guillain-Barré syndrome: An update. *J Neurosci* [Epub ahead of print]. Available at http://www.ncbi.nlm.nih.gov/pubmed/19356935?ordinalpos=3anditool=EntrezSystem2.PEntrez.Pubmed.Pubmed_ResultsPanel.Pubmed_DefaultReportPanel.Pubmed_RVDocSum. Accessed April 20, 2009.

73. Pritchard J. What's new in Guillain-Barre syndrome? (Reprint). *Postgrad Med J* 84:532–538, 2008.

74. Durand MC, Porcher R, Orlikowski D, et al. Clinical and electrophysical predictors of respiratory failure in Guillain-Barre syndrome: A prospective study. *Lancet Neurol* 5(12):1021–1028, 2006.

75. National Institute of Neurological Disorders and Stroke, National Institutes of Health: Office of Communications and Public Liaison. Clinical Practice Corner. Guillain-Barre Syndrome. *Can J Neurosci Nurs* 30(2):20.

76. Gilhus NE. Autoimmune myasthenia gravis. *Exp Rev Neurotherapeut* 9(3):351–358, 2009.

77. Meriggioli MN. Myasthenia gravis with anit-acetylcholine receptor antibodies. *Frontiers Neurol Neurosci* 26: 94–108, 2009. Available at http://www.ncbi.nlm.nih.gov/pubmed/19349707?ordinalpos=5andito ol=EntrezSystem2.PEntrez.Pubmed.Pubmed_ResultsPanel.Pubmed_DefaultReportPanel.Pubmed_RVDocSum. Accessed March 15, 2009.

78. George-Gay B, Chernecky CC. *Clinical Medical Surgical Nursing: A Decision Making Reference*. Philadelphia: Saunders; 2002.

79. Kusner LL, Puwanant A, Kaminski HJ. Ocular myasthenia: Diagnosis, treatment and pathogenesis. *Neurologist* 12(5):231–239, 2006.

80. Juel V. Myasthenia gravis: Management of myasthenic crisis and perioperative care. *Semin Neurol 24*(1):75–80, 2004.

81. Bachmann K, Burkhardt D, Schreiter I, et al. Thymectomy is more effective than conservative treatment for myasthenia gravis regarding outcome and clinical improvement. *Surgery 145*(4):392–398, 2009.

82. Hermanns M. Parkinson's focus. *RN 71*(10):25–28, 2008.

83. National Parkinson Foundation. About Parkinson's Disease. Available at http://www.parkinson.org/Page.aspx?pid=225. Accessed April 20, 2009.

84. Scherzer CR, Eklund AC, Morse LJ, et al. Molecular markers of early Parkinson's disease based on gene expression in blood. Available at http://www.pnas.org/content/104/3/955.long. Accessed March 31, 2009.

85. Jankovic J. Parkinson's disease: Clinical features and diagnosis. *J Neurol Neurosurg Psychiatry 79*:368–376, 2008.

86. Friedman JH. Fatigue in Parkinson's disease patients. *Curr Treatment Opt Neurol 11*(3):186–190, 2007.

87. National Parkinson Foundation. Treatment options. Available at http://www.parkinson.org/Page.aspx?pid=227. Accessed April 21, 2009.

88. Holden K. Ten nutrition tips for living well with Parkinson's disease. *Parkinson Report: Official J Nat Parkinson Fdn 20*(1):9, 2009. Available at http://www.parkinson.org/Document.Doc?id=420. Accessed March 31, 2009.

89. Flensmark J. Physical activity, eccentric contractions of plantar flexors, and neurogenesis: Therapeutic potential of flat shoes in psychiatric and neurological disorders. *Med Hypoth* [Article in press]. Available at http://www.sciencedirect.com.libproxy.uams.edu/science?_ob=ArticleURLand_udi=B6WN2-4W232DT-1and_user=1496715and_rdoc=1and_fmt=and_orig=searchand_sort=dandview=cand_acct=C000053083and_version=1and_urlVersion=0and_userid=1496715andmd5=343cfbb5e3a4c3dc3f6aa781c530ab8d. Accessed April 15, 2009.

90. Alzheimer Foundation of America. Alzheimer facts. Available at http://www.alzfdn.org/AboutAlzheimers/warningsigns.html. Accessed April 21, 2009.

91. Tarzian AJ, Marco CA. Responding to abusive patients: A primer for ethics committee members. *HEC Forum 20*(2):127–136, 2008.

92. Porth CM. *Pathophysiology: Concepts of Altered Health States.* 8th ed. Philadelphia: Lippincott Williams & Wilkins; 2008.

93. Leypold BG, Flanders AE, Schwartz ED, Burns AS. The impact of methylprednisolone on lesion severity following spinal cord injury. *Spine 32*(3):373–378, 2007.

94. Hogan MA, Hill K. *Pathophysiology: Reviews and Rationales.* Upper Saddle River, NJ. Prentice Hall Nursing; 2004.

95. Centers for Disease Control and Prevention. Information on arborviral encephalitides. Available at http://www.cdc.gov/ncidod/dvbid/arbor/arbdet.htm. Accessed April 12, 2009.

CHAPTER

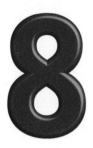 **8** # Renal and Urologic Disorders

OBJECTIVES

In this chapter you will review:

- The pathophysiology associated with common urinary tract and renal disorders.
- The key concepts and priorities associated with nursing care of the patient with urologic or renal dysfunction.
- Technologic advances that improve the quality of life when renal and urologic function is threatened or compromised.
- The effects of renal and urologic dysfunction on elimination, acid–base balance, erythropoiesis, physical safety, and comfort.
- Treatment modalities to promote restoration of optimal urologic and renal function.
- Patient teaching to enhance self-care while *recovering* from a urologic or renal disorder, or while living with a *chronic* renal dysfunction.

INFECTIONS OF THE URINARY TRACT

Urinary tract infections (UTIs) are classified as:

- Upper UTI: Infection of the ureters and/or kidney (pyelonephritis)
- Lower UTI: Infection of the bladder and/or urethra (cystitis, urethritis)
- Complicated
- Uncomplicated
- Acute
- Chronic

Let's get the normal stuff straight first!

- The lower urinary tract is susceptible to infection because of microbial invasion, urinary stasis, or reflux leading to cystitis or urethritis.
- The lower urinary tract consists of the bladder and the urethra.
- A number of intrinsic defense mechanisms help protect the lower urinary tract against bacterial invasion:
  - The bladder is lined with an adherent, protective mucin layer.
  - Epithelial cells become enmeshed within the mucin layer and produce protective substances that reinforce the antimicrobial mucin layer.
  - Shedding of bladder epithelial cells into the urine is another means of eliminating bacteria.
  - With each voiding, any invading bacteria are flushed from the bladder and urethra.
  - The normal urethral flora of females *(Lactobacillus)* prevents foreign bacteria from colonizing the urinary tract.
  - Hydrophilic protein glycosaminoglycan (GAG) forms a water barrier between urine and the bladder wall to keep bacteria from adhering, and thereby halting its colonization in the mucin layer.[1]
  - Acidic vaginal pH (4.0) of healthy premenopausal women inhibits urethral contamination from the rectal area.[2]
  - The male urethra is protected by antimicrobial prostatic fluid to hinder growth of microorganisms.[3]
- Infections of the lower urinary tract can occur for a variety reasons.

  Urinary tract infections can also be classified as uncomplicated or complicated.

- Uncomplicated: Infections that occur in a person who has a normal healthy urinary tract and usually involves only the bladder
- Complicated: Infections that occur in the presence of coexisting factors:
  - Diabetes
  - Obstruction (stones, congenital stenosis)

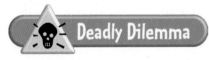

Deadly Dilemma

Urosepsis is a UTI that has evolved into a systemic infection. It is a medical emergency and must be treated promptly.

- Neurologic diseases
- Pregnancy
- Indwelling catheter
- Recurrent infections

LOWER URINARY TRACT INFECTIONS

Two lower urinary tract infections arise from the initial inflammatory response to trauma or uropathogens:

- **Cystitis** is inflammation of the urinary bladder, commonly occurring in sexually active women and menopausal women.
- **Urethritis** (also called urethral syndrome) is inflammation of the urethra, which is more common in women and has the same clinical presentation as cystitis.[4]

Prostatitis is inflammation of the prostate gland, which occurs in adult men of all ages. Prostatitis, the most frequently occurring prostate problem (more than prostate cancer or hyperplasia) affects half of the male population at some time. It can contribute to a UTI but is not classified as a UTI.

✛ Cystitis

What is it?

Cystitis is an infection of the urinary bladder, also known as a lower urinary tract infection (UTI).

Causes and why?

UTI is caused by coliform bacteria (most commonly *E. coli* and enterococci). Children can get viral cystitis caused by adenovirus, but this is rarely seen in adults. In men, cystitis is usually related to bacterial invasion of the urethra that spreads upward and to the prostate.

✛ Urethritis

What is it?

Urethritis is an infection of the urethra and can occur in both men and women.

Causes and why?

- Viral infections
- Bacterial infections
- Organisms that cause sexually transmitted diseases/infections (gonorrhea, chlamydia, etc)

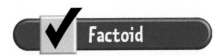

Cystitis can occur without bacterial contamination. Radiation to the bladder and interstitial cystitis are characterized by sterile urine.

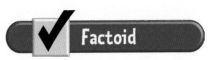

Male patients with gonococcal urethritis present with purulent urethral discharge. This is a urinary tract infection caused by the bacteria that causes gonorrhea, and also a sexually transmitted disease/infection.

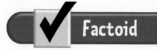

Factoid

Men who have chronic bacterial prostatitis may never actually be completely cleared from the infection because prostatic tissue is difficult to penetrate with antibiotics; therefore, the prostate continues to reinfect the bladder.

- Large families of gram-negative bacilli (Enterobacteriaceae, primarily *E. coli*) as well as gram-positive organisms are implicated in urinary tract infections.
- "Smart bugs" have developed means of overcoming the intrinsic defenses of the urinary tract with such distinctiveness as adhesins pili/fimbriae, and hemolysins for gaining access and colonizing.[2]
- Additionally, certain conditions enhance the development of lower urinary tract infections (Table 8-1).

Table 8-1 Conditions that enhance the development of lower urinary tract infections

Causes	Why
Transmission of microorganisms	*E. coli* and other organisms travel from the urethra to the bladder. Bacteria attack and colonize the epithelium of the urinary tract making urination painful and emptying of the bladder difficult. The urethra is short in women and is located in close proximity to the vagina and anus. Sexual intercourse can introduce bacteria from around the vagina (which is normally colonized) and the anus to the bladder through the urethra. Wiping back to front can also cause transmission of bacteria to the urethra in women (Fig. 8-1). The most frequent cause of UTIs in men is obstructions of the urinary tract caused by benign prostatic hyperplasia.
Pregnancy	Cystitis is common in women, especially during reproductive years. Pregnancy can cause incomplete emptying of the bladder because of the size and location of the uterus in proximity to the bladder, and possibly because of hormonal influences and changes in pH, which can alter normal flora.
Stasis of urine flow related to obstruction anywhere in the urinary tract	Kidney stones and/or an enlarged prostate can partially obstruct the flow of urine. The urine can't flow, leading to the multiplication of organisms in stagnant urine.
Stasis of urine flow related to structural abnormality (drooping uterus and bladder)	Prevents complete bladder emptying.
Stasis of urine flow related to reflux	Reflux occurs when urine moves from the urethra into the bladder (urethrovesical reflux) or from the bladder into the ureters (vesicoureteral). Urethrovesical reflux can occur during normal activities (in women), such as coughing or squatting. Vesicoureteral reflux can occur as a result of congenital defects of the ureters.
Impaired immune system	*Candida,* which tends to overgrow in those with impaired immune systems, can attack the bladder.
Procedures of the urinary tract (catheterization, cystoscopic procedures)	Organisms are introduced by way of invasive procedures with instruments or other equipment, such as catheters.
Diaphragm use	Diaphragms and spermicides (especially used together) can alter the normal flora, allowing other microorganisms to take over.
Diabetes	Hyperglycemia encourages bacterial growth in the urinary tract because bacteria love to live in a high glucose environment.
Inadequate voiding	Not taking the time to let the bladder completely empty allows bacteria to remain in the bladder and multiply, causing inflammation and infection.

Source: Created by the author from References 1, 2, 3, and 6.

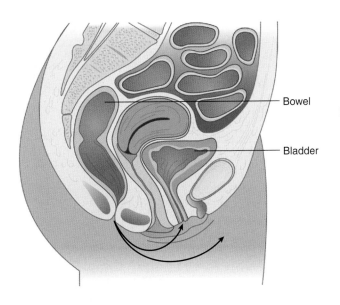

▶ Figure 8-1. Perianal contamination of urethra.

— Bowel

— Bladder

Factoid

UTIs can be caused by a fungal or parasitic infection; however, it is rarely seen in patients with a normal immune system. Patients with diabetes mellitus, AIDS, and recurrent UTIs are at greater risk.

Signs and symptoms and why?

Symptoms vary somewhat based on whether the condition is *acute* or *chronic*.

✦ Cystitis/urethritis

Cystitis and urethritis have nearly the same clinical presentation (Table 8-2):

- Pelvic pain and pressure with suprapubic localization
- Dysuria: Urinary frequency, urgency, and burning
- Unaccustomed nocturia (nighttime awakenings to void)
- Mild incontinence
- Cloudy urine with an offensive smell
- Hematuria (blood in the urine)

Table 8-2 Testing, testing, testing

Test	Clinical significance	Nursing care	Common interfering factors
Dipstick (for uncomplicated cases)	Based on the presence of nitrites, leukocytes, and/or blood in the urine.[5]	Obtain history related to signs and symptoms of LMP.	A menstruating woman may have a positive dipstick.
Urinalysis	Will reveal bacteria, RBCs, and casts	Instruct the client (especially females) to clean the labia minora and the area around the urethral meatus.	Bacteria from the vaginal area may contaminate the urine specimen.
C&S (urine culture and sensitivity)	Will identify the causative organism and anti-infectives to which the organism is sensitive or resistant.[2]		

(Continued)

Table 8-2 Testing, testing, testing (*Continued*)

Test	Clinical significance	Nursing care	Common interfering factors
Imaging CAT scan (CT)	Rules out obstructions caused by calcifications, tumors, hypertrophy, strictures, etc, which could be causing urinary stasis.		
Intravenous pyelogram (or CT)	Helpful for ruling out an infected stone when the patient has chronic cystitis, recurring infection with the same organism, or a history of childhood or to determine causation for children experiencing frequent urinary tract infections.		
Voiding cystourethrogram (or MRI)	Rule out the presence of urinary diverticulum.		
Cystourethroscopy	This is indicated for asymptomatic patients who have blood in the urine to rule out urinary tract stones or prostate calcifications, polyps, tumors, or anatomical abnormalities.[2]		
Prostate specific antigen (PSA)	This is indicated in men >50 and if suspiciously high will be followed by a transrectal ultrasound for needle biopsy to rule out prostate cancer.		
Meares-Stamey four glass test	Collection of urine before and after prostate massage can pinpoint the prostate as the site of a UTI.		

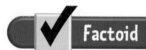

Bacteria can be present in the urine even if the patient is asymptomatic (especially the elderly patient).

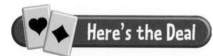

Elderly patients as well as diabetics may be asymptomatic because of decreased pain sensitivity related to neuropathy. Prior to any urinary tract surgery or instrumentation, a C&S is performed to detect bacteria in the urine (bacteriuria). Treating the infection before mucosal trauma will prevent spread of the infection.

Interventions and why?

- The treatment plan is formulated based on whether the urinary tract infection is acute, chronic, or complicated (Table 8-3).
  - An acute condition may require 10 days of antimicrobial therapy.
  - A chronic infection may necessitate treatment of 6 weeks or longer.
- The first uncomplicated infection is effectively treated with a three-day course of antibiotics not requiring urine culture and sensitivity.
- If symptoms recur after an appropriate antibiotic for an appropriate length of time, the entire urinary tract (upper as well as lower) must be re-evaluated with more extensive testing in case underlying pathology was overlooked.[6]
- The complicated infection (refer to Predisposing Factors) must be closely monitored. The rule is: If the antibiotic isn't working in two weeks, it should be discontinued.[5]
- If urodynamic testing determines that the underlying cause of recurrent lower urinary tract infections is a neurogenic bladder (which could be secondary to conditions such as multiple sclerosis, Parkinson's disease, diabetes mellitus, or spinal cord injury), a bladder retraining program and intermittent catheterizations will be prescribed to promote bladder emptying.

Table 8-3 Treatment for lower urinary tract infections

Lower urinary tract infection	Recommended treatment plan	Hurst hints
Acute uncomplicated cystitis or urethritis	**Antibiotics** • Nitrofurantoin (Macrobid) or • Trimethoprim/sulfamethoxazole (TMP-SMX) (Bactrim, Septra) **Short-term urinary analgesics** • Phenazopyridine (Pyridium) • Urised (Orasept) **Rest** **Rehydration**	• Nitrofurantoin turns the urine brown. • The most common bacteria causing lower UTIs is *E. coli.* • If not responding to Bactrim or Septra (TMP-SMX), the bacteria may be resistant. • *Ofloxacin* or *Floxin* belong to the category of drugs known as fluoroquinolones. • Macrobid (nitrofurantoin) is tough on lower urinary tract pathogens but gentle on normal flora. • The antibiotic should have a high concentration in the bladder and bowel and a lower concentration in body tissues. • Acidity of urine inhibits bacterial growth.
Chronic or recurrent cystitis	Culture and sensitivity of urine • Antibiotics based on sensitivity report. • Vaginal estrogen replacement may be indicated for postmenopausal women. • Postcoital antibiotics for sexually active premenopausal women. Prophylaxis may be indicated for 6 months (one dose nightly) with periodic reculture. • Nitrofurantoin (Macrobid) • Cephalexin (Keflex) • Trimethoprim/sulfamethoxazole (TMP-SMX) (Bactrim, Septra)	Be supportive and encouraging. Chronic cystitis interferes with daily living, job responsibilities, and relationships.

PATIENT TEACHING

• Women have a short, straight urethra that is close to the anal opening. This puts them at a higher risk for UTIs.

• Advise women to void after coitus to flush the urethra.

• Ask the patient to keep track of fluid intake and frequency of urination.

• Report pain (use scale of 1–10).

• Warn the patient that her urine will turn red if she is taking Pyridium (urinary analgesic); otherwise, she will think that she is hemorrhaging!

• Women of childbearing age should use contraception while taking a quinolone derivative such as ciprofloxacin (Cipro). This drug is contraindicated in pregnant or breastfeeding women.

• Antibiotics kill the pathogens causing infection as well as normal vaginal flora. Without vaginal flora, the patient may develop a yeast infection.

  • Eat yogurt.

  • The doctor or nurse practitioner may prescribe medication to prevent yeast infection, especially if the patient is prone to yeast infections when taking antibiotics.

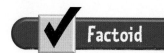

- Wipe front to back to avoid contaminating the urethra with bacteria from the anal area.
- Avoid bubble baths, scented soaps, and feminine hygienic sprays and wipes, all of which are irritating. Showers are preferred over tub bathing.
- Wear clean cotton undergarments and always wash new briefs before wearing.
- Drink 8 to 10 glasses of clear fluid daily.
- Avoid caffeine, alcohol, and soda (which cause bladder irritation).
- Void regularly, at least every two to three hours while awake, to flush the bladder.
- Avoid food items that decrease the activity of glycosaminoglycan (GAG) such as: diet drinks (aspartame, saccharin), alcohol, caffeine, and vinegar.
- Void before and after coitus to flush the urethra.
- Reconsider birth control methods. Stop the use of diaphragms and spermicides for acceptable alternatives.
- If a condom catheter with gravity drain is used, the tubing and bed position should not allow standing urine to contaminate the urethra.
- If suprapubic catheter is in place, remove any urine contaminated gauze, clean the site, and apply a sterile dressing as needed.

What can harm my patient and why?

- Hold Pyridium if the patient is allergic to sulfa.
- Discontinue nitrofurantoin immediately for any sign of peripheral neuropathy: numbness, tingling, or muscle weakness.
- Any infection of the lower urinary tract can ascend to the upper urinary tract, leading to:
  - Sepsis
  - Pyelonephritis
  - Acute nephritis with inflammation anywhere in the kidney
  - Chronic nephrosis, which leaves large holes in the glomerulus
  - Decreased renal function, uremia, and hypoalbuminemia
  - Edematous blockage of ureters and hydronephrosis

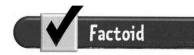

Cutting edge

Device manufacturers have antimicrobial Foley catheters on the market to reduce catheter-related urinary tract infections in adults! Silver alloy-coated Foley catheters effectively reduce bacteria in the urine, eliminating the reservoir that could lead to UTI and urosepsis.[8]

PROSTATITIS

What is it?

Prostatitis is a group of inflammatory and noninflammatory conditions affecting the prostate gland.

Signs and symptoms and why?

- Pelvic and peritoneal pain
- Pain in the testicles, groin area, penis, and scrotum radiating to the low back
- Urinary hesitancy with a weak stream when voiding
- Sexual dysfunction with painful ejaculation and postejaculatory pain in the rectum and anus
- Systemic symptoms: chills, fever, hypotension[9]

When prostatitis is chronic, there are urinary and nonurinary signs and symptoms:

- Dribbling of urine
- Inguinal and perineal pain
- Urethral burning
- General signs: Diaphoresis, fatigue, and cold feet.[5]

What can harm my patient and why?

Any infection of the lower urinary tract can ascend to the upper urinary tract, leading to:

- Sepsis
- Pyelonephritis
- Acute nephritis with inflammation anywhere in the kidney
- Chronic nephrosis which leaves large holes in the glomerulus
- Decreased renal function, uremia, and hypoalbuminemia
- Edematous blockage of ureters and hydronephrosis
- Acute bacterial prostatitis may result in blocked urine flow because of the edematous prostate requiring catheterization for immediate relief of urinary retention (Table 8-4).[8]

Here's the Deal

Stopping the burning, frequency, and urgency with a urinary analgesic (eg, phenazopyridine) gives the patient symptomatic relief with the first voiding because the drug is excreted in the urine.

Priority Nursing Care for All Patients with Indwelling Urinary Catheters:

- Secure the catheter to the thigh with a tension loop to prevent tension on the urethra.
- Routinely clean around the catheter using aseptic technique.
- Monitor urine for cloudiness and foul odor. Obtain urine for C&S from the injection port or via a fresh sterile catheter, but NEVER from the drainage bag!
- Avoid unnecessary catheterizations and advocate for removal of urinary catheters as soon as possible.
- Fluid intake of 1.5 L/day is required to flush out the bladder.
- Monitor output and check for bladder distention if there is no increase in output in excess of 4 hours.
- Administer prescribed urinary antibiotics based on culture and sensitivity report.

Interventions and why?

Table 8-4   Treatment for prostatitis

Acute and chronic prostatitis	Treatment	Associated nursing care
Acute prostatitis	Prostate massage may be indicated to drain occluded ducts, allowing better penetration of antibiotics: • Prulifloxacin (active metabolite ulifloxacin penetrates prostate tissue) Antiinflammatory agents (NSAIDs) to reduce pain Alpha-adrenergic receptor antagonists (alpha-blockers) for urinary symptoms Agents to decrease androgens: 5-alpha-reductase inhibitors[10] to shrink the prostate: • Glycosaminoglycans or • Quercetin or • Cernilton (CN-009) • Saw palmetto (botanical)	Prepare patient in advance that prostate massage is uncomfortable, but that he will feel better afterward. Premedicate if PRN medication is available. Monitor for side effects of prulifloxacin: GI upset, nausea, diarrhea, and skin rash.[11]
Chronic prostatitis	Causative organism *E. coli* responds favorably to one month of fluoroquinolone therapy: • Norfloxacin (Noroxin) • Cipro Floxin (Cipro) An alternate therapy is three months of therapy with Trimethoprim/sulfamethoxazole (TMP-SMX) (Bactrim, Septra)	Question patients about sensitivity to fluoroquinolones or history of seizure disorders. Do not administer fluoroquinolones within 2 hours of iron preparations or antacids because these drugs reduce absorption. Administer fluoroquinolones on an empty stomach and make sure the patient is well hydrated before and during therapy to prevent formation of crystals in the urine.

Source: Created by the author from References 2 and 5.

▶ Figure 8-2. Enlarged prostate.

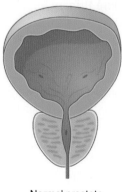
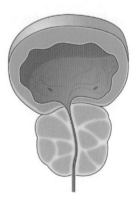

Normal prostate   Enlarged prostate

- The most popular surgery today is a transurethral prostatectomy (TURP) to relieve urinary symptoms and urinary retention.
- A TURP may be performed for symptomatic benign prostatic hypertrophy (BPH), especially if the patient has recurrent UTIs because of stasis of urine.
- The most important things to remember about post-TURP are:
  - We expect bleeding, but hemorrhage is the main concern!
  - Patients have painful bladder spasms afterward.
  - Usually three-way catheters are in place for continuous "through and through" irrigation with sterile GU irrigant to flush out blood clots and maintain patency of the three-way catheter.
  - Monitor I&O, keeping close track of urinary output.
- Remember … when continuous GU irrigation is in progress, subtract the GU irrigant from the output to determine how much of the total is urine.

PATIENT TEACHING

- Drink 8 to 10 glasses of clear fluid daily, avoiding caffeine, alcohol, and acidic foods/beverages that cause bladder irritation.
- Void regularly, at least every two to three hours while awake, to flush the bladder.
- Avoid food items that decrease the activity of GAG, such as diet drinks (aspartame, saccharin), alcohol, caffeine, and vinegar.
- If a condom catheter with gravity drain is used, the tubing and bed position should not allow standing urine to contaminate the urethra.
- If suprapubic catheter is in place, remove any urine-contaminated gauze, clean the site, and apply a sterile dressing as needed.

UPPER URINARY TRACT INFECTIONS

Let's get the normal stuff straight!

The upper urinary tract includes the kidneys and the ureters. The ureters are simply drainage tubes from the kidneys to the bladder; however, the matching pair of kidneys are incredibly complex organs. They are responsible for seven activities that are essential to health and well-being.

The following acronym (A-WET-BED) has been devised by nurses Hall and Esser[12] to help you remember functions of the normal kidney:

- **A**cid–base balance: Reabsorption or excretion (whichever is needed) of hydrogen and bicarbonate to maintain pH 7.35 to 7.45.
- **W**ater balance (fluid balance): Excretion or reabsorption of water as dictated by antidiuretic hormone (ADH) secretion. In dehydration, more water will be reabsorbed to help counteract the effects of fluid volume deficit. With fluid volume excess (FVE) more water is excreted to counteract the effects of fluid volume excess.

- **Electrolyte regulation:** To maintain tight control of sodium, potassium, calcium, magnesium, and phosphorus.
- **Toxin removal:** Excretion of waste and end products of metabolism (creatinine) or drugs.
- **Blood pressure regulation:** Activation of the renin-angiotensin system as needed when blood volume or cardiac output drops.
- **Erythropoietin:** Production of erythropoietin in response to hypoxemia for manufacture of healthy mature RBCs.[13]
- **D vitamin (vitamin D activation):** Changes vitamin D from the inactive to the active form for used by the body (with PTH, calcium, and phosphorus) for maintenance of strong bones.

The functional unit of the kidney is the nephron, and each kidney has about a million nephrons. Each nephron is comprised of the glomerulus, which is a tuft of tiny capillaries all intertwined. Blood leaving the glomerulus has been filtered and is normally free of protein (albumin) because large molecules do not normally cross the glomerular wall.[3]

- Bowman's capsule is a double-walled membrane that further filters and surrounds the glomerulus and routes the glomerular filtrate to the proximal convoluted tubule.
- The proximal convoluted tubule drains Bowman's capsule. It is at this site that 65% of all tubular reabsorption takes place.

✚ Glomerulonephritis

Glomerulonephritis is also referred to as *nephritis*.

What is it?

Glomerulonephritis is *inflammation* of the glomerulus, which affects the kidney's ability to filter urine. Note: Inflammation can occur anywhere in the kidney:

- Glomerulus, the most common site of inflammation
- Tubules
- Surrounding interstitial tissues

What causes it and why?

- The most common cause is a streptococcal infection that usually starts as a sore throat (strep), progressing to nephritis 7 to 12 days later.[3] Glomerulonephritis caused by a streptococcal (strep) infection usually resolves with treatment. Other forms of acute glomerulonephritis eventually progress to chronic glomerulonephritis.
- Following infection with certain viruses (measles, mumps, and/or chickenpox), the patient can develop glomerulonephritis.

Signs and symptoms and why?

- The patient may be asymptomatic if disease progression is slow.
- Hematuria (blood in the urine) and proteinuria (an abnormal amount of protein in the urine). Inflammation causes damage of the

glomerular membrane, leading to enlarged openings, allowing blood and protein to leak out. The damage with glomerulonephritis isn't as severe as with nephrosis and is treatable.

- Edema of hands and face from sodium and water retention can lead to fluid volume overload. Monitor for weight gain.
- Malaise and headache: Malaise may be a symptom of anemia related to decreased erythropoietin production OR from retention of toxins.
- Nausea and vomiting may be related to retention of toxins.
- Increased blood pressure related to fluid volume excess. Kidney function is impaired, leading to ineffective urine production.
- Symptoms of fluid volume overload include:
  - Dyspnea (related to pulmonary edema)
  - Engorged neck veins
  - Periorbital edema
  - Edema of hands, face, ankles, and feet
- Dark urine (coffee or cola colored).
- Oliguric phase followed by a diuretic phase.
- Diureses should begin 1 to 2 weeks after onset of glomerulonephritis, but blood and protein may stay in the urine for months.
- An onset of diuresis indicates the beginning of the recovery phase!

Testing, testing, testing

- Urinalysis is positive for blood and protein.
- 24-hour urine to determine creatinine clearance. Observing the creatinine clearance determines the glomerular filtration rate (GFR), which indicates how the kidneys are functioning. It may be <50 mL/min.
- Elevated serum BUN and creatinine related to impaired kidney function.
- Imaging studies to get a closer look at the kidney
  - Renal ultrasound
  - X-ray of the kidneys, ureters, and bladder (KUB)
  - Both studies may show kidney enlargement.
- Renal biopsy to determine the health of the renal tissue
- Antistreptolysins, O titer: This checks for the strep antibody and determines if there has been a recent infection. Remember, strep can lead to glomerulonephritis.
- Tests to determine the presence of autoimmune disorders (eg, ANA)

Interventions and why?

- Urea is not being excreted, so BUN goes up. Restrict protein in the diet to prevent a further rise in BUN.
- Sodium restriction: Sodium causes fluid retention.

- Monitor fluid intake to control edema.
- Monitor output to prevent complications from fluid volume excess. When the output drops, diuretics can be given to prevent circulatory overload.
- Monitor weight.
- Give diuretics to stimulate excretion of excess sodium and water.
- Phosphate-binding drugs (Amphojel) decrease phosphorus in the blood and increase serum calcium. Phosphorus is not being excreted with impaired renal function.
- Treatment of stress ulcers with H$_2$ blockers or proton pump inhibitors (eg, Zantac, Nexium).
- Steroids decrease inflammation of the glomerulus if the cause is auto-immune related.
- Treatment of the strep infection (if the cause).
- Bed rest decreases the metabolic demand and induces diuresis. The supine position increases kidney perfusion followed by increased urine production.
- Increase carbohydrates in the diet for energy and to prevent the body from breaking down muscle for protein, which leads to muscle wasting.
- When permanent damage occurs, as in chronic glomerulonephritis, dialysis is initiated. A kidney transplant may be considered.
- Administer albumin as ordered.
- Administer Lasix as ordered:
  - At least two venous accesses are required for the simultaneous infusions of Lasix and albumin.
  - The albumin infusion pulls fluid into the vascular space from the edematous tissues and the furosemide induces diuresis to eliminate the excess fluid once it's pulled into the vascular space. Therefore, if albumin is given **ALONE,** it will cause fluid volume excess, and if Lasix is given **ALONE,** it will produce shock because the patient is already in a fluid volume deficit.
- Prioritize activities and space them out to conserve energy and prevent fatigue.
- Provide meticulous skin care and frequent position changes because edematous tissue is at risk for breakdown.
- Administer prednisone to reduce the inflammatory response in the glomerulus and hopefully shrink the openings where the protein is leaking out.
- Auscultate lungs every two hours. The oliguric phase (not excreting fluid) causes FVE.
- Monitor for rhythm changes:
  - There is a risk for hyperkalemia during the oliguric phase. No urine output means decreased potassium excretion.

- There is a risk for hypokalemia during the diuretic phase. Increased urinary output can lead to excessive loss of potassium.
- Monitor and record I&O.
- Monitor and record daily weights.
- Diet:
  - Low sodium, because increased aldosterone causes sodium retention
  - Increase carbohydrates to support energy requirements. This prevents protein from being used to meet the energy requirements.
  - For glomerulonephritis, decrease proteins if the BUN is elevated.
  - For nephrosis, this renal patient CAN have protein because he or she is losing it through the damaged glomerulus.

What can harm my patient and why?

- Acute glomerulonephritis can progress to chronic glomerulonephritis with permanent damage to or even failure of the kidney.
- Too much protein in the diet.
- Hypertension.
- Circulatory overload, leading to pulmonary edema and congestive heart failure.
- Hypertensive encephalopathy, leading to seizures (medical emergency).
- Electrolyte imbalances (eg, hyperkalemia leads to arrhythmia).
- Increased serum phosphorus (which means decreased serum calcium) because of decreased renal excretion.
- Metabolic acidosis: Decreased excretion of hydrogen and decreased generation of bicarbonate.

PATIENT TEACHING Take antibiotics as prescribed to fully eradicate the organism (strep) and prevent complications.
  Educate the patient about the signs and symptoms of renal failure.

- Malaise
  - Headache, Anorexia, Nausea, Vomiting, Weight Gain, Oliguria
  Teach patient to avoid nephrotoxic substances.

✚ Nephrotic syndrome

What is it?

Significant **damage** to the glomerulus, leading to severe protein loss. Severe protein loss leads to hypoalbuminemia (insufficient protein in the blood).

Causes and why?

- Diabetes is the most common cause. It leads to diabetic nephropathy.
- Autoimmune diseases such as lupus erythematosus. Autoimmune diseases cause the body to attack itself. Antigen-antibody complexes are formed that damage the kidney.
- Medications such as NSAIDs, aminoglycosides, "mycin" antibiotics, amphotericin B, chemotherapy, lithium, IV contrast dye.

- Some illnesses damage the capillary membrane of the glomerulus. Examples include:
  - Hodgkin's disease
  - Syphilis
  - Hepatitis
  - HIV
  - Allergic reaction

Signs and symptoms and why?

Note: Many of the symptoms of glomerulonephritis and nephritic syndrome are the same. Notice that with nephrotic syndrome there are a few differences, such as **severe** edema because fluid is leaving the vascular space caused by hypoalbuminemia from the massive protein loss. The fluid leaves the vascular space and enters the interstitial space, leaving a fluid volume deficit and *hypotension*. Remember with glomerulonephritis one of the symptoms is *hypertension* because the fluid builds up in the vascular space. The difference is that with glomerulonephritis there is **not** a severe loss of protein causing the fluid to shift out of the vascular space but the kidneys still aren't functioning well enough to remove the excess fluid from the body.

- Severe fluid retention
  - Ascites
  - Periorbital edema
- Muscle atrophy and wasting owing to loss of nutrients and/or protein.
- Dyspnea related to pulmonary edema, ascites causing pressure on the diaphragm.
- Anemia related to decreased erythropoietin production. This leads to malaise.
- Retention of toxins also leads to malaise and anorexia.
- Pale skin color related to edema and/or anemia and malnutrition.

  Erythropoietin is produced by the kidney and is needed to stimulate production and maturation of red blood cells.

- Malaise and headache caused by the buildup of toxins.
- Flank pain and costovertebral tenderness caused by the renal inflammatory response.
- Oliguria—no urine output.

Interventions and why?

- Angiotensin-converting enzyme (ACE) inhibitors to:
  - Decrease proteinuria (how?)
  - Decrease lipid levels (how?)
- Restrict sodium to prevent further fluid retention.
- Restrict saturated fat in the diet because the patient is hyperlipidemic.
- Avoid medications that are nephrotoxic, which prevents further renal damage.

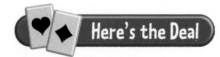

Here's the Deal

Impaired kidney function for any reason results in decreased erythropoietin production.

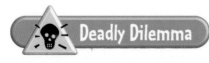

Deadly Dilemma

ACE inhibitors can increase the potassium level in patients with renal disease.

- Employ dialysis if indicated.
  - Hemodialysis
  - Peritoneal dialysis
- The patient may receive a renal transplant for renal failure.
- Encourage the patient with ascites to avoid large meals. Rather, small frequent meals should be encouraged to prevent abdominal fullness.
- Anticoagulants to prevent blood clots.
- If allergens are the culprit, allergy shots may be indicated.
- Restrict protein in the diet depending on the GFR. Once dialysis is initiated, the protein may be increased according to the patient's needs.
- Administer steroids to decrease damage to the kidney if an autoimmune disease is the culprit.
- Administer an albumin infusion to pull fluid back into the vascular space.
- Diuretics stimulate diuresis to rid the body of excess fluid.

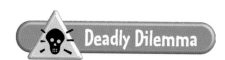

Diuretics increase the risk for blood clots caused by increased viscosity of the blood (blood is thicker).

Testing, testing, testing

- Urinalysis reveals sediment, protein, and hematuria with red cell casts.
- Decreased GFR.
- Elevated BUN (normal, 6–20 mg/dL).
- Elevated serum creatinine (normal, male: 0.6–1.3 mg/dL; female: 0.5–1.0 mg/dL).
- Anti-DNase B level (antideoxyribonuclease B) detects antigens produced by strep.
- ASO titer (normal findings adult/elderly <160 Todd units/mL) reveals strep antibodies from recent strep infection. This is helpful in the diagnosis of a poststreptococcal disease.[14]
- Imaging studies to help determine the degree of damage.
- Serum and urinary electrophoresis differentiate among normal renal function, glomerular proteinuria, and tubular proteinuria.
- Note: Tubular proteinuria indicates damage to the proteinuria rather than the glomerulus. Remember that damage can occur in the glomerulus, the tubules, or the interstitial tissues.
- Lipid levels: LDL and triglycerides will be elevated in an attempt to compensate for albumin loss, but increased lipids ALSO lead to atherosclerosis in the nephritic client.

What can harm my client and why?

- Massive loss of proteins in the urine may lead to more frequent infections. Immunoglobulins (proteins) are responsible for fighting infection. Think of them as being like antibodies.
- Loss of binding proteins causes decreased ions such as iron, copper, and zinc, and decreased levels of hormones (thyroid and sex hormones).

- Because many drugs bind to proteins for transport, the patient is at risk for overdose owing to insufficient protein.
- Retinopathy (why?)
- Untreated hypertension leads to further kidney damage and enlargement of the heart.
- Blood clots
  - Pulmonary embolism
  - Deep vein thrombosis (DVT)
  - Renal vein thrombosis
- **Anasarca**
  - Low blood volume to the kidneys causes them to respond as if the body were in shock. Therefore, the renin-angiotensin system is activated to restore volume and raise the blood pressure. The adrenal glands respond by producing more aldosterone, causing retention of sodium and water to increase circulating volume. Because there is insufficient protein (albumin) to keep the fluid in the vascular space, it shifts into the interstitial space! The result is **anasarca** (total body swelling).

Table 8-5 Quick comparison of nephritis and nephrosis

Glomerulonephritis (nephritic syndrome)	Nephrotic syndrome
Inflammation of the glomerulus	*Damage* to the glomerulus
Inflammation of the glomerulus, causing protein and blood to leak into the urine.	Large openings are formed in the glomerulus owing to **significant damage.**
Acute onset can lead to permanent renal damage, especially in vulnerable populations.	The main difference between nephrosis and nephritis is the massive protein loss that occurs with nephrotic syndrome which results in hypoalbuminemia and anasarca.
Antigen-antibody complexes lodge in the glomerulus and cause damage.	
Most common in boys ages 3–7.	Nephrosis is characterized by low serum albumin with loss of fluid from the vascular space with total body swelling.
Treatable with high recovery rate.	
With acute onset the patient will experience an oliguric phase and later on a diuretic phase.	

Source: Created by the author from Reference 3.

✚ Pyelonephritis

Let's get the normal stuff straight!

Organisms from the urethra can ascend into the bladder (common in women), and then the woman sneezes or squats or strains to lift something and bladder pressure pushes urine backward into the ureters, where the organism (probably *E. coli*) ascends and colonizes the pelvis of the kidney.

What is it?

Acute pyelonephritis is characterized by a patchy interstitial infection with inflammation in the **tubules** and the **interstitium** with formation of abscesses. Remember we said inflammation can occur in the glomerulus, tubules, or interstitial tissues.

Inflammation damages the tubules; therefore, the kidneys become unable to concentrate urine, regulate electrolyte balance, and eliminate waste products.[3]

Causes and why?

The most common cause is vesicoureteral reflux, which causes bacteria to ascend to the pelvis of the kidney. The most common organisms are *E. coli* and *Staphylococcus aureus*.

Interventions and why?

Treat infection:

- Obtain specimens (blood and urine) for cultures.
- Administer the prescribed antibiotic to which the pathogen is sensitive.
- If the patient develops nephrosis related to tubular damage in pyelonephritis, he or she may develop anasarca.
- Advise bed rest to reduce metabolic demand. Bed rest also induces dieresis.
- Monitor temperature.

PATIENT TEACHING   When long-term steroids are prescribed, teach the patient to:

- Expect changes in physical appearance (eg, moon face, buffalo hump, acne, truncal obesity).
- Take medication with meals or a snack to decrease gastric irritation.
- Avoid alcohol, which will increase gastric acidity and the risk for ulcerations (and is harmful to the kidney as well).
- Monitor capillary glucose more frequently (if diabetic) because steroids raise blood sugar.
- Perform blood pressure checks more frequently (if hypertensive) and restrict sodium because steroids increase circulating volume.
- Never abruptly stop taking medication! Steroids must be gradually tapered down before discontinuation to avoid adrenal gland (Addisonian) crisis.
- Wear a medic alert bracelet declaring long-term steroid therapy.
- Because glomerulonephritis can lead to renal failure, educate the patient about the signs and symptoms of renal failure:
  - Malaise
  - Headache

- Anorexia
- Nausea
- Vomiting
- Weight gain
- Oliguria
- Teach patient to avoid nephrotoxic substances (see Table 8-6).

Cutting edge

- Lupus erythematosus is a systemic disease that often leads to renal failure because of an autoimmune response in the kidney.
- Investigators in Boston have discovered help for lupus and a new role for T cells in reducing the incidence of inflammatory glomerulonephritis![13,15]
- Oral anti-CD3 induces a regulatory T cell to secrete high levels of another substance (TFG-β), which suppresses autoantibodies.
- What a find! We want to thank all the little mice who gave themselves to medical science to help rescue our lupus patients from dialysis!

Diabetic patients also have a huge incidence of renal failure, because sugar destroys vessels just like fat!

- There may be help on the horizon for preventing diabetic nephropathy! Researchers in Chapel Hill, NC and Ontario, Canada chose to study the relationship between matrix metalloproteinases (MMPs) and tissue inhibitors of this enzyme (TIMP3) because their effect on renal cells has been poorly understood.
- A balance of these two substances (MMPs and TIMP3) is important in renal tissue integrity.[16]
- Mice with higher levels of TIMP3 developed fibrosis of renal interstitial tissue and tubules.
- Patients with diabetic nephropathy have an increase of TIMP3 in the renal artery and proximal tubules.
- If inhibiting TIMP3 protects the little mouse kidney from damage, hopefully there will soon be a way to regulate this substance to decrease renal damage in our diabetic patients!

Nephritis or nephrosis compromises renal function, so treatment is aimed toward:

- Supporting failing renal function while correcting the cause (usually strep)
- Reducing the inflammatory response with administration of steroids
- Dialysis (see renal failure), which may be indicated if renal function is severely compromised

RENAL FAILURE

What is it?

The majority of nephrons of BOTH kidneys are no longer functional. Renal failure is said to occur when the GFR suddenly diminishes by 50% or more. This leads to oliguria and anuria with accumulation of metabolic wastes in the blood (azotemia).[13]

Renal failure can be acute or chronic. Acute renal failure can be reversed if treated quickly and effectively.

Define time

Oliguria describes a total urine output between 100 and 400 mL/24 hours. Anuria is a total urine output of <100 mL/24 hours.[17]

The patient with one functional kidney may not realize the other one is nonfunctional. The healthy kidney will take over all of the normal functions:

- Remove fluid and toxins
- Maintain electrolyte/acid–base balance
- Maintain levels of vitamin D and erythropoietin production

Clinical application

I was allowed to observe a dead kidney that had been discovered and removed by the surgeon during a routine hysterectomy. It looked like a ballet slipper (bean-shaped and "hollowed out"), with one dangling shoe string (the ureter). Lodged inside the ureter was a big stone. The patient was shocked after being informed. She had no idea there was a problem with one of her kidneys!

What causes it and why?

- Acute renal injury can lead to acute renal failure (ARF). Renal injury may be related to a variety of reasons:
  - Decreased perfusion
  - Internal (intrinsic) damage
  - Obstruction to urine flow (eg, stones)

Renal failure is classified according to the location of injury and the pathophysiologic process (Fig. 8-3).

- *Prerenal failure:* Caused by **decreased renal perfusion.** This is the most common form affecting critically ill patients and carries a high mortality rate for intensive care patients.[13]
- *Intrarenal failure:* Caused by **death of nephrons** within the kidney (intrinsic).
- *Postrenal failure:* Caused by **obstructed outflow** anywhere along the urinary tract.
  - Obstruction of urine outflow can lead to hydronephrosis.

▶ Figure 8-3. Pathophysiology of nephritis and nephrosis.

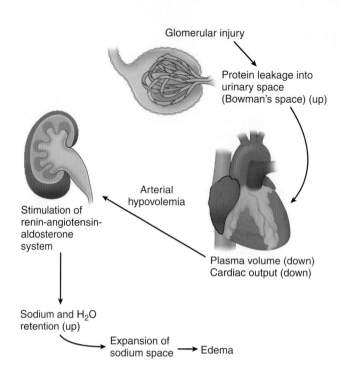

Define time

Hydronephrosis literally means kidney damage caused by water pressure, implying that the ureter and the renal pelvis are distended with urine, which creates a back pressure because of obstructed urine outflow. The pressure causes atrophy of the nephron with cyst formation. Refer to Table 8-6 for examples of various types of ARF and its causes.

Table 8-6   Types of renal failure and causes

Prerenal failure Caused by any condition that drops the cardiac output and reduces renal perfusion	Intrarenal failure caused by damage from trouble, toxins, or trauma within the kidney	Postrenal failure Caused by conditions that obstruct urine flow out of the kidneys, ureters, or urethra
Conditions that lead to pre-renal failure because blood cannot get into the kidney: • Shock • Hypovolemia (FVD) from any cause (including third spacing) • Hemorrhage • Hypotension • Heart attack • Heart failure • Arrhythmias (bradycardia or tachycardia)	Intrinsic damage and destruction of nephrons happens when there is: • Hypoxia of the nephron caused by unrelieved pre-renal causes • Hypoxia caused by obstruction • Sludge within the nephron • Pressure from masses and nephrotoxins Specific causes include: • Bacterial toxins (strep in particular) • Crushing injuries or hemolysis of cells with severe burns because free hemoglobulins and myoglobulins plug up renal tubules	Causes of postrenal failure include all mechanical or functional obstructions that reduce or halt urinary outflow: • Ureteral strictures • Enlarged prostate • Blood clots (ie, after transurethral prostatectomy) • Kidney stones • Tumors (masses) compressing ureters • Edematous ureteral stomas and obstructed ureteral or urethral catheters

(Continued)

Table 8-6 Types of renal failure and causes (*Continued*)

Prerenal failure Caused by any condition that drops the cardiac output and reduces renal perfusion	Intrarenal failure Caused by damage from trouble, toxins, or trauma within the kidney	Postrenal failure Caused by conditions that obstruct urine flow out of the kidneys, ureters, or urethra
Cardiac tamponade Sepsis Note: Stenosis of the renal arteries is a cause of renal failure unrelated to decreased CO. If the arteries are occluded with plaque, obviously there will be decreased renal perfusion.	• Longstanding hypertension and PIH (pregnancy-induced hypertension) damages the fragile capillary tufts within the glomerulus. • Nephrotoxic drugs, particularly loop diuretics, NSAIDs, aminoglycosides, penicillin derivatives, and the "mycins." • Dietary toxins: caffeine, alcohol. • Radiopaque (X-ray) dye used with imaging studies. • Disseminating intravascular coagulation (DIC) plugs up renal tubules with micro clots. • Organic substances such as ethylene glycol (antifreeze). • Heavy metals (mercury, copper). • Diseases such as diabetes, nephritis, nephrosis, pancreatitis or SLE (systemic lupus erythematosus).	• Crystallization within the glomerulus or renal tubules (upper urinary tract obstruction) Note: Nerve damage that keeps the bladder from emptying or hinders voiding can promote retention of urine just like the obstructional causes of postrenal failure.

Source: Created by the author from References 16 and 24.

Testing, testing, testing

The glomerular filtration rate (GFR) is a reflection of how the kidneys are functioning:

- The amount of creatinine filtered out by the kidneys equals the amount excreted in the urine.
- When the serum creatinine level rises, the GFR is falling.
- Protein metabolism produces urea, which should also be filtered out by healthy kidneys. The BUN measures blood urea nitrogen levels, which are increased in renal failure.
- BUN alone is not a reliable indicator of renal failure. BUN can be affected by other variables. Examples include:
  - Serum urea (reflected by the BUN level) is increased in the presence of dehydration.
  - BUN is increased during catabolism of muscles.
- When BOTH the serum urea and creatinine levels rise, the kidneys are in trouble.
- ABGs will reveal metabolic acidosis because the kidneys can't regulate acid–base balance:
  - Low pH <7.35
  - Base deficit > +2

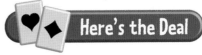
Here's the Deal

Reduced mean arterial pressure (MAP) causes the kidneys to respond by kicking in the renin angiotensin system to raise the blood pressure and (hopefully) restore renal perfusion. If renal blood flow is compromised for 20 minutes or longer, renal tissue may suffer irreparable hypoxemic damage.

- Hyperkalemia will be evidenced by:
  - Serum electrolytes: K^+ >5.0 mEq or 5.0 mmol/L
  - EKG: the T wave will be peaked and tall reflecting elevated serum potassium
- Urinalysis and urine specific gravity:
  - Depending on the stage of failure (diuretic versus oliguric phase), the urine will either be dilute or concentrated.
  - Normally, when a patient with normal kidneys is given a fluid bolus, the specific gravity decreases because the kidneys diurese and the fluid to particle ratio is increased (or diluted).
  - The specific gravity of the patient with renal failure who receives a 250-mL fluid bolus of NS will be unchanged because the nonfunctional kidneys have forever lost the ability to dilute.
  - Looking for fixed specific gravity is helpful in the diagnosis of renal failure.
- A "fixed" specific gravity is determined by administration of a fluid bolus, which should normally decrease the specific gravity; however, in renal failure (when the kidneys have lost their ability to concentrate and dilute) the urine specific gravity will remain unchanged.

Signs and symptoms and why?

Acute renal failure has an initial oliguric phase and later diuretic phase:

- During the oliguric phase, urine output is decreased, and the patient may develop fluid volume excess.
- During the oliguric phase, the patient is retaining potassium (hyperkalemic), because normally the kidneys excrete potassium.
- Hyperkalemia leads to arrhythmias.
- During the diuretic phase, the urine output is increased and the patient may develop fluid volume deficit.
- Polyuria during the diuretic phase leads to increased excretion of potassium (hypokalemia) and the patient may develop a fatal arrhythmia.
- Headache, malaise, nausea, and vomiting (retaining toxins).
- Weight gain, decreased urine output, signs/symptoms of FVE (retaining fluid)
- Anorexia, stomatitis, and metallic taste because of urea in the saliva with bacterial breakdown of urea to ammonia causing mucosal ulcerations.
- Symptoms of acid–base imbalance (metabolic acidosis).
- Symptoms of electrolyte imbalance: hyperkalemia, hyperphosphatemia, and hypocalcemia.
- Symptoms of anemia.
- Signs of osteoporosis.
- **Uremic frost:** Highly irritating urea crystals on the surface of the skin (Fig. 8-4).

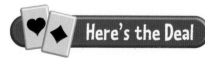

Here's the Deal

Any time the serum calcium drops, PTH will pull calcium from the bone to raise the serum calcium; however, the bones will become brittle and porous from calcium depletion, and now the patient has renal failure AND osteoporosis!

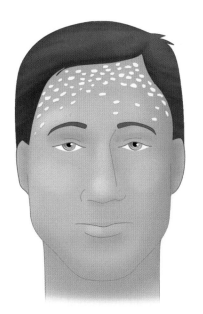

▶ Figure 8-4. Uremic frost.

- Change in color of urine (reddish, brown, or black) because of red blood cell casts (looks like cola).

What can harm my patient and why?

- Arrhythmias caused by potassium imbalance.
- Anemia caused by decreased production of erythropoietin.
- Metabolic acidosis caused by decreased excretion of hydrogen by the failing kidneys.
- The brain is NOT happy when the pH deviates from the normal range of 7.35 to 7.45!
- Hypertension is caused by fluid volume excess.
- Heart failure is caused by increased preload and afterload, leading to heart failure.
- Acute renal failure (ARF) can lead to tubular necrosis with irreversible death of the kidneys if not corrected promptly.
- Whether renal failure is acute or chronic, when the kidneys fail, the patient is at risk for:
  - Progression to end-stage renal disease (ESRD) and uremia
  - Multisystem organ failure
  - Increase in overall mortality rate by 50%[13]
- Early recognition and aggressive treatment of any condition that drops the cardiac output is priority because it only takes 20 minutes of low or absent perfusion for acute renal failure (ARF) to occur.
- Monitor blood pressure and urinary output frequently in susceptible patients. Be alert to trends of decreasing BP and falling urine outputs. Don't wait for these parameters to reach critical ranges before intervening.

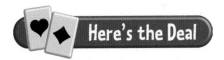

Here's the Deal

When the kidneys are sick (metabolic acidosis), who has to compensate? The lungs! With what chemical? (The only one they have is CO_2!) So will the respirations become more rapid? Or slower? You know the answer! If your patient is in metabolic acidosis, should he or she keep the CO_2 or blow it off? (Refer to Chapter 3 if necessary.)

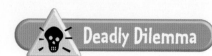

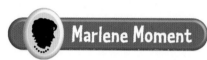

- The more severe the existing renal disease, the greater the incidence of "nonrecovery" of renal function after an insult from acute renal failure during hospitalization.
- A high of incidence of these patients who do seemingly recover from the largely preventable acute renal failure during hospitalization die later or progress to ESRD.[18]
- Notify the physician immediately of the following:
  - Increased BUN
  - Increased creatinine
  - Decreased urinary output

  Screen physician orders and medications for any nephrotoxic agents.
- Check BUN and creatinine before any procedure using radiopaque dye. Radiopaque dye is excreted by and nephrotoxic to the kidney.
- Evaluate all prescribed medications for renal (versus regular) dosing.
- Fluid volume depletion requires immediate fluid bolus to restore renal perfusion.
- Blood transfusion is required for massive hemorrhage, which drops the blood pressure and reduces renal perfusion.
- After a bad burn or a crushing injury, the nurse monitors for brown or red urine and notifies the doctor immediately, so that fluids and osmotic diuretics can be initiated quickly to flush out the kidneys before sludge can plug up the tubules.[19]
- In all hospitalized patients, decreased cardiac output should be treated promptly by administering inotropics, antiarrhythmics, etc. (Refer to Chapter 4 for cardiac protocols and Chapter 5 for shock protocols.) This prevents renal failure caused by decreased renal perfusion.

Interventions and why?

- Bed rest induces diuresis.
- Frequent, effective mouth care: Urea in saliva leads ulcerative stomatitis and anorexia.
- Frequent skin care when uremic frost is present gets irritating urea off the skin surface.
- Fluid restriction: Daily fluid allowance is based on the patient's losses plus 600 mL. An additional 600 mL are added to the patient's losses to compensate for insensible loss (respirations, perspiration, metabolic processes). For example:
  - The 24-hour urine output is 280 mL. Gastric suction is 200 mL. The TOTAL loss is 480 mL. The daily allowance should be 480 + 600 = 980 mL for the next 24 hours.
- Administer prescribed Epogen (erythropoietin) as prescribed to stimulate red blood cell production because the failing kidney cannot produce erythropoietin.

- Prepare the patient for dialysis (explaining options with attention to physical and psychosocial aspects) when the decline in renal function makes some form of dialysis inevitable.

- With 85% to 90% loss of renal function, the nephrologist will encourage placement of a permanent vascular access device in preparation for hemodialysis. Planning ahead prevents the inconvenience and expense of a temporary graft, while allowing time for the new vascular access to mature (Fig. 8-5).

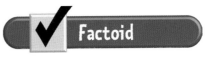

Factoid

Provide factual information the patient can understand so he or she can make appropriate decisions based on what is right for that individual. Patients are more confident with their health care decisions if given time to examine the risks versus the benefits associated with procedures and treatments.

▶ Figure 8-5. Vascular access.

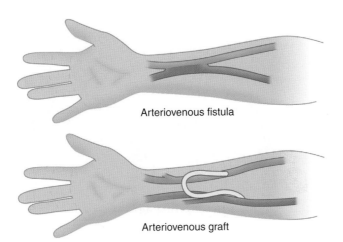

Arteriovenous fistula

Arteriovenous graft

- Provide appropriate nutritional support.

✚ Nutritional considerations

- The following guidelines are commonly prescribed for chronic renal failure and dialysis patients between treatments:
  - Decrease sodium intake (usually 2 g/day) because more rapid fluid gain is "normal" for renal patients.
- Limit intake of potassium (fruits, tomatoes, potatoes), because potassium is not being excreted and can build up in the blood.
- Limit phosphorus-containing foods (milk, cheese, colas, any food high in protein), because the kidneys have lost the ability to regulate phosphorus levels.
- Limit protein, which reduces nitrogenous byproducts of urea and creatinine.[11]
- An option for malnourished dialysis patients is intradialytic parenteral nutrition (IDPN). IDPN is a mode of alimentation that does not depend on patient compliance, feeding tubes, or vascular access,

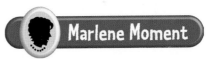

Marlene Moment

There is no such thing as "normal" unless you are talking about the setting on your washing machine. "Normals" vary for different patients! For example, it is "normal" for renal patients to retain fluid! We still worry about it, though! (So much for "normal!")

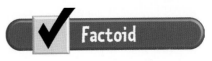

Factoid

High protein intake is avoided in chronic renal failure (not on dialysis), but protein malnutrition must be avoided. The death rate increases when serum albumin levels are <4.0 g/dL.[20]

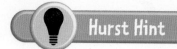

Turn the patient from side to side and change positions to allow pockets of fluid to drain out if all the dialysate fluid does not return.

because nutritional support is accomplished during dialysis with ultra-filtration for fluid management.[20]

- Chronic metabolic acidosis in renal insufficiency contributes to protein malnutrition because of increased breakdown of proteins and decreased synthesis of albumin.[21]

- The most consistent indicator of well-being of dialysis patients is the serum albumin. When serum levels are <4.0 g/dL, there is increased mortality.

- When the decline in renal function mandates dialysis, there are options: hemodialysis or peritoneal dialysis. Refer to Table 8-7 for a comparison of hemodialysis and peritoneal dialysis (Figs. 8-6 and 8-7).

▶ Figure 8-6. Hemodialysis. The dialyzer becomes the kidney!

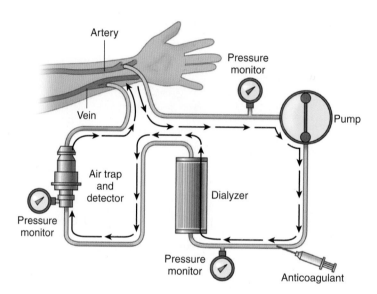

Table 8-7   Comparison of hemodialysis and peritoneal dialysis

Hemodialysis	Peritoneal dialysis
What is it?	**What is it?**
• A method for removing excess fluid and toxins as the patient's blood circulated through an artificial kidney (the dialyzer).	• Peritoneal dialysis accomplishes the same goals as hemodialysis (removal of excess fluid and toxins).
• The process of diffusion moves solutes (eg, excess potassium) from the blood across the semipermeable membrane (the dialyzer filter) into the dialysate for excretion from the body.	• The process of diffusion is the means by which toxins, wastes, and excess fluid moves from the blood into the dialysate.
• The goal is correction of fluid and electrolyte imbalance, removal of toxins and waste products of metabolism, and control blood pressure.[19]	• The peritoneum (rather than the dialyzer) becomes the semipermeable membrane.
• Continuous renal replacement therapy (CRRT) and ultrafiltration are other forms of hemodialysis.	• Perineal dialysis can be accomplished by either continuous ambulatory peritoneal dialysis (CAPD) or continuous cycle peritoneal dialysis (CCPD).

(Continued)

Table 8-7 Comparison of hemodialysis and peritoneal dialysis (*Continued*)

Hemodialysis	Peritoneal dialysis
What is required for hemodialysis?	**What is required for peritoneal dialysis?**
• Emergency dialysis for acute renal failure, acidosis, major drug overdose, hyperkalemia, or FVE unresponsive to conservative measures will require insertion of a central venous catheter inserted into the femoral, jugular, or subclavian vein.	• A catheter is surgically placed into the peritoneal cavity just below the umbilicus.
• Surgical creation of an arteriovenous (AV) fistula to bring the radial artery together with the cephalic vein, causing the vein to bulge outward with arterial pressure.	• The catheter is accessed multiple times each day for CAPD and accessed only twice a day to connect and disconnect lines for CCPD.
• A temporary catheter (eg, Asch catheter) must be used until the AV fistula matures, dilates, and toughens in response to increased pressure and turbulence (usually 2–6 weeks).	The patient must be active in the treatment and possess these essential qualifications:
• Temporary catheters are rarely used beyond 90 days because of the risk for infection.[16]	• Energy and motivation for self-care
• Surgical placement of a synthetic AV graft when AV fistula is contraindicated because of vascular disease (diabetes or peripheral vascular disease).	• Ability to learn and follow instructions
• The patient and the machine must be anticoagulated because of turbulent blood flow and the possible formation of clots.	
When is it performed?	**When is it performed?**
• Hemodialysis may be performed daily when the patient has acute renal failure.	• CAPD involves four gravity flow exchanges performed daily, seven days a week!
• It is usually prescribed two to three times weekly for chronic renal failure.	• The dialysate (2000–2500 mL of warmed hypertonic glucose solution) is instilled and left in the abdomen for a length of time (dwell time), usually 4–6 hours.[22]
• Hemodialysis is more appropriate for hemodynamically stable patients who can tolerate the more aggressive fluid shift over 3–4 hours[22] with approximately 300 mL of blood in the filter at a given time.[16]	• Fluid and toxins are drained off when the dialysate is drained.
• CRRT is indicated when the patient has a fragile cardiovascular status and cannot tolerate a large shift in intravascular volume. Because this form of dialysis pulls fluid over a 24-hour period (continuously) with only about 80 mL of blood is in the filter at any time, there is a much smaller (and gentler) shift of vascular fluid with less incidence of hypotension.	• The patient goes to bed after the last exchange of the day and drains upon arising from sleep.
• Ultrafiltration (which follows the same principle as hemodialysis, except that the semipermeable membrane is only permeable to water) is used alone or in conjunction with hemodialysis or peritoneal dialysis when more water needs to be pulled off.	• CCPD is usually performed at night. The patient connects the peritoneal dialysis catheter to a cycler at night, and the machine warms and exchanges the dialysate all night (in and out) while the patient sleeps.
	• CCPD is discontinued each morning, so the patient has more freedom.
What are disadvantages of hemodialysis?	**What are disadvantages of peritoneal dialysis?**
• Planning vacations around dialysis centers (many of which cannot take extra patients).	• A constant sweet taste in the mouth caused by the hypertonic glucose dialysate.[16]
• Body image change (big distended AV fistula or graft visible on the arm).	• Frequent exchanges with CAPD interrupt activities of daily living.

(*Continued*)

Table 8-7   Comparison of hemodialysis and peritoneal dialysis (*Continued*)

Hemodialysis	Peritoneal dialysis
What are complications of hemodialysis? • Hypotension (most common) • Hemorrhage at the site after hemodialysis induced by anticoagulation • Infection at the venous access site • Allergy to heparin requiring an alternate solution with anticlot property (sodium citrate) • Depression with suicidal ideation • Failed dialysis access: Most often it is "clotted off" (thrombosed).[23] • Change in LOC or seizures if BUN and creatinine are decreased too rapidly[11]	**What are complications of peritoneal dialysis?** • Infection (peritonitis), as evidenced by abdominal pain and cloudy effluent when dialysate is drained. • Hernia (separated abdominal wall with protrusion of internal organ), because of increased abdominal pressure from the dialysate fluid. • Altered body image and sexuality.

▶ Figure 8-7. Peritoneal dialysis.

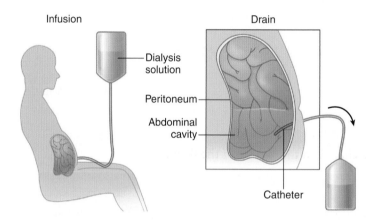

Infusion — Dialysis solution — Peritoneum — Abdominal cavity

Drain — Catheter

✚ Hemodialysis

• After insertion of a vascular access device, perform frequent neurovascular checks below the site. Look for the "5 Ps" and immediately report any pain, pallor, pulselessness, paresthesia (tingling sensation), paralysis (loss of movement), or poikilothermy (cold). And don't forget to check capillary refill!

• Monitor bruit (auscultate the "whoosh" of blood over the access device) and feel the thrill (palpate the vibrations created by turbulent blood flow) each time you assess the patient.

• Never allow anyone to use the venous access device for IVPBs or obtaining blood samples. This site is dedicated only to hemodialysis!

• Place signs above the bed to mandate protection of the vascular access arm: no blood pressures, no venipunctures, no constriction of any kind. Constriction can cause clotting within the graft or fistula, necessitating intervention to save it.

• The dialysis nurse minimizes risk for infection at the venous access site during hemodialysis by using aseptic technique and allowing the

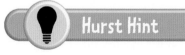

Hurst Hint

A weak or absent bruit or thrill means diminished blood flow and a probable clot in the vascular access device. Notify the nephrologist or surgeon immediately!

antiseptic solution to dry for 3 minutes before puncturing into the site.[11]

● After dialysis, the pressure dressing is left in place over the access site for 10 to 20 minutes.

✚ Peritoneal dialysis

● Warm the dialysate to promote vasodilation and bring more blood flow into the peritoneum. Warming the dialysate to bring more blood flow into the peritoneum will result in more fluid and toxins being drawn out and drained off.

● If all the dialysate fluid does not return, turn the patient from side to side and change positions to allow pockets of fluid to drain back out.

● Record amount of dialysate instilled, the dwell time, the amount of dialysate returned, and the color and clarity of the fluid.

● If cloudy effluent, abdominal pain, or fever is present, notify the doctor and obtain specimen for culture and sensitivity. Cloudy effluent and abdominal pain when fluid is instilled means infection!

PATIENT TEACHING   The patient with a prosthetic arteriovenous graft (AVG) or an arteriovenous (AV) fistula needs to know how to protect the AVG and check daily to see if it is working properly.

● Feel over the site for the vibrating sensation (called a "thrill") caused by turbulent blood flow within the graft, which indicates patency.

● Notify the health care provider or the hemodialysis nurse immediately if there is a change in the quality of the thrill.[24]

● Avoid any pressure or constriction on the access arm. Don't let anyone take a blood pressure or draw blood! And don't wear tight clothing (elastic sleeves), wear a watch, carry a purse, or sleep on the access arm, either!

● Adhere to the diet (see previous nutritional considerations), so that between treatments waste products won't build up in your blood too quickly.

● Peritoneal dialysis patients should increase fiber in the diet to offset constipation owing to decreased peristalsis. (The intestines are floating in a hypertonic dialysate solution.)

● Peritoneal dialysis patients must strictly adhere to handwashing and asepsis, and follow guidelines for accessing the abdominal catheter.

● Epogen (erythropoietin) injections (subcutaneous or IV) as prescribed increase energy and endurance because increased RBCs means better oxygenation and less fatigue.

Cutting edge

Using a novel quality of life tool, a new study finds that quality of life (with variables of health and family being most important) is reportedly improved with dialysis regardless of the modality (hemodialysis versus peritoneal dialysis) as opposed to living with chronic renal failure.[25]

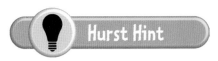

Hurst Hint

A postdialysis pressure dressing that is too tight or left in place too long can jeopardize patency of the graft or fistula.

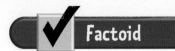

Five stages of kidney failure based on estimated glomerular filtration rate provide guidelines for monitoring and treatment,[20] depending on the severity of renal failure.

- Stage 1 = kidney damage with normal or increased GFR >90 mL/min
- Stage 2= kidney damage with mild decrease in GFR 60 to 89 mL/min
- Stage 3 = moderate decrease in GFR 30 to 59 mL/min
- Stages 4 = severe decrease in GFR 15 to 29 mL/min
- Stage 5 = renal failure <15 mL/min

It is based on existing renal damage and the estimated glomerular filtration rate. The patient's needs will vary.

The individualized treatment plan for the patient with renal failure is also based on other variables:

- Renal Failure, whether acute or chronic, and severity of renal dysfunction
- Mutually agreed upon care pathways, which may or may not include dialysis
- Coexisting cardiovascular disease (ie, hypertension and right heart failure)

The cardiovascular problems may dictate the following interventions:

- Tight control of hypertension with sodium restriction, antihypertensives, and loop diuretics as indicated. (The target blood pressure is based on the urine protein/creatinine ratio.)
- Initiation of ACE inhibitors and angiotensin receptor blockers as indicated. (These drugs are discontinued when hyperkalemia is problematic.)
- Erythropoietin-stimulating agents (ie, Epogen) initiated early in the predialysis state help delay progression of renal failure and development of right ventricular failure.
- Antilipidemics, smoking cessation, weight loss, and limiting alcohol are also indicated (see Chapter 4).

Management of fluid and electrolyte problems may mandate the use of:

- Phosphorus binding agents (eg, Renagel, Phos Lo, Os-Cal)
- Calcium supplements (usually calcium carbonate—definitely NOT calcium phosphate) and vitamin D

Other general treatment guidelines include:

- Regular measurements of renal function and other tests (hemoglobin, PTH)
- Periodic evaluation of electrolytes (potassium, calcium, and phosphorus) with frequency according to severity of renal failure
- Regular review of all medications to re-evaluate and revise renal dosages as necessary according to current laboratory data

✚ Nephrolithiasis

Kidney stones and urinary stones can obstruct and infect the urinary tract.

Let's get the normal stuff straight!

Urine manufactured in the million tiny glomeruli drain into the pelvis of the kidney, which drains into the ureter attached to that kidney. The pair of ureters drain into the bladder to be thoroughly evacuated with each voiding. The proximal and distal convoluted tubules perform their respective jobs of reabsorbing water and electrolytes as needed by the body to maintain constant stable levels as well as acid–base balance.

What is it?

Nephrolithiasis (kidney stones) are a solidification of mineral salts around organic material that can occur in the collecting duct of the urinary system to be deposited in any part of the renal network: the pelvis of the kidney (stag horn calculus) or as a single kidney or bladder stone or the urethra (Fig. 8-8). The majority of kidney stones are made of calcium; however, any other dissolved mineral can precipitate out to create a stone: cystine, ornithine, arginine, lysine, xanthine (gout patients), or uric acid (people who eat a lot of purines (meat or yeast).[22]

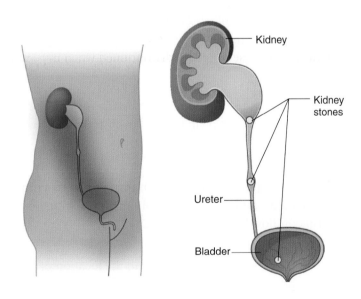

Kidney

Kidney stones

Ureter

Bladder

► Figure 8-8. Nephrolithiasis with referred pain demonstrated.

What causes it and why?

The pH of the urine contributes directly to the formation of renal calculi:

● Acid urine predisposes to formation of uric acid and cystine stones.

● Alkaline urine predisposes to formation of calcium phosphate and struvite stones.

Any condition that increases the concentration of calcium in the blood (hyperparathyroidism plus added risk factors),[27] or decreases the blood volume (dehydration) can lead to concretion of mineral salts and formation of nephrolithiasis.

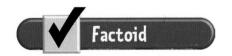

Factoid

Most kidney stones are calcium (in combination or with traces of phosphate, oxalate, or struvite).

The following patient conditions increase the risk for development of kidney stones:

- There is 50% greater incidence of nephrolithiasis in men, but when women do develop nephrolithiasis, the age is at around 30 years.[27]
- History of having had a previous kidney stone.
  - Side effects of medications (eg, diuretics, which can lead to dehydration or magnesium-containing antacids), which set the stage for concretion of mineral salts.
  - Obesity, because increased body weight may be implicated in increased urinary excretion of calcium, oxalates, and uric acid, which are the principal components of stones.[26]
  - Anatomical deformity of the urinary tract that allows elements such as calcium, phosphates, or oxalates to precipitate out and stick together, creating stones.

Testing, testing, testing

The clinical presentation (renal colic) will provide the first diagnostic clue. When the urinalysis reveals the presence of RBCs, a kidney stone is present, so the next step will be radiologic interventions to identify the size and location of the stone with various forms of X-rays and imaging (with or without contrast media) to visualize the kidneys and urinary tract:

- KUB (kidneys, ureters, bladder): Plain X-ray of abdomen while lying flat and sitting upright
- IVP (intravenous pyelogram): X-ray using injection of contrast media (radiopaque dye) showing urine flow through the upper urinary tract
- IVU (intravenous urogram): X-ray using injection of contrast media (radiopaque dye) showing urine flow through the lower urinary tract

Clinical alert

IVP or IVU requires injection of contrast media (nephrotoxic dye) and must be used cautiously when renal function is impaired (ie, obstruction of urine outflow because of a stone)!

- CT (computed tomographic) scanning reveals the structure and size of the kidney and the obstruction, and the location of the stone.
- Renal ultrasound imaging also identifies structural changes, the size of the kidney, and the presence and location of a stone.

What's wrong with my patient?

Symptoms begin when the stone starts to move through the urinary pathway, causing severe spasmodic pain called *renal colic,* which begins in the affected ureter. The excruciating pain (which radiates to the pelvic floor, groin, testicles, or labia) can trigger reflex nausea and vomiting. Other signs and symptoms are:

- Hematuria, which can be microscopic (occult) or gross (readily visible) because of trauma as the stone moves through the urinary tract

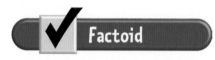

Factoid

Stones made of uric acid are not radiopaque and will not show up on the KUB.[28]

- White cells in the urine caused by the local inflammatory response secondary to trauma
- Difficulty passing urine (dysuria) when the stone reaches the bladder

What can harm my patient and why?

Any blockage of the upper or lower urinary tract can lead to postrenal failure:

- Nephrolithiasis can produce a backache (flank pain) that goes away when the stone stops moving, but the stone is still there and has lodged, so renal colic subsides, making the patient think that he or she is "okay now."
- But if the calculi is blocking urine flow out of the kidney, hydronephrosis can occur, causing the death of that kidney.
- Localized infection may occur secondary to trauma (scratching as the spines on the stone move through the urinary tract), which can become systemic (urosepsis).
- The source of infection may be an infected stone, which also can lead to a systemic infection.

Interventions and why?

The nurse assesses the patient and his or her pain (using scale of 1–10) and collects a urine specimen to be check for RBCs. Gross hematuria may also be visible when the stone is moving and "clawing" its way down the ureters.

- Establish IV access for administration of rapid onset medication and IV fluids if prescribed.
- Administer analgesia: Dilaudid, Toradol, Morphine, or Demerol as prescribed.
- Administer alpha-blocker medication (eg, tamsulosin), hopefully to relax the smooth muscle of the ureter and aid in spontaneous passage of the stone.[27]
- Administer IV fluids as prescribed, based on physician assessment of the size of the stone and the probability of being spontaneously passed.

  Saving the kidney is the top priority, so the nurse will prepare the patient for diagnostic tests and imaging to locate and evaluate the stone. Pain control with potent analgesics will require continued monitoring:

- Monitor respirations: maximum doses of opiates and potent analgesics are often required to relieve the severe pain of renal colic.
- Notify the physician for unrelieved pain, recurring pain, or a drop in urine output, as this may mean that pressure in the affected kidney is increasing (because urine cannot get out).
- Notify the physician about hematuria that persists >48 hours or gross hematuria (really red stained urine).

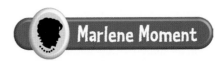

Marlene Moment

People just don't die from kidney stones! You know you've never heard anybody say, "Poor Uncle George, just 'up and died' of a kidney stone." No! That doesn't happen, but the pain is so bad the patient may think he or she is going to die. So don't delay medicating the patient who has renal colic!

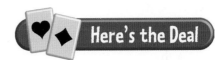

Here's the Deal

You always assess before you intervene, don't you? Pain is rated by the patient on a scale of 1 to 10, and characteristics of pain are noted. The urinalysis is also an assessment. Blood in the urine plus renal colic points directly to nephrolithiasis! Therefore IV access is a necessary first intervention before analgesia, because the IV route is commonly used when the patient is in severe pain needing immediate relief.

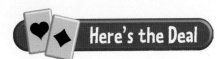

Here's the Deal

IV fluids are contraindicated if the stone is too big to be spontaneously passed because the added fluid volume increasing urine output also increases the patient's pain if it can't get out of the kidney. Even worse, urine produced by the IV fluids could back up in the obstructed kidney and cause permanent renal damage if urine can't get out! However, with administration of tamsulosin (an alpha blocker), the hydrostatic force of urine behind the stone can help to push the stone down the ureter and into the bladder (unless of course the stone is too large). This decision is the physicians' call! Either way the nurse had better be monitoring urinary output!

▶ Figure 8-9. JJ stent with nephrostomy tube placement.

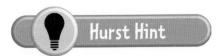

Hurst Hint

If fluid goes in, it is supposed to come out!

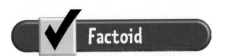

Factoid

The portal of entry for infection can be invasive procedures, tubes, or surgery as well as trauma from the stone.

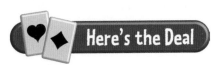

Here's the Deal

If a nephrostomy tube is inserted to drain the kidney this can also be a portal for entry of organisms, which can go directly to the kidney.

Hydration is important during the acute stage of nephrolithiasis as well as the lifetime of the patient because kidney stones tend to recur (refer to patient teaching later in this section).

- Keep fluids available at the bedside.
- Monitor hourly output if the patient is receiving IV fluids.
- Monitor and record 24-hour intake and output.

Monitor for infection because the moving stone has caused trauma to the urinary tract:

- Obtain a mid-stream urine specimen or catheter specimen for microscopic examination.
- Check the temperature every 4 hours and monitor WBC.
- Notify the doctor if the temperature spikes so that cultures can be obtained in a timely manner.
- Administer prophylactic antibiotic therapy as prescribed.

Clinical alert

If the output from a nephrostomy tube ever diminishes in quantity, the doctor must be notified immediately because the kidney can be at risk for hydronephrosis.

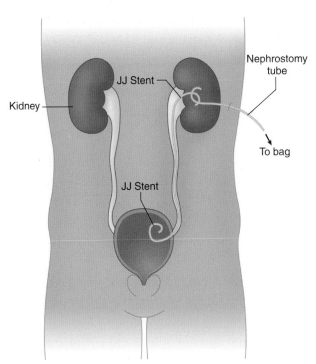

Fluid intake should always result in fluid output! When the patient returns from extracorporal lithotripsy, the nurse must:

- Monitor urinary output hourly.
- Notify the physician for any continued renal colic.

- Observe the urine for the gritty, fine, sandlike sediment that should appear in the tubing and drainage collection bag of the indwelling catheter.

PATIENT TEACHING The patient who forms a kidney stone is at high risk for development of future calculi, so the patient is taught to:

- Force fluids (lifelong) to keep the urine dilute.
- Avoid dehydration at all times: rehydrating in hot weather, replacing losses of body fluids during times of illness.
- Maintain a daily urine output of 2000 to 3000 mL/d.
- Reduce or avoid foods known to contain elements commonly implicated in the formation of stones:
  - Calcium phosphate: milk, dairy products, spinach, whole grains
  - Calcium oxalate: chocolate, nuts, berries, tofu and soy products, beer, tea
  - Uric acid: animal proteins, whole grains, legumes

Cutting edge

There are options for extracorporal lithotripsy. Based on the doctor's preference, you can chose the "spa" treatment, in which you go to the "tub" in your nylon Nike shorts (so the Foley catheter tubing can come out the leg hole) as you are submerged in warm water, or you can have lithotripsy in the nephrologist's office with a CRNA (certified nurse anesthetist) available with the Versed drip and have the shock waves over the affected kidney or ureter go through a large prewarmed bag of GU irrigant to bust up the stone that is too large to be passed!

Most stones are passed spontaneously; however, extracorporal lithotripsy or surgical intervention may be required for stones >4 to 5 mm.[27]

- Ureteroscopy is used when lithotripsy is ineffective in relieving the obstruction to break up the stone so it can be passed.
- Basket extraction (in conjunction with ureteroscopy) is used to manually remove the stone.
- Nephrostomy is the insertion of a tube directly into the affected kidney to allow urine to exit from the renal pelvis, thereby reducing hydrostatic pressure within the kidney. (This procedure may be indicated prior to lithotripsy.)[27]
- Litholapaxy is the passage of an instrument through the urethra to crush the stone into small fragments that can be flushed out by catheter irrigation.
- A ureteral stent (Fig. 8-9), JJ stent is inserted into the affected ureter to dilate the ureter and enhance spontaneous passage of the stone into the bladder.

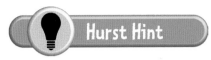

Hurst Hint

When there is nothing that the nurse can do to help the patient, the doctor must be notified at the first indication of trouble. If the JJ stent has moved, or edema closes off the ureter or the nephrostomy tube, this is a medical emergency that only the doctor is prepared to handle! Don't ever delay treatment by continuing to monitor the patient when you see urine output trending down. And don't wait till the urine output is at a critical level either! The NCLEX lady wants you to intervene EARLY rather than LATE (Fig. 8-9).

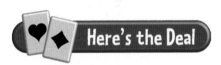

Here's the Deal

When you see sediment in the drainage bag or catheter tubing following lithotripsy, you know the treatment has been effective! This is "true grit," which gives evidence of the disintegrated stone!

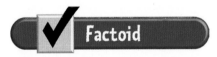

Factoid

If urine pH is alkaline, the patient needs an acid/ash diet.

PRACTICE QUESTIONS

1. A male patient who has been treated for recurrent urinary tract infections now complains of back pain. Which of the following nursing actions is most appropriate?

   A. Advise him to drink cranberry juice.

   B. Check for costovertebral tenderness.

   C. Obtain a midstream urine specimen.

   D. Inquire about any recent back strain or injury.

2. Which patient teaching is priority when a fluoroquinolone prescription is given on discharge?

   A. Take the medication with meals.

   B. Stay well hydrated before and during therapy.

   C. Do not be alarmed when your urine changes color.

   D. Notify your doctor immediately if visual changes occur.

3. A patient who has been in acute pre-renal failure has received aggressive treatment to restore circulating volume and adequate blood pressure, but the urine output is still only 25 to 35 mL/h. When evaluating this patient situation, the nurse correctly understands the following:

   A. Intracellular dehydration is causing the kidneys to reabsorb water.

   B. Once tubular necrosis occurs, better cardiac output does not improve urine output.

   C. Pre-renal failure has progressed to post-renal failure requiring further treatment.

   D. It takes a minimum of three days before the kidneys will be able to excrete water.

4. Given the following data in report, the nurse should immediately check on which patient (first) and then call the doctor?

   A. The burn patient who has developed dark and smoky, almost black urine.

   B. The myocardial infarction patient who required sublingual nitroglycerin for chest pain.

   C. The postpartal woman who saturated a V-pad with lochia rubra in one hour.

   D. The postoperative thyroidectomy patient whose systolic blood pressure is 100 mm Hg.

5. Which of the following is the most positive indicator of acute renal failure?

    A. The blood pressure is stable at 92/58.

    B. The serum BUN and creatinine are stable.

    C. The serum potassium is 5.8, down from 6.2.

    D. The urine specific gravity is fixed after a fluid bolus.

6. When teaching a patient with diabetic nephropathy to perform self-CAPD (continuous ambulatory peritoneal dialysis), which of the following concepts is priority?

    A. Medical asepsis

    B. Catheter site care

    C. Dietary compliance

    D. Activity restrictions

7. Which of the following complaints by a continuous cycle peritoneal dialysis (CCPD) patient would be of greatest concern to the home health nurse?

    A. Abdominal pain

    B. Low-grade fever

    C. Obstinate constipation

    D. Cloudy dialysate return

8. Which of the following is the priority nursing assessment when the patient has a diagnosis of nephrolithiasis (renal calculi) high in the left ureter?

    A. Monitor for presence of pain.

    B. Measure I&O, straining all urine.

    C. Observe urine and dipstick test for hematuria.

    D. Monitor temperature and check for CVA tenderness.

9. A patient returns to the med-surg unit after having extracorporeal lithotripsy. Which of the following is the best indicator that the treatment has been effective?

    A. The patient is totally relieved of the pain (renal colic).

    B. The urine is straw colored and free of RBCs per dipstick test.

    C. The urinary output (per Foley catheter) has doubled since return to the unit.

    D. There is sediment in the Foley catheter tubing and in the bedside drainage bag.

10. Your patient usually loses 5 to 6 lb after each hemodialysis, but today near the end of dialysis, only 4 lb is lost and the blood pressure is still somewhat elevated. Even though the dialysis procedure and time on the machine was the same, the serum sodium is 133 mEq/L. Which of the following additional interventions should the nurse expect the nephrologist to prescribe?

A. Ultrafiltration to follow hemodialysis

B. CRRT (continuous renal replacement therapy)

C. A repeat of hemodialysis until blood pressure and weight are normal

D. Peritoneal dialysis (one exchange) before the next scheduled hemodialysis

References

1. Smeltzer SC, Bare BG, Hinkle JL, Cheever KH. *Brunner & Suddarth's Textbook of Medical-Surgical Nursing.* 11th ed. Philadelphia: Lippincott Williams & Wilkins; 2008.

2. Nicolle LE, Bradley S, Colgan R, et al. Infectious Diseases Society of America guidelines for the diagnosis and treatment of asymptomatic bacteriuria in adults. *Clin Infect Dis 40*(5):643–654, 2005.

3. Lobel B, Rodriguez A. Chronic prostatitis: What we know, what we do not know, and what we should do. *World J Urol 21*(2):57–63, 2003.

4. Rahn DD. Urinary tract infections: Contemporary management. *Urol Nurs 28*(5):333–341, 2008.

5. Little P, Turner S, Rumsby K, et al. Dipsticks and diagnostic algorithms in urinary tract infection: Development and validation, randomized trial, economic analysis, observational cohort and qualitative study. *Health Technol Assess 13*(2):iii–iv, ix–xi, 1–73, 2009.

6. Katchman EA, Milo G, Paul M, et al. Three-day vs. longer duration of antibiotic treatment for cystitis in women: Systematic review and meta-analysis. *Am J Med 118*(11):1196–1207, 2005.

7. George-Gay B, Chernecky CC. *Clinical Medical Surgical Nursing: A Decision Making Reference.* Philadelphia: Saunders; 2002.

8. Ciavarella DJ, Ritter J. Strategies to prevent catheter-associated urinary tract infections. *Infect Control Hosp Epidemiol 30*(4):404–405, 2009.

9. Murphy AB, Maceiko A, Taylor A, Nadler RB. Chronic prostatitis: Management strategies. *Drugs 69*(1):71–84, 2009.

10. Mark LS. Use of 5 alpha-reductase inhibitors to prevent benign prostatic hypertrophy disease. *Curr Urol Rep 7*(4):293–303, 2006.

11. Giannarini G, Tascini C, Selli C. Prulifloxacin: Clinical studies of a broad-spectrum quinolone agent. *Future Microbol 4*:13–24, 2009.

12. Hall G, Esser E. Challenges of care for the patient with acute kidney injury. *J Infus Nurs 31*(3):150–156, 2008.

13. Wu H, Center E, Tsokos G, Weiner H. Suppression of murine SLE by oral anti-CD3: Inducible CD4+CD25-Lap+ regulatory T cells control the expansion of IL-17+ follicular helper T cells. *Lupus 18*(7): 586–596, 2009.

14. Pagana KD, Pagana TJ. *Mosby's Diagnostic and Laboratory Test Reference*. 6th ed. St. Louis: Mosby; 2003.

15. Kim AH, Markiewicz MA, Shaw AS. New roles revealed for T cells and DCs in glomerulonephritis. *J Clin Invest 119*(5):1074–1076, 2009.

16. Kassiri Z, Oudit GY, Kandalam V, et al. Loss of TIMP3 enhances interstitial nephritis and fibrosis. *J Am Soc Nephrol* [Epub ahead of print]. Available at http://www.ncbi.nlm.nih.gov/pubmed/19406980?ordinalpos=14&itool=EntrezSystem2.PEntrez.Pubmed.Pubmed_ResultsPanel.Pubmed_DefaultReportPanel.Pubmed_RVDocSum. Accessed May 12, 2009.

17. Hurst M. *Hurst Review's NCLEX-RN Live Review*. Brookhaven, MS: Hurst Review Services; 2009.

18. Hsu CY, Chertow GM, McCulloch CE, et al. Nonrecovery of kidney function and death after acute on chronic renal failure. *Clin J Am Soc Nephrol* [EPub ahead of print]. Available at http://www.ncbi.nlm.nih.gov/pubmed/19406959?ordinalpos=4&itool=EntrezSystem2.PEntrez.Pubmed.Pubmed_ResultsPanel.Pubmed_DefaultReportPanel.Pubmed_RVDocSum. Accessed May 04, 2009.

19. Castner D. Patient education: Kidney dialysis. *Nursing 2007 39*(9):45, 2007.

20. National Kidney Foundation. KDOQI Clinical practice guidelines for chronic kidney disease guidelines: Part 4. Definition and classification of stages of chronic kidney disease. Available at http://www.kidney.org/professionals/kdoqi/guidelines_ckd/p4_class_g1.htm. Accessed May 26, 2009.

21. Moore E. Challenges of nutrition intervention for malnourished dialysis patients. *Art Sci Infusion Nurs 31*(6):361–366, 2008.

22. Steggall JM, Omara M. Urinary tract stones: Types, nursing care and treatment options. *Br J Nurs* (Continence Supplement) *17*(9): S20–S23, 2008.

23. Berger AD, Wu W, Eisner BH, et al. Patients with primary hyperparathyroidism—why do some form stones? *J Urol 181*(5):2141–2145, 2009.

24. Castner D, Ball LK. Action stat: Failed dialysis access. *Nursing2007 37*(8):72, 2007.

25. Abdel-Kader K, Myaskovsky L, Karpov I, et al. Individual quality of life in chronic kidney disease: Influence of age and dialysis modality. *Clin J Am Soc Nephrol 4*(4):711–718, 2009.

27. Taylor EN, Stampfer JJ, Curhan GC. Obesity, weight gain and the risk of kidney stones. *JAMA 293*(4):455–462, 2005.

CHAPTER

9 Gastrointestinal Disorders

OBJECTIVES

In this chapter you will review:

- The pathophysiology associated with common gastrointestinal disorders.
- The key concepts and priorities associated with nursing care of the patient with gastrointestinal dysfunction.
- Nursing intervention to improve the quality of life when gastric, hepatic, or pancreatic function is threatened or compromised.
- The effects of hepatic and pancreatic dysfunction related to priority needs of circulating volume, nutrition, physical safety, and comfort.
- Treatment modalities to promote restoration of optimal gastrointestinal function.
- Components of a teaching plan to enhance self-care and monitoring when the patient is recovering from or living with an acute or chronic dysfunction of the GI tract.

**Let's Get The Normal Stuff
Straight First!**

▶ Figure 9-1. Anatomy of the Gastrointestinal System. (Reproduced from Saladin K. *Anatomy and Physiology: The Unity of Form and Function.* New York: McGraw-Hill Higher Education; 2007.)

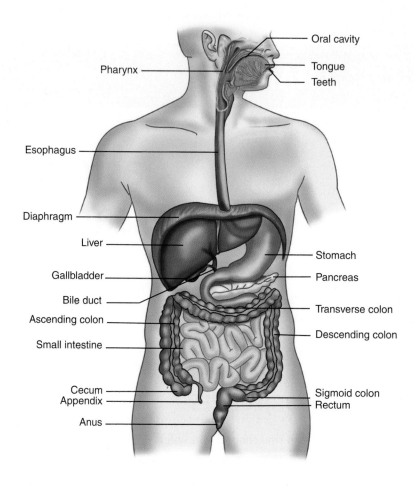

The GI system consists of a muscular tube that extends from the mouth to the anus (Fig. 9-1). The primary organs of the GI system include the:

- Oral cavity (mouth)
- Throat (pharynx)
- Esophagus
- Stomach
- Small intestine
- Large intestine
- Rectum
- Anus

   The accessory organs of digestion include the:

- Liver
- Gallbladder
- Pancreas

Specifically, the GI system:

- Aids ingestion, mastication, and salivation of food in the oral cavity
- Transports and digests food material from the oral cavity through the esophagus into the stomach and small intestine
- Absorbs nutrients in the small intestine that are transported by the bloodstream to the liver for metabolism
- Reabsorbs water from digested food and eliminates indigestible material (chyme) in the large intestine
- Stores chyme in the rectum for defecation through the anal canal[1,2]

The accessory organs of digestion are not actual sites of digestion:

- The liver produces digestive secretions (bile).
- The gallbladder stores bile for use in the small intestine.
- The pancreas produces digestive enzymes.

✚ Gastritis

Let's get the normal stuff straight!

Segment	Organ	Functions
Upper GI system	Oral cavity (mouth)	Mechanical digestion, chewing (mastication)
		Production of saliva, which moistens food
		Start of carbohydrate breakdown
	Throat	Transport of food from oral cavity
	Esophagus	Movement of food from throat to stomach by peristalsis
		Prevention of a backflow of stomach contents
	Stomach	Reservoir for digestion by gastric secretion and mechanical movement Cardia (holding area for food in the top of stomach)
		Substances (gastric juices) produced in stomach:
		• Mucus
		• Hydrochloric acid
		• Pepsinogen
		Pyloric sphincter regulates passage of contents from stomach into small intestine.

Gastritis occurs when the protective stomach mucosa is overwhelmed by toxins or irritating substances. It can be acute (lasting a few days) or it can be chronic. This irritation can lead to mucosal bleeding, edema, and erosion.

Causes and why?

Causes	Why
Infection	*Helicobacter pylori* cause gastric lining inflammation. Immunocompromised clients may develop viral or fungal gastritis.
Irritation (medication, alcohol, food, corrosive substances)	Aspirin, corticosteroids, NSAIDs, excessive alcohol consumption, spicy foods, ingestion of corrosive substances or chemicals
Stress	Causes hypersecretion of gastric acids
Radiation	Causes gastric lining irritation
Gastrectomy	Inflammation may occur at incision site

Signs and symptoms and why?

Signs and Symptoms	Why?
Pain or discomfort	Occurs because of inflammation or necrosis of gastric mucosa
Dyspepsia (heartburn)	Caused by erosion of the stomach lining
Gnawing or burning in upper abdomen	Caused by the inflammation
Nausea and vomiting	Caused by the inflammation and erosion
Loss of appetite	Food intake may aggravate symptoms
Bloating, belching	Caused by increased acid production
Weight loss	Caused by anorexia
Bleeding	Caused by acute or prolonged irritation of the stomach lining

Testing, testing, testing

- Esophagogastroduodenoscopy (EGD) to check for inflammation of the gastric area and confirm the diagnosis; a biopsy sample determines the specific type of gastritis
  - Explain procedure and confirm that a signed consent form has been obtained.
  - Assure NPO 8 to 12 hours prior to test.
  - Record name of person responsible for driving client home after test, if outpatient.
  - Have patient remove jewelry, dentures, glasses, or contacts.
  - Have client empty bladder prior to procedure.
  - Take vital signs and start IV for sedation.
  - Instruct client that there may be a sensation of fullness or pressure because of insertion of air.

- Blood tests to check for anemia if bleeding is present
- Blood, urea breath, and stool test to check for *H. pylori*

Interventions and why?

Treatment of gastritis varies, depending on the underlying cause and the degree of symptoms. Antacids and drugs that decrease acid production may be used:

- Proton-pump inhibitors—such as omeprazole (Prilosec), lansoprazole (Prevacid), esomeprazole (Nexium), and pantoprazole (Protonix)—to inhibit gastric acid formation
- H_2-receptor blockers—such as nizatidine (Axid), ranitidine (Zantac), and famotidine (Pepcid)—to inhibit gastric acid secretion
- Antacids—such as aluminum magnesium combinations (Mylanta, Maalox)—to neutralize existing gastric acid
- Mucosal barrier fortifiers—such as sucralfate (Carafate) to protect the mucosal barrier

    Infection with *H. pylori* requires a two-week course with three drugs. The most common combinations are bismuth subsalicylate (Pepto-Bismol) or a proton-pump inhibitor and metronidazole (Flagyl) and tetracycline (Achromycin) or clarithromycin (Biaxin) and amoxicillin (Amoxil).

PATIENT TEACHING

- Avoid aspirin and NSAIDs.
- Avoid foods that aggravate: spicy, hot foods; fatty foods; caffeine.
- Eliminate or decrease alcohol consumption and tobacco use.
- Eat small, frequent meals; avoid eating within four hours of bedtime.
- Lose weight (for overweight or obese clients).
- Participate in a regular exercise program such as walking daily.
- Avoid tight waistbands or belts.
- If conservative measures are unsuccessful or major bleeding occurs, surgery may be needed.

What can harm my patient and why?

Complications	Why?
Myocardial infarction	Chest pain can be mistaken for upper gastric pain, causing delay of treatment.
Ulcers, stomach cancer, perforation of stomach wall	Chronic irritation and inflammation can lead to serious damage to the stomach lining.
Resistant *Helicobacter pylori*	Failure to complete antibiotic regimen can cause resistant strains to develop.

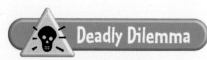

Life-threatening hemorrhage can occur as a result of gastritis. Carefully monitor vital signs and report new or increased hematemesis or melena. Hemorrhage can lead to intravascular volume depletion and shock!

Cutting edge

Be aware that clients undergoing major surgeries, suffering from severe burns, or being cared for in an intensive care setting are at increased risk of developing stress gastritis. Many physicians order medication to prevent complications of gastritis.

✚ Gastroenteritis

Let's get the normal stuff straight!

Lower GI system	Small intestine (longest portion of GI tract: 16–19 feet in adults) Consists of: • Duodenum • Jejunum • Ileum	Completion of digestion Absorption of nutrients Pancreatic enzymes and bile enter through Sphincter of Oddi
	Large intestine (5–6 feet long) Consists of: • Cecum • Ascending colon • Transverse colon • Descending colon • Sigmoid colon	Reabsorption of water Passage of indigestible material to rectum
	Rectum	Holds fecal material until an urge to defecate occurs
	Anus	Opening through which stool leaves the body. Anal sphincter provides closure of anus

What is it?

Gastroenteritis (better known as the stomach flu) is an inflammation of the GI tract. Although gastroenteritis can occur at any age, infants and older adults are at risk of having more severe symptoms.

Causes and why?

Causes	Why?
Pathogens • Parasitic organisms (*Entamoeba histolytica* and *Cryptosporidium* and *Giardia* species) • Bacterial organisms (*Escherichia coli, Vibrio cholerae,* and *Campylobacter, Salmonella,* and *Shigella* species) • Viral organisms (astroviruses, Norwalk virus, rotaviruses) Chemical toxins (lead, arsenic, mercury, poisonous mushroom, exotic seafood)	Direct Contact • Infected person passes organism to another person. • Unwashed or inadequately washed hands after a bowel movement. • Diaper changes (in a daycare) without cleaning between infants. • Use of dirty eating utensils (glasses, plates, silverware). Food • Undercooked or unpasteurized food does not kill microorganisms. Water • Water contaminated with infected stool of animals or people is ingested.

Source: Created by the author from Reference 5.

Signs and symptoms and why?

Signs and symptoms	Why?
Diarrhea (hallmark symptom of gastroenteritis)	Infected large intestine looses the ability to retain fluids
	Diarrhea may last 24 hours or as long as 7–10 days depending on the underlying cause
Nausea and vomiting	Defense mechanisms try to rid the body of invading agent
Abdominal cramps	Occurs because of GI inflammation
Loss of appetite	Occurs because of GI inflammation
Fever and chills	Body's compensatory reaction to infection
Dehydration	Occurs because of prolonged diarrhea, elevated temperature, nausea, and vomiting
	Fluid and electrolyte imbalances require fluid replacement
Weakness, fatigue	Occurs because of fluid and electrolyte imbalances

Source: Created by the author from References 4 and 5.

Testing, testing, testing

- Onset of symptoms.
- Recent travel, especially to another country and tropical regions. Traveler's diarrhea is a common problem during visits to countries with poor sanitation.
- History of foods consumed, especially foods with mayonnaise, undercooked foods, or seafood.
- Stool culture to identify organism responsible for symptoms.
- Blood tests to evaluate cause and potential problems (if symptoms are severe or persist). If the client is dehydrated, tests may include chemistry profile to assess potassium, sodium, and other electrolyte levels.
- GI studies to determine the presence of underlying disease (if the symptoms persist).

Interventions and why?

- Replacing fluids and electrolytes is the most important treatment. Fluid intake should continue, even if vomiting occurs. The amount consumed depends on the client's age.
- Oral rehydration therapy (eg, Pedialyte, Resol) may be needed for infants, children, and older adults.
- Antibiotics may be ordered, if the infecting agent is bacterial. Often antibiotics are not used because they can cause further diarrhea and lead to antibiotic-resistant organisms.

418 MARLENE HURST ✚ Hurst Reviews: Medical-Surgical Nursing Review

- Antiparasitics may be ordered, if the infecting agent is parasitic.
- Antidiarrheals are not recommended because they can prolong the effects of the infection by preventing elimination of the organism.
- If severe vomiting occurs, suppositories or injectable medications may be ordered to decrease episodes of vomiting.
- If vomiting and diarrhea persist, intravenous (IV) fluids may be administered. Generally hypotonic IV fluids are ordered and may include a potassium supplement if serum potassium level is low.

PATIENT TEACHING

- Avoid carbonated, caffeinated, and high-sugar drinks, which can increase diarrhea.
- First, use clear liquids with electrolytes (Pedialyte); then use clear broths and gelatin.
- Diet should progress, as tolerated. As the symptoms begin to subside, bland foods (cream soups, crackers, toast, rice, yogurt, custards) can be introduced into the diet. Spicy foods, dairy products, vegetables, fruits, high-sugar foods, and alcohol should be avoided for the first two to three days.
- Skin irritation can occur from frequent diarrhea stools. Cleansing should include use of a washcloth with warm water. PAT THE AREA; avoid wiping. Barrier creams and ointments may prevent further irritation. Witch hazel compresses (tucks) may be indicated to relieve discomfort.

What can harm my patient and why?

Complications	Why?
Dehydration	Occurs because of persistent vomiting and diarrhea - Monitor your client for: decreased urination, dark concentrated urine, decreased blood pressure, dry skin and mucous membranes, extreme thirst, weakness, sunken cheeks or eyes, low potassium and sodium levels, and elevated BUN - Assess infants for sunken fontanels, the separations in the skull that are present at birth
Spread of infection	Lack of knowledge of transmission - Education should include: handwashing after using bathroom and when handling food, cleaning areas used to prepare raw meat and eggs with disinfectant, and avoiding raw or improperly cooked meat and eggs
Exposure to contaminant	Traveling, especially to other countries - Education should include: Drink bottled water and other beverages from original container without using a straw. - Avoid raw meat, fruit, and vegetables. If poor sanitation is present, avoid using water from tap to brush teeth or clean dishes and eating utensils; avoid ice cubes.

✚ Gastroesophageal reflux disease (GERD)

See Figure 9-2.

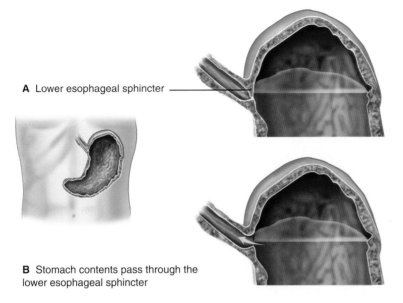

A Lower esophageal sphincter

B Stomach contents pass through the lower esophageal sphincter

◀ Figure 9-2. Gastroesophageal Reflux Disease (GERD). GERD is a condition in which the gastric contents flow backwards into the esophagus.

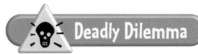

Deadly Dilemma

If dehydration becomes severe, the client will be at risk for experiencing shock and/or a life-threatening electrolyte imbalance.

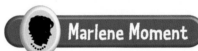

Marlene Moment

Avoid using water to replace fluids, because it does not contain electrolytes lost with diarrhea and vomiting.

What is it?

GERD is a condition in which gastric contents reflux (move backward) into the esophagus.

Causes and why?

Causes	Why?
Insufficient closure of lower esophageal sphincter (LES)	Abdominal cavity pressure is greater than thoracic cavity pressure, causing gastric contents to push through a weakened sphincter, resulting in oral and esophageal burning. Commonly occurs in pregnancy and obesity.
Gastric distention	Excessively high pressures in the abdominal cavity lead to gastric reflux into the esophagus through the normal sphincter. Causes of distention include consumption of large meals, pregnancy, obesity, or clothing that binds the abdomen.
Hiatal hernia (protrusion of part of the stomach into the esophagus)	Pressure pushes part of the stomach into the esophagus, causing reflux of stomach contents that irritates the esophageal lining.
Lifestyle	Smoking can weaken the LES and lead to reflux. Dietary factors (including high-fat diet; increased intake of caffeine, chocolate, alcohol, and spicy foods; and excessively large meals) can lead to GERD.
Medications	NSAIDs and some drugs to treat cardiovascular conditions (nitrates, calcium channel blockers) place a person at risk for developing GERD.

Source: Created by the author from References 4, 6, and 7.

Signs and symptoms and why?

Signs and symptoms	Why?
Dyspepsia (heartburn)	Acid irritation of esophageal tissue.
	Repeated exposure to high pH leads to a burning sensation in the throat that can radiate into the chest.
	Dyspepsia may intensify with bending and lying flat.
Regurgitation (may be described as bitter or sour tasting)	Warm food particles and fluid reflux because of an inability of the LES to prevent backflow.
Hypersalivation	Reflux triggers salivary glands to increase saliva production.
Nausea	Prolonged reflux can lead to nausea, especially in the morning.
Pain	Caused by acid irritation of the mucosal lining.
	Usually occurs 30 minutes after meals or when lying down at night.
Hoarseness, wheezing, throat clearing	Acid irritation and backflow of gastric contents irritate the throat.
Dysphasia (difficulty swallowing)	Scarring from long-term exposure to acid irritation can cause narrowing in esophagus.
Odynophagia (painful swallowing)	From spasms in the esophagus caused by irritation of tissue.

Source: Created by the author from References 4, 6, and 7.

Testing, testing, testing

- Esophageal pH monitoring: A pH probe is inserted nasally and positioned 5 cm above the lower esophageal sphincter. The client is monitored for 18 to 24 hours while the client eats normally and engages in usual activities. A pH drop below 4 is considered to be a reflux episode.

- Tubeless pH monitoring: During an endoscopic procedure a small device is attached to the wall of the esophagus. The client is monitored for 10 to 14 days for episodes of reflux.

- Endoscopy: This procedure accurately documents the type and extent of mucosal injury. It cannot, however, determine the nature or severity of reflux.

  - Explain procedure and confirm that a signed consent form has been obtained.

  - Assure NPO 8 to 12 hours prior to test.

  - Record name of person responsible for driving client home after test, if outpatient.

  - Have patient remove jewelry, dentures, glasses, or contacts.

  - Have client empty bladder prior to procedure.

  - Take vital signs and start IV for sedation.

  - Instruct client that there may be a sensation of fullness or pressure because of insertion of air.

  - Keep NPO until gag reflex returns.

- Biopsy: May be performed during an endoscopy procedure to confirm or eliminate the presence of Barrett's epithelium or cancer.
- Esophageal manometry: Used to measure pressure of esophageal wave motility and identify LES pressure sufficiency. It is performed by inserting a water-filled catheter through the nose and into the esophagus; pressures and peristalsis are measured as the catheter is withdrawn. Keep NPO until gag reflex returns.
- Other tests:
  - Barium swallow may be used to document the presence of a hiatal hernia.

    Keep client NPO for 6 hours prior to test. Barium preparation is in a milkshake form, which may cause nausea; serve cold to make more palatable. The client must take a laxative afterward to ensure the elimination of the barium; if the barium is not expelled, it will harden and cause a fecal impaction.
  - Acid perfusion (Bernstein) test links acid levels and heartburn symptoms.

    The test reproduces the pain of heartburn. Hydrochloric acid is instilled into the distal esophagus via NG tube; causation of pain produces a positive test. The esophagus is then rinsed and antacids are administered.

Interventions and why?

- Proton-pump inhibitors—such as omeprazole (Prilosec), lansoprazole (Prevacid), esomeprazole (Nexium), and pantoprazole (Protonix)—to inhibit gastric acid formation

  Proton-pump inhibitors are typically the most effective treatment for GERD.
- H$_2$-receptor blockers—such as nizatidine (Axid), ranitidine (Zantac), and famotidine (Pepcid)—to inhibit gastric acid secretion.
- Antacids—such as aluminum magnesium combinations (Mylanta, Maalox)—to neutralize existing gastric acid.
- Mucosal barrier fortifiers—such as sucralfate (Carafate) to protect the mucosal barrier.
- Endoscopic intervention to tighten the LES and prevent reflux.
- Surgical intervention to correct LES weakness. May be needed if client does not respond to medical management or problem is complicated by a hiatal hernia. Laparoscopic Nissen fundoplication (LNF) is the most common procedure. Some people choose to undergo surgery to prevent lifelong use of medication to treat GERD.

PATIENT TEACHING
- Lose weight if overweight or obese.
- Eat a low-fat, high-protein diet to reduce acid production.
- Limit or avoid chocolate, fatty foods, and mints to ease LES pressure.

- Eat small frequent meals (four to six a day) to help reduce abdominal pressure.
- Avoid carbonated beverages, which can increase stomach pressure.
- Avoid meals within three hours of going to bed to reduce reflux caused by larger meals.
- Avoid spicy and high-acid foods, which can irritate the esophageal lining.
- Avoid alcohol, especially late at night before bedtime.
- Increase fluid intake to help wash gastric contents out of the esophagus.
- Discontinue NSAIDs, as ordered by physician.
- Elevate the head of the bed (HOB) 6 to 12 inches or more to prevent reflux during sleep.
- Smoking cessation to improve pressure on the LES.
- Avoid constrictive clothing (tight clothes increase intra-abdominal pressure).

What can harm my patient and why?

Complications	Why?
Esophagitis	Long-term untreated GERD causes acidic burning of tissue.
Stricture	Narrowing of the esophagus caused by scar tissue can lead to swallowing difficulties.
Barrett's esophagus	Long-term untreated GERD can cause a precancerous change in the tissue of the esophagus that can lead to esophageal cancer.

+ Hiatal hernia

See Figure 9-3.

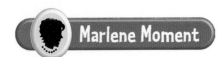

Marlene Moment

Cimetidine (Tagamet) can inhibit the elimination of other drugs, such as warfarin (Coumadin) and phenytoin (Dilantin) and is used less frequently than the other H_2-receptor blockers.

▶ Figure 9-3.Hiatal Hernia. With a hiatal hernia, part of the stomach protrudes through the esophageal hiatus, which can potentially lead to bleeding of the hernia lining.

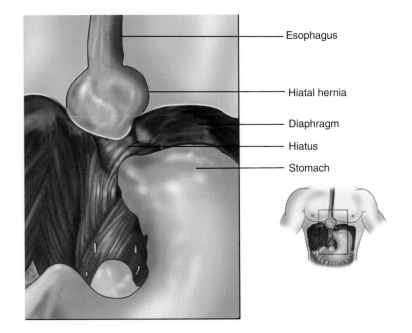

What is it?

A hiatal hernia occurs when part of the stomach protrudes through the esophageal hiatus. There are two major types of hiatal hernias:

- Sliding (Direct): The upper segment of the stomach including the esophageal-stomach junction slides through the opening in the diaphragm.
- Paraesophageal (Rolling): The upper segment of the stomach moves into the chest; the esophageal-stomach junction remains in normal position.

Causes and why

Causes	Why?
Malformation	Larger-than-normal esophageal hiatus that allows a portion of the stomach to enter the thorax.
Muscle weakness of the esophageal hiatus	Muscle weakening allows a portion of stomach to move into the thorax.
Esophageal shortening	Caused by tissue scarring from gastric acids.
Obesity	Increased pressure variations between thoracic and abdominal cavities causes stomach protrusion into diaphragm.

Source: Created by the author from References 7 and 8.

Signs and symptoms and why?

Small hiatal hernias are usually asymptomatic (without symptoms). Signs and symptoms are usually related to reflux.

Signs and symptoms	Why?
Feeling of fullness, smothering, or suffocation after meals	Occurs more with paraesophageal hiatal hernia because part of the stomach is in the thorax. Eating distends the stomach, leading to a decreased ability of the lungs to expand.
Anemia	Bleeding of the hernia lining may occur with both types of hernias.

Source: Created by the author from References 5 and 6.

Testing, testing, testing

- Barium swallow may be used to document the presence of a hiatal hernia.

  Keep the client NPO for 6 hours prior to the test. Barium preparation is in a milkshake form, which may cause nausea; serve cold to make more palatable. The client must take a laxative afterward to ensure the elimination of the barium; if the barium is not expelled, it will harden and cause a fecal impaction.

- Upper endoscopy.

Interventions and why?

Surgical repair may be needed if symptoms persist after instituting dietary and medical management:

- Surgery is more common for large paraesophageal hernias.
- The most common technique is the LNF.

PATIENT TEACHING

- Remind the client to SIT UP after eating to keep the stomach down.
- Lose weight if overweight or obese.
- Eat small frequent meals (four to six a day) to help reduce abdominal pressure.
- Avoid carbonated beverages, which can increase stomach pressure.
- Avoid meals within three hours of going to bed to reduce reflux caused by larger meals.
- Avoid spicy and high-acid foods, which can irritate the esophageal lining.
- Avoid alcohol, especially late at night before bedtime.
- Increase fluid intake to help wash gastric contents out of the esophagus.
- Discontinue NSAIDs, as ordered by your physician.
- Elevate the head of the bed 6 to 12 inches or more to prevent reflux during sleep.
- Smoking cessation to improve pressure on LES.
- Avoid constrictive clothing (tight clothes increase intra-abdominal pressure).

What can harm my patient and why?

Complications	Why?
Strangulation	The hernia can become pinched causing it to lose blood supply; immediate surgical intervention is required.
Esophagitis, esophageal ulceration	Chronic reflux (GERD) causes irritation, inflammation.

✚ Peptic ulcer disease (PUD)
What is it?

Peptic ulcer disease is an erosion of the lining of the stomach, pylorus, duodenum, or esophagus caused by exposure to hydrochloric acid, pepsin, and *H. pylori*. *Helicobacter pylori* causes damage to the mucosa of the GI tract. Ulcers are named according to the area where they occur. Duodenal ulcers are more common than gastric ulcers. PUD is more common in the elderly and Caucasians. When you hear the term PUD, usually this is referring to either a stomach or duodenal ulcer.

- Gastric ulcers (referred to the "laboring ulcer"; clients are malnourished in appearance; pain occurs one-half hour to one hour after meals; food doesn't help but vomiting does; clients tend to vomit blood (hematemesis). Frequent vomiting after meals leads to loss of weight.
- Duodenal ulcers are common in executive-type personalities (type A); clients are well nourished in appearance; pain occurs at night and two to three hours after meals. Eating relieves pain so the client with this type of ulcer eats frequently which often leads to weight gain.; It is not uncommon for blood to appear in the stool (melena). Duodenal ulcers are the most common ulcer to rupture.

Causes and why

Causes	Why?
Infection (*Helicobacter pylori* accounts for 90% of duodenal and 80% of gastric ulcers).	*Helicobacter pylori* produces substances that damage the gastric mucosa leading to irritation and inflammation.
Medications • Aspirin • Nonsteroidal anti-inflammatory drugs (NSAIDs) • Theophylline • Caffeine • Prednisone	Aspirin and NSAIDs irritate the stomach and duodenum lining, exposing it to acid and digestive enzymes that can damage the epithelium and lead to ulcer formation. Theophylline and caffeine stimulate acid production, which can damage the GI tract lining and lead to ulceration.
Smoking	Decreases gastric blood flow and delays ulcer healing; nicotine causes vasoconstriction.
Stress	Increases acid production that can lead to erosions and ulcerations.

Source: Created by the author from References 7, 8, and 9.

Signs and symptoms and why?

Signs and symptoms	Why?
Dyspepsia (indigestion): gnawing or burning in the left epigastric or upper abdominal area May be described as sharp, burning, gnawing Some clients say they feel hungry.	Stomach acid and digestive juices erode the stomach lining. Gastric—pain mainly in the left epigastric area. Duodenal—pain mainly in the right epigastric area.
Nausea, vomiting after eating. Belching and bloating	GI tract is inflamed (dyspeptic symptoms). Ulcers can affect pyloric sphincter, which could delay gastric emptying.

(Continued)

Signs and symptoms	Why?
Weight loss	Gastric ulcers: Chronic nausea and vomiting can cause weight loss.
Pain one to two hours after eating	Gastric ulcers: Eating promotes motility of the stomach and decreases acids and digestive enzymes on eroded areas. After eating, an increase in acids and enzymes and a swelling of tissue leading to the small intestine make food passage difficult.
Burning or cramping pain in right epigastric or upper abdominal area	Duodenal ulcers: Caused by high acid concentrations.
Pain two to four hours after meals or during the night	Duodenal ulcers: Eating buffers stomach acids for the first two hours. Pain returns when the stomach is empty.
Weight gain	Duodenal ulcers: Increased food consumption decreases burning and cramping.
Relief from food, milk, antacids	Duodenal ulcers: Food, milk, and antacids buffer acids produced in the stomach.

Source: Created by the author from References 7, 8, and 9.

Testing, testing, testing

- Urea breath test or (serum) to detect *H. pylori*. Carbon dioxide excreted in client's breath is measured before and after client drinks carbon-enriched urea solution.

- Serum IgG antibody screening (enzyme-linked immunosorbent assay; ELISA) to detect immunoglobulin response to *H. pylori*. Blood test identifies antibodies to *H. pylori*. Cannot confirm cure.

- Serial stool specimens (stool for occult blood × 3) to detect occult (hidden) blood.

- Stool HpSA to measure *H. pylori* in the stool. Can be used to confirm cure.

- Complete blood count to detect low hemoglobin level and hematocrit from bleeding.

- String test to obtain organisms for culture. A string is swallowed and recovered; test is less expensive than endoscopy.

- Upper GI endoscopy with tissue biopsy and cytology for microscopic examination. PyloriTek is a biopsy urea test used to detect *H. pylori* per upper GI.

- Upper GI (barium swallow) to visualize changes in GI tract structure and function (peptic ulcers).

  Keep client NPO for six hours prior to the test. Barium preparation is in a milkshake form, which may cause nausea; serve cold to make it more palatable. The client must take a laxative afterward to ensure the elimination of the barium; if the barium is not expelled, it will harden and cause a fecal impaction.

- Esophagogastroduodenoscopy (EGD) to confirm presence of ulcers. Flexible tube (endoscopy) is inserted through the mouth and into the stomach and duodenum. A tissue sample is taken to test for *H. pylori* and gastric cancer.

- Gastric secretory studies (gastric acid secretion test and serum gastric level test); this will be elevated in some syndromes such as Zollinger-Ellison syndrome (a condition associated with high levels of gastric acid).

Interventions and why?

- Proton-pump inhibitors—such as omeprazole (Prilosec), lansoprazole (Prevacid), esomeprazole (Nexium), and pantoprazole (Protonix)—to inhibit gastric acid formation
- H_2-receptor blockers—such as nizatidine (Axid), ranitidine (Zantac), and famotidine (Pepcid)—to inhibit gastric acid secretion
- Antacids—such as aluminum magnesium combinations (Mylanta, Maalox)—to neutralize existing gastric acid
- Mucosal barrier fortifiers—such as sucralfate (Carafate)—to protect the mucosal barrier

PATIENT TEACHING

- Eat a bland diet with no spicy or high-acid foods that could cause irritation.
- Avoid irritants such as caffeine, tea, cola, alcohol, and smoking because these substances irritate the lining of the stomach or cause increased release of gastric acid. Coffee stimulates gastrin release and irritates the stomach.
- Meditation to relieve stress.
- Herbs and vitamins to increase healing.
- Avoid bedtime snacks because they increase gastric secretions.
- Avoid NSAIDs and salicylates (eg, aspirin). Misoprostol (Cytotec) may be given to reduce the incidence of NSAID-induced ulcers.
- Decrease GI bleeding if applicable (may require surgery to do so).

What can harm my patient and why?

Complications	Why?
Bleeding (hemorrhage) May be controlled by cauterization (endoscopy), H_2-receptor blockers or proton pump inhibitors, saline lavage, NPO to rest the gut, or surgery	Gastric secretions can cause ulcers to bleed.
Perforation Requires IV fluid and electrolyte replacement, NG suctioning, and surgery	Severe ulcers can advance through the gastric mucosa.
Penetration May be treated with drugs or surgery	Ulcer penetrates the stomach or duodenum and continues into adjacent organs.
Obstruction NG suctioning and ulcer treatment regimen	Edema (swelling) or scarring of tissue around an ulcer can decrease the passageway and cause a feeling of fullness, vomiting, regurgitation, and a loss of appetite.

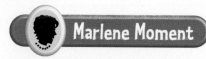

Barium studies should not be used if a perforation (tear in the lining) is suspected. Generally, abdominal X-rays are performed to check for free air (a sign of perforation) before these studies.

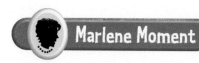

Calcium carbonate (Tums) causes rebound acid secretion by triggering gastrin release and thus is not recommended for ulcer disease.

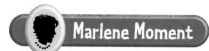

Flavored antacids should be avoided because the flavoring increases the emptying time of the stomach.

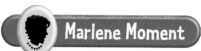

Infection with *Helicobacter pylori* requires a two-week course with three drugs. The most common combinations are bismuth subsalicylate (Pepto-Bismol) or a proton-pump inhibitor and metronidazole (Flagyl) and tetracycline (Achromycin) or clarithromycin (Biaxin) and amoxicillin (Amoxil).

+ Malabsorption disorders

What is it?

Malabsorption disorders are disorders in which nutrients are not digested or absorbed properly.

Causes and why?

Causes	Why?
Bile salt deficiencies	Inadequate production of enough bile salts prevents fats and fat-soluble vitamins from adequate absorption.
Lactase deficiency (can be genetic or be caused by bacterial overgrowth or viral hepatitis)	Inadequate lactase prevents lactose breakdown for use by the body.
Pancreatic enzyme deficiency (can be caused by destruction or obstruction of the pancreas)	Pancreatic enzymes are needed for proper absorption of B_{12}.
Infections (viral, bacteria, or parasitic)	Infection injures the intestinal lining and leads to decreased absorption of nutrients.
Gastric surgery	Removal of a section of the stomach (the most common cause of malabsorption) prevents adequate mixing of digestive enzymes and acids with food, decreasing digestion of nutrients.
Intestinal surgery	Intestinal surgery leads to a loss of surface area for absorption.
Lymphatic system blockage from conditions such as lymphoma (cancer of the lymph system) and Crohn's disease	Blockage of lymph flow can lead to a loss of vitamin B_{12}, folic acid, minerals, and lipids.
Decreased blood supply	Inadequate blood supply to the GI system reduces the absorption of nutrients.
Crohn's disease	The inflammation of Crohn's disease decreases bile salt absorption and leads to fat malabsorption.
Ulcerative colitis	The inflammation of ulcerative colitis decreases bile salt absorption and leads to fat malabsorption.
Celiac sprue (genetic intolerance to gluten that causes damage to the lining of the small intestines)	Damage to the lining of the small intestines leads to decreased absorption of iron, protein, vitamin B_{12}, and calcium.
Tropical sprue (a disease of unknown cause occurring in people who live in tropical areas)	Tropical sprue may be caused by an infectious agent and leads to decreased absorption of vitamin B_2, prothrombin (substance needed for normal blood clotting), folic acid, vitamin B_{12}, and iron.

Source: Created by the author from References 4 and 8.

Signs and symptoms and why?

Signs and symptoms	Why?
Weight loss	The body is unable to absorb needed nutrients.
Steatorrhea (light-colored, bulky, foul-smelling stool)	Fat is inadequately absorbed and eliminated in waste.
Diarrhea, flatulence (gas)	Inadequate absorption of nutrients.
Increased bruising	Clotting factors such as prothrombin are decreased.
Edema (swelling)	Results from decreased protein absorption.
Anemia	Results from vitamin B_{12}, folic acid, or iron deficiencies.

Source: Created by the author from References 6, 7, and 8.

Testing, testing, testing

- Decreased mean corpuscular volume (MCV), mean corpuscular hemoglobin (MCH), and mean corpuscular hemoglobin concentration (MCHC) indicate an iron deficiency. (Elevated MCV may indicate vitamin B_{12} and folic acid deficiencies.)
- Iron level—Low iron level may indicate protein malabsorption.
- Cholesterol—Low level may result from decreased fat digestion.
- Calcium—Low level may indicate decreased vitamin D absorption.
- Albumin—Low albumin level indicates protein loss.
- Vitamin A and carotene—Low levels may indicate bile salt deficiencies.
- A lactose tolerance test—Less than a 20% rise in glucose levels above fasting levels indicates lactose intolerance.
- Biopsy and microscopic examination of the lining of the small intestine to detect abnormalities that may cause malabsorption. Observe for signs of bleeding post biopsy.
- Stool sample to assess for undigested food, indicating an inability to break down and absorb nutrients.
- Ultrasonography to detect tumors that might be causing malabsorption.
- Barium enema to detect changes in the mucosal lining and determine the underlying cause of malabsorption. Keep client NPO for six hours prior to test. Barium preparation is in a milkshake form, which may cause nausea; serve cold to make more palatable. The client must take a laxative afterward to ensure the elimination of the barium; if the barium is not expelled, it will harden and cause a fecal impaction.

Interventions and why?

- Gastrectomy clients should maintain a high-protein and high-calorie diet and eat small, frequent meals.

- Clients should take nutritional supplements for their specific deficiencies.
- Clients with tropical sprue or other disorders caused by infection should take prescribed antibiotics.
- Clients with decreased gastric motility should take antidiarrheal agents.

PATIENT TEACHING

- For lactose intolerance, the client should avoid dairy products.
- For celiac disease, the client should maintain a gluten-free diet.
- For gallbladder disease and pancreatic insufficiency, the client should maintain a low-fat diet.

What can harm my patient and why?

Complications	Why?
Bleeding, bone pain, fractures, hypocalcemia, anemia, glossitis, cheilosis, muscle tenderness, peripheral neuritis, dermatitis	Fat-soluble vitamin deficiency
Hypoalbuminemia, edema, loss of muscle mass	Protein deficiency

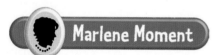

Calcium supplements should be taken to prevent a deficiency of calcium.

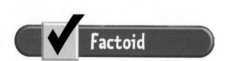

Adenomas are considered precancerous polyps. Generally, the larger the polyp, the greater the chance it is precancerous.

✚ Polyps

What is it?

Polyps are small growths along the lining of the intestinal tract. They are classified according to tissue type (adenomas, hyperplastic, or hamartomatous) and appearance (sessile or pedunculated).

Causes and why?

Causes	Why?
Familial polyposis	Polyps develop during childhood in the large intestine and rectum and can lead to colorectal cancer.
Gardner's syndrome (a rare, inherited disorder characterized by multiple growths (polyps) in the colon)	In addition to precancerous polyps, nonmalignant tumors develop on various parts of the body.
Peutz-Jeghers syndrome (characterized by the development of growths called hamartomatous polyps in the gastrointestinal tract—particularly the stomach and intestines)	In utero (before birth), polyps develop in the stomach, small intestines, large intestines, or rectum. Typically, they are noncancerous.

Source: Created by the author from References 5, 8, and 9.

Certain groups of people are more prone to polyps. Clients over age 50, those with a positive family history, those who eat a high fat/low calcium diet, smokers, and those who exercise little/none seem to have a higher frequency of polyps.

Signs and symptoms and why?

Signs and symptoms	Why?
Bleeding	Polyp becomes irritated from the passage of intestinal contents and bleeds.
Abdominal pain and cramping	Large polyps may obstruct the flow of GI contents, causing pain and cramping.
Diarrhea or any change in bowel habits	Some polyps can excrete water and salts that lead to excessive watery stools. Some clients may have constipation, increased frequency of bowel movements, or a change in appearance of stool.

Source: Created by the author from References 5, 8, and 9.

Testing, testing, testing

- Digital examination (inserting a gloved finger into the rectum and palpating) to locate a rectal polyp.
- Flexible sigmoidoscopy (examining the lower large intestine through a flexible tube) to detect a polyp

  Bowel preparation is required; sedation is not used.
- Colonoscopy (examining the entire large intestine through a flexible tube) to determine the number of polyps and allow biopsy of one or more

  This is considered the gold standard for diagnosis of colon cancer. It requires a thorough bowel preparation and sedation. If done in an outpatient setting, clients must not drive themselves home.
- Fecal occult blood test (FOBT). Blood could be an indicator of cancer.

  Eliminate red meat, aspirin, NSAIDs, turnips, horseradish, and vitamin C from the diet for two days before and throughout sample collection.
- Barium enema may be done to visualize the polyp.

  Bowel preparation must be done. Laxatives must be administered following the procedure to ensure elimination of barium. If barium is not expelled, it will harden and cause a fecal impaction.
- A molecular marker test detects known deoxyribonucleic acid mutations associated with colorectal cancer.
- CT or virtual colonoscopy—air is pumped into the colon to distend it prior to a spiral CT scan. A bowel preparation is required prior to this test; no sedation is required.

Interventions and why?

- Removal of polyps (polypectomy) because of the risk of that they will become cancerous. It is usually done during colonoscopy. If removal is not possible with colonoscopy, abdominal surgery is performed.
- Removal of a section of the intestine because cancerous polyps may have spread to the area. If familial polyposis is present, the entire large intestine and rectum may be removed.

PATIENT TEACHING

- Increase calcium intake (studies seem to show calcium can decrease reoccurrence).
- NSAIDs/ASA (seems to decrease reoccurrence; can be very irritating to GI tract).
- Exercise, stop smoking, decrease alcohol, eat a low-fat/high-fiber diet.
- Routine colorectal screenings.

What can harm my patient and why?

Complications	Why?
Excessive rectal bleeding	Excessive polyp irritation from passage of intestinal contents
Intestinal obstruction	Large or numerous polyps may obstruct the flow of GI contents.
Colorectal cancer	Potential outcome of polyps, especially if tissue type is adenoma

✚ Hemorrhoids

What is it?

Hemorrhoids are varicose (twisted/knotted)/distended veins of the anal canal. External hemorrhoids are located below that anorectal junction; internal hemorrhoids form above this junction.

Causes and why?

Causes	Why?
Chronic constipation	Increased intra-abdominal pressure increases pressure in the veins when straining during bowel movements.
Pregnancy	Increased circulating fluid volume and increased constipation put more pressure on the veins of the anal canal.
Obesity	Can cause increased pressure in the veins of the anorectal area and lead to hemorrhoid development.
Heavy lifting, straining, standing for long periods of time	Pressure increases in the venous system with continued heavy lifting or straining.

Source: Created by the author from References 5 and 6.

Signs and symptoms and why?

Signs and symptoms	Why?
Bleeding, usually bright red	Stool passing through the rectum and anus irritates the hemorrhoids, causing them to bleed
Itching	Can occur if adequate cleaning of the anal area cannot be performed because of hemorrhoid protrusion
Pain	Results from swelling and irritation of the hemorrhoid

Source: Created by the author from References 5 and 6.

Testing, testing, testing

- Inspection and digital examination (inserting a gloved finger into the rectum and palpating) to locate hemorrhoids. No bowel preparation is necessary.
- Anoscopy and flexible sigmoidoscopy (examining structures of the rectum and sigmoid colon through a flexible tube) to detect hemorrhoids. Bowel preparation is required for sigmoidoscopy.

Interventions and why?

- Sclerotherapy (injection of material to remove hemorrhoids) to treat bleeding hemorrhoids.
- Band ligation (tying off hemorrhoids with rubber bands) if sclerotherapy is not successful or the hemorrhoids are internal.
- Cryosurgery and photocoagulation (exposure of hemorrhoid tissue to liquid nitrogen), radiation, or another agent. The treated tissue necroses and sloughs off. Fecal discharge is foul smelling for several days.
- Surgery (hemorrhoidectomy) for hemorrhoids that do not respond to less invasive treatments.
- Sitz bath to relieve symptoms. (Sitz bath is a device that looks like a small basin and is placed between the lids of the toilet. Warm water runs from a bag through a small tube into the basin. The warm water gently sprays and soaks the hemorrhoids.) Some clients prefer to sit in a warm bathtub.
- Nonprescription creams and ointments such as Dibucaine to reduce swelling and pain associated with hemorrhoids.
- Compress pads of witch-hazel (Tucks™) to control symptoms.

PATIENT TEACHING

- Clean anal area by blotting not wiping with a moistened wipe. (Sometimes baby wipes are used to reduce abrasion caused by toilet paper.)
- Increase dietary fiber and fluids to manage constipation (client needs to decrease straining with bowel movements).

- Use stool softeners to manage constipation.
- Establish a regular time for defecation; do not ignore the urge to defecate.
- Avoid nuts, coffee, and spicy foods that can further irritate hemorrhoids. Use stool softeners, such as docusate, to help prevent straining during defecation.
- Avoid long periods of sitting, which can put more pressure on already irritated hemorrhoids.

What can harm my patient and why?

Complications	Why?
Bleeding with bowel movements	Irritation of hemorrhoids caused by fecal passage
Disruption of daily activities	Pain and swelling inhibit activities
Exacerbation of symptoms	Straining with constipation

✚ Dumping syndrome

What is it?

Early dumping syndrome is the rapid movement of food from the stomach into the jejunum after a meal. Late dumping syndrome is the release of an increased amount of insulin causing hypoglycemia. The term refers to vasomotor and GI symptoms that occur in 50% of patients after gastric resection and vagotomy surgery.

Causes and Why?

Causes	Why?
Gastric surgery • Gastrectomy (removal of some or all of the stomach) • Gastric bypass surgery (creation of a smaller stomach pouch to decrease intake of food in obese clients) • Gastroenterostomy, gastrojejunostomy (direct connection of stomach to small intestines, bypassing the pylorus) • Fundoplication (surgery to reduce reflux of gastric contents into the esophagus) • Vagotomy (cutting of nerves to stomach to decrease acid production)	These surgeries alter mucosal function and decrease acid, enzyme, and hormone secretions, leading to accelerated gastric emptying. Also, the stomach is structurally altered with surgery and may not have the capacity it once did.
Zollinger-Ellison syndrome (rare disorder involving peptic ulcer disease and gastrin-secreting tumors in the pancreas)	Can lead to damage of the pylorus and changes in the production and release of enzymes, resulting in dumping syndrome.

Source: Created by the author from References 7 and 8.

Signs and symptoms and why?

Signs and Symptoms	Why?
Systemic • Sweating (diaphoresis) • Extreme fatigue and strong desire to lie down • Palpitations • Lightheadedness and syncope • Flushing	Early dumping syndrome: Systemic signs and symptoms occur because rapid gastric emptying causes fluid shifts from the intravascular area into the intestinal lumen.
Abdominal • Nausea and vomiting • Abdominal cramping • Bloating and fullness • Diarrhea • Stomach growling (borborygmi)	Early dumping syndrome: Abdominal signs and symptoms occur because of distension of the small intestine and increased contractility.
Systemic • Tremors • Inability to concentrate • Sweating (diaphoresis) • Decreased level of consciousness • Hunger • Hypotension (low blood pressure) • Increased heart rate	Late dumping syndrome: Systemic signs and symptoms occur because of a low glucose level brought on by a pronounced release of insulin.

Source: Created by the author from References 7 and 8.

Testing, testing, testing

Use the client history to identify past surgeries that could be causing the dumping and to determine the onset and duration of symptoms. If the client has a history of gastric surgery (which they usually do), no further tests are needed because the cause is already known.

Interventions and why?

• Anticholinergic drugs (dry up secretions in stomach; gastric contents will become less moist and therefore empty more slowly out of stomach)

• Antisecretory agents to delay gastric emptying and inhibit insulin and hormone release

• Surgery to repair or reconstruct the underlying problem

PATIENT TEACHING

• Eat six small, frequent meals daily.

• Restrict fluid intake during and at least one half hour after meals (fluids should be taken in between meals).

• Decrease carbohydrate intake and increase fat and protein intake (carbs tend to move through the GI tract fast).

- Lie flat (preferably on left side to keep food in stomach longer) after meals to delay gastric emptying and increase venous return.
- Use dietary fiber supplements to delay glucose absorption.

What can harm my patient and why?

Complications	Why?
Malnutrition and weight loss	Accelerated gastric emptying
Anxiety and fear of food (sitophobia)	Fear of embarrassment; desire to control diarrhea
Social isolation	Fear of embarrassment

✚ Hernia

See Figure 9-4.

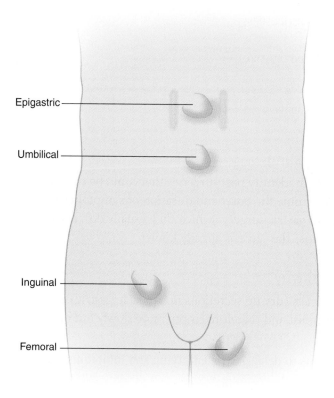

► Figure 9-4. Hernia. A hernia is an abnormal protrusion of a bowel loop through the muscular wall of the abdomen.

What is it?

Hernias are an abnormal protrusion of a loop of bowel through the thin muscular wall of the abdomen. Hernias can be classified as:

- Reducible hernias. Can be placed back into the abdominal cavity with gently pressure

- Irreducible (incarcerated) hernias. Cannot be placed back into the abdominal cavity
- Strangulated hernia. Blood supply cut off by pressure from the muscle around the hernia

Four types of hernias

Hernia type	Description
Inguinal	• Protrusion of the spermatic cord (male) or round ligament (female) through the inguinal canal of the abdominal wall • Can be direct (passes through weakness in the wall) or indirect (pushes into the inguinal canal) • Most common type of hernia
Femoral	• Occurs in the upper part of thigh region, below the groin • More common in females • Femoral canal (area where the femoral artery, vein, and nerve leave the abdominal cavity) enlarges and allows a portion of the intestines to enter
Umbilical	• Orifice of the umbilicus does not close, allowing protrusion • Most common in infants • Usually closes by age two • Can recur later in life because of weakness of the wall at this site
Incisional (ventral)	• Weakness in the abdominal wall, secondary to abdominal surgery

Source: Created by the author from the References 5, 8, and 9.

Causes and Why?

Causes	Why?
Congenital	Weakness or incomplete closure of abdominal wall at birth.
Increased abdominal pressure	May lead to bulging of contents into the weaker areas of the abdomen. Conditions that increase this risk are obesity, straining, heavy lifting, prolonged coughing, chronic lung problems, fluid accumulation in the abdomen, and pregnancy.
Abdominal surgery	Abdominal surgery leads to weakness in the affected portion of the abdominal wall, which can lead to hernia formation.

Source: Created by the author from References 5, 8, and 9.

Signs and symptoms and why?

Signs and symptoms	Why?
Bulging in abdominal cavity	Occurs when intestine and intestinal contents protrude into weakened area of the abdominal wall. Bulging is worse when standing or lifting, but usually is reduced when lying down.
Pain	May precede discovery of bulge. Pain caused by pressure created by protrusion.

Source: Created by the author from References 5, 8, and 9.

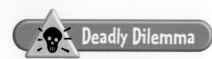

Deadly Dilemma

New onset of pain and tenderness at the bulge may signal strangulation (cutting off of blood supply to intestines) and is a surgical emergency.

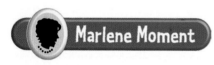

Marlene Moment

Incarcerated hernias should be reduced before applying a truss.

Testing, testing, testing

- Use the client history to determine events that may have led to hernia development (weight lifting, bronchitis with extreme coughing, or smoking history leading to chronic coughing) and to obtain a past history of hernias.
- A physical examination can help determine the location and size of the hernia and the need for immediate surgery.
- If the hernia is strangulated, a complete blood count may be ordered to determine the presence of infection and to prepare for surgical correction.
- Minimally invasive inguinal hernia repair (MIIHR) or herniorrhaphy involves placing a synthetic mesh inside the abdominal wall. A laparoscope (fiberoptic tube to view the herniation) is used, when possible.
- Hernioplasty involves placing a mesh patch on the weakened outside wall.
- Traditional surgery involves placing the contents of the hernia back into the abdomen and closing the opening.

PATIENT TEACHING

- Explain why and how to avoid increased abdominal pressure: avoid lifting heavy objects, stop smoking, prevent constipation, and use deep-breathing exercises to decrease chronic cough.
- Explain the signs and symptoms of strangulation.
- Suggest the client use a truss (elastic belt) to hold abdominal contents and prevent herniation. It should be applied before getting out of bed. Never forcibly reduce a hernia! It could cause an intestinal rupture.

What can harm my patient and why?

Complications	Why?
Bowel obstruction and necrosis	Incarceration (inability of contents to return to the abdominal cavity)
Infection, peritonitis	Gangrene (death of intestinal wall)
Intestinal rupture	Forcible reduction of a hernia

+ Intestinal obstruction

What is it?

An intestinal obstruction, which may be mechanical or nonmechanical, is a blockage of the flow of intestinal contents. If not treated, the lining swells with contents and can rupture.

A mechanical obstruction is caused by adhesions (bands of fibrous tissue that can connect intestines to intestines, organs, or the abdominal wall), twisting of the intestines, or strangulated hernias creating pressure in the abdominal cavity.

A nonmechanical obstruction (paralytic ileus) is caused by impaired peristalsis from abdominal surgery, trauma, and mesenteric ischemia. There is no physical obstruction, just decreased or absent peristalsis.

Causes and why?

Causes	Why?
Birth Defects • Volvulus (twisting of the intestines) • Intussusception (portion of the intestines slides over another area of the intestines)	Mechanical obstruction: Birth defects of the GI system can lead to an inability to move contents through the GI tract.
Obstruction of small intestine	Mechanical obstruction: Obstruction may occur from scarring of tissue as a result of ulcers and abdominal surgery. Adhesions (tissue of one area sticks to another area) can lead a collapse of a portion of the intestines.
Obstruction of large intestine	Mechanical obstruction: Obstruction can result from stool impaction, inflammatory bowel disease (IBD), or diverticulitis (from scar tissue or adhesions).
Cancer	Mechanical obstruction: The growth of malignant cells can block the intestinal tract.
Parasites	Mechanical obstruction: A large number of parasitic worms in the GI tract can form an obstruction.
Surgery	Nonmechanical obstruction: Handling of the intestines leads to temporary loss of function.
Electrolyte imbalance	Nonmechanical obstruction: Hypokalemia can increase the risk of paralytic ileus.
Peritonitis (inflammation of the abdominal wall)	Nonmechanical obstruction: Irritation from contents leaking into abdominal cavity can lead to inflammation with decreased or absent peristalsis.
Decreased blood flow to the bowel	Nonmechanical obstruction: Can lead to ischemia and decreased or absent peristalsis.

Source: Created by the author from References 6 and 9.

Signs and symptoms and why?

Signs and symptoms	Why?
Abdominal cramping and pain	GI system passageway can be partially or completely blocked. Pain may be intermittent.
Abdominal distention with peristaltic waves	Results from an inability of food, gas, or digestive enzymes to pass through the obstruction. Peristaltic wave (the abdomen visibly moves up and down). This is the intestine trying to move bowel contents past the obstruction.
Bowel changes	Obstipation (absence of stool) occurs with complete blockage because contents cannot pass. Diarrhea (ribbon-like stools) may occur with a partial obstruction because liquids can pass but solid contents cannot.

(Continued)

Signs and symptoms	Why?
Bowel sound changes	High-pitched bowel sounds proximal to the obstruction (called borborygmi) and absent bowel sounds distal to obstruction; as obstruction worsens, bowel sounds will become absent.
Vomiting and anorexia (lack of interest in eating)	Occurs because of accumulation of contents.
	The higher the obstruction is in the GI tract, the quicker vomiting occurs. The further down the GI tract the obstruction is, the more food, gas, and fluids can accumulate before the body begins to rid itself of them.
Fluid and electrolyte imbalances	Can occur because of the body's inability to absorb nutrients to maintain balance; vomiting and diarrhea.
Fever	If an obstruction leads to a rupture, infection can quickly develop in the abdominal cavity (bacterial peritonitis). Fever occurs as the body tries to fight the infection and is usually low grade.
Hiccups	Seen in all types of obstructions; may be caused by stimulation of the phrenic nerve.

Source: Created by the author from References 6 and 9.

Testing, testing, testing

- Abdominal computed tomography (CT) scan to show the location and cause of the obstruction and air in the abdomen (an indication of rupture).
- Abdominal x-ray (flat and upright X-ray) to show distention above obstruction and free air below the diaphragm, indicating perforation of the intestines.
- Complete blood count (CBC) to detect bleeding (low hemoglobin and hematocrit) and infection (elevated white blood cell count).
- Chemistry studies to assess for fluid imbalances (elevated creatinine and blood urea nitrogen levels) and electrolyte imbalances (decreased sodium, chloride, and potassium levels).
- Arterial blood gases to determine acid–base imbalance.
- Endoscopy or barium enema to determine the cause of lower bowel obstruction. Bowel preparation is required for either test. A laxative must be administered after a barium enema to ensure the elimination of the barium. If barium is not expelled, it will harden and cause a fecal impaction.

Interventions and why?

- Keep NPO.
- NG tube to suction to remove contents blocked by the obstruction.
  - Confirm proper tube placement with X-rays.
  - Ensure that the nares are cleaned; monitor for skin breakdown at tube-insertion site.
  - Ensure the tube is secured to nares, using tape or foam patch.
  - Check patency of tube at least every 4 hours (may be flushed with 30 mL of saline if GI contents are thick and plug tube).

- Monitor contents being suctioned (documenting color, consistency, and amount).
  - Assess suction equipment to ensure correct settings (Levin tubes require low intermittent suction, and Salem pump tubes are set on low continuous suction.).
- Fluid (NS, lactated Ringer's) and electrolyte replacement administered by intravenous (IV) route to replace those lost due vomiting and NG suctioning.
- Correction of acid base imbalance.
- Pain management including assessment of character, intensity, and location. Analgesics may be withheld until it is known if the client has a perforation or peritonitis.
- Antibiotic therapy if perforation has occurred.
- Antiemetic therapy to prevent further vomiting.
- Exploratory surgery to find and correct mechanical obstruction. Obstruction can be removed sometimes using barium enemas or passing an endoscope into the lower colon.
- Temporary or permanent colostomy, depending on severity and location of obstruction.

PATIENT TEACHING

- Explain the rationale for limited analgesic administration; encourage requests for nonpharmacologic comfort measures (linen changes, back rubs, repositioning, distraction).
- Encourage semi- to high Fowler's position to relieve abdominal pressure.
- Encourage frequent position changes and ambulation when able to reestablish peristalsis.

What can harm my patient and why?

Complications	Why?
Necrosis, perforation, and peritonitis	Strangulation of an intestinal segment: change in pain can be an indication. Barium enemas are not used if perforation of the intestinal wall is suspected.
Arrhythmias	Severe electrolyte, especially potassium imbalances.
Acid–base imbalances: metabolic alkalosis	If blockage is high in small intestine then the client will vomit hydrochloric acid from the stomach because the secretions cannot go forward.
Acid–base imbalances: metabolic acidosis	If the obstruction is lower in the GI tract, then the client will vomit the HCL acid first, then intestinal secretions, which are alkalotic. Because the client has lost a lot of base, this leaves the client in metabolic acidosis.
Shock or death	Bowel perforation.
Pulmonary complications	Caused by decreased lung expansion related to abdominal bloating and pressure pressing on diaphragm.

✚ Appendicitis

See Figure 9-5.

▶ Figure 9-5. Appendicitis. Appendicitis is the acute inflammation of the appendix, a nonessential digestive organ.

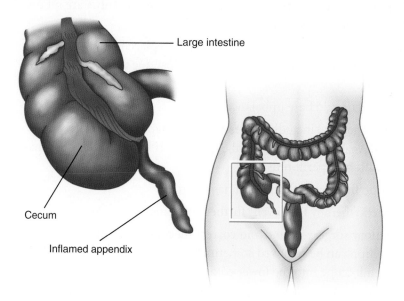

Large intestine

Cecum

Inflamed appendix

What is it?

Appendicitis is an acute inflammation of the appendix, which is not an essential organ in the digestive process. The appendix is a little sac on the intestine that can get filled with bowel contents, become inflamed and possibly rupture. Surgery for appendicitis is one of the most common abdominal surgeries.

What causes it and why?

Cause	Why?
Obstruction	When the appendix opening becomes obstructed, inflammation and infection can occur. Obstruction can be a result of fecal mass, tumor, stricture, worms, and viral infections.

Source: Created by the author from References 7 and 9.

Signs and symptoms and why?

Signs and symptoms	Why?
Pain • Usually around the umbilical area; increasingly intense, becoming more constant and severe	Pain results from swelling caused by inflammation. Rupture of appendix can lead to increased pain.

(Continued)

Signs and symptoms	Why?
• Pain will progress to the right lower quadrant, known as McBurney's point (one-third of the distance from the anterior superior iliac spine to the umbilicus), where the base of the appendix typically lies. Remember the appendix can be in different anatomical locations for different people resulting in a variation of clinical presentations (ie, rectal and low back pain for retroperitoneal appendicitis). • Rebound tenderness (pain after the abdomen is pressed and released suddenly) occurs at this location. • Pain increases with cough or sudden movement, which could be suggestive of peritoneal irritation. • Fetal position can help alleviate symptoms, which is a strong clue for appendicitis.	
Abdominal rigidity	Related to abdominal guarding or appendix perforation with peritonitis.
Nausea and vomiting	May result from pain or the inflammatory process in the GI tract. Nausea and vomiting are most likely during the onset of umbilical pain.
Increased white blood cell (WBC) count and fever	As bacteria lodge in the appendix, inflammation and infection develop. Fever may start as low grade but if it elevates above 101°F, we think peritonitis.
Loss of appetite	Caused by pain, nausea, and vomiting.

Source: Created by the author from References 7 and 9.

Testing, testing, testing

- Client history and physical examination can reveal when symptoms began and if the client has pain at McBurney's point.
- Complete blood count (CBC) to determine if the white blood cell (WBC) count is greater than 10,000/mL, which indicates an infection.
- Computed tomography (CT) scan or ultrasonography to determine if the appendix is inflamed.
- Urinalysis to rule out a urinary tract infection, which can have similar symptoms.

Interventions and why?

- NPO (nothing by mouth) order on admission to acute care facility.
- Intravenous (IV) fluids to prevent dehydration and electrolyte disturbances.
- To avoid masking changes in symptoms, pain medication is usually held until the definitive diagnosis is made.

- Immediate surgery for removal of appendix (appendectomy). Rupture can occur within 24 to 48 hours making the need for surgery immediate.
- Antibiotic therapy if appendix ruptures to prevent peritonitis.

PATIENT TEACHING

- Avoid using heat for pain management because heat will increase blood flow to the appendix and increase inflammation.
- Do not use laxatives or enemas for a client with appendicitis; this can cause perforation of the appendix.
- Elevate the HOB to keep bowel contents down in one area in case of perforation.
- Maintain NPO status.

What can harm my patient and why?

Complication	Why?
Peritonitis	Rupture of the appendix causing a leakage of pus into abdominal cavity

Worst case scenario

If rupture of the appendix occurs, mass infection can spread rapidly throughout the body. This is a medical emergency.

✚ Peritonitis

What is it?

Peritonitis is an acute inflammatory disorder of the peritoneum (lining of the abdominal cavity).

Causes and why?

Cause	Why?
Rupture (perforation) of organs This is the most common cause	Rupture of the appendix, intestines, stomach, or gallbladder allows bacteria to enter the peritoneal cavity.
Infection	Inflammation of other organs (pancreas) or other inflammatory processes (pelvic inflammatory disease) can irritate the cavity and lead to peritonitis.
	Fluid accumulation (ascites) from liver disease and complications of surgery could also lead to infection of the peritoneum.
	Peritoneal dialysis can introduce bacteria into the abdominal cavity through drains used during the procedure.
Wound	Penetrating wounds can allow foreign material to enter the abdominal cavity.

Source: Created by the author from References 7, 8, and 9.

Signs and symptoms and why?

Signs and symptoms	Why?
Pain • Generalized pain progressing to more localized pain is common. • Rebound tenderness (pain after the abdomen is pressed and released suddenly) is common and occurs as quick movement of peritoneal fluid occurs when pressure is released.	From the inflammation of the lining of the peritoneal cavity
Abdominal rigidity aggravated by movement (board-like abdomen) Abdomen distention	Caused by widespread inflammation and increased fluid in the abdominal cavity
Decreased peristalsis leading to decreased bowel sounds	Results from absence of normal movement of contents through the GI tract
Increased pulse	Occurs as fluid leaves the GI tract and moves into the peritoneal cavity (hypovolemia)
Decreased urinary output	Kidneys begin to retain fluid because of decreased fluid in the vascular system
Elevated white blood cell (WBC) count and fever (heart rate goes up as fever increases especially in the pediatric population)	Results from bacterial infection development
Nausea and vomiting	Inflammation, infection, and irritation of GI tract. Remember, the peritoneum covers the entire abdominal cavity.
Fluid and electrolyte imbalances	Dehydration caused by vomiting or leakage of GI contents into the abdominal cavity
Hiccups	Results from irritation to the diaphragm

Source: Created by the author from References 7, 8, and 9.

Testing, testing, testing

- A client history and an assessment of the abdomen can reveal the signs and symptoms of peritonitis.
- Abdominal X-rays (to identify perforated bowel or abnormal air patterns in the bowel).
- Fluid biopsy and blood samples for culture to determine the type of infection and determine best treatment option (obtain prior to initiation of antibiotic therapy).
- Complete blood count (CBC) to determine if the white blood cell (WBC) count is elevated, which indicates an infection.
- Chemistry profile to determine fluid and electrolyte imbalances.
- ABGs need to be monitored. Remember, abdominal problems can lead to pulmonary complications that can alter the ABGs.

- Peritoneal lavage to assess for bleeding and presence of infection by gram stain (RBCs and WBCs will be present in fluid).

Interventions and why?

- NPO to ensure no further leakage of contents into the peritoneal cavity (applicable only if bowel perforation is the cause).
- Fluid and electrolyte replacement (IV) to replace the fluids lost in the peritoneum.
- Antibiotic therapy to treat infection.
- NG tube insertion to decompress stomach and intestine (See Intestinal obstruction for care of a nasogastric tube.)
- Pain management with IV medications. A patient-controlled analgesia (PCA) pump may be used to administer continuous low doses of analgesics and allow the client to initiate bolus doses according to regulated settings.
- Surgical excision, repair, or resection of perforated section or organ and drainage of abscess. If peritonitis is caused by pelvic inflammatory disease or acute pancreatitis, surgery is usually withheld, and the underlying problem is treated. Wound care will be needed after surgery. Surgery doesn't "fix" peritonitis; it only eradicates the source..
- Temporary colostomy (applicable only if perforated intestine is the cause).
- Oxygen if needed depending on respiratory status.
- Semi-Fowler's position to promote drainage of peritoneal contents downward and localized in one area. Also facilitates adequate respiratory function because abdominal contents could be pressing on diaphragm, which could impede respirations.

PATIENT TEACHING

- Routine respiratory care
- Movement and ambulation when tolerated

What can harm my patient and why?

Complications	Why?
Renal failure	Decreased circulating volume because of hemorrhage resulting in decreased renal perfusion
Septicemia, leading to multi-organ failure	Delay of antibiotic therapy; inappropriate antibiotic therapy
Shock	Hypovolemia caused from fluid leaking into the abdominal cavity
Respiratory distress	Increasing pressure placed on the diaphragm from fluid leaking into the abdominal cavity

✚ Crohn's disease

What is it?

A type of chronic inflammatory bowel disease (IBD) that can affect the entire alimentary system but typically involves a portion of the small intestine (ileum). In the affected area, the intestine thickens, narrowing the lumen. Crohn's disease involves all layers of the small intestine and is characterized by regional segments of involvement. Onset is between ages 15 and 30, and the condition affects more women than men. Crohn's disease is characterized by remissions and exacerbations. It's also referred to as regional enteritis.

Causes and why?

The etiology of Crohn's disease is unknown, but it is thought to be an autoimmune response.

Causes	Why?
Smoking	Has been proposed as a risk factor in the disease development. May also facilitate exacerbations.
A familial or genetic predisposition such as immunoregulation of inflammation in the intestinal tract	The disease affects Caucasians, Jews, and upper middle class, urban populations. Family members tend to develop the disease with similar patterns and age of onset.

Source: Created by the author from References 5, 6, and 7.

Signs and symptoms and why?

Signs and symptoms	Why?
Pain • Crampy abdominal pain most often in the right lower quadrant (Ileum is the typical area of involvement) • Periumbilical pain before and after bowel movements	Pain results from inflammatory process
Weight loss and malnutrition	From lack of eating, malabsorption, and chronic inflammatory process
Chronic diarrhea	Associated with inflammatory process
Elevated temperature	From severe inflammatory process
Fluid and electrolyte imbalances	From malabsorption of food and fluid

Source: Created by the author from References 5, 6, and 7.

Testing, testing, testing

• The client history may reveal a family history of the disorder, characterized by the client's ongoing bouts of diarrhea associated with abdominal cramping.

- Upper GI barium swallow or barium enema to detect areas with cobblestone appearance. A laxative must be administered following the test to ensure the expulsion of the barium. If the barium is not expelled, it will harden and cause a fecal impaction. Barium studies should be withheld if risk of perforation is high. The increased pressure in the GI tract can increase the risk of perforation.
- Colonoscopy to diagnose the disorder if barium swallow does not. A bowel preparation is required.

Interventions and why?

- Bowel rest; NPO, NG tube.
- Dietary supplements and total parenteral nutrition during severe exacerbations. Fish oil may help maintain remission.
- Corticosteroids to decrease inflammation, pain, and diarrhea. Corticosteroids can also increase appetite.
- Immunosuppressants (other than corticosteroids) to suppress response to antigens
- Antidiarrheal to decrease diarrhea and control fluid and electrolyte loss.
- Sulfasalazine to reduce inflammation.
- Antibiotic therapy to treat abscess (accumulation of pus from infection) and fistula (abnormal passageway between organs or vessels) and to help induce remission.
- Opioid analgesics or antispasmodics to control pain and decrease diarrhea.
- Surgery if obstruction or perforation occurs.
- I&Os.
- Daily weight.

PATIENT TEACHING

- Implement a low-residue, low-fat diet when acute episode is over, that is high in calories, protein, and carbohydrates, with vitamin and mineral supplements. This should include decreasing intake of foods that can irritate GI tract (spicy foods, caffeinated beverages, and alcohol) and taking nutritional supplements to provide needed nutrients.

What can harm my patient and why?

Complications	Why?
Severe dehydration with electrolyte imbalances	Malabsorption and dehydration
Anorexia	Malabsorption
Peritonitis, sepsis	Severe inflammatory process; transfer of bacteria
Obstruction	Strictures caused from inflammation and scarring
Hemorrhage, bowel perforation	Damaged tissue because of severe inflammatory process
Fistulas	Commonly occur in acute episodes. To promote fistula healing, the client may need 3000 or more calories per day

✦ Ulcerative colitis

See Figure 9-6.

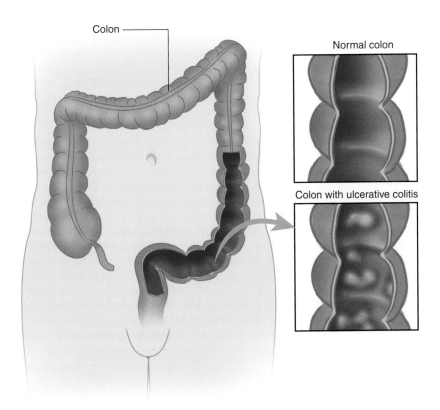

Colon

Normal colon

Colon with ulcerative colitis

◀ Figure 9-6. Ulcerative Colitis. The inflammation of ulcerative colitis leads to eroded lesions along the lining of the large intestine.

What is it?

Ulcerative colitis is a chronic inflammatory bowel disease that affects the mucosal layer of the large intestine and rectum. Inflammation leads to eroded lesions (Lieberkühn's crypts) along the lining of the large intestine. The disease most often begins in the rectum and moves toward the cecum. Onset typically occurs between ages 15 and 40.

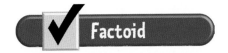
✓ **Factoid**

When only the rectum is involved, it is called ulcerative proctitis.

Causes and why?

The etiology is not fully understood.

Causes	Why?
Infection, allergy, or overactive immune response (autoimmunity)	Environmental factors such as viral or bacterial infections, dietary insults. Immunologic problems are suspected but have not been definitively identified.
Familial (genetic) predisposition	Predisposition for illness is increased among nuclear family members. A person has a 10 times greater risk of developing this disorder if he or she has a first-degree relative who has it.
	It is most common in Americans of Jewish descent, occurring four to five times more frequently within the Jewish population. While it is significantly less prevalent in other populations, the incidence is increasing in African Americans and Hispanics. Caucasian women appear to be at particular risk.

Source: Created by the author from References 6, 7, and 8.

Signs and symptoms and why?

These signs and symptoms are intermittent; flare-ups can occur gradually or quickly.

Signs and symptoms	Why?
Left-quadrant abdominal pain (may be cramping)	Multiple ulcerations, diffuse inflammation with continuous involvement of large intestine
	Pain increases with severity of illness
Fecal urgency and/or diarrhea	Ulceration of the colon and rectum
Painful straining (tenesmus)	Bowel scarring diminishes or eliminates the sensation of the urge to defecate leading to anal seepage
Frequent, painful bowel movement (up to 20 liquid bloody stools daily with pus and mucus)	
Rectal bleeding	
Increased bowel sounds	
Anorexia (lack of desire to eat)	May occur because of the pain associated with consumption of food and fear of diarrhea
Weight loss	From frequent diarrhea and anorexia
	Can lead to fluid and electrolyte imbalances as flare-ups become more frequent and severe

Source: Created by the author from References 5, 6, and 7.

Testing, testing, testing

- Sigmoidoscopy or colonoscopy to detect the presence and extent of ulcerations. Bowel preparation required prior to procedure.
- Barium enema to differentiate Crohn's disease from ulcerative colitis. Bowel preparation required prior to procedure. A laxative must be administered following the procedure to ensure the evacuation of the barium. If the barium is not expelled it will harden and cause a fecal impaction.
- Stool sample to rule out infectious agent and detect blood.
- Complete blood count (CBC) to determine if the white blood cell (WBC) count is elevated, which indicates an infection. Hemoglobin and hematocrit may be low because of bleeding.
- Chemistry profile to detect decreased sodium, chloride, and potassium levels resulting from chronic diarrhea.
- Serum albumin measurement to detect decreased level.
- Erythrocyte sedimentation rate (ESR) to detect an increase in response to inflammation.
- Rectal biopsy to differentiate ulcerative colitis from other diseases such as cancer.

Interventions and why?

- NPO or clear liquids to allow the bowel to rest.
- Bed rest.
- IV fluid replacement for hypovolemia and/or electrolyte deficiency because of severe diarrhea.
- Total parenteral nutrition (TPN) may be given to restore nitrogen balance in cases of severe diarrhea with dehydration.
- Use of sulfasalazine (sulfonamide antibiotic). It cannot be used during pregnancy; patients allergic to sulfa may be sensitive. It is the oral drug of choice for acute and maintenance therapy.
- Corticosteroids to decrease inflammation and frequency of flareups.
- Immunomodulators such as azathioprine (AZA) may be used instead of corticosteroids for immunosuppression. A 4-month continuous therapy regimen is required for optimum effects to be evident. Bone marrow suppression may occur; therapy should be discontinued if leucopenia or thrombocytopenia occur.
- Immunosuppressant to maintain remission of symptoms.
- Antidiarrheals to control frequency and consistency of stools.
- Iron supplements or blood transfusions for treatment of anemia because of excessive bleeding.
- Surgery may be indicated if other treatments are unsuccessful. Removal of large intestines and rectum will cure the disorder. This can be accomplished in three ways:
  1. Removing the colon, rectum, and anus and placing an ileostomy. A pouch system is attached to the abdomen for drainage of GI contents.
  2. Removing the colon, rectum, and anus and forming a pouch from the terminal ileum. Stool is stored in this reservoir until it is drained with a catheter. The reservoir is connected to a stoma flush with the skin with a nipple-like valve that prevents the use of an external pouch and decreases skin irritation caused by the external pouch.
  3. Removing the colon and rectum, suturing the ileum to the anal canal, creating an ileoanal reservoir, and preserving the rectal sphincter. A temporary ileostomy is performed to allow healing of the surgical site.

PATIENT TEACHING

- Dietary modifications to decrease or eliminate high-bulk foods (raw fruits and vegetables) and use a low-residue diet. Foods such as milk products, alcohol, and caffeinated beverages may further aggravate the disorder.

What can harm my patient and why?

Complications	Why?
Increased risk for colon cancer	Diffuse inflammation, multiple ulcerations
Malnutrition and anemia	Anorexia, frequent bloody diarrhea
Perforation, hemorrhage	Diffuse inflammation, multiple ulcerations
Electrolyte imbalances, hemorrhoids	Frequent bloody diarrhea
Toxic megacolon (extreme dilation of affected segment of the colon)	May occur after diagnostic tests such as Barium enema or from the use of opioid narcotics or anticholinergic drugs
Toxic colitis	Damage to the intestinal wall that leads to an absence of contractions to move contents through the GI tract
Growth retardation in children	Inadequate absorption of nutrients and vitamins because of anorexia and frequent diarrhea
Risk of infertility in women	Inadequate absorption of nutrients and vitamins because of anorexia and frequent diarrhea

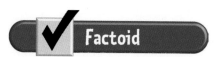

Factoid

IBS is not an inflammatory condition, and anatomic abnormalities are not present. It does not lead to inflammatory bowel disease and is not a life threatening disorder. IBS symptoms can manifest as predominantly diarrhea, predominantly constipation, or a combination of the two. It is marked by periods of remission followed by exacerbation when exposed to causative factors.

Cutting edge

Genetic tests, though not widely used, are available for use in conjunction with other tests. Perinuclear antineutrophil cytoplasmic antibodies (pANCA) are present in 60% to 80% of patients with ulcerative colitis.

✚ Irritable bowel syndrome (IBS)

What is it?

Irritable bowel syndrome (IBS) is a chronic intestinal disorder characterized by altered intestinal motility and an increase in visceral sensations.

Causes and why?

Cause	Why?
Emotions	The digestive system is controlled by the brain, and emotions, such as stress and fear, can lead to abnormal contractions of the GI tract.
Food	Certain foods (coffee, tea, raw fruits and vegetables, dairy products, and fatty foods) can trigger an abnormality of the contraction-relaxation cycle of the GI system. Eating too quickly can trigger for IBS.
Hormones	Changes in hormonal levels during menstruation can trigger IBS. IBS affects women three times more frequently than men.

Source: Created by the author from References 4 and 9.

Signs and symptoms and why?

The primary manifestation of irritable bowel syndrome can be either diarrhea, constipation, or both.

Signs and symptoms	Why?
Left lower quadrant abdominal pain	The pain of IBS generally begins after eating and is relieved with defecation. It occurs with colon spasms.
Bloating, flatulence (gas), constipation	Abnormal contraction and relaxation of the digestive tract traps gas and stool. Constipation leads to a feeling of fullness, and abdominal distention may occur.
Diarrhea (possibly with mucus in the stool and possibly alternating with constipation)	Eating triggers dumping of contents into the large intestines; diarrhea typically starts within a few minutes of eating. Mucus in the stool results from mucosal irritation. Pain and cramping may occur with onset of diarrhea and resolve after a bout of diarrhea.
Anxiety, depression	Related to fears of a loss of bowel control and an IBS episode in public. Viscous circle begins as these emotions further increase episodes of IBS.

Source: Created by the author from References 4 and 9.

Testing, testing, testing

- The client history reveals the onset of symptoms, precipitating factors, and frequency of episodes. The physical exam is typically normal, although the lower abdomen may be tender.
- Sigmoidoscopy to rule out inflammatory bowel disorders, such as Crohn's disease and ulcerative colitis. Findings for IBS are normal because it does not affect the anatomy of the digestive tract. A bowel preparation is required prior to the exam.
- Stool examination to rule out other disorders.
- Upper GI barium swallow or barium enema to rule out other disorders with similar symptoms. The onset of colon spasm during the test supports the diagnosis of IBS. A bowel preparation is required prior to the exam. A laxative must be administered following the test to ensure the excretion of the barium. If the barium is not expelled, it will harden and can cause fecal impaction.
- Lactose intolerance testing to determine if IBS are related to milk ingestion.

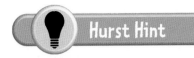
Hurst Hint

Because IBS doesn't change the appearance of the bowel mucosa, the GI testing is done to rule out other disorders. Generally, these test results are normal with IBS, though colon spasms may occur during testing.

Interventions and why?

- Treatment for IBS varies, depending on precipitating factors and the type of IBS (predominantly constipation, predominantly diarrhea, or a combination of the two).
- Antidepressants, analgesics such as Tylenol or Ultram to manage pain
- Stress management (relaxation strategies and antianxiety drugs)
- Antidiarrheals, such as loperamide (Imodium) for diarrhea-predominant IBS
- Bulk-forming laxatives, such as psyllium (Metamucil) for constipation-predominant IBS
- Anticholinergics or antispasmodics, such as dicyclomine (Bentyl), to treat cramping

PATIENT TEACHING

- Increase intake of fiber foods (30–40 g/day) and osmotic laxatives if constipation is the primary clinical manifestation.
- Increase fluids to 8 to 10 cups/day.
- Take antidiarrheals to improve stool consistency in those whose primary clinical manifestation is diarrhea.
- Avoid caffeine, alcohol, fructose, and foods that can trigger an IBS episode.
- Avoid dairy foods, if lactose intolerance is the problem.
- Consume smaller meals to help decrease episodes of IBS.

What can harm my patient and why?

Complications	Why?
Depression, social isolation, sexual dysfunction, interference with work and sleep, decreased quality of life	Fear of embarrassment from accidents, pain, discomfort, limited spontaneity
Unnecessary surgery (cholecystectomies, appendectomies, or partial colectomies)	Misdiagnoses

✚ Diverticulitis

See Figure 9-7.

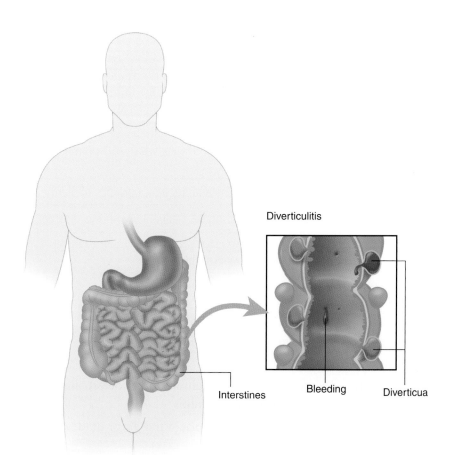

◀ Figure 9-7. Diverticulitis. Diverticulitis is characterized by blind pouches (diverticula) in the bowel mucosa that become inflamed or infected.

Diverticulitis

Interstines   Bleeding   Diverticua

What is it?

Diverticulitis is an acute inflammatory bowel disease characterized by inflammation or infection of blind pouches (diverticula) in the bowel mucosa. Diverticula are pouch-like herniations that can occur anywhere along the intestinal tract. They tend to occur at weakened areas of the intestinal wall and most commonly appear in the sigmoid colon.

Causes and why?

Cause	Why?
Low-fiber diet	A low-fiber diet often leads to constipation that increases the pressure on the colon wall and traps bacteria-rich stool in diverticula.
Decreased colon motility	Decreased colon motility slows the passage of GI contents and increases the risk of food and bacteria being trapped in diverticula.

Source: Created by the author from References 7, 8, and 9.

Signs and symptoms and why?

Signs and symptoms	Why?
Pain in the left lower abdominal quadrant that may be intermittent at first but becomes progressively steady	Occurs from irritation and inflammation of the diverticulum
Fever	From bacterial infection in the diverticula, which can even lead to abscess formation
Weakness and fatigue	From the inflammatory process and frequent episodes of diarrhea.
Elimination changes, alternating between constipation and diarrhea	An unexplained problem that occurs frequently with this disorder
Anemia	May occur with rupture of diverticula
Rectal bleeding	May occur with rupture of diverticula

Source: Created by the author from References 7, 8, and 9.

Testing, testing, testing

- CT (computed tomography) scan or ultrasound to detect abscesses or thickening of the bowel from diverticulitis
- Abdominal X-rays to detect the presence of free air or fluid, which indicates perforation
- CBC (complete blood count) to detect an increased white blood cell (WBC) count caused by inflammation and infection and to detect low hemoglobin and hematocrit that would indicate bleeding caused by perforation
- Colonoscopy to diagnose diverticulitis and determine the extent of the disease. Bowel preparation is necessary prior to the exam. Sedation may be used.
- Barium enema to detect diverticula. Bowel preparation is necessary prior to the exam. A laxative should be administered following the exam to facilitate expulsion of barium. If the barium is not expelled, it can harden and cause a fecal impaction.

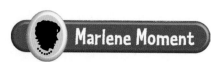

Marlene Moment

Colonoscopy and barium enema are not performed during acute inflammation because of the risk of perforation of sensitive diverticula.

Interventions and why?

- IV (intravenous) antibiotics to treat severe infections
- Oral antibiotics to treat mild diverticulitis
- Pain control, including rest and analgesics (pain medications)
- Surgery (colon resection with removal of involved area), if symptoms persist after typical treatment

PATIENT TEACHING

- Liquid diet initially.
- Progress to a soft diet in two to three days.
- Low-fiber diet and stool softeners for several weeks after acute episode.
- After healing, a high-fiber diet and increased fluid intake to prevent constipation.

- Avoid laxatives, which increase the motility of intestines and enemas, which increase pressure in the intestines.

What can harm my patient and why?

Complications	Why?
Hemorrhage	Perforation of diverticula
Bowel obstruction	Decreased colon motility
Fistula formation	Inflammatory process
Septicemia	Microperforation and mucosal damage permit spread of bacteria through blood
Absess	Bacterial infection in the diverticula, which can even lead to abscess formation
Pain	Inflammation and/or infection

✛ Cirrhosis

See Figure 9-8.

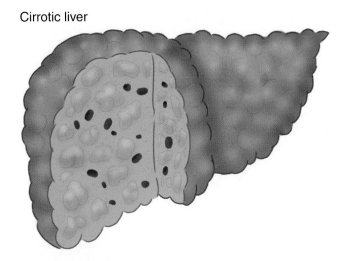

Cirrotic liver

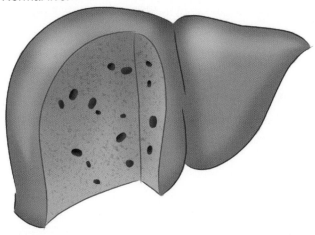

Normal liver

◄ Figure 9-8. Cirrhosis. Cirrhosis of the liver is characterized by potentially fatal scarring and fibrosis of liver tissue.

Let's get the normal stuff straight!

Accessory organ	Liver (has many important functions not related to digestion)	Production of bile (breaks down fat)
		Processing of absorbed nutrients before circulation throughout body
		Storage of some minerals and vitamins

Source: Created by the author from References 1, 2, and 3

What is it?

Cirrhosis is severe, potentially fatal scarring and fibrosis of liver tissue.

Causes and why?

Causes	Why?
Chronic alcoholism	By-products of alcohol metabolism act as a toxin, leading to inflammation. Scar tissue develops with prolonged use and the liver is unable to function properly.
Viral or autoimmune hepatitis	Immune and inflammatory responses are stimulated, leading to hepatocyte damage and eventually scarring of the liver tissues.
Inherited or genetic disorders (hemochromatosis and alpha$_1$-antitrypsin)	Hemochromatosis is an excess iron buildup in the body; iron is stored in organs such as the liver and eventually destroys the liver cells. Alpha$_1$-antitrypsin is a genetic defect that results in deficient liver protein, leading to liver cell destruction.
Bile duct obstruction	Bile builds up and leads to a rupture of the canaliculi.
Right-sided heart failure	The liver becomes engorged with venous blood as the heart's ability to pump weakens. This congestion prevents nutrient-rich blood from entering the liver, leading to hepatic cell death and fibrosis.
Drugs and toxins	Exposure of the liver to some drugs and environmental toxins can lead to hepatic cell damage.

Source: Created by the author from References 5, 6, and 9.

Signs and symptoms and why?

In the early or mild stage of cirrhosis, a person may be asymptomatic. Late-stage symptoms result from the overall deterioration of liver function.

Signs and symptoms	Why?
Jaundice	Normally, bilirubin is carried in bile to the small intestines and removed. If the liver cannot excrete bilirubin into bile or if bile flow is obstructed, bilirubin accumulates in the blood and is deposited in the skin. This leads to the yellow discoloration of the skin and sclera of jaundice (seen in sclera first).
	Skin deposits may cause itching.
	Urine becomes dark because the kidneys are excreting larger amounts of bilirubin.
Fluid in the abdomen (ascites)	One of the major functions of the liver is to synthesize albumin. If the liver is sick, then albumin cannot be made so the serum albumin level goes down. As a result, fluid leaves the vascular space and can move into the peritoneum (ascites).
Hepatomegaly (enlarged liver)	Caused by inflammation and interstitial swelling.
Nausea, anorexia, and abdominal discomfort	Any time liver is not functioning properly, toxins cannot be metabolized and accumulate. The liver will be probably be enlarged, with the capsule surrounding it stretched. This capsule is filled with nerves and causes discomfort/pain. This same capsular stretching occurs in the pancreas (ie, pancreatitis).
Malnutrition	Decreased production and release of bile impairs the absorption of fat and fat-soluble vitamins.
Spider angiomas (lesions with red centers radiating outward into branches), ecchymosis (bruising), and petechiae (pinpoint, red-purple rash)	Skin changes result from decreased absorption of vitamin K. The lack of vitamin K prevents sufficient production of clotting factors, leading to increased risk of bleeding and bruising.
Increased medication sensitivity	This is because the liver is unable to metabolize medications.
Splenomegaly (enlarged spleen)	Blood flow to the liver may become obstructed by fibrosis and scarring, leading to portal hypertension. This diverts blood flow to the spleen where it is removed from the general circulation, resulting in: • Anemia (decreased red blood cells) • Thrombocytopenia (decreased platelets) • Leukopenia (decreased white blood cells)
Esophageal varices	These result from portal hypertension, which causes back pressures through the esophagus that causes vessels to distend.
Neurologic effects • Confusion, mood changes, behavioral changes, and agitation • Hepatic encephalopathy • Asterixis (rapid back and forth movement of the wrist), sometimes called a flapping tremor	Inability of the liver to remove toxins from the blood results in accumulation, leading to deterioration of brain processes and neurologic symptoms. The major toxin that accumulates in the blood with liver problems is ammonia. Ammonia can affect neurologic status of the client in many ways.
Shortness of breath	Increased fluid in the abdomen places pressure on the thoracic cavity, leading to decreased lung expansion.

Source: Created by the author from References 5, 6, and 9.

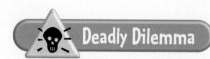

Deadly Dilemma

Esophageal varices may abruptly begin to bleed, leading to hemorrhage and death. This is a medical emergency!!!

Testing, testing, testing

- Ultrasound or computed tomography (CT) scan to show shrinkage or an abnormal appearance of liver. If radioactive isotopes are used, the scan can show level of liver function.
- Laboratory studies—bilirubin, albumin, alanine transaminase (ALT), aspartate transaminase (AST), prothrombin time, and serum ammonia—to check for elevated values, which indicate hepatic cell destruction. These are the common lab values elevated with almost any type of liver disease.
- Liver biopsy to confirm the diagnosis microscopically.
- Esophagoscopy to determine the presence of esophageal varices. Keep client NPO until gag reflex resumes.
- Paracentesis for examination of ascetic fluid for cell, protein, and bacterial count.
- Monitoring of client for hypovolemia and electrolyte imbalance.

Interventions and why?

- No known medical cure is available. The goal of treatment is to prevent the progression of the disease by treating causes and complications.
- Diuretic administration to help with excess fluid. If diuretics are non-potassium sparing, the client may need potassium supplements.
- Paracentesis for relief of ascites. Monitor the client for hypovolemia and electrolyte imbalance.
- Albumin administration to help maintain osmotic pressure.
- Pain management if indicated.
- Monitor medications that are usually metabolized in the liver.
- Elevate the head of the bed at least 30 degrees to decrease shortness of breath.
- Esophagogastric intubation (balloon placed into the esophagus and inflated to put pressure on bleeding sites) or endoscopic sclerotherapy (placing a flexible tube into the esophagus and using an agent that causes sclerosing of the bleeding area) for bleeding esophageal varices. If sclerotherapy is unsuccessful, endoscopic banding may be performed.
- Blood transfusions for significant bleeding.
- Hepatitis A vaccine (HAV) and Hepatitis B vaccine (HBV) because the client is more susceptible to hepatitis.
- Liver transplant (possible depending upon the cause).

PATIENT TEACHING

- Immediately stop alcohol consumption to slow the progression of cirrhosis.
- Take vitamins (thiamine, folate) and nutritional supplements for malnutrition to correct nutritional deficiencies.

- Decrease sodium intake (<2 g/d) to control fluid accumulation/ascites.
- Restrict fluid intake to 1000 to 1500 mL daily, if serum sodium levels are decreased.
- Use frequent rest periods or periods of bedrest to help conserve energy depleted from decreased nutritional intake, and induce diuresis.

What can harm my patient and why?

Complications	Why?
Esophageal varices	Portal hypertension causes back pressures through the esophagus that causes vessels to distend.
Coagulopathies	Inadequate liver circulation can result in anemia, thrombocytopenia, or leukopenia.
Peritonitis	Infection resulting from ascites, increased permeability of peritoneum.
Liver failure	Liver engorgement from right-sided heart failure leads to liver necrosis and fibrosis.
Liver cancer	Cellular changes related to disease process.
Hepatitis A or B	Increased susceptibility because of disease process.
Hepatic encephalopathy	Accumulation of toxins (ammonia) can affect neurologic status.
Hepatorenal syndrome	Renal vasoconstriction resulting in azotemia.

✚ Cholecystitis

Let's get the normal stuff straight!

Gallbladder	Storage and concentration of bile until its release is triggered by food entering the duodenum

What is it?

Cholecystitis is an inflammation of the gallbladder. About 90% of cases result from gallstones obstructing the cystic duct. If cholecystitis occurs without gallstones, it is usually after a major illness or injury (acalculous cholecystitis). Cholecystitis affects about 1 million new clients annually. It can be acute (sudden onset of inflammation) or chronic (long-term inflammation with repeated gallbladder attacks [attacks of pain]). Cholecystitis is more common among women and Mexican-American clients.

Causes and why?

Causes	Why?
Acute cholecystitis: edema, inflammation, and impaction of gallstones in cystic duct	Responses to obstruction of bile duct; buildup of bile in gallbladder causes irrigation and pressure.
Chronic cholecystitis: fibrotic thickening of gallbladder wall and incomplete emptying	Responses to repeated acute attacks or chronic irritation of gallstones.

Source: Created by the author from References 3, 7, and 8.

Signs and symptoms and why?

Signs and symptoms	Why?
Severe acute right upper quadrant (RUQ) and epigastric pain (4–6 hours after eating a fatty meal) radiating to shoulder and right scapula and aggravated by breathing movement Pain usually lasts >12 hours, and abdominal muscles become rigid within a few hours of the onset of pain.	Pain occurs from the obstruction of the cystic duct of the gallbladder or a spasm as the stone moves through the duct.
Nausea and vomiting	Because of severity of pain occurring during the attack.
Fever	An elevated temperature may occur in response to inflammation.
Indigestion (dyspepsia), gas (flatulence), and belching (eructation)	A lack of bile decreases the ability of the GI tract to breakdown meals that are high in fat, disrupting the normal digestion process.
Steatorrhea (fatty stools)	A lack of bile leads to decreased absorption of fats and steatorrhea.

Source: Created by the author from References 3, 6, and 8.

Testing, testing, testing

- Complete blood count (CBC) to detect an elevated white blood cell count (WBC), which indicates inflammation and infection.
- Serum amylase and lipase levels to detect an elevation, which occurs with common bile duct stone or pancreas involvement.
- AST and ALT levels to assess for liver injury as a result of bile duct obstruction.
- Ultrasound to check for gallstones in the gallbladder and thickening of the gallbladder wall (from chronic inflammation).
- X-ray to identify gallstones as calcium versus cholesterol.
- ERCP (endoscopic retrograde cholangiopancreatography) to visualize the pancreatic and bile ducts for presence of stones. Consent is necessary for the procedure. Client will be NPO for six to eight hours prior to exam. Sedation will be used. Client must remain NPO following the procedure until gag reflex returns.

Interventions and why?

- NPO (nothing by mouth) order and administration of intravenous (IV) fluids and electrolytes. NPO status allows the GI tract time to rest.
- Progression to a low-fat diet after acute symptoms subside.
- Pain control (opioids and comfort measures to reduce the intensity of pain). Morphine typically is not ordered because it can cause biliary spasms.
- Antispasmodics or anticholinergics to reduce biliary colic.
- Antibiotic therapy to prevent infection.

- Laparoscopic cholecystectomy (removal of gallbladder through tubes inserted through the abdomen).

PATIENT TEACHING

- Exercise for 30 minutes daily
- Obtain and maintain ideal body weight
- Eat a well-balanced, low-fat, low-calorie diet
- Maintain normal lipid levels, through medication administration if necessary
- Maintain normal glucose levels, through medication administration if necessary

What can harm my patient and why?

Complications	Why?
Perforation of gallbladder	Build up of bile, inflammatory process.
Gangrene	Necrosis caused by vasoconstriction, inflammatory process.
Abscess	Infection develops because of bile collection and inflammation.
Ileus	Bowel movement inhibited by the presence of one or more gallstones that have passed into the small bowel, impacting and causing an obstruction.
Pancreatitis	Obstruction of the pancreatic duct.

✦ Pancreatitis

Let's get the normal stuff straight!

Pancreas	Produces digestive enzymes and hormones
	Digestive enzymes
	• Amylase-carbohydrate digestion
	• Lipase-fat digestion
	• Trypsin-protein digestion
	Hormones
	• Glucagon
	• Insulin
	• Somatostatin

What is it?

Pancreatitis is an acute or chronic inflammation of the pancreas. Acute pancreatitis results when pancreatic enzymes are activated while still in pancreas, instead of waiting until they get to the small intestines, Because the purpose of a digestive enzyme is to digest, the pancreatic enzyme that is trapped in the pancreas begins to eat the pancreas. This leads to a cascade effect of inflamed cells releasing additional enzymes. The process of the pancreas eating itself, is called autodigestion.

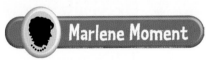

Marlene Moment

You may have learned about the "4 Fs" that signal you to be alert for clients at increased risk for cholecystitis. These are the ladies who present to the hospital with a new onset of pain. The 4 Fs (female, fertile, forty [and over], and fat) are a way to remember the most commonly diagnosed population. So remember when you are assessing a client with an acute onset of pain, if the 4 Fs apply, you may very well be dealing with cholecystitis.

Chronic pancreatitis results when progressive, recurring episodes of acute pancreatitis cause structural changes, and functional capabilities of the pancreas become damaged.

Causes and why?

Causes	Why?
Toxic metabolic processes (alcoholism, medications)	Scar tissue forms throughout the GI tract. This causes blockages in the pancreas resulting in trapped pancreatic enzymes. These trapped enzymes start eating the pancreas.
Biliary obstruction (gallstones, stenosis of sphincter of Oddi)	A gallstone can fall and block the pancreatic duct leading to autodigestion.
Trauma	Blunt trauma or penetrating wounds can damage the pancreas. Endoscopic and surgical procedures can also cause damage.
Viral infections	Some viral infections, such as mumps, can lead to an inflammation of the pancreas.
Cancer	Pancreatic cancer can lead to an inability of the pancreas to function normally, resulting in inflammation.
Unknown origin	Chronic pancreatitis can occur from unknown etiology; tropical countries have an increased incidence.

Source: Created by the author from References 7, 8, and 9.

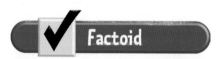
Factoid

Alcohol use accounts for 80% of chronic pancreatitis; however, do not automatically assume that someone who has pancreatitis is an alcoholic.

Signs and symptoms and why?

Remember, the GI tract is one system. When one organ gets sick, another organ in the system can be affected as well. For example, a sick pancreas can lead to a sick liver and vice versa. A sick liver can lead to a sick esophagus (esophageal varices).

Signs and symptoms	Why?
Pain	Severe left upper abdominal pain that may radiate to the back, epigastrium, or the left shoulder or back. It occurs because of the inflammatory process in the pancreas. Movement, coughing, or lying supine may intensify the pain. The abdomen may become rigid because of guarding, peritonitis, or hemorrhaging.
Nausea and persistent vomiting	GI tract is upset.
Decreased or absent bowel sounds	From decreased motility of intestines and possible ileus. Any time the GI system gets sick, it can shut down. Electrolyte imbalances can cause a paralytic ileus.
Respiratory distress Atelectasis	Atelectasis, effusion, and pneumonia can result because of escaping pancreatic enzymes from the peritoneum to the pleural cavity.

(Continued)

Signs and symptoms	Why?
Fluctuation in blood pressure (typically low)	Vasodilation frequently occurs because of chemicals that are released. Also, proteins are leaking into the peritoneal space related to tissue destruction, which leads to a circulating loss of protein in the vascular space. Volume in vascular space goes down as does the blood pressure.
Fever	Inflammatory process.
Malaise and decreased level of consciousness	Accumulation of toxins released during pancreatic digestion; decreased oxygenation; shock; if liver is involved ammonia level could go up, leading to LOC.
Steatorrhea (fatty, frothy, foul-smelling stools)	Decreased pancreatic enzymes.
Cullen's sign (bluish discoloration around naval)	Bleeding.
Turner's sign (grayish-blue discoloration of flank area)	Hemorrhaged blood settles to flank area when supine. Pancreatic enzymes are leaking.
Ascites (possibly)	Pancreatic duct can rupture causing fluid to leak into the peritoneum; pancreas is digesting itself, so fluid could leak out of the pancreas.

Source: Created by the author from References 7, 8, and 9.

Testing, testing, testing

- Serum amylase and lipase (enzymes produced in the pancreas) may be elevated. Amylase increases hours after disease onset to 2 to 3 times normal level. It may be normal in chronic pancreatitis. Lipase usually elevates rapidly and remains elevated up to two weeks; it is considered a more specific indicator of acute pancreatitis than amylase.
- AST and ALT; increased liver is involved.
- Electrolytes—imbalances related to dehydration.
- White blood cell (WBC) count elevation (leukocytosis) related to inflammation or possible infection.
- Serum albumin—decreased related to sick liver.
- Glucose levels—(may or may not be elevated) because the pancreas is unable to produce and release insulin. Remember, think of glucose problems with pancreas problems.
- Urine amylase—may be elevated.
- Bilirubin—increased with compression or obstruction of the common duct.
- Alkaline phosphatase—elevated when anything is going on in the gut.
- C-reactive protein (CRP) elevates after 48 hours—possible pancreas necrosis.
- Calcium—may be elevated in 25% of clients; however, many clients have hypocalcemia (pancreas loses calcium into the peritoneal space when it digests itself). Monitor for seizures.
- Abdominal ultrasound to identify gallstones, mass, or pseudocyst.

- Endoscopic ultrasonography can detect pancreatic changes related to chronic pancreatitis. Consent is necessary. Sedation may be used. Client must be NPO prior to procedure and must be kept NPO following procedure until gag reflex is involved.

- Abdominal X-rays may show pancreatic calcifications or gallstones. This could suggest alcohol or liver problems as the cause.

- CT (computed tomography) scan to detect structural changes and size of pancreas (may be enlarged) and calcification of ducts; will show perfusion deficits in areas of necrosis.

- ERCP (endoscopic retrograde cholangiopancreatography) to locate obstructions and ductal leaks. Can help to diagnose chronic pancreatitis. Will also differentiate inflammation and fibrosis from carcinoma. Consent must be obtained. Client must be NPO for 6 to 8 hours prior to procedure. Sedation will be used. Keep the client NPO following procedure until the gag reflex returns.

- Percutaneous fine-needle aspiration biopsy—to differentiate chronic pancreatitis from cancer of the pancreas by examining cells. Consent must be obtained. Client must be NPO four to six hours prior to procedure. Aspirin and/or other anticoagulants should be stopped 24 to 48 hours prior to procedure. Prophylactic antibiotics may be administered.

Interventions and why?

Pain management, typically includes narcotics such as meperidine (Demerol), as well as proper positioning (fetal positioning). A PCA pump may be used. Morphine is generally avoided because it can cause spasms of the sphincter of Oddi.

- Anticholinergic drugs to dry up secretions.

- Replacement of pancreatic enzymes for chronic pancreatitis. These are typically taken orally with meals.

- Antacids, H_2-receptor blockers, or proton pump inhibitors to decrease gastric acid content or prevent gastric enzyme production. Prevents stress ulcer formation, which is a common complication related to acute illnesses.

- Sodium bicarbonate to reverse metabolic acidosis.

- Insulin to treat hyperglycemia if present.

- Prevention of complications (ie, pulmonary)—cough and deep breathing to improve respiratory function.

- Vital signs, I&O, daily weight.

- Daily abdominal girth if pancreatic ascites is suspected.

- Surgical intervention to treat the underlying cause, such as surgical repair of trauma or incision and drainage of a pseudocyst (a collection of tissue and fluid that can enlarge and become infected or rupture); debridement or pancreatectomy to remove pancreatic necrotic tissue; cholecystectomy for pancreatitis related to gallstones.

- ERCP (endoscopic retrograde cholangiopancreatography) to remove gallstones.

- Oral hygiene.
- NPO to decrease gastric secretions; when secretions go into the stomach, the pancreas thinks its time to make more enzymes, which increases pain.
- Administration of intravenous (IV) fluids and electrolytes to prevent or treat dehydration, electrolyte imbalances, and shock from decreased circulating volume.
- Nutritional support using total parenteral nutrition (TPN). This involves placement of an access device in a large vein to administer lipids and other nutritional components.
- Prophylactic antibiotic therapy to avoid infection or treat existing infection.
- Nasogastric placement and suctioning to keep stomach empty and dry.
- Oxygen administration using nasal cannula or, in severe cases, a ventilator. Oxygen deprivation may be present because of pain, anxiety, acidosis, abdominal pressure, or pleural effusions.

PATIENT TEACHING

- Once acute pancreatitis is resolved, gradually resume a low-fat, low-caffeine diet as tolerated.
- Rest, with gradual increase in activity.
- Minimize stress to prevent recurrent acute attacks that could lead to chronic pancreatitis.
- Avoid alcohol.

What can harm my patient and why?

Complications	Why?
Seizures	Pancreas loses calcium into the peritoneal space when it digests itself—hypocalcemia
Arrhythmias	Electrolyte imbalance caused by dehydration
Pancreatic ascites	Fluid leak into peritoneum caused by disease process
Pancreatic abscess; infection; sepsis	Inflammation; infection caused by leaking
Pulmonary infiltrates, pleural effusion, ARDS	Escaping pancreatic enzymes from the peritoneum to the pleural cavity
Peritonitis	Inflammation, infection of peritoneum because of fluid leak
Ileus	Decreased motility of intestines because of insult to GI system
Shock	Movement of fluid from vascular space
Hemorrhage	Bleeding caused by liver dysfunction
Acute renal failure	Inadequate blood flow because of hemorrhage and/or hypovolemia

Cutting edge

Magnetic resonance cholangiopancreatography (MRCP) is a noninvasive imaging test that may replace the ERCP.

PRACTICE QUESTIONS

1. Which statement by the patient with GERD would indicate a need for further patient teaching?

   A. I will be particularly alert to portion control with all meals.

   B. I plan to reduce my dietary intake of pizza, spaghetti, and ravioli.

   C. I will lie on my right side for 30 minutes after eating to promote gastric emptying.

   D. I will take my prescribed proton pump inhibitor 30 minutes before breakfast each morning.

2. Which of the following would most likely precipitate painful symptoms when the patient has a hiatal hernia?

   A. Eating a large meal

   B. Eating a fatty meal

   C. Drinking alcohol with a meal

   D. Engaging in physical activity after a meal

3. A geriatric patient with arthritis who regularly takes large doses of an NSAID became "dizzy" and fell, breaking a hip. Which question by the nurse during the admission history will give a clue to the underlying cause of this injury?

   A. "What were you doing when you fell?"

   B. "Do you have a history of inner ear trouble?"

   C. "Have you been having any black or tarry stools?"

   D. "What additional medications do you regularly take?"

4. Which of the following will most effectively prevent transmission of *H-pylori* causing iatrogenic infection?

   A. Proper sterilization of equipment used for endoscopy.

   B. Placing patients with active *H. pylori* infection in reverse isolation.

   C. Using safety needles (no recapping) with disposal in sharps containers.

   D. Wearing a mask when in direct contact with an infected patient or contaminated equipment.

5. Upon discharge post-endoscopic retrograde cholangiopancreatography (ERCP) for removal of a gallstone blocking the common bile duct, all vital signs are normal. Which complaint by the patient may represent a serious complication of this procedure, necessitating that discharge be cancelled?

   A. The stool I just passed was very pale.

   B. My upper abdomen feels tender to touch.

   C. I felt dizzy when I arose from the chair suddenly.

   D. My gums bled just now as I was brushing my teeth.

6. Following severe acute pancreatitis, the alcoholic patient with previously chronic pancreatitis returns to the doctor's office for a follow-up visit. Which of the following assessments is priority for communicating to the physician?

   A. Weight loss of 10% and stools that float on top of the water.

   B. Reports of having experienced a series of terribly frightening dreams.

   C. Normal blood pressure and pulse, but a decrease in pulse pressure by 20%.

   D. "Bloodshot" eyes (injected sclera) and warm rosy nose with spider angiomas.

7. Which of the following strategies by the dialysis nurse would have the greatest impact on preventing peritonitis in a continuous ambulatory peritoneal dialysis (CAPD) patients who perform four exchanges per day?

   A. Hold yearly classes in medical-surgical asepsis.

   B. Teach handwashing before the CAPD decision is made.

   C. Collaborate with the physician for prophylactic antibiotics.

   D. Regularly monitor exchange technique with constructive suggestions.

8. Which of the following nursing intervention(s) or assessments is/are priority when the patient has inflammatory bowel disease (IBD)?

   A. Monitor BP, I&O, and weigh daily.

   B. Administer prescribed antidiarrheal medications.

   C. Monitor temperature, bowel sounds and check for rebound tenderness.

   D. Administer prescribed analgesics (codeine sulfate) for abdominal cramping.

9. Which discharge teaching is most important when a woman is discharged following diagnosis of hepatitis A virus?

   A. Wear gloves when changing your baby's diaper.

   B. Wash your hands before preparing food for the family.

   C. Do not kiss your baby or your husband until you test negative for HAV.

   D. Do not have unprotected sexual relations until your jaundice has subsided.

10. Which first intervention is priority when the patient with cirrhosis coughs and experiences sudden severe hemorrhage with copious amounts of bright red blood bubbling from his mouth?

   A. Call for any doctor to respond to this emergency.

   B. Administer 100% oxygen by tight fitting face mask.

   C. Stay with the patient and hold a basin to catch the blood flow.

   D. Raise the head of the bed and apply pressure to the external carotids.

References

1. Beers MH, ed. *The Merck Manual of Medical Information. Digestive Disorders.* Whitestation, NJ: Merck Research Laboratories; 2003.

2. Vela MF. The clinical usefulness of high-resolution manometry for the management of achalasia. *Curr Gastroenterol Rept 11*(3):170–172, 2009.

3. Kraichely RE, Farrugia, G, Pittock SJ, et al. Neural autoantibody profile of primary achalasia. *Dig Dis Sci 55*(2):307–311, 2009 [Epub ahead of print]. Available at http://www.ncbi.nlm.nih.gov/pubmed/19499338?ordinalpos=2&itool=EntrezSystem2.PEntrez.Pubmed.Pubmed_ResultsPanel.Pubmed_DefaultReportPanel.Pubmed_RVDocSum. Accessed June 16, 2009.

4. Smeltzer SC, Bare BG, Hinkle JL, Cheever KH. *Brunner & Suddarth's Textbook of Medical-Surgical Nursing.* 11th ed. Philadelphia: Lippincott Williams & Wilkins; 2008.

5. Tatum, RP, Wong JA, Figueredo EJ, et al. Return of esophageal function after treatment for achalasia as determined by impedance-manometry. *J Gastrointest Surg 11*(11):1403–1409, 2007.

6. Go, MR, Dundon JM, Darlowicz DJ, et al. Delivery of radiofrequency energy to the lower esophageal sphincter improves symptoms of gastroesophageal reflux. *Surgery 136*(4):786–794, 2004.

7. Schneider JH, Juper M, Konigsrainer, A, Brucher B. Transient lower esophageal sphincter relaxation in morbid obesity. *Obes Surg 19*(5):595–600, 2009.

8. Robertson L. A new horizon: Recommendations and treatment guidelines for Barrett's esophagus. *Gastroenterol Nurs 32*(3):202–210, 2009.

9. Moazzez R, Bartlett D, Anggiansah A. The effect of chewing sugar-free gum on gastro-esophageal reflux. *J Dent Res 84*(11):1062–1065, 2005.

10. Avidan B, Sonnenberg A, Schnell TG, Sontag SJ. Walking and chewing reduce postprandial acid reflux. *Aliment Pharmacol Ther 15*(2):151–155, 2001.

11. Ganz RA, Fallon E, Wittchow T, Klein D. A new injectable agent for the treatment of GERD: Results of the Durasphere pilot trial. *Gastrointest Endosc 69*(2):318–323, 2009.

12. Broeders JA, Draaisma WA, deVries DR, et al. The preoperative reflux pattern as prognostic indicator for long-term outcome after Nissen fundoplication. *Am J Gastroenterol 104*(8):1922–1930, 2009. [Epub ahead of print]. Available at http://www.ncbi.nlm.nih.gov/pubmed/19491839?ordinalpos=10&itool=EntrezSystem2.PEntrez.Pubmed.Pubmed_ResultsPanel.Pubmed_DefaultReportPanel.Pubmed_RVDocSum. Accessed June 16, 2009.

13. Tseng EE, Wu TT, Yeo CJ, et al. Barrett's esophagus with high-grade dysplasia: Surgical results and long-term outcome-an update. *J Gastrointest Surg 7*(2):164–171, 2003.

14. Hurst M. *A Critical Thinking and Application NCLEX Review.* Brookhaven, MS: Hurst Review Services; 2008.

15. National Digestive Diseases Information Clearinghouse. Heartburn, gastroesophageal reflux (GER) and gastroesophageal reflux disease

(GERD). Available at http://digestive.niddk.nih.gov/ddiseases/pubs/gerd/index.htm. Accessed June 18, 2009.

16. Sihvo EI, Salo JA, Rasanen JV, Rantanen TK. Fatal complications of adult paraesophageal hernia: A population-based study. *J Thorac Cardiovasc Surg* 137(2):419–424, 2009.

17. Salvador R, Dubecz A, Polomsky M, et al. New era in esophageal diagnostics: The image-based paradigm of high-resolution manometry. *J Am Coll Surg* 208(6):1035–1044, 2009.

18. Bawahab M, Mitchell P, Church N, Debru E. Management of acute paraesophageal hernia. *Surg Endosc* 23(2):255–259, 2009.

19. National Digestive Diseases Information Clearinghouse. NSAIDs and peptic ulcers. Available at http://digestive.niddk.nih.gov/ddiseases/pubs/nsaids/index.htm. Accessed June 21, 2009.

20. The Helicobacter Foundation. Epidemiology. Available at: http://www.helico.com/h_epidemiology.html. Accessed June 24, 2009.

21. Mandeville KL, Krabshuis J, Nimzing GL, et al. Gastroenterology in developing countries: Issues and advances. *World J Gastroenterol* 15(23):2839–2854, 2009.

22. Vakil N, Zullo A, Ricci C, et al. Duplicate breath testing to confirm eradication of *Helicobacter pylori*: incremental benefit and cost in 419 patients. *Aliment Pharmacol Ther* 28(11–12):1304–1308, 2008.

23. Pagana KD, Pagana TJ. *Mosby's Diagnostic and Laboratory Test Reference.* 6th ed. St. Louis: Mosby; 2003.

24. Mayo Clinic staff. Peptic ulcer treatment and drugs. Available at http://www.mayoclinic.com/health/peptic-ulcer/DS00242/DSECTION=treatments-and-drugs. Accessed June 24, 2009.

25. Hurst M. Pharmacology in a nutshell. *Hurst Review's NCLEX®-RN Review.* New York: McGraw-Hill; 2008.

26. De Vries R, Klok RM, Brouwers JR, Postma MJ. Cost-effectiveness of a potential future *Helicobacter pylori* vaccine in the Netherlands: The impact of varying the discount rate for health. *Vaccine* 27(6):846–852, 2009.

27. Aebischer T, Bumann D, Epple H J, et al. Correlation of T cell response and bacterial clearance in human volunteers challenged with *Helicobacter pylori* revealed by randomized controlled vaccination with Ty21a-based Salmonella vaccines. *Gut* 57(8):1065–1072, 2008.

28. The Helicobacter Foundation. Treatment. Available at http://www.helico.com/faq_treatment.html#Q32. Accessed June 24, 2009.

29. Sung JJ, Barkun A, Kuipers EJ, et al. Intravenous esomeprazole for prevention of recurrent peptic ulcer bleeding: A randomized trial. *Ann Intern Med* 150(7):455–464, 2009.

30. Cheung FK, Lau JY. Management of massive peptic ulcer bleeding. *Gastroenterol Clin North Am* 38(2):231–243, 2009.

31. Isai JJ, Hsu YC, Perng CL, Lin HJ. Oral or intravenous proton pump inhibitor in patients with peptic ulcer bleeding after successful endoscopic epinephrine injection. *Br J Clin Pharmacol* 67(3):326–332, 2009.

32. Olsen M, Christensen S, Rils A, Thomsen RW. Preadmission use of systemic glucocorticoids and 30-day mortality following bleeding peptic ulcer: A population-based cohort study. *Am J Ther* [Epub ahead of print]. Available at http://www.ncbi.nlm.nih.gov/pubmed/19531935?ordinalpos=1&itool=EntrezSystem2.PEntrez.Pubmed.Pubmed_ResultsPanel.Pubmed_DefaultReportPanel.Pubmed_RVDocSum. Accessed June 21, 2009.

33. MedicineNet.com. Online medical dictionary. Available at http://www.medterms.com/script/main/art.asp?articlekey=25631. Accessed June 25, 2009.

34. Marschall HU, Einarsson C. Gallstone disease. *J Intern Med* *261*(6):529–542, 2009.

35. Ziessman HA. Interventions used with cholescintigraphy for the diagnosis of hepatobiliary disease. *Semin Nucl Med 39*(3):174–185, 2009.

36. The Merck Manual of Medical Information. *Periodontal Disease.* Beers MH, ed. Whitestation, NJ: Merck Research Laboratories; 2003.

37. Wang D Q-H, Cohen DE, Carey MC. Biliary lipids and cholesterol gallstone disease. *J Lipid Res 50*(4):S406–S411, 2009.

38. Duke University Medical Center Research. (2009). A randomized, double-blind, prospective trial of oral administration of aprepitant for prevention of post-endoscopic retrograde cholangiopancreatography (ERCP) pancreatitis. M. Poleski principal investigator: (now recruiting for study). Available at http://www.clinicaltrials.gov/ct2/show/NCT00736073?term=pancreatitis&recr=Open&rank=12. Accessed June 27, 2009.

39. Swaroop VS, Chari ST, Clain JE. Severe acute pancreatitis. *JAMA 291*(23):2865–2868, 2004.

40. Tonsi AF, Bacchion M, Crippa S, et al. Acute pancreatitis at the beginning of the century: The state of the art. *World J Gastroenterol 15*(24):2945–2959, 2009.

41. Lindberg DA. Acute pancreatitis and hypertriglyceridemia. *Gastroenterol Nurs 32*(2):75–82, 2009.

42. Lieb JG 2nd, Forsmark CE. Review article: Pain and chronic pancreatitis. *Aliment Pharmacol Ther 29*(7):706–719, 2009.

43. Pancreatic Cancer Action Network. Pancreatic enzyme supplements. Available at http://www.pancan.org/Patient/Pancreatic/Diet/PancreaticEnzymes.htm. Accessed June 27, 2009.

44. Westlund KN. Gene therapy for pancreatitis pain. *Gene Ther 16*(4):483–492, 2009.

45. Porth CM. *Pathophysiology: Concepts of Altered Health States.* 7th ed. Philadelphia: Lippincott Williams & Wilkins; 2007.

46. Poortman P, Oostvogel HJM, Bosma E, et al. Improving diagnosis of acute appendicitis: Results of a diagnostic pathway with standard use of ultrasonography follow by selective use of CT. *J Am Coll Surg 208*(3):434–441, 2009.

47. George-Gay B, Chernecky CC. *Clinical Medical Surgical Nursing: A Decision Making Reference.* Philadelphia: Saunders; 2002.

48. Tabutsadze T, Kipshidze N. New trend in endoscopic surgery: Transvaginal appendectomy NOTES (Natural Orifice Transluminal Endoscopic Surgery). *Georgian Med News 168*:7–10, 2009. Available at http://www.ncbi.nlm.nih.gov/pubmed/19359710?ordinalpos=5&itool=E ntrezSystem2.PEntrez.Pubmed.Pubmed_ResultsPanel.Pubmed_ DefaultReportPanel.Pubmed_RVDocSum. Accessed June 6, 2009.

49. Song S, Itawi EA, Saber AA. Natural orifice transluminal endoscopic surgery (NOTES). *J Invest Surg 22*(3):214–217, 2009.

50. Mintz Y, Horgan S, Cullen J, et al. NOTES: A review of the technical problems encountered and their solutions. *J Laparoendosc Adv Surg Tech 18*(4):583–587, 2008.

51. Garg CP, Vaidya BB, Chengalath MM. Efficacy of laparoscopy in complicated appendicitis. *Int J Surg 7*(3):250–252,2009 [Epub ahead of print]. Available at http://www.ncbi.nlm.nih.gov/pubmed/1939377 6?ordinalpos=8&itool=EntrezSystem2.PEntrez.Pubmed.Pubmed_ ResultsPanel.Pubmed_DefaultReportPanel.Pubmed_RVDocSum. Accessed June 6, 2009.

52. Alcaraz M, Brzostowicz M, Moran J. Decreasing peritonitis infection rates. *Nephrol Nurs J 35*(4):421–423, 2008.

53. Riche FC, Dray X, Laisne MJ, et al. Factors associated with septic shock and mortality in generalized peritonitis: Comparison between community-acquired and postoperative peritonitis. *Crit Care 13*(3):R99, 2009.

54. Lochbuhler H, Sachs J, Raute-Kreinsen U. The pharmacological effect of sodium phosphate after absorption from the peritoneal cavity. *Eur J Pediatr Surg 5*(2):84–87, 1995.

55. Shah SB, Hanauer SB. Treatment of diarrhea in patients with inflammatory bowel disease: Concepts and cautions. *Rev Gastroenterol Disord 7* Suppl(3):S3–S10, 2007.

56. Comerford KC, Labus D, eds. *Nursing2010 Drug Handbook.* Philadelphia: Lippincott Williams & Wilkins; 2010.

57. Behm BW, Bickston SJ. Tumor necrosis factor-alpha antibody for maintenance of remission in Crohn's disease. *Cochrane Database Syst Rev (on line) 23*(1):CD006893, 2008. Available at http://www.ncbi. nlm.nih.gov/pubmed/18254120?ordinalpos=1&itool=EntrezSystem2. PEntrez.Pubmed.Pubmed_ResultsPanel.Pubmed_DiscoveryPanel. Pubmed_Discovery_RA&linkpos=1&log$=relatedreviews&logdbfro m=pubmed. Accessed June 28, 2009.

58. Yun L, Hanauer S. Selecting the appropriate anti-TNF agent in inflammatory bowel disease. *Expert Rev Gastroenterol Hepatol 3*(3):235–248, 2009.

59. Center for Disease Control and Prevention. Viral hepatitis. Available at http://www.cdc.gov/hepatitis/index.htm. Accessed June 29, 2009.

60. Lam W.-Y, Rickjason CW, Chan J, et al. Genotype distribution and sequence variation of hepatitis E virus, Hong Kong. *Emerg Infect Dis 15*(5):792–794, 2009.

61. Shackel NA, Jamis J, Rahman W, et al. Early high peak hepatitis C viral load levels independently predict hepatitis C-related liver failure post-liver transplantation. *Liver Transpl* 15(7):709–718, 2009.

62. Friedman SL, McQuaid KR, Grendell JH, eds. *Current Diagnosis and Treatment in Gastroenterology.* 2nd ed. New York: Lange Medical Books/McGraw-Hill; 2003.

63. Lucidarme D, Foucher J, Le Bail B, et al. Factors of accuracy of transient elastography (fibroscan) for the diagnosis of liver fibrosis in chronic hepatitis C. *Hepatology* 49(4):1083–1089, 2009.

64. Saab S, Hernandez JC, Chi AC, Tong MJ. Oral antibiotic prophylaxis reduces spontaneous bacterial peritonitis occurrence and improves short-term survival in cirrhosis: A meta-analysis. *Am J Gastroenterol* 104(4):993–1001, 2009.

65. Garcia-Tsao G, Lim J. Management and treatment of patients with cirrhosis and portal hypertension: Recommendations from the Department of Veterans Affairs Hepatitis C Resource Center Program and the National Hepatitis C Program. *Am J Gastroenterol* 104(7):1802–1829, 2009 [Epub ahead of print]. Available at http://www.ncbi.nlm.nih.gov/pubmed/19455106?ordinalpos=46&itool=EntrezSystem2.PEntrez.Pubmed.Pubmed_ResultsPanel.Pubmed_DefaultReportPanel.Pubmed_RVDocSum. Accessed June 28, 2009.

66. National Institute of Health. What I need to know about cirrhosis. *The National Digestive Diseases Information Clearinghouse.* Available at http://digestive.niddk.nih.gov/ddiseases/pubs/cirrhosis_ez/WINTKAcirrhosis.pdf. Accessed June 29, 2009.

67. Mullens W, Abrahams Z, Francis,GS, et al. Prompt reduction in intra-abdominal pressure following large-volume mechanical fluid removal improves renal insufficiency in refractory decompensated heart failure. *J Card Fail* 14(6):508–514, 2008.

68. Umgelter A, Reindl W, Franzen M, et al. Renal resistive index and renal function before and after paracentesis in patients with hepatorenal syndrome and tense ascites. *Intensive Care Med* 35(1):152–156, 2009.

69. Nobili V, Bedogni G, Alisi A, et al. A protective effect of breastfeeding on progression of nonalcoholic fatty liver disease. *Arch Dis Child* 94(10):801–805, 2009 [Epub ahead of print]. Available at http://www.ncbi.nlm.nih.gov/pubmed/19556219?ordinalpos=2&itool=EntrezSystem2.PEntrez.Pubmed.Pubmed_ResultsPanel.Pubmed_DefaultReportPanel.Pubmed_RVDocSum. Accessed June 28, 2009.

70. Garcia-Tsao G, Parikh CR, Viola A. Acute kidney injury in cirrhosis. *Hepatology* 48(6):2064–2077, 2009.

71. Vere CC, Streba CT, Streba LM, et al. Psychosocial stress and liver disease status. *World J Gastroenterol* 15(24):2980–2986, 2009.

72. National Institute of Health. Adult to adult living donor liver transplant. Available at http://www.nih-a2all.org/. Accessed June 29, 2009.

73. Kantola T, Koivusalo AM, Paramanen S, et al. Survival predictors in patients treated with a molecular adsorbent recirculating system. *World J Gastroenterol* 15(24):3015–3024, 2009.

10 Metabolic and Endocrine Dysfunction

OBJECTIVES

In this chapter you will review:

- The pathophysiology associated with selected metabolic and endocrine disorders.
- The key concepts and priorities associated with management of care for patients having acute complications and lifelong compensation for metabolic and/or endocrine dysfunction.
- The effects of metabolic and endocrine dysfunction related to the priority needs of nutrition, fluid and electrolyte balance, tissue perfusion, and physical safety.
- Treatment modalities and nursing care to promote attainment of maximum metabolic and endocrine function.
- Pharmacology and technology that improves quality of life and reduces threat to life when normal metabolic/endocrine function is compromised.
- The impact of age, nutritional status, lifestyle choices, genetics, and comorbidities that alter health when coupled with endocrine dysfunction.
- Components of a teaching plan to enhance self-care and monitoring when the patient has an alteration in normal function of the endocrine system.

THE ENDOCRINE SYSTEM

Let's get the normal stuff straight!

The endocrine hormones are chemical messengers, which are secreted by the endocrine organs and transported to target cells, where they bind to specific receptor sites and act on the cell. Hormones do not cause reactions; instead, they regulate tissue responses. Hormone levels are controlled by the pituitary gland and a series of feedback systems, both negative and positive.

✚ Endocrine dysfunction

What is it?

Metabolic and endocrine disorders present many commonly occurring health issues; of these, diabetes mellitus and complications from diabetes affect more individuals than all other endocrine conditions combined.

✚ Diabetes mellitus

Diabetes mellitus is a leading cause of death and disability in the United States.

Let's get the normal stuff straight!

The body has energy needs that require fuel comprised primarily from glucose produced from carbohydrates and fatty acids derived from fats and proteins.

- Metabolizing these ingredients for energy requires oxygen, which is supplied by the lungs and heart.
- Utilization of glucose is dependent upon a functional endocrine pancreas to produce an adequate and effective supply of insulin.
- The Islets of Langerhans within the endocrine pancreas contain specialized beta cells, which secrete insulin, and alpha cells, which secrete glucagon.
- The brain has the greatest need for glucose and the least resources! It can neither manufacture nor store glucose, yet a continuous supply is needed.
- The brain cannot function properly in the presence of glucose deprivation, and severe or prolonged glucose lack can result in brain death.
- Dietary glucose passes through the liver before getting into the systemic circulation.[1]

The liver has a crucial role in regulating serum glucose through three mechanisms:

- Glucogenesis: forming and storing glycogen for when the body needs it.
- Glycogenolysis: breaking down glycogen (stored form) to use as glucose.
- Gluconeogenesis: making new glucose from noncarbohydrate sources.

Marlene Moment

Back in the first century AD when an early physician described diabetes (which is Greek, meaning *going through*), it was noted that the urine was "honey sweet" (hence the Greek word, *mellitus*) and that volume was greatly increased (polyuria)! I'm surely glad health care providers don't have to taste test urine anymore!

- When blood sugar increases above normal requirements, the liver removes excess glucose from the circulation, converts it to glycogen, and stores it for later use (Fig. 10-1).[1]

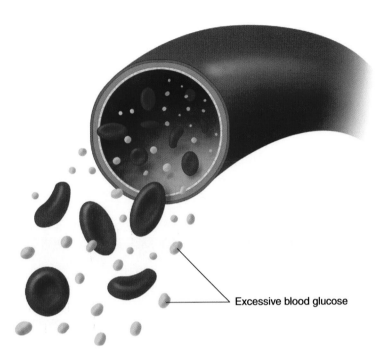

◀ Figure 10-1. Excessive blood glucose.

Excessive blood glucose

- When blood sugar levels fall, the liver retrieves stored glycogen, converts it to glucose, and transports it to the circulation quickly.

  Fats can be used for energy and provide 9 kcal/g, more than double that of proteins and carbohydrates (4 kcal/g).

- There is only one problem: The end product of fat metabolism is ketones!

- Ketones can get a diabetic in trouble, because ketones are acid!

- The brain can't convert fatty acids to glucose, so fat energy won't do the brain any good.

  Proteins can also be used for energy but only after retrieving amino acids from muscle storage!

- Excess amino acids (not needed for building or repairing something) are converted from storage and used as ingredients for fuel (not actual fuel).

- The liver uses stored ingredients to make new sugar (gluconeogenesis), because the brain can't use anything for energy except sugar![1]

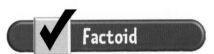

Factoid

All the sugar in the world won't do the body any good without insulin! Insulin is the key that signals "Glut4 (glucose transporter 4) to open the door" (Fig. 10-2). This allows glucose to enter the cell!

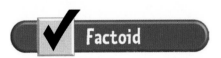

Factoid

The main way that insulin gets glucose into muscle and fat cells is by signaling the movement of Glut4 (glucose transporter 4) to the cell surface. The door has to open from the inside![2]

▶ Figure 10-2. Glut4. Insulin signals "Glut4 to open the door!"

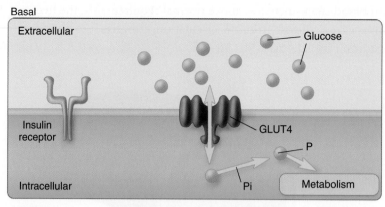

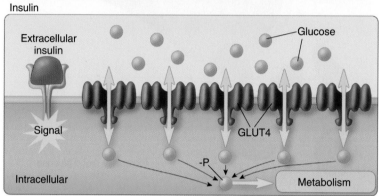

What is it?

Diabetes is a disorder of carbohydrate metabolism wherein the supply of insulin is absent, insufficient, or ineffective because of insulin resistance. Therefore, even though glucose is present in the blood, it cannot get into the cell. There are five types of adult diabetes:

- Type 1 formerly called insulin dependent diabetes mellitus (IDDM).

- Latent autoimmune diabetes in adults (LADA) also called Type 1.5 (alias "double diabetes") has characteristics of both Type 1 and Type 2 because it occurs after 30 years (like Type 2), but may be a slow onset variety of Type 1.[3]

- Type 2, formerly called non-insulin dependent diabetes mellitus (NIDDM).

- Gestational diabetes, which occurs during the course of pregnancy.

- Diabetes that results from other illnesses, such as Cushing's disease (too many steroids) or pancreatitis (autodigestion of pancreas).

The most common forms of diabetes are Type 1 and Type 2 diabetes and are the primary focus of this chapter. In addition, "prediabetes" is briefly explored. Prediabetes is a condition that usually precedes the development of Type 2 diabetes.[4] Refer to Table 10-1 for a comparison of Type 1 and Type 2 diabetes mellitus.

- The patient with prediabetes (fasting plasma glucose 100–125 mg/dL) has impaired glucose metabolism, causing serum glucose to be higher than normal, but not high enough to be diagnostic of diabetes mellitus.

● It is important to identify persons at risk for prediabetes early because this condition can be prevented or delayed with dietary and lifestyle modifications.[3]

Table 10-1 Comparison of Type 1 and Type 2 diabetes mellitus

Type 1 diabetes mellitus	Type 2 diabetes mellitus
Juvenile onset: usually occurs before age 30.	Adult onset can occur at any age, but usually occurs after age 30.
Abrupt onset usually presents as DKA (diabetic ketoacidosis), which is a medical emergency.	Slow and progressive onset over years or decades. It is usually discovered by "accident" during a doctor's visit for an infection.
Comprises 5%–10% of all cases of diabetes.	Comprises the majority of all cases of diabetes (90%–95%)
The pancreas produces little or no insulin: 90% of insulin producing beta cells are permanently destroyed, requiring lifelong insulin therapy.	The pancreas produces some insulin, but not enough to keep up with the glucose load consumed.
Patients are usually thin because the body is unable to utilize or store glucose. This excess glucose is lost through the urine. Constant starvation triggers the metabolism of fat and muscle tissue for energy.	Patients are usually obese because metabolic syndrome delays the normal glucose-induced insulin secretion. More teens are developing metabolic syndrome, causing the incidence of Type 2 diabetes to increase in the "under 30" age group.

Source: Created by the author from References 4 and 5.

Type 1 diabetes is primarily characterized by nonfunctional beta cells in the pancreas. These nonfunctional beta cells fail to produce insulin, and this lack of insulin results in an inability of the body to maintain normal blood sugar levels. Unlike the Type 2 diabetic, who produces some insulin, Type 1 diabetics are characterized by a complete deficiency of insulin. Remember, insulin is the key that signals Glut4 "to open the door." Without insulin glucose cannot get to the cells, resulting in hyperglycemia and diabetic ketoacidosis.[6]

Causes and why?

Destruction of insulin producing beta cells in Type 1 diabetes is caused by a combination of factors:

● Genetic predisposition: human leukocyte antigen (HLA)

● Viruses and toxins are being investigated as potential initiators of autoimmune destruction

● Autoimmune response (autoantibodies against islet cells)[1]

The exact cause of Type 2 diabetes is unknown; however, there is a strong genetic correlation between insulin resistance and impaired insulin secretion.

The pathophysiology of Type 2 diabetes includes:

● Reduced pancreatic beta cell responsiveness to glucose

● Defective insulin receptors in the cells

● Impaired processing of glucose by the liver [1]

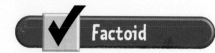

Factoid

Urine glucose can be influenced by a high carbohydrate meal or a number of drugs (ASA, vitamin C, sulfonamides, loop diuretics, estrogens, isoniazid, dextrothyroxine).[7]

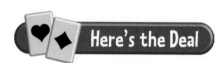

Here's the Deal

The kidneys are trying to help the diabetic patient get rid of the high blood sugar, but there is a big problem. Fluid is pulled into the vascular space because of the hypertonicity of sugary blood, but all that volume came from the cells, leaving them dehydrated. And because polyuria depletes the fluid volume in the vascular space, your patient's blood pressure (and cardiac output) will be dropping, as heart rate is increasing. Once the patient gets cold and clammy, the sympathetic nervous system has kicked in, causing vasoconstriction in an attempt to raise the blood pressure and shunt blood flow to the vital organs.

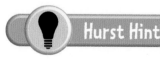

Hurst Hint

When your patient has polyuria (regardless of the cause), always think SHOCK first!

Testing, testing, testing

Serum and urine are tested for glucose:

* Qualitative urine glucose (screening test only) is a component of routine urinalysis. Random specimen should be negative for glucose.
* Fasting (8 hours) plasma glucose (normal, <99 mg/dL): Results of 100 to 125 mg/dL indicate prediabetes and >125 mg/dL indicate diabetes.[8]
* Oral glucose tolerance test can confirm diabetes and prediabetes, even when the fasting blood sugar is normal. Seventy-five grams of glucose is given PO and blood is drawn 2 hours later. Results of 140 to 199 mg/dL indicate prediabetes, whereas 2-hour plasma glucose of 200 mg/dL or greater indicates diabetes.[9]

Signs and symptoms and why?

Remember the "three Ps" associated with hyperglycemia:

* Polyuria is an excessive volume of sweet urine! The renal threshold for "spilling" sugar particles from the blood into the urine is around 180 mg/dL.[10] Once the blood sugar reaches approximately 180 mg/dL, the kidneys can no longer reabsorb it, resulting in glucose excretion in the urine. The kidneys begin excreting sugar particles, but when sugar is excreted, fluid volume goes with it, resulting in polyuria.
* Polydipsia is excessive thirst! Thirst is a compensatory mechanism that accompanies the polyuria. The body is trying to replace the volume lost from excessive diuresis.
* Polyphagia is excessive hunger! The brain cells are very hungry because the sugar in the blood cannot move from the serum into the cell and brain cells require a constant supply of glucose!

Hurst rule

Illness + Diabetes = DKA

Table 10-2 Hyperglycemia and hypoglycemia: signs and symptoms

Hyperglycemia	Why are these symptoms occurring?
Hunger	Cellular starvation resulting from catabolism and depletion of stored carbohydrates, fats, and proteins produces a corresponding increase in hunger.
Changes in urine output: • Polyuria • Oliguria • Anuria	Glucose particles in the blood result in particle-induced diuresis (PID). Body fluid is pulled into the vascular space to dilute the glucose particles for urinary excretion. Initially large volumes of urine are produced, but as fluid volume decreases, urinary output decreases. As cardiac output and blood pressure continue to drop, renal perfusion is critically diminished and urine output ceases.
Dry mouth and thirst	Osmotic diuresis leads to excessive loss of body fluid. Thirst is a compensatory mechanism for dehydration. Thirst results from intracellular dehydration.

(Continued)

Table 10-2 Hyperglycemia and hypoglycemia: signs and symptoms

Hyperglycemia	Why are these symptoms occurring?
Blurred vision	Hyperosmotic effects of elevated glucose levels alter water balance (aqueous humor) within the eye, changing the shape and position of the lens and the light reflected to the retina.
Flushed, warm skin	Blood vessels dilate as tissue and cellular fluid is pulled into the vascular space in response to hyperglycemia.
Lethargy, somnolence	Brain cells require a constant glucose source. Neurological dysfunction results because glucose from the blood cannot be transported to brain cells. Body cells require glucose for production of adenosine triphosphate (ATP). Deficient ATP means deficient cellular energy!
Increased fatigue	When body cells cannot metabolize glucose due to the lack of insulin, body fat is metabolized for energy. Metabolizing fat consumes more energy than readily available glucose; therefore, the negative calorie effect leaves little reserve energy for ADLs.
Coma	When blood glucose is unavailable to brain cells, proteins and fats are metabolized for energy. However, brain cells cannot utilize this form of energy. Fat metabolism produces acidic ketones, which are toxic to the brain. The brain does not like it when the pH is out of balance.

Hypoglycemia	Why are these symptoms occurring?
Headache	A "hungry headache" may be the first warning sign. Brain cells are sending the message that they are hungry for glucose.
Cold and clammy	Vasoconstriction (autonomic response to hypoglycemia) diverts blood flow away from the skin to the vital organs. Decreased perfusion of warm blood leaves the skin cool to touch. Perspiration does not evaporate readily on cold skin; hence, the skin will feel clammy.
Moodiness, impaired judgment, agitation, mental confusion, fainting, and all manifestations of decreased LOC	Glucose is the main energy source of the brain. When glucose (fuel for metabolism) is lacking, the brain quickly begins to become dysfunctional!
Nervous, irritable (subjective feelings)	Psychological response to altered cerebral function. Low glucose levels create an energy deficit within the cells, leading to a sense of unease as the body senses something is wrong.
Tremulous and shaky (behavioral signs)	Neurologic manifestation of sympathetic stimulation.
Tachycardia	Activation of the sympathetic nervous system results in a bolus of epinephrine, which causes the heart to race.

Source: Created by the author from References 1 and 5.

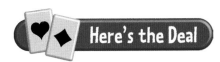

If there is no available insulin for transport of glucose into the cells, the brain keeps screaming, "I'm hungry! I'm starving! Feed me quick!" But if you ate everything in sight (plus the legs off the table) and the serum glucose is 800 mg/dL, would any of this glucose be available to the brain? No! Why? Because there is no insulin to facilitate transport into the cell, so glucose remains in the blood stream and unavailable to the cells.

When diabetic patients are seen in the hospital, their blood sugar (which may normally be well controlled) can go really high in response to a stressor such as illness.

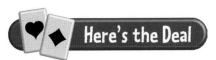

Physiologic stress produces a natural increase in the blood sugar to help us handle the stressor. The normal pancreas can handle fluctuations in blood sugar during times of stress, but when a diabetic patient gets sick, he or she is headed straight for hyperglycemia and DKA (Table 10-2).

What can harm my patient?

Extremes of blood glucose present acute problems that result in life-threatening medical emergencies (Table 10-3):

- Hyperglycemia/hypoinsulinism
- Diabetic ketoacidosis (DKA)
- Hypoglycemia/hyperinsulinism
- Brain dysfunction, coma, and death
- Cardiac arrest (pulseless electrical activity, PEA) because of profound acidosis[10]

Table 10-3   Causes and complications of hypoglycemia and hyperglycemia

Hyperglycemia: What causes DKA (diabetic ketoacidosis) and hypertonic hyperosmolar nonketotic syndrome (HHNK)?	Hypoglycemia: What causes low blood sugar and insulin reaction (shock)?
• Too much to eat! When excessive food (carbohydrates) is metabolized, sugars are released into the blood.	• Not enough to eat! Possibly because of skipping meals (busy young adults) or delaying meals after having taken short-acting insulin. • Consuming meals or snacks that are too small. • Financial limitations and/or decreased appetite (both common in the elderly) can result in not enough to eat.[11]
• Not enough insulin; therefore, glucose cannot get out of the serum and into the cells. Insulin is the key that signals Glut4 "to open the door" and allow glucose entry into the cell.	• Too much insulin. May occur because of visual deficits that predispose to incorrectly drawing up too much insulin in the syringe, or confusion regarding whether a dose was given (leading to a repeat dose).
• Strenuous exercise when blood sugar is high and ketones are present (blood or urine) causes blood sugar to go even higher. Exercise becomes a stressor under these circumstances.	• Increased physical activity. Exercise supports the transport of glucose out of the blood and into muscle cells.
• Fever, infectious processes, and/or illness (stress) raise the blood sugar. This is not accompanied by a corresponding increase in insulin owing to the dysfunctional pancreatic beta cells.	• Consuming alcoholic beverages. Alcohol blocks the release of glucose from the liver. • Alcoholism or binge drinking in combination with Metformin (Glucophage). Excessive drinking can increase drug effects.[12]
Anytime the blood sugar goes really high, the patient is headed straight for: • Diabetic ketoacidosis (DKA); more common in Type 1 diabetes • Hyperosmolar hyperglycemic nonketosis coma HHNK or hyperosmolar hyperglycemic nonketosis coma (HHNC); more common in Type 2 diabetics	• Hypoglycemia unawareness (hypoglycemia-associated autonomic failure) may occur after repeated episodes of hypoglycemia. The person does not know that hypoglycemia is happening in time to respond before the blood glucose drops dangerously low. • Severe hypoglycemia can cause loss of consciousness and death.[3]

Source: Created by the author from References 3 and 13.

Vascular problems and neuropathies associated with diabetes develop over time and pose health problems that lead to loss of quality life, disability, and death.[14] These health problems can include:

- Sexual dysfunction (impotence/decreased sensation)
- Gastroparesis with risk for aspiration
- Amputations necessary because of necrosis/gangrene
- Retinopathy and blindness
- Nephropathy and chronic renal failure
- Cardiovascular disease (CAD and heart attack)
- Stroke[5]

> More diabetics die from heart attacks and strokes (65%) resulting from long-term vascular pathology than from glucose emergencies.[3]

Interventions

Prediabetes (incorrectly called "borderline" diabetes by laypersons) can be halted, or progression to Type 2 diabetes can be delayed if the patient is committed to diet and exercise: 150 minutes of exercise per week is recommended and will result in a 7% weight loss.[8] The general diabetic treatment plan should include:

- Lifestyle modifications, including avoidance or moderation of marijuana and alcohol
- An individualized daily exercise plan after achieving target blood glucose
- Antihyperglycemic medications and/or insulin injections
- Monitoring of hemoglobin A1C (every three months) to gauge long-term control, extending testing times to every six months after target goals are attained

Type 1 diabetes mellitus is often diagnosed following an initial episode of DKA, which is generally treated in the emergency room. Once the patient has been stabilized, the treatment plan will include:

- Multiple daily insulin injections: basal bolus long-acting insulin with rapid-acting insulin given at meal times to cover the prandial glucose load.
- Premixed formulations with both rapid- and intermediate-acting insulins work well for patients who have established routines of eating and exercise.[15]
- Continuous insulin delivery per insulin pump is an option for patients needing greater flexibility of insulin dosing.[15]

When the patient has a diagnosis of Type 2 diabetes mellitus, the treatment plan will begin with lifestyle modifications: carbohydrate control, exercise, and a weight loss program.

- Oral antidiabetic agents (Table 10-4): monotherapy or combined drugs as indicated by the degree of glycemic control.
- Rather than using multiple oral antidiabetic agents, insulin may be added to the pharmacologic regimen to more efficiently and cost-effectively achieve glycemic control.[16,17]

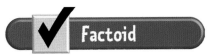

Factoid

Hypoglycemia unawareness (also called hypoglycemia-associated autonomic failure, or HAAF) occurs most commonly in Type 1 diabetics who have frequent episodes of low blood glucose. These frequent hypoglycemic episodes cause the body to stop releasing stress hormones and epinephrine; therefore, no warning symptoms of hypoglycemia occur.[3]

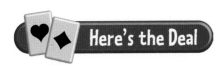

Here's the Deal

Poor circulation develops because of vessel damage. Sugar irritates the vessel lining (tunica intima) and leads to inflammatory changes, these inflammatory changes decrease the size of the vessel lumen and result in decreased blood flow.

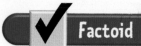

Type 2 diabetics may perceive that the addition of insulin is a punishment for noncompliance, they have failed in self-management, or the severity of their diabetes is increasing.

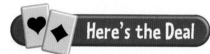

Introduction of insulin earlier in the medication regime for Type 2 diabetics can be a positive rather than a negative step when glycemic control and avoidance of neuropathic complications is the goal, especially when it means less cost (multiple oral agents) and more normal patterns of glycemic control.[15]

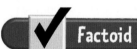

Cookies, cake, whole milk, and other high-fat sources of sugar are not appropriate for treatment of hypoglycemia because the fat content slows metabolism, and when the patient is hypoglycemic, glucose is needed in a hurry![11]

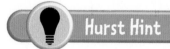

After pushing IVP hypertonic glucose (50%) you had better back up! When the patient starts waking up, he or she will be scared, disoriented, and possibly combative. (You do NOT want to be in the direct line of fire.)

Goals for glycemic control for all diabetics have been established by the ADA:

- Hemoglobin A1C <7%
- Capillary plasma glucose before meals: 90–130 mg/dL
- Peak postprandial capillary plasma glucose <180 mg

When symptoms of hypoglycemia occur, the brain needs glucose immediately!

If the symptomatic patient is conscious (able to swallow), a fast-acting sugar is needed:

- Juice (fructose), glucose tablets, or skim milk (galactose) to raise the blood sugar quickly
- Check blood sugar in 15 minutes (Accu-Chek), if <70 mg/dL repeat the simple sugar (above). (If >70 mg/dL, serve the scheduled meal or provide a snack if mealtime is not imminent.)
- A complex carbohydrate and a protein snack must always follow a simple sugar to prevent rebound hypoglycemia.

If the diabetic patient cannot be aroused:

- 50% glucose IVP is given immediately and hopefully the patient will wake up!
- Glucagon can be given by the IM route if venous access is not immediately attainable.

Clinical alert

The patient who is hypoglycemic because of alcohol intoxication must have IVP glucose: glucagons will not work! Alcohol blocks the liver from being able to release sugar when glucagon is given.[18]

When the patient has hyperglycemia and acidosis (DKA), the priorities are to get the blood sugar down, replenish circulating blood volume, and restore cardiac output through rehydration:

- Obtain venous access (large-gauge catheter in the antecubital site) and prepare for fluid resuscitation.
- Insert a Foley catheter to monitor urine output prior to and during rehydration therapy.
- Initiate continuous cardiac monitoring, because potassium levels will be changing as insulin is given to reduce serum glucose.

Clinical alert

It is possible that when the patient in DKA is catheterized, no urine returns and you are positive that the catheter is in the bladder! When this happens you had better hurry up and rehydrate the patient because of the risk for acute renal failure.

- Isotonic IV fluids such as NS are given to combat dehydration secondary to polyuria.
- Insulin per continuous IV infusion is initiated while monitoring hourly blood glucose and serum potassium.

- Monitor the ABGs and update the physician of reports (pH, CO_2, and base deficit).
- Keep the physician informed of hourly serum glucose and serum potassium.
- D5W with KCl may be initiated (in place of one of the NS infusions) when blood sugar comes down to around 300 mg/dL. This is to counteract potential iatrogenic hypoglycemia because the insulin infusion is still in progress.[5]

DANGER: DKA

If the admitting diagnosis is DKA, after initially getting the blood glucose down from critically high levels, the next task is to find the cause:

- Is there illness, infection, or fever? Specimens for blood, urine, sputum, or wound cultures may be obtained as indicated before the initial antibiotic.
- Has the patient experienced unusual stress or trauma? Blacking out at the wheel could have caused the MVA, or the MVA could have caused the DKA!
- Has the patient skipped an insulin dose or indulged in too many carbs? A focused interview and patient teaching may be indicated!

The patient will need a calorie-controlled diet comprised of:

- Carbohydrates (50%–60% of caloric intake)
- Fats (20%–30% of caloric intake)
- Proteins (10%–20% of caloric intake)

Implement the prescribed treatment algorithms:

- Administer oral antidiabetic agents before meals or with meals as indicated (Table 10-4).

Table 10-4 Oral antidiabetic agents

Oral antidiabetic agents: name and classification	Mechanism of action	Nursing implications
Glipizide (Glucotrol): second-generation sulfonylurea with decreased incidence of side effects compared with first-generation (Diabinese).	Stimulates release of insulin from the pancreas and increases sensitivity to insulin.	• Extended release is available for once-daily dosing. • Advise the patient not to take any OTCs without consulting the doctor. • Caution against alcohol-induced hypoglycemia.

(Continued)

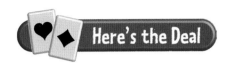

Here's the Deal

The patient in DKA has polyuria caused by PID (particle-induced diuresis), and guess what? The particle is sugar! They may be "dry" (FVD) upon admission to the emergency department, and when the vascular space is empty, the patient goes from polyuria to oliguria to anuria as circulating volume drops. When cardiac output is critically low following polyuria, blood flow may be diverted away from the renal circulation in an attempt to salvage the other three vital organs (heart, brain, and lungs) at the expense of the kidneys.

Hurst Hint

If there is a shortage of blood flow for any reason, the kidneys will be the first of the vital organs to be "voted off the island." Be on the alert for oliguria and anuria, which can signal decreased renal perfusion and the onset of acute renal failure.

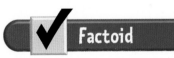

Factoid

Insulin results in two "hypos": hypoglycemia and hypokalemia!

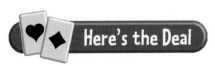

Here's the Deal

At some point, potassium (KCl) will be added to one of the IVs to combat hypokalemia because the insulin infusion (in progress to lower the blood glucose) also drives potassium from the serum (blood) into the cell.

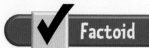

Factoid

Carbohydrates affect blood sugar level more than any other nutrient consumed.[12]

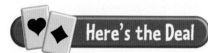

Here's the Deal

Comparing carbohydrates and proteins: only half of consumed meats, fish, and poultry are converted to glucose, as opposed to 100% of sugars and starches. The end product of protein metabolism (nitrogen) places added workload on the kidneys, and diabetic patients tend to have renal dysfunction secondary to vascular complications. High blood sugar destroys blood vessels in the kidneys and everywhere else, just like fat does!

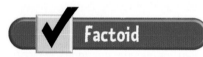

Factoid

Sugar destroys blood vessels just like fat!

Table 10-4   Oral antidiabetic agents (*Continued*)

Oral antidiabetic agents: name and classification	Mechanism of action	Nursing implications
Glyburide (DiaBeta®, Glynase®): second-generation sulfonylurea; contains drug in smaller particle size (micronized glyburide), which is NOT the same as regular glyburide tablets!	Stimulates release of insulin from the pancreas and increases sensitivity to insulin.	• Administer with breakfast or the first main meal. • Report episodes of low blood sugar to the doctor immediately because a severe episode can be fatal (which has occurred with doses as low as 2.5–5 mg daily).
Glimepiride (Amaryl®): sulfonylurea; adjunct to diet and exercise. Used in conjunction with metformin or insulin when Type 2 diabetes can't be managed with glimepiride alone.	Stimulates release of insulin from functioning beta cells and can lead to increased sensitivity to insulin.	• Discourage concurrent use of alcohol owing to hypoglycemic reaction. • Administer with the first meal of the day. • Monitor labs: can increase AST, BUN, and creatinine; may decrease hemoglobin, sodium, and WBC counts.
Metformin (Glucophage®): biguanide	Alters glucose uptake by tissues and changes rate of hepatic gluconeogenesis.	• Monitor renal function: Elevated BUN and creatinine may require a different antidiabetic agent. • The risk of lactic acidosis is low but can be fatal. The risk increases with renal impairment and age. • Stop the drug for any illness causing hypoxemia or dehydration because of the danger of lactic acidosis.
Acarbose (Precose®) and miglitol (Glyset®): alphaglucosidase inhibitors; adjunct to diet and exercise; used in conjunction with a sulfonylurea or insulin.	Delays absorption of glucose from the GI.	• Give with the first bite of each of the three main meals. • Adverse effects occur early in treatment and diminish over time. • Keep glucose tablets readily available in the event of hypoglycemia.

(*Continued*)

Table 10-4 Oral antidiabetic agents (*Continued*)

Oral antidiabetic agents: name and classification	Mechanism of action	Nursing implications
Pioglitazone (Actos®): Thiazolidinedione; can be used alone, with a sulfonylurea, metformin, or insulin	Increases glucose uptake in muscles, decreases insulin resistance, and decreases hepatic glucose production.	• May administer without regard to meals. • Monitor liver enzymes and stop the drug if ALT increases to three times normal or jaundice occurs. • Monitor daily weight and I&O for signs of fluid retention, which could indicate heart failure.
Nateglinide (Starlix®): meglitinide derivative; used alone (monotherapy) or with Metformin or a thiazolidinedione.	Stimulates beta cells in the pancreas to increase insulin secretion (onset 20 minutes, peak 1 hour, duration 4 hours).	• Take 1–30 minutes before each meal. • Patient must have the meal immediately after the dose. • For NPO patients, do not administer if the meal is skipped.
Sitagliptin phosphate (Januvia®): dipeptidyl peptidase-4 (DDP-4); most recently added to the ADA/EASD algorithm for management of Type 2 diabetes.[19]	DDP-4 is an enzyme that renders incretin hormones ineffective. Incretins are a group of gastrointestinal hormones that stimulate the beta cells in the pancreas to secrete insulin. By blocking this enzyme (DDP-4), the pancreas can produce more insulin.	• May be taken without regard to food. • Monitor for hypersensitivity reaction. • Monitor labs (BUN and creatinine) to assess renal function, especially in elderly patients.

Source: Created by the author from Reference 20.

Clinical alert

Avandia® (rosiglitazone), an oral antidiabetic agent of the thiazolidinedione class, which increases glucose uptake in muscles and decreases endogenous glucose production, is no longer a part of the ADA recommended algorithm because of increased risk for cardiovascular disease and liver failure.[21]

• Administer metoclopramide hydrochloride (Reglan®) before meals and at bedtime as prescribed for diabetic gastroparesis to remedy delayed gastric emptying.

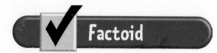

Factoid

Sliding scale insulin has historically been the means by which rapid- or short-acting insulin is given in response to elevations in blood glucose before meals and at bedtime.

The ADA endorses constant "tight" glycemic control through use of basal or basal-bolus insulin therapy with evidenced-based algorithms that improve outcomes of hospitalized patients.[22]

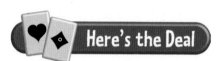

Here's the Deal

Tight glycemic control means that nurses must be on the alert for hypoglycemia, which is a risk when maintaining blood glucose levels <110 mg/dL (fasting) and <180 mg/dL (nonfasting). Some patients by virtue of their potential for instability (elderly patients, patients with comorbidities, or previous severe hypoglycemia) are not candidates for tight control.[20]

▶ Figure 10-3. Insulin sites. Insulin site rotation chart: sites A–J.

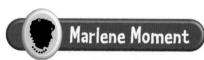

Marlene Moment

The "roller coaster" phenomenon is what tight glycemic control is supposed to avoid. It is the highs and lows that lead to cellular death and vascular damage.

• Monitor blood glucose (Accu-Chek) as indicated with insulin coverage as prescribed.

Define time

Insulin allows the body to use glucose for energy. Insulin may be administered either via basal and/or bolus therapy. Basal insulin therapy uses intermediate or long-acting insulins to provide a continuous supply of insulin to meet the energy needs of metabolism and maintain basic functions during periods of fasting. Bolus insulin therapy uses rapid- or short-acting insulin given before meals to cover carbohydrate ingestion.[20]

Define time

Comorbidities for the diabetic patient means that in addition to having diabetes, other diseases such as heart failure, renal failure, thyroid disease, or cancer could be present. These additional stressors complicate glycemic control. A high percentage of diabetics (40%) have as many as three comorbid conditions.[18]

Hurst rule

Extremes in blood sugar (high or low) = vascular damage!

• Administer and record time and consumption (%) of prescribed between-meal and bedtime snacks (usually administered at 10 AM, 1 PM, and 10 PM).

    Administer prescribed daily doses of SQ insulin (Table 10-5).

• Pinch up the skin and administer insulin into subcutaneous tissue without aspirating.

• Rotate sites of insulin. Review existing patient schedule, or collaborate to revise as needed if all available sites are not being utilized (Fig. 10-3, sites A–J) or if SQ tissue appears hard, nodular, or lumpy.

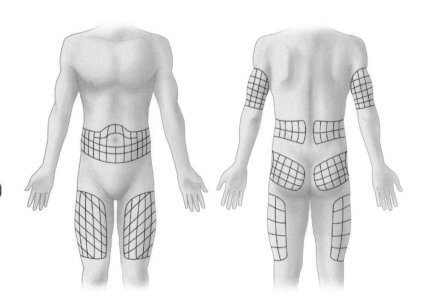

Clinical alert

Do not aspirate insulin because aspiration causes subcutaneous tissue trauma leading to scar and connective tissue damage, which inhibits the absorption of insulin. This is the same reason we also do not aspirate heparin or Lovenox (Table 10-5).

Table 10-5 Comparison of insulins: onset, peak, and duration

Generic name	Trade name	Onset	Peak	Duration
Rapid-acting insulins: Insulin aspart	NovoLog®	15 minute	1–3 hour	3–5 hour
Insulin lispro	Humalog®	15 minute	30 minute–1½ hour	3–4 hour
Short-acting insulins: Insulin glulisine (rDNA origin: cannot be mixed with other insulins)[13]	Apidra®	IV = immediate SQ = 15 minute	IV = unknown SQ = 55 minute	Unknown Unknown
Regular human Insulin	Humulin R®	30 minute	2–4 hour	6–8 hour
	Novolin R®	30 minute	2½–5 hour	8 hour
Intermediate-acting insulins: Human insulin isophane suspension	NPH®	1½ hour	4–12 hour	24 hour
Human insulin zinc suspension	Lente®	2½ hour	7–15 hour	22 hour
Human insulin extended zinc suspension	Ultralente®	4 hour	8–20 hour	28 hour
Basal long-acting insulins: Insulin glargine (rDNA origin)	Lantus®	1 hour	None	24 hour
Insulin detemir (rDNA origin)	Levemir®	Unknown	6–8 hour	6–23 hour
Combination insulins: 70% insulin aspart protamine suspension/30% insulin aspart	NovoLog Mix 70/30®	15 minute	1–4 hour	24 hour

(Continued)

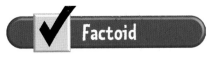

The Type 2 diabetic has excessive amounts of stored glycogen in the liver. During the night, some of this glycogen is changed back into glucose for release into the blood. This is what causes their morning fasting glucose levels to be elevated.[16]

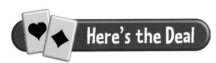

A bedtime snack for some Type 2 diabetics will actually increase the morning fasting glucose levels. The diabetic patient who takes insulin at the evening meal must have a bedtime snack to cover the insulin peak during the night. Additionally, patients with hypoglycemia unawareness (hypoglycemia-associated autonomic failure, HAAF) should also never miss a snack because they will have no warning symptoms if blood glucose levels fall. The snack must contain a minimum of 100 calories (15 g) for the average adult; more may be needed for an active adult.[16]

Table 10-5   Comparison of insulins: onset, peak, and duration (*Continued*)

Generic name	Trade name	Onset	Peak	Duration
75% insulin lispro protamine suspension/25% insulin lispro	Humalog mix 75/25®	15 minute	1–2 hour	24 hour
70% human insulin isophane suspension (NPH)/30% regular insulin	Humulin 70/30®	30 minute	2–12 hour	24 hour
	Novolin 70/30®	30 minute	2–12 hour	24 hour
50% human insulin isophane suspension (NPH)/50% regular insulin	Humulin 50/50®	30 minute	3–5 hour	24 hour

Source: Created by the author from References 5 and 12.

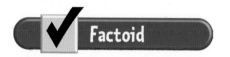
Factoid

Insulin is the only hormone that lowers the blood glucose![5]

Clinical alert

When insulin is peaking, your patient's blood sugar is at its lowest!

Clinical alert

Don't confuse NovoLog Mix 70/30 with Novolin 70/30. They are NOT the same drug (see Table 10-5).

* Awaken the sleeping diabetic patient to monitor for early morning fluctuations in blood glucose related to the Somogyi effect or dawn phenomenon.

Define time

The Somogyi (pronounced so-MO-gee) effect occurs in the Type 1 diabetic whose blood glucose is normal or elevated at bedtime but drops between 2 and 3 AM. Hypoglycemia triggers the release of hormones (epinephrine, ACTH, glucagon, and growth hormone) that raises the blood glucose level, producing rebound hyperglycemia. Somogyi effect is corrected by increasing the caloric content of the bedtime snack (adding a protein) and decreasing the insulin (NPH® or Lente®) dosage.

Define time

The dawn phenomenon occurs in the Type 1 diabetic who has normal blood glucose, which begins to rise around 3 AM because of a surge of nocturnal growth hormone and cortisol. These surges cause a decrease in tissue sensitivity to insulin and result in early morning hyperglycemia (5–8 AM). The problem can be resolved by administering the evening dose of intermediate-acting insulin (NPH® or Lente®) later in the evening.

Symptomatic relief from peripheral neuropathies (burning, numbness, prickling, tingling) may be obtained with the use of pregabalin (Lyrica®) or gabapentin (Neurontin®) and tricyclic antidepressants taken at bedtime.[14] Neuropathy increases the risk for accidental injury and resultant infections; therefore, instructions for close monitoring are indicated.

- Foot wounds don't heal properly because patients with neuropathy keep traumatizing the foot owing to the fact that they don't have normal sensation.[23]
- A large number of diabetic hospitalizations are caused by foot infections that fail to heal because of limb ischemia.[24]
- Often ulcers are concealed underneath thick calloused hard tissue and are discovered between toes when probing.

Salvaging infected and necrotic distal extremities is a matter of urgency because of the risk of sepsis and exacerbation of other chronic illnesses (cardiovascular and renal).

- Rapid stabilization and surgical intervention cannot be delayed in excess of 48 hours because of the risk of gas gangrene and necrotizing fasciitis.
- Broad-spectrum antibiotics and agents to treat methicillin-resistant *Staphylococcus aureus* (MRSA) should be initiated quickly.[25]
- Collaboration with a vascular lab for evaluation can assist in determining if arterial blood flow is sufficient to heal a foot ulcer.[23]

Many times multiple surgeries with the use of negative pressure wound healing (vacuum-assisted closure therapy)[26] is employed along with skin grafting. This provides wound coverage.

Amputations are performed at the most distal site that will heal. All efforts are employed to preserve joints when possible and enable a more normal gait.[5] After surgical healing of an amputation, physical rehab is employed to desensitize the stump for weight bearing. The stump is shaped by compression (limb socks) to conform to the prosthesis.

PATIENT TEACHING Self-care and monitoring are critical components of diabetic patient teaching. The patient must know the signs and symptoms of hyperglycemia and hypoglycemia and quickly initiate corrective actions!

- Refer to Table 10-2 for teaching signs and symptoms of hyperglycemia and hypoglycemia.
- Teach the importance of adhering to diet, exercise, and prescribed medications.
- Carry glucose (dextrose) tablets/gel or other form of simple sugar to take at the first sign of hypoglycemia.[12]

Clinical alert

If the patient is taking the oral antidiabetic agent miglitol (Glyset), table sugar or fruit juice (sucrose/fructose) will not be effective. Therefore, glucose tablets must be available as treatment for hypoglycemia.[12]

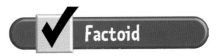

Patients with diabetic neuropathy can walk around with a needle buried in their foot and never feel it!

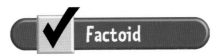

Diabetic foot ulcers have delayed healing because of vascular insufficiency and neuropathy, boosting the cost for an average 2-year treatment in the United States to $37,000, and that is only the monetary cost![27]

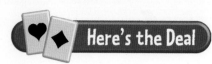

Here's the Deal

Alpha-glucosidase in the small intestine converts carbohydrates to usable glucose. Alpha-glucosidase inhibitors (eg, miglitol or acarbose) delay digestion of carbohydrates, but oral glucose (dextrose) does not require digestion because it is ready for immediate use.[12]

Hurst Hint

Technology can be overwhelming and challenging, but studies have shown that patients adapt well with nursing support and encouragement, along with assistance in selecting just the right device to match patient needs.[22]

Factoid

Diabetic patients learn to gauge food servings that equal 15 carbohydrate grams per serving and should plan to include the appropriate number of prescribed carbohydrates with each meal; that is, four servings equal 60 grams, or five servings equal 75 grams (Fig. 10-4).[2]

Clinical alert

Hypoglycemia may be hard to recognize in elderly patients who are taking beta blockers (autonomic neuropathy) concurrently with oral antidiabetic agents.

- "Mealtime" insulins (given to cover ingested carbs) such as Humalog are so rapid-acting that they must be given within 15 minutes before or within 20 minutes after starting a meal. There is no defensible excuse for not having a meal or food readily available before administering rapid-acting insulin. In other words, don't administer rapid-acting insulin before the meal trays arrive!

- A variety of insulin pens are available that are suited to needs and lifestyles, including prefilled cartridges and dial-a-dose.[22]

- Insulin pumps provide a continuous SQ basal infusion of insulin. The pumps require one needle stick every three days when the site is rotated. Many pumps have carb counters and safety alarms with the capability of delivering insulin boluses in response to carbohydrate intake.[18]

- Wear (or carry on your person) medical identification at all times.

- Rotate SQ insulin injection sites within the area (using all of one area before moving to the next site) to prevent lipodystrophy, which will interfere with absorption of insulin. Refer to Figure 10-3 for anterior/posterior sites A–J.

- Seek medical advice promptly during times of illness, fever, or trauma because these stressors raise blood sugar.

- Alcohol alters glycemic control and increases the risk for hypoglycemia. Patients should not drink unless well controlled, and even then, they should monitor their blood glucose frequently and always have a snack before bedtime (see additional alcohol warnings with diet teaching).

- Teach patients that marijuana may increase glucose levels, and smoking not only increases glucose levels, but also decreases response to insulin.[12]

Diabetic patient teaching can make life-changing (and limb-saving) differences in long range outcomes! Diet, exercise, and foot care are essential components of the teaching plan. Dietary teaching is specific to prescribed calories and follows the ADA guidelines:

- Evenly space out meals and snacks throughout the day.

- Use the method of choice for calorie/carbohydrate control, estimating serving size or carbohydrate grams.

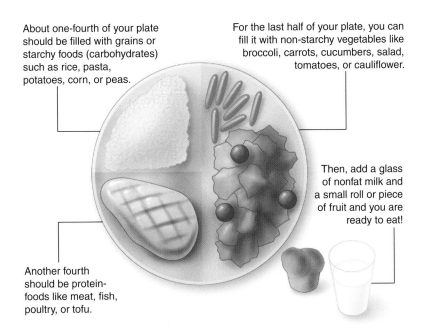

About one-fourth of your plate should be filled with grains or starchy foods (carbohydrates) such as rice, pasta, potatoes, corn, or peas.

For the last half of your plate, you can fill it with non-starchy vegetables like broccoli, carrots, cucumbers, salad, tomatoes, or cauliflower.

Then, add a glass of nonfat milk and a small roll or piece of fruit and you are ready to eat!

Another fourth should be protein-foods like meat, fish, poultry, or tofu.

◄ Figure 10-4. Diabetic servings.

- Choose polyunsaturated and vegetable oils rather than fats from animal sources to reduce cholesterol levels and the risk for coronary artery disease.

- Eat more nonanimal sources of protein (legumes, whole grains). This will help to reduce cholesterol and saturated fats.

- Gradually increase fiber in the diet to 25 g daily for satiety. This enhances weight loss and lowers blood glucose and lipid levels.

Clinical alert

Make sure your diabetic patients don't try to achieve 25 g of fiber the first day! They will have horrible abdominal cramps and may have hypoglycemia because of the decreased absorption of glucose. Fiber should be introduced gradually, once the ideal recommendation is achieved, insulin and/or oral agents may be gradually decreased.

- Use moderation with alcohol and choose drinks with fewer calories; that is, light beer and dry wines.

- Never drink on an empty stomach! Always consume food along with alcohol!

Patient teaching regarding exercise:

- Don't begin a new exercise program until diabetes is well controlled and avoid exercise during times of hyperglycemia (ie, illness).

- Establishing a routine is important. Exercise at the same time and in the same amount every day.

- Wear proper footwear and any other gear appropriate for a particular exercise.

- Have a snack (a complex carbohydrate and a protein) pre-exercise to avoid hypoglycemia and wait for the snack to peak before exercising.

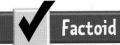

Factoid

Dietary fiber in the form of whole grain breads and cereals helps keep the blood sugar steady by slowing down the absorption of glucose in the intestine.

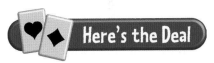

Here's the Deal

Alcohol consumption by the diabetic can be very dangerous because it can cause a hypoglycemic episode. Alcohol is not dependent on insulin and is rapidly absorbed, thereby reducing the liver's ability to make new sugar (gluconeogenesis). In addition, alcohol is a toxin and your body reacts like you just consumed a poison. The liver tries to clear it from the blood quickly, not releasing any glucose until all alcohol has been detoxified and excreted. If your blood glucose level is falling, you can quickly wind up with very low blood sugar.

- Wear water shoes to protect the feet from rocks in streams or shells at the beach.
- Always remove moist, sweaty socks and inspect the feet after exercise.

Clinical alert

Patients with diabetic neuropathy are more apt to experience preventable activity-related foot injuries.[28]

Last but not least—diabetic foot care!

- Avoid all harsh chemicals on the feet, such as Betadine, bleach, and perfumed soaps.
- Inspect the feet (morning and evening)[29] using a mirror or get a friend or family member to assist.
- Inspect footwear daily. Feel inside for worn areas or rough places.
- Soak and wash feet daily with mild soap and dry well between toes.
- Do not use lotion or powder between the toes. (Nonperfumed emollient cream may be applied to dry heels only.)
- Never self-treat corns or calluses. This is a job for the podiatrist!
- Never use any form of external heat, heating pads, or hot water bottles.
- Wear rounded-toe, low-heeled shoes that fit well with plenty of toe room.[14]
- Never go barefoot, even in the home, because trauma can occur unknowingly owing to decreased sensation.
- Visit the podiatrist periodically for professional foot care and to have toenails cut straight across.[5]

Cutting edge

Continuous blood glucose monitoring with intensive insulin therapy reduces the incidence of long-range complications associated with diabetes. However, there is always the danger of hypoglycemia to consider. The new concept of an "artificial pancreas" for management of Type 1 diabetes matches the normal tight control of a healthy pancreas with minute-by-minute responsiveness to real-time blood glucose levels, much like a real biological pancreas! Patients will have a glucose monitor, a prescribed control algorithm, and an insulin pump that communicate together to deliver the exact dose of insulin and thereby maintain blood sugar.[15]

Even though pancreatic and islet cell transplants have been available since the 1990s when new immunosuppressive drugs made insulin independence a reality,[9] suitable organ donations are still limited and long-term results have been disappointing. (Only 10%–15% are free from insulin injection after five years.) Current stem cell research may be the future cure for diabetes with the focus on producing functional beta cells within the diabetic pancreas from existing pancreatic precursor cells for a limitless and renewable insulin supply. At present there are safety concerns (formation of teratomas) and technical considerations that must be addressed, but the future holds tremendous promise (Fig. 10-5).[30]

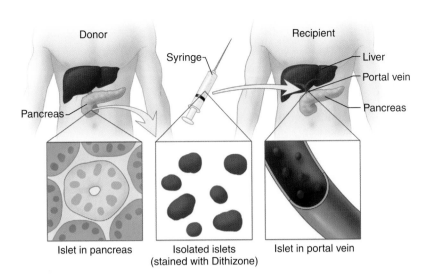

◀ Figure 10-5. Islet cell transplantation.

✚ Pituitary disorders

Let's get the normal stuff straight!

The two-lobed pituitary gland is often called the "master" gland of the body. The pituitary gland receives messages from the hypothalamus regarding blood levels of endocrine hormones and regulates glandular activity by sending out messenger hormones targeted to particular glands to increase hormone production as needed (Fig. 10-6).

◀ Figure 10-6. The pituitary gland.

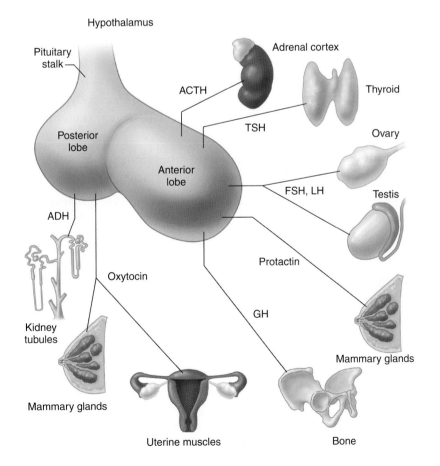

Here's another way to look at it:

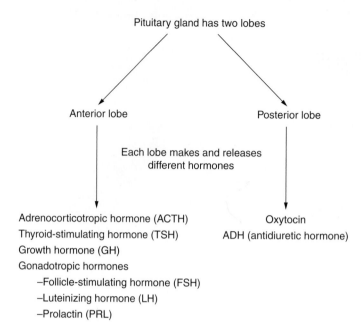

The posterior pituitary—also known as neurohyphosis—secretes:

- Oxytocin—important for cervical dilatation prior to birth and helps the uterus to contract during labor and delivery, especially during the second and third stages.

  - In breastfeeding (lactating) mothers, oxytocin causes milk to be "let down" into an area of the breast where the baby can suckle and receive milk.

  - Which diseases are seen with oxytocin problems? There really aren't any diseases or disorders associated with endogenous (made by the body) oxytocin. However, oxytocin can be given as a drug in the exogenous form called Pitocin. Pitocin is used frequently to induce labor and is associated with serious side effects such as uterine rupture resulting from overcontraction.

- Vasopressin—also known as antidiuretic hormone (ADH)—when ADH is secreted, **WATER** is retained in the vascular space.

Antidiuretic hormone (ADH), also called vasopressin, is manufactured in the hypothalamus and routed to the posterior pituitary gland for circulatory distribution.[1]

- When blood volume is low, ADH is secreted to cause fluid to be retained.

- Changes in levels of ADH (increased or decreased) can occur in response to physical and chemical stressors.

- Increased ADH secretion causes the kidneys to reabsorb more water, resulting in very concentrated urine and increased free water within the vascular space.

- Decreased ADH secretion causes more water to be excreted by the kidneys, resulting in very dilute urine and hemoconcentration.

- Pituitary problems and stressors can cause alterations in hypothalamic synthesis and pituitary release of ADH.

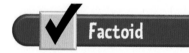

ADH is against diuresis! This hormone is all about retaining fluid!

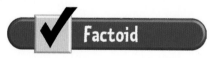

Alcohol inhibits the synthesis and release of ADH.

- Excessive ADH secretion causes free water to be retained and coupled with inappropriate renal excretion of sodium (SIADH); symptoms of hyponatremia occur.[1,9,25]

- When water is excreted (insufficient ADH), the serum sodium is concentrated and symptoms of hypernatremia occur.

✦ Diabetes insipidus: SIADH (syndrome of inappropriate antidiuretic hormone)

What is it?

Diabetes insipidus (DI) is a condition related to insufficient or ineffective renal response to ADH, causing inability of the kidneys to concentrate urine, and resulting in excessive urine output and hemoconcentration.

The syndrome of inappropriate antidiuretic hormone (SIADH) is a condition of excessive ADH production, causing renal reabsorption of excessive free water, which expands the vascular space and causes hemodilution.

Causes and why?

DI and SIADH can be attributed to neurogenic, nephrogenic, and carcinogenic causes.

- With neurogenic causes there is an excess or a deficit of ADH production and release by the pituitary gland, which can result in diabetes insipidus or SIADH depending on whether there is a deficit or excess.

Hurst rule

Key words to make you suspect ADH problems resulting from neurogenic causes are craniotomy, head injury, pituitary tumor, sinus surgery, increased intracranial pressure, and the "biggie"—TRANSSPHENOIDAL HYPOPHYSECTOMY!

Define time

Transsphenoidal hypophysectomy is a surgical procedure through (trans) the sphenoid sinus (sphenoidal) to remove (ectomy) a portion (hypophysis) of the pituitary gland.

- With kidney disease the ADH level can be normal, but the kidney tubules are less sensitive to ADH stimulation.

- Certain tumors (oat cell carcinoma of the lung and other malignancies) can produce excessive secretion of ADH.

- Other endocrine disorders (Addison's disease, hypothyroidism) can lead to ADH excesses and deficiencies.

The syndrome of inappropriate antidiuretic hormone secretion (SIADH) is one big mouthful of words! That's why we just say SIADH!

Other causes of SIADH include viral infections causing autonomic dysfunction (Guillain-Barré syndrome) and other CNS infections. Additionally, some medications may elevate ADH levels and cause SIADH. Refer to Table 10-6 for drugs that increase ADH secretion.

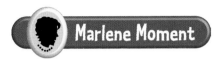

Marlene Moment

If you guzzle a six-pack of beer, you can expect to pee, pee, pee! Alcohol suppresses ADH.

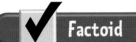

Factoid

Narcotics such as meperidine (Demerol) and morphine increase ADH levels.

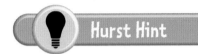

Hurst Hint

Water = H_2O. Antidiuretic hormone = ADH. ADH causes the patient to retain water, only water! Not water and sodium, only water and more water!

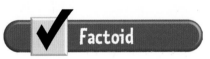

Factoid

Too much ADH = SIADH
Too little ADH = Diabetes insipidus

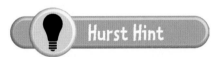

Hurst Hint

ADH problems are usually secondary to other things!

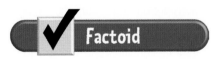

Factoid

Renal disease can cause the kidney to be unresponsive to ADH stimulation, resulting in nephrogenic DI.[7]

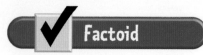

Diabetes insipidus (DI) shares a common characteristic with diabetes mellitus (polyuria), but unlike diabetes mellitus, the dilute urine of diabetes insipidus has nothing whatsoever to do with blood sugar!

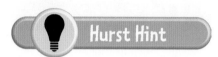

SIADH = too many letters, too much water!

Table 10-6   Drugs affecting ADH secretion

Drugs that elevate ADH levels	Drugs that decrease ADH levels
• Acetaminophen	• Alcohol
• Oxytocin	• Beta adrenergic agents
• Vincristine	• Morphine antagonists
• Narcotics	• Dilantin (phenytoin)
• Thioridazine (phenothiazine class)	
• Thiazide diuretics	
• Tricyclic antidepressants (amitriptyline)	
• Estrogens	
• Oral hypoglycemic agents	
• Cholinergic agents	
• Cyclophosphamide®	

Source: Created by the author from References 5, 7 and 31.

Testing, testing, testing

Urine specific gravity and urine and serum osmolality give indication of fluid and electrolyte balance. Refer to Table 10-7 for DI and SIADH lab findings.

Table 10-7   Laboratory findings: DI and SIADH

Laboratory findings and normal ranges	Diabetes insipidus	Syndrome of inappropriate antidiuretic hormone
Serum sodium (135–145 mEq/L)	Increased >145 mEq/L owing to hemoconcentration	Decreased <35 mEq/L and may be as low as 100 mEq/L because of hemodilution
Urine osmolality (12- to 14-hour fluid restriction ≥850 mOsm/kg H$_2$O) Supper is eaten without fluids the evening before the test and no fluids are permitted until urine is collected. The patient is instructed to void at 6 AM and test urine is collected at 8 AM. Random urine (first voided specimen) normal = 50–1200 mOsm/kg H$_2$O depending on fluid intake.	Decreased osmolality (dilute urine)	Increased osmolality (concentrated urine)
Serum osmolality (280–295 mOsm/kg H$_2$O)	Increased serum osmolality (hemoconcentration)	Decreased serum osmolality (hemodilution)
Osmolar gap (particles expected to be in urine versus actual measure of osmolality) normal = 80–100 mOsm/kg of H$_2$O.	Low (dilute urine)	High (concentrated urine)

(Continued)

Table 10-7 *Laboratory findings: DI and SIADH (Continued)*

Laboratory findings and normal ranges	Diabetes insipidus	Syndrome of inappropriate antidiuretic hormone
Water deprivation ADH stimulation test (differentiates between neurogenic DI and nephrogenic DI). Water intake is restricted and urine osmolality is measured before and after administration of vasopressin.	Neurogenic DI: • No increase in urine osmolality with water restriction • Increased urine osmolality after vasopressin administration. Nephrogenic DI (primary renal disease) • No rise in urine osmolality after either fluid restriction or vasopressin administration	Increased osmolality regardless of water restriction and vasopressin administration because there is already too much ADH (vasopressin) which causes water to be retained in the vascular space and inappropriate excretion of sodium in the concentrated urine.
ADH suppression test (also called the "water load" test) differentiates between SIADH and other causes of hyponatremia. Normal values: 65% excretion of water load at 4 hours. 80% of water load excreted at 5 hours.	• Not applicable	• None or very little of the water load is excreted. • Patients with non-ADH causes of hyponatremia will excrete up to 80% of the fluid load.

*ADH is *against* diuresis and will not allow the kidney tubules to filter out water.

Source: Created by the author from Reference 7.

Signs and symptoms and why?

SIADH is the same thing as fluid volume excess (FVE) and dilutional hyponatremia; therefore, the patient will display these signs and symptoms:

• Decreased urine output: Oliguria/anuria

• Weight gain but without peripheral edema

• Hyponatremia (owing to sodium loss and water gain) causes cerebral dysfunction, which produces neurologic symptoms: headache, altered mental status, lethargy, confusion, seizure, and coma.

• Hypotension occurs because the hypotonic intravascular fluid is pulled from the extracellular space into the cell, causing swelling and lysis of cells.

The neurologic signs associated with SIADH result from hyponatremia which causes movement of hypotonic fluid into the cells, producing

• Cerebral edema and increased ICP

• Cerebral herniation and death[27]

• Osmotic demyelination with too rapid correction of hyponatremia

• Permanent, irreversible brain damage because of neural compression (ICP) and osmotic demyelination

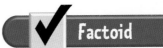

Factoid

Concentration makes numbers go UP and dilute makes numbers go DOWN. This applies to serum sodium, hematocrit, and urine specific gravity.

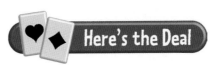

Here's the Deal

When the patient has SIADH (retaining water, water, and more water) the weight will go up, but because the excess fluid is in the vascular space, there is no peripheral edema. However, the associated hyponatremia causes the cells to swell as water is pulled in from the extracellular fluid, causing a "fingerprinting" effect over bony prominences.[11]

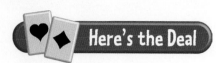

Here's the Deal

"Fluid" volume excess or deficit means that water and sodium in approximately equal parts are gained or lost within the vascular space. If the patient has a pituitary dysfunction, he or she retains or loses only water: not sodium and water! Therefore, SIADH is actually water intoxication (see Chapter 2).

Deadly Dilemma

In diabetes insipidus, the amount of urine output can be anywhere from 4 to 30 L a day! Get fluid replacement started quickly!

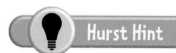

Hurst Hint

If DI occurs as a result of some type of brain injury, the symptoms usually occur three to six days postinjury and can last for up to 10 days. Therefore, be very watchful of the vital signs and urine output during this time.

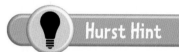

Hurst Hint

1000 mL = 2.5 lb

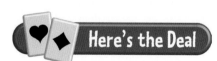

Here's the Deal

Diabetes insipidus has NOTHING to do with your blood sugar. So don't pick Accu-Cheks Q4 hours on a test!

✚ Diabetes insipidus

Signs and symptoms	Why?
Thirst and polyuria (sudden onset)	Not enough ADH; water is excreted by the kidneys in large amounts; thirst is your body's way of saying, "Drink fluids, you've lost too much."
Dehydration (You had better review all the signs and symptoms of dehydration, because they are very applicable here.)	Excessive loss of water from the vascular space.
Polydipsia (excessive thirst)	Polyuria causes dehydration. The osmoreceptors relay the message (dehydration) to the brain, so that it will trigger the sensation of thirst. (The patient needs increased water intake.)
Hypotension	Excessive loss of water from the vascular space (less volume = less pressure) and decreased peripheral resistance.
Tachycardia	The heart rate increases. The heart is trying to pump the decreased volume to perfuse vital organs.
Decreased central venous pressure (CVP)	If the vascular volume is decreased, then the volume inside the heart chambers is decreased, so CVP goes down (less volume = less pressure).
Irritability	Brain changes are associated with dehydration and sodium imbalances. Your brain doesn't like it when the volume is too low or sodium is out of balance.
Changes in LOC: lethargy to possible coma	Hypernatremia because so much water has been lost. The brain doesn't like it when sodium is too high or too low. Neurologic changes begin as a result.
Vision changes	If a tumor is causing DI, the tumor might be pressing on the optic nerve.
Weight loss	When water is lost, weight is lost.
Headache	Cellular dehydration of brain.

Source: Created by the author from References 2, 4, and 6.

Interventions and why?

Identify patients at risk for the development of DI or SIADH.

- Neurosurgic patients
- Patients following simple sinus surgery

- Traumatic brain-injured patients[31]
- Any patient with increased ICP
- Patients with other endocrine disorders (hypothyroidism, Addison's disease)

   Be alert to changes in urinary output:

- Diuresis occurs with DI.
- Oliguria/anuria occurs with SIADH.

   When ADH excess and deficit are diagnosed, rarely is the condition (SIADH or DI) a primary problem, so initially the priority is to remedy the sodium imbalance and restore circulating volume. Imaging studies may be indicated to find the source of the problem (ie, CNS or lung tumors or infections) as well as a careful drug history to identify any drugs that might be increasing or suppressing ADH production (see Table 10-6). Additional testing may be in order to differentiate various causes of the DI or SIADH (see Table 10-7).

- All traumatic brain-injured patients are monitored closely for the onset of polyuria, which may precede mild hypernatremia.
- Electrolytes are monitored on an ongoing basis when patients are at risk for conditions that could precipitate DI or SIADH.
- Because of the risks associated with the administration of hypertonic saline, dietary sodium is the first-line therapy if the patient can eat and drink.
- Thereafter, lactated Ringers solution and isotonic saline are indicated to raise the serum sodium.
- Only severe hyponatremia accompanied by neurologic manifestations warrants the use of hypertonic saline with a loop diuretic.
- Sodium imbalance must be corrected slowly to avoid serious and possibly irreversible or fatal neurologic sequelae.[11,31,32]

   Diabetes insipidus responds well to slow correction of hypernatremia with hypotonic electrolyte solutions (1/4 NS) or D5W plus the administration of DDAVP (desmopressin acetate) a synthetic vasopressin.[11,34,35]

   Monitor serum electrolyte levels for imbalances and report to physician:

- Hyponatremia occurs with SIADH.
- Hypernatremia occurs with DI.

   Monitor fluid volume status, being alert for signs of:

- Water intoxication with SIADH
- FVD and shock with DI

   When the patient has a fluid problem, these interventions are always indicated:

- Monitor intake and output.
- Weigh daily and record.
- Monitor vital signs frequently as indicated.
- Monitor serum sodium levels, being alert to trends.

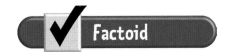

Early recognition and treatment of DI or SIADH can avert serious consequences.

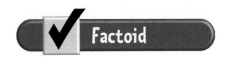

Polyuria causes shock!

Diabetes insipidus (DI) requires the nurse to:

• Initiate sodium poor IV fluid (ie, D5W) as prescribed.

Clinical alert

Serum sodium must be decreased slowly to prevent cerebral edema. While diluting the patient with prescribed IVF, the serum sodium is monitored at regular intervals and must not be decreased any greater than 1 to 2 mEq/L per hour.[11,31]

• Administer prescribed vasopressin (DDAVP).

Syndrome of inappropriate antidiuretic hormone (SIADH) mandates:

• Restrict fluids (800 mL/24 hours) as prescribed.[11]

• Auscultate lung fields (anterior and posterior) for moist rales.

• Auscultate heart sounds for gallops (S3 or S4).

• Administer prescribed hypertonic sodium (3% or 5%) in conjunction with furosemide (Lasix) for severe hyponatremia accompanied by neurologic signs.

• Monitor serum sodium throughout IV sodium replacement therapy at one- to two-hour intervals.[32]

Clinical alert

Hypertonic sodium is administered very slowly per pump with close monitoring. Too rapid correction of the hypotonic state can cause osmotic demyelination (Fig. 10-7).[32]

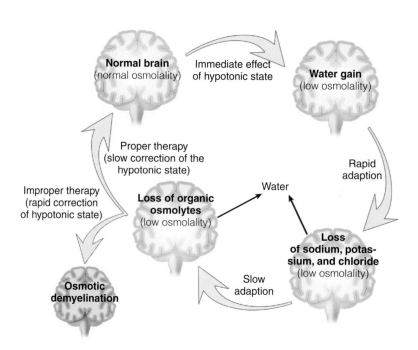

▶ Figure 10-7. Physiology of hypotonicity: adaption and correction.

PATIENT TEACHING   Any patient who is discharged from the emergency department after having any head trauma, or discharged from the outpatient department following sinus surgery should be taught to:

* Notify your doctor immediately for any increase (or decrease) in urinary output.

* Family members are to return you to the emergency department immediately for any change in neurologic status (alteration in mental status, unusual sleepiness, or confusion).

What can harm my patient?

The excessive urinary output of dilute urine and hemoconcentration associated with DI can lead to

* Hypotension and decreased organ perfusion

* Shock with multisystem organ failure

* Hypernatremia, which produces neurologic changes

Cutting edge

A large retroactive study of traumatic brain injured patients (Glasgow score <8) treated in an ICU setting with mechanical ventilation revealed that hypernatremia was independently related to increased (threefold) risk for death. More than half of the patients received desmopressin acetate (DDAVP) upon onset of polyuria and mild (mean 150 mEq/L) hypernatremia when central diabetes insipidus was suspected. Many received mannitol an osmotic diuretic to reduce brain swelling. DDAVP was noted to modify the risk for death significantly.[33]

✛ Thyroid disorders
Let's get the normal stuff straight!

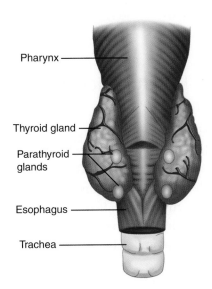

◀ Figure 10-8. The thyroid gland and parathyroid glands.

Pharynx

Thyroid gland

Parathyroid glands

Esophagus

Trachea

The **thyroid gland** lies under the larynx and takes iodine from the blood to make thyroid hormones (Fig. 10-8). When thyroid hormone levels get low, the hypothalamus is triggered to release thyroid-releasing hormone (TRH) → TRH triggers the anterior pituitary to release thyroid-stimulating hormone (TSH) →TSH stimulates the thyroid gland to produce thyroid hormone that is released into the blood → metabolism increases and energy levels increase.

- The thyroid produces three hormones:
  - T3 = triiodothyronine increases metabolic rate and growth of cells and tissues; and indirectly increases blood glucose levels.
  - T4 = thyroxine increase metabolic rate of cells and tissues; precursor to T3; and indirectly increases blood glucose levels.
- Calcitonin:
  - Decreases intestines ability to absorb calcium
  - Decreases osteoclast activity in the bones, reducing calcium release
  - Decreases calcium reabsorption from the kidney tubules, causing excretion
- When thinking about thyroid hormones, think energy and metabolism! You either have too much or not enough.

How does thyroid hormone affect the body?
- Increases the metabolism of protein, fat, and glucose
- Increases body temperature as metabolism increases
- Increases oxygen use as metabolism increases
- Aids in neural and skeletal system development of fetuses
- Helps regulate secretion of growth hormone; aids in normal growth and development
- Aids in red blood cell production
- Affects respiratory rate: too much thyroid hormone increases respiratory rate and too little decreases respiratory rate

---

✚ Hyperthyroidism

What is it?

Hyperthyroidism is caused by an overactive thyroid that leads to increased levels of thyroid hormone, increasing the body's metabolism. Sometimes the terms Graves' disease and hyperthyroidism are used interchangeably. Graves' disease is an autoimmune disorder that **causes** hyperthyroidism. If you come across a test question on Graves' disease, think hyperthyroidism! Hyperthyroidism is mainly seen in women, and is most common after childbirth or during menopause.

What causes it and why?

Causes	Why?
Graves' disease.	A gene causes antibodies to stimulate the thyroid to produce and secrete excess thyroid hormones.
Infected thyroid: viral or bacterial thyroiditis	Virus or bacteria invade the thyroid, causing a release of more thyroid hormones.
Thyroiditis: acute, inflammatory problem. The thyroid does return to normal with treatment.	Inflammation causes the thyroid gland to release stored thyroid hormone.
Toxic nodules (adenoma), tumors, thyroid cancer.	Tumors and nodules can produce too much thyroid hormone.
Overactive pituitary: very rare cause.	Produces too much TSH, which triggers thyroid gland to release thyroid hormone.
Any severe illness.	The body's natural response is to produce more hormones for energy.
Toxic substances and radiation exposure.	It causes inflammation that releases stored thyroid hormone.

Source: Created by the author from References 1, 2, and 4.

Signs and symptoms and why?

Signs and symptoms	Why?
Goiter	Overstimulated and overworked thyroid; thyroid hypertrophy.
Thyroid may be palpable; may auscultate a bruit	Enlarged thyroid; increased circulation to area causes bruit.
Nervousness, jitteriness, tremor	Too much energy; stimulation of sympathetic nervous system; muscles react more vigorously because of an increased effect on neural synapses.
Heat intolerance, sweating	Increased metabolism.
Weight loss in the presence of increased appetite	Increased metabolism.
Increased bowel movements; hyperactive bowel sounds	Hyperactive GI system.
Exophthalmos (protrusion of eyeball): only seen with Graves' disease	Fluid accumulates behind the eye, which pushes the eye forward; increased fat deposits around the eye.
Decreased concentration, mood swings	Hyperstimulated central nervous system.
Clumsiness	Increased spinal cord activity.
Moist, smooth, flushed warm skin	Increased metabolism causing sweating and warmth; vasodilation helps body heat escape.

(*Continued*)

Signs and symptoms	Why?
Fine, soft hair Premature graying Hair loss; weak nails	Dermal layer of skin is affected; increased circulation causes increased growth and brittleness of hair and nails.
Normal blood pressure; increased pulse (90–160 beats/min at rest); bounding pulse; arrhythmia; palpitation (atrial fibrillation in clients over age 50)	Increased cardiac output; systemic vasodilation effect to help the body rid of heat. The two counteract each other keeping the BP in a close to normal range. BP will go up if the client begins to go in to thyroid storm; arrhythmias and palpitations caused by stimulation of nervous system.
Increased cardiac output	Increased work load; however, if it continues over a period of time, then heart failure (left ventricular hypertrophy) can begin, which would result in a decreased cardiac output; depends on length of untreated hyperthyroidism.
Increased respiratory rate	Increased oxygen demand owing to hypermetabolic state; client breathes faster to get more oxygen.
Dyspnea on exertion	Hypermetabolic uses more oxygen. Heart failure causes decreased cardiac output preventing forward blood flow, which results in backward blood flow into the lungs.
Menstrual problems (amenorrhea); fertility problems	Thyroid hormone controls FSH and LH, which aid in regulation of ovulation and menses. Excess TH alters the function.
Decreased libido	The thyroid gland influences all hormones.
Gynecomastia in men (rare)	The thyroid gland influences all hormones; may cause an increase in estrogen.

Source: Created by the author from References 1 and 7.

Testing, testing, testing

- Thyroid stimulating hormone (TSH): Low or undetectable; non-fasting; recent administration of radioisotopes for other diagnostic tests may affect results.

- T3 and T4: Increased; may be affected by recently administered radio-isotopes, selected drugs, pregnancy.

- Radioactive iodine uptake test (scan): Increased; NPO status for procedure. Question physician if and when the following preparations should be stopped: iodized salt, thyroid hormone replacements, anti-thyroid medications, or medications containing iodine such as multi-vitamins, cough syrups, or some heart medications, such as amiodarone. The procedure is contraindicated for women who are pregnant or breastfeeding.

- Thyroid scan: Increased iodine uptake with hyperthyroidism; contraindicated with pregnancy, breastfeeding, or allergy to iodine.

- Thyrotropin-releasing hormone (TRH) test: TSH increase within 30 minutes after receiving TRH; administered via IV bolus.

- Thyroid ultrasound: Differentiates cystic form from solid nodules; may be used to assist needle biopsy.
- Pregnancy test: Hyperthyroidism can occur during the first four months of pregnancy when hCG levels are high; pregnancy can cause hyperthyroidism.
- CT or MRI of the eye orbit if client has exophthalmos, especially if it is unilateral: Monitor for pressure on the optic nerve or orbital contents. Clients should wear loose clothing without zippers or metallic implements, remove all jewelry, eyeglasses, hearing aids, and removable dental appliances; may be asked to abstain from eating or drinking for 1 hour prior to procedure.
- Antinuclear antibody (ANA): Presence of autoimmune marker because Graves' disease is an autoimmune disease affecting the thyroid gland.
- Fine needle biopsy: Etiology of nodular lesions. This is the preferred approach to clients with thyroid masses.

Interventions

Euthyroid is the desired goal of treatment; however, patients may develop the opposing thyroid condition after thyroidectomy or gland irradiation and with administration of thyroid to treat hypothyroidism!

- Notify your doctor for recurrence of any signs of hypothyroidism or hyperthyroidism. (Refer to table for teaching signs and symptoms.)
- Consult with your doctor before taking health food supplements or other medications because these may interact with thyroid hormones.
- Lifelong thyroid replacement therapy is required. Symptoms of hypothyroidism will recur if the medication is stopped.
- Avoid extremes of temperature (hot or cold) until a normal thyroid level (euthyroid state) is achieved.
- Wear medic-alert identification and carry medical information card.
- Keep regular follow-up visits with your doctor to monitor return to normal thyroid and/or the need for adjustment of medication.
- Client specific; depends on the severity of the disease.
- Monitor for arrhythmias; maintain pulse at 80 beats/min; manage CHF if it occurs.
- Propylthiouracil (Propyl-Thyracil) and methimazole (Tapazole): inhibits thyroid hormone synthesis.
- Potassium iodide (Pima), Lugol's solution, sodium iodide (Iodotope): inhibits synthesis and release of hormone.
- Beta blockers, atenolol (Tenormin), propranolol (Inderal): decrease effects of thyroid hormone; decrease tachycardia and nervousness.
- Acetaminophen: Decrease fever; aspirin is contraindicated because it displaces thyroid hormone from thyroglobulin, causing thyroid hormone levels to increase.

- Radioactive iodine: Treatment of choice for Graves' disease; given slowly until the client is euthyroid (normal thyroid function). Only a single oral dose of I^{131} is needed. Contraindicated in pregnancy and clients are informed to not become pregnant for 3 months after treatment; pregnancy test prior to initiation of treatment. Antithyroid drugs are sometimes given before and after radioiodine treatment.
- Propylthiouracil (Propyl-Thyracil): Preferred drug during pregnancy and breastfeeding.
- Surgery (thyroidectomy): When the client continues to relapse or has a large goiter.
  - All or part of the thyroid may be removed in an effort to drop the serum thyroid hormone levels.
  - Monitor for hypocalcemia postop: Parathyroids may be removed during surgery; IV calcium should be readily available.
  - Iodine compounds such as potassium iodide (Pima), Lugol's solution, and SSKI may be given preoperatively. They decrease vascularity in order to prevent bleeding prior to surgery. They must be given with milk or juice with straw because they stain the teeth.
  - Monitor for tracheal swelling or respiratory distress; have tracheostomy set readily available.
- Thyroid storm treatment: Antithyroid drugs prevent the conversion of T4 to T3; beta blockers decrease sympathetic effects such as increased blood pressure and tachycardia; corticosteroids decrease conversion of T4 to T3; increase fluids and caloric intake to hydrate and maintain strength; monitor for congestive heart failure and stroke; administer oxygen; decrease body temperature; sedate for comfort.
- Client may require referral to specialist for high doses of prednisone, orbital irradiation, or decompression of the orbit by surgery in order to save vision.

PATIENT TEACHING   The radioactive iodine recipient should:

- Avoid kissing and close personal contact, interaction with children, and food preparation for others for a period of days.
- Drink large amounts of fluid to flush radioactive material.
- Flush the toilet twice after each use.
- Avoid pregnancy and breastfeeding until cleared by physician.
- Nothing by mouth two hours prior to or following the procedure to decrease nausea.
- Salivary gland swelling may occur; suck on hard candy to decrease severity.
- Sore throat may occur; use acetaminophen (Tylenol) as an analgesic.
- Ophthalmologic treatment:
  - Employ eye lubricants such as artificial tears, petrolatum, and Lacri-Lube.
  - Use sunglasses when outdoors.

- Elevate the bed at night (to decrease fluid retention behind the eyes).
- Eye protectors during sleep can be helpful to protect the protruding eye.
- Consume a well-balanced diet of adequate calories to prevent weight loss.

Clinical alert

- The most important concept regarding levothyroxine administration is that the patient develop a consistent routine for taking the medication at the same time each day (in the morning to avoid insomnia) 1/2 to 1 hour before breakfast to maintain a constant hormone level.

What can harm my patient and why?

Complications	Why?
Extreme tachycardia; arrhythmias	Increased metabolic rate and oxygen demand; dehydration and hypovolemia
Hyperpyrexia	Increased metabolic rate
Respiratory alkalosis	Increased respiratory rate results in loss of CO_2
Hypocalcemia	May occur post thyroidectomy
Thyroid storm	Untreated or inadequately treated hyperthyroidism
Rebound thyroid effect	Surge of thyroid hormone release owing to drop in hormone levels post thyroidectomy

Cutting edge

In a recent study TSH levels were monitored in patients whose daily levothyroxine (T4) was administered "with breakfast," "before breakfast," and "at bedtime." Keeping in mind the inverse relationship between TSH levels and circulating thyroid hormone (TH) levels, it was found that taking the medication in a fasting state produced higher hormone levels (lower TSH levels). Because there is a fine line between therapeutic and toxic levels of TH, it is recommended that levothyroxine be taken on an empty stomach to maintain consistent levels and avoid fluctuations.[34]

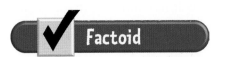

Factoid

A thyroid storm can be precipitated by any physical or psychological stress.

✛ Hypothyroidism

What is it?

Hypothyroidism is characterized by underactivity of the thyroid gland. As a result, the thyroid does not produce enough thyroid hormone, which slows all body functions and metabolism.

- Low levels of thyroid hormone lead to a decreased metabolic rate; everything slows down.

- An insufficient amount of thyroid hormone causes abnormal lipid metabolism, with increased cholesterol and triglyceride levels. These two things increase the presence of atherosclerosis and cardiac disease. The etiology of this particular aspect of hypothyroidism is not well understood.

  - The terms *myxedema* and *hypothyroidism* are frequently used interchangeably. Different sources explain myxedema different ways. Some sources say myxedema is a condition of edema that results from prolonged hypothyroidism. Other sources say that when hypothyroidism becomes severe, it is called myxedema. The fluid associated with myxedema is made of mucins that trap water in the interstitial space. Pleural, cardiac, and abdominal effusions are a result of this process.

  - Myxedema coma is a rare presentation of untreated hypothyroidism. It is usually seen in elderly women with chronic hypothyroidism. It is an end-stage manifestation of hypothyroidism.

- Cretinism is hypothyroidism present at birth. This is very dangerous if not detected early because it can lead to slowed mental and physical development. A baby's thyroid level is checked in the hospital. If the baby does not develop appropriately, sleeps a lot, or gains an unusual amount of weight, a thyroid panel may be repeated. Once detected, treatment is immediate.

Causes and why?

Causes	Why?
Hashimoto thyroiditis (most common cause of hypothyroidism)	The thyroid is gradually destroyed, producing decreased amounts of thyroid hormone.
Congenital defects	Poor or absent thyroid development in utero.
Thyroidectomy (surgically induced hypothyroidism)	If you do not have a thyroid, you cannot make thyroid hormone.
Radiation therapy used in treatment for cancers of the head and neck	Loss of thyroid tissue decreases hormone output.
Antithyroid medications (drug induced)	Decreased thyroid hormone production.
Thyroiditis	Bacterial or viral infection causes decreased thyroid hormone.
Pituitary failure (very rare)	Cannot produce TSH, so thyroid hormone levels drop.
Pregnancy	Immune system response; antibodies attack the thyroid decreasing output of thyroid hormones.
Iodine deficiency	Dietary iodine is necessary for thyroid hormone production. This is only seen in certain parts of the world (in the United States, dietary iodine is added to table salt.)

(Continued)

Causes	Why?
Medications (aka drug goitrogen)	Can cause a decreased output of thyroid hormones.
Lithium carbonate (Eskalith)	
Iodide	
Propylthiouracil (Propyl-Thyracil)	
Methimazole (Tapazole)	
Sulfonamides	
Amiodarone (Cordarone)	
Interferon alpha (Alferon N)	
Interleukin 2 (Proleukin)	

Source: Created by the author from References 2 and 4.

Signs and symptoms and why?

Signs and symptoms	Why?
Slowed thinking, decreased attention span, clumsiness, slowed movements, slurred speech	Low energy.
Decreased heart rate leading to low cardiac output; decreased temperature	Metabolism is slowed leading to a decreased temperature.
Fluid volume excess	If cardiac output is decreased (from low heart rate), then renal perfusion is compromised, leading to decreased fluid excretion. If fluid is not excreted, it remains in the body and builds up, causing volume excess.
Fatigue	Low energy.
Puffy hands, feet, and eyes	Fluid retention.
Intolerance to cold temperatures; cold hands and feet	Decreased metabolic rate and decreased heat production; client is already cold and can't tolerate being colder.
Increased weight	Slowed metabolism; weight gain owing to slowed metabolism, not increased intake.
Decreased caloric requirements	When metabolism is slowed, fewer calories are needed.
Constipation (can lead to megacolon)	Slowed GI tract related to low metabolism.
Change in reproductive function (no ovulation—also called anovulation)	When the thyroid is sick, the reproductive system is usually affected; and the thyroid has an effect on FSH, LH, and prolactin levels.
Dry, flaky skin; thinning hair; may lose outer third of eyebrows; brittle fingernails	Lack of nutrients.
Prolonged deep tendon reflex (especially ankle jerk); ataxia, nystagmus	TH affects neural control of muscle tone. A decrease in TH causes muscles to react slowly.

Source: Created by the author from References 2 and 4.

Testing, testing, testing

- Newborn screening is performed after delivery in all states and prior to leaving the hospital. Infants can still develop hypothyroidism several weeks later, even though they had a normal TSH while hospitalized.
- TSH is elevated. Thyroid tissue says to the brain, "We need stimulation in order to produce thyroid hormone. Send MORE. Send MORE!" This occurs in primary hypothyroidism. In pituitary insufficiency, the TSH may be decreased or normal. If the pituitary is the main problem, then it may have difficulty secreting TSH.
- Serum T3 and T4 is decreased, especially T4.
- The thyroid antibody test is done to confirm the presence of chronic thyroiditis. (Hashimoto's thyroiditis is an autoimmune problem.)
- Serial ultrasound studies detect changes in the thyroid over time.
- A thyroid scan or sonogram detects structural abnormalities.
- CT and MRI detects pituitary or hypothalamic lesions, causing secondary hypothyroidism. The patient may be asked to refrain from eating or drinking for one hour prior to the procedure. Clients should wear loose clothing; remove jewelry, eyeglasses, hearing aid, and removable dental work. Contrast is contraindicated for those with previous reaction or allergy to shellfish.
- Cholesterol is elevated.
- An EKG shows varying degrees of bradycardia.

Interventions

- Levothyroxine (Synthroid) is the treatment of choice even in pregnant women. Watch for cardiac problems, especially in the elderly because of increase in heart rate and work load. Remember, too, most hypothyroid clients have high cholesterol and triglycerides.
- Women who take estrogen may require higher doses of thyroid supplement.
- Levothyroxine must be continued for life and may need to be adjusted periodically throughout the client's life by testing TSH levels and monitoring clinical status.
- IV levothyroxine is given for myxedema in the hospital. These clients will need warm blankets because of hypothermia. Sometimes intubation is needed for assisted mechanical ventilation.

PATIENT TEACHING

- Lifelong hormone replacement is necessary. Do not manipulate hormone replacement dosage without consultation with a physician. Because of variable bioavailability, do not change the brand of drug without the physician's knowledge and consent.
- Avoid extremely cold environments.
- Consume adequate fluids and a high-fiber diet to encourage GI tract motility.

- Synthetic hormone replacements should be taken on an empty stomach to stabilize absorption. Four hours should separate this medication from antacids, iron, or vitamin/mineral supplements.

What can harm my patient and why?

Complications	Why?
Sedation	Decreased metabolic rate places patient at risk. Sedation can further depress metabolism.
Myxedema coma	Severely depressed metabolism can cause stupor, hypoventilation, hypoglycemia, hyponatremia, hypotension, and hypothermia.*
Chest pain, myocardial infarction, heart failure	Decreased metabolic rate causes decreased heart rate and cardiac output, resulting in inadequate blood supply to the heart muscle. Heart failure can result if heart cannot sustain adequate forward blood flow.
Megacolon	Slowed GI motility and peristalsis can result in large collection of colon content, stretching the colon.
Replacement therapy reactions	Replacement hormone therapy should be initiated carefully. As metabolism increases, the client is at risk for cardiovascular complications.

*Major symptoms include cardiovascular collapse, hypoventilation, hyponatremia, hypoglycemia, and lactic acidosis. The death rate for myxedema coma is extremely high and is a life-threatening emergency. Severe hypothyroid clients are at risk for myxedema coma when exposed to the following conditions: acute illness, anesthesia, surgery, hypothermia, chemotherapy, sedatives, rapid withdrawal of thyroid medications, and untreated or undertreated hypothyroidism.

✚ Parathyroid disorders

Let's get the normal stuff straight!

The parathyroid glands are attached to the bottom of and behind the thyroid. We have four parathyroids, each about the size of a pea. The parathyroid glands regulate calcium in the blood. The parathyroid glands secrete parathyroid hormone (PTH), which **makes the serum calcium level go up.** PTH works by pulling calcium from the bone, then placing it in the blood. It decreases calcium excretion from the kidneys and stimulates calcium reabsorption through the gastrointestinal tract.

- Too much PTH = hyperparathyroidism = hypercalcemia, hypophosphatemia, bone damage, and renal damage
- What causes an increase in PTH secretion? Low blood calcium. When blood calcium is low, PTH secretion increases which causes calcium to be pulled from the bone. This causes bone breakdown and the serum calcium to go up.

✚ Hyperparathyroidism

What is it?

Hyperparathyroidism is overactivity of the parathyroid glands resulting in excess production of PTH, leading to increased serum calcium (hypercalcemia). Remember, when PTH is secreted, it pulls calcium from the bone and places it in the blood; therefore, serum calcium goes up.

Causes and why?

Causes	Why?
Dysfunction of the parathyroid gland (eg, adenoma of one of the four parathyroid glands) which is considered a primary dysfunction	Adenoma is a benign tumor. These adenomas secrete PTH and are responsible for hypercalcemia.
Renal failure: example of secondary cause of hyperparathyroidism	Certain medical conditions can cause the parathyroids to produce too much PTH in response to chronically low levels of serum calcium. In renal failure, phosphorus is not excreted, causing hyperphosphatemia; therefore causing hypocalcemia (owing to the inverse relationship). Hypocalcemia stimulates the parathyroids to produce more PTH.
Vitamin D deficiency	Without vitamin D, calcium isn't absorbed well. As a result, the parathyroids produce PTH to get the serum calcium back up.
Pregnancy and lactation	Hormones stimulate the parathyroid glands predisposing them to tumor. This is why it is more common in women than men and children.

Source: Created by author from References 1, 2, and 6.

Signs and symptoms and why?

Signs and symptoms	Why?
Neurologic: Depression, confusion, lethargy, decreased level of consciousness (LOC)	Too much calcium has a sedative effect
Arrhythmias	Calcium is essential in the function of muscles. Any and all muscles can be affected by calcium problems, and your heart is definitely a muscle.
Gastrointestinal: nausea, vomiting, weight loss, constipation

These are the most common symptoms seen in mild cases of hyperparathyroidism | Sedative action of calcium causes everything to be slowed down. If everything is slowed, the small intestine (smooth muscle) is slowed, decreasing peristalsis. Calcium is essential in nerve function. |
| Kidney stones (renal calculi): extreme tendency for renal calculi | Most kidney stones are made from calcium. Hyperparathyroidism is caused by too much calcium in the blood. |
| Muscular: atrophy of muscles with weakness and fatigue, decreased deep tendon reflexes (DTRs), fractures, and kyphosis (curvature) of the spine | Calcium is essential to muscle function and affects muscle tone. Too much calcium causes sedation of the muscles.

Calcium is pulled from the bone into the blood. |
| Osteoporosis puts the client at risk for fractures | Calcium is pulled from the bone into the blood. |

Source: Created by the author from References 1, 2, and 6.

Testing, testing, testing

- PTH hormone is elevated.

- Serum calcium: Elevated (hypercalcemia) – serum calcium above 10.5 mg/dL or ionized calcium >5.4 mg/dL.

- Serum phosphate: low, <2.5 mg/dL (hypophosphatemia). Why? When PTH is increased, calcium is pulled from the bone, as is phosphate. However, PTH stimulates renal excretion of phosphate.

- Urinalysis: Elevated phosphate due to excessive loss of phosphate in the urine

- 24-hour urine collection tests kidney function and measures the amount of calcium excreted in the urine. Instruct the patient to empty the bladder and discard the urine at the time the test starts. Save all urine from each voiding into a separate container to prevent contamination from bowel movement. Provide specific instructions for container storage. At the time to end the test, instruct the patient to void, saving the urine. Label the container and submit to the laboratory.

- Serum phosphate level: Serum phosphate increases because the kidneys can't secrete phosphorus if hyperparathyroidism is caused by renal failure.

- Alkaline phosphatase increases because calcium is being pulled from the bone. Any time the bone is significantly disturbed, osteoblasts are active, and alkaline phosphatase is elevated. Alkaline phosphatase goes up (ie, bone cancer, multiple myeloma, etc) because when osteoblasts are active, they secrete large quantities of alkaline phosphatase.

- A bone mineral density test or X-ray determines the degree of osteoporosis.

- Imaging studies detect the presence of a tumor or abnormal parathyroid gland, identify its location prior to surgery, and identify possible kidney stones.

Interventions and why?

- Parathyroidectomy: calcium, phosphorus, and magnesium levels must be monitored closely and treated promptly. Serum calcium will drop during the first five postop days.

- Treat severe hypercalcemia with hospitalization and intense hydration with IV saline to flush out the calcium. Monitor for secondary congestive heart failure. Check lung sounds frequently to prevent fluid volume excess and pulmonary edema.

- Bisphosphonates for hypercalcemia: Some are given PO to elevate the phosphorus level in the blood; therefore, decrease the serum calcium.

- Drugs to inhibit bone resorption: calcitonin (SQ Calcimar).

- Glucocorticoids decrease calcium absorption in the intestines and increase renal excretion of calcium as well.

- Dialysis removes excess calcium. It is also used in clients who are in renal failure.

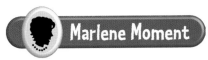
Marlene Moment

Hypercalcemia often will cause no signs and symptoms, but those who are symptomatic often complain of problems with "bones, stones, abdominal groans, psychic moans, with fatigue overtones!" (Source: McPhee, and Papadakis. *CMTD*. McGraw-Hill; 2005.)

- If the client is on digoxin (Lanoxin), be very cautious because toxicity to digoxin is likely.
- Avoid thiazide diuretics because they slow calcium excretion.
- Strain the urine for stones.
- Turn the patient gently, as he or she is at high risk for pathologic fractures.
- Watch for the development of a peptic ulcer. High serum calcium causes the stomach to produce excessive acid.
- Watch for arrhythmias.
- Provide an acidotic diet.
- Acidic drugs are frequently used for treatment of renal stones.

PATIENT TEACHING

- Avoid calcium-containing antacids or supplements.
- Limit foods high in calcium.
- Drink cranberry juice to lower the pH of the urine.
- Initiate mobility as tolerated—rocking chair to walking.
- Use stool softeners as needed to prevent or decrease constipation.

What can harm my patient and why?

Complications	Why?
Kidney stones; renal failure	Excess calcium in the blood contributes to kidney stones.
Osteoporosis leading to fractures	Excess PTH causes calcium to be pulled from the bone, leaving it brittle.
Hypoparathyroidism postop	Removal of parathyroid glands results in severe decrease in serum calcium the first five days.
Cardiac problems	Abnormal calcium levels.
Peptic ulcer disease; hemorrhage, perforation	When serum calcium is high, the stomach produces too much acid, which irritates tissues, and promotes bleeding or perforation.
Fluid volume overload	Owing to rapid IV saline administration.

Cutting edge

In lieu of removing the parathyroid gland using general anesthesia, a minimally invasive, radioguided parathyroidectomy is now available using local anesthesia. This surgical approach reduces the risk of hemorrhage and vocal cord damage.

Chronic renal failure is the most common etiology for secondary hyperparathyroidism. A recently approved drug, paricalcitol (Zemplar), may be administered orally or by injection during hemodialysis. Serum plasma levels of PTH are tested at two-week intervals for three months, then monthly for three months. Determine the individual dosage. Stable patients may be checked every three months. Large amounts of aluminum, such as Maalox, Mylanta, Gaviscon, and Amphojel, should be avoided.

✛ Hypoparathyroidism

Let's get the normal stuff straight!

Too little PTH = hypoparathyroidism, hypocalcemia, hyperphosphatemia, hyperreflexia, and cognitive changes (altered sensorium).

What causes a decrease in PTH secretion? High serum calcium or high serum magnesium. Magnesium is chemically similar to calcium. If serum calcium is high, then PTH is not released. PTH is only released when more calcium is needed in the blood.

What is it?

Hypoparathyroidism results from decreased activity of the parathyroid gland, which leads to inadequate production of PTH. As a result, the serum calcium goes down and the serum phosphorus goes up because PTH normally stimulates renal excretion of phosphate. In hypoparathyroidism, the bones remain intact.

Causes and why?

Causes	Why?
Damage to or accidental removal of the parathyroid glands during a thyroidectomy or surgery for throat or neck cancer; most common cause of hypoparathyroidism	Decreased amounts of PTH cause serum calcium levels to drop.
Autoimmune destruction of the parathyroid gland	Decreased amounts of PTH cause serum calcium levels to drop.
Radiation treatments of face and neck	Parathyroids are destroyed, leading to decreased PTH secretion.
Hypomagnesemia: as seen in alcoholism because of poor nutrition and increased excretion by kidneys	Must have adequate magnesium levels for the parathyroid to secrete PTH.

Source: Created by the author from References 2 and 4.

Signs and symptoms and why?

Signs and symptoms	Why?
Neurologic: hyperactive reflexes, irritability, seizure activity, anxiety, stridor, laryngospasm.	Calcium is essential to muscle function. Hypoparathyroidism causes low calcium, thus preventing a sedative effect on the body.
Arrhythmias.	The heart is made of muscle, and calcium is essential for muscle function.
Musculoskeletal: tetany, positive Chvostek's and Trousseau's signs, increased DTRs. The bones remain intact.	With hypoparathyroidism there is not enough calcium. Nonsedative = hyperactivity, excitability.
	In regard to the calcification of bones, this occurs because the calcium moves from the serum and blood into the bones.

(Continued)

Signs and symptoms	Why?
Carpal pedal spasm	Lack of calcium, which is necessary for proper neuromuscular function (not enough sedative).
Tingling of the mouth or extremities	Lack of calcium, which is necessary for proper neuromuscular function (not enough sedative).
Integumentary: skin is dry, nails are brittle, alopecia (thinning of the hair), and malformation of the teeth	Hair loss and skin changes can occur as calcium has a role in nutrition that is crucial for hair growth and skin cell development. Low calcium can also cause a defect in cellular immunity that can affect hair and skin cell development. If a client is hypocalcemic, then the client is also hyperphosphatemic. Phosphorus plays a role in cell division; therefore, too much phosphorus can affect the cells of the skin and hair.

Source: Created by the author from References 2 and 4.

Testing, testing, testing

- Serum calcium: low
- Serum phosphate: high
- PTH: decreased
- Urine calcium: decreased
- Serum alkaline phosphatase: normal
- EKG changes associated with hypocalcemia

Interventions and why?

- IV calcium.
- Calcium acetate given with meals to bind phosphate: lowers the serum phosphorus and increases serum calcium.
- Medications to decrease seizures and relax muscles: used until calcium level normalizes.
- Increased dietary intake of calcium.
- PO calcium supplements.
- Quiet, nonstimulating environment.
- Estrogen replacement in postmenopausal women: reduces hypercalcemia.
- Avoid digitalis preparations in the presence of calcium imbalances, which could cause toxicity.
- Vitamin D added to the diet to enhance calcium absorption.
- Thiazide diuretics to enhance calcium retention.
- Monitor for and treat arrhythmias.
- Phosphorus-binding drugs (Maalox, Mylanta, Amphojel) lower serum phosphorus.
- PTH is given only occasionally because of the extreme expense, and it has not been shown to be very effective.

PATIENT TEACHING

- Avoid carbonated soft drinks, which contain phosphorus.
- Consume a high calcium, low phosphorus diet.

What can harm my patient and why?

Complications	Why?
Arrhythmias	Heart is made of muscle, and calcium is essential for muscle function. Imbalance causes dysrhythmias.
Laryngospasm	Larynx is made of muscle, and calcium is essential for muscle function. Imbalance causes spasm.
Seizures	With hypoparathyroidism there is not enough calcium. Nonsedative = hyperactivity, excitability.
Kidney stones	Calcium is excreted through the kidneys, so stone formation is possible.
Rapid administration of calcium	Use caution with calcium administration or replacement. Monitor for hyperparathyroidism.

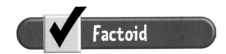

Factoid

Milk, milk products, and egg yolks are excluded from the diet; while high in calcium, they are also high is phosphorus. Spinach is excluded because of the presence of oxalate, which causes the formation of insoluble calcium.

✦ Adrenal disorders

Let's get the normal stuff straight!

There are two adrenal glands. They live in the penthouse of the kidney (the top floor, that is) and have an inner layer and an outer layer. The inner layer is called the *adrenal medulla*, which is functionally related to the sympathetic nervous system, secreting epinephrine and norepinephrine in response to sympathetic stimulation. The outer layer is called the *adrenal cortex*, which produces glucocorticoids, mineralocorticoids, and sex hormones, hormones called *corticosteroids*. The pituitary secretes ACTH, which then stimulates the adrenal cortex to release hormones (Fig. 10-9).

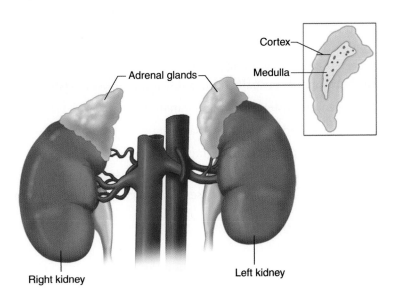

◄ Figure 10-9. The kidneys, adrenal glands, adrenal cortex, and adrenal medulla with cross-section.

Adrenal cortex

The hormones the adrenal cortex produces are frequently called *steroids*. The first major steroid is aldosterone, which is the principal mineralo-corticoid, and the second is cortisol, which is the principal glucocorti-coid. Steroids are produced naturally in the body, but synthetic steroids are also administered as drugs (eg, cortisone, prednisone, Solu-Medrol, Solu-Cortef, hydrocortisone).

Glucocorticoids

- Stimulate gluconeogenesis—the formation of carbohydrates from proteins and other substances by the liver.
- Provide amino acids and glucose during times of stress.
- Suppress the immune system because of powerful immunosuppressive and anti-inflammatory properties.
- Stimulate fat breakdown for energy production. Glucocorticoids are considered to be catabolic steroids because they break down the body's stored resources during times of need.

Mineralocorticoids

- There is one major mineralocorticoid—aldosterone. Aldosterone causes sodium and water retention in the vascular space and potassium excretion from the body. Therefore, aldosterone plays a major role in body fluid regulation.
  Aldosterone secretion is increased by:
- Low fluid volume levels in the vascular space (shock or hypovolemia)
- High blood levels of potassium (inverse relationship with sodium)

✚ Sex hormones

Sex hormones are actually made by the adrenal cortex and the gonads, which include the ovaries and testes.

Gonadocorticoids is one name for sex hormones. Another name is androgens—think masculine characteristics.

Sex hormones are usually broken down into three categories:

1. Androgens, testosterone being the main one

2. Estrogens, estradiol being the main one

3. Progestogens, progesterone being the main one

The majority of testosterone in males is produced during puberty; therefore, this is when we see secondary sexual characteristics begin to form.

✚ Addison's disease

What is it?

Addison's disease is the same as adrenal hypofunction or adrenal insufficiency.

- Primary Addison's disease is caused by the adrenal gland itself.
- Secondary Addison's disease is caused by a problem outside of the adrenal gland.

If there is not enough aldosterone, the body cannot hold on to sodium and water anymore and begins to excrete sodium and water, causing a drop in the vascular volume.

Causes and why?

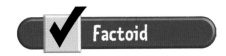

Causes	Why?
Primary cause is an immune problem	Antibodies kill the adrenal tissue, decreasing steroid secretion.
Bilateral adrenalectomy: primary cause, if you want to get picky	Lack of adrenal glands makes it impossible to produce adrenal (steroid) hormones.
Hypopituitarism: secondary cause, if you want to get picky	If the pituitary is not functioning, then the adrenals can't be triggered to secrete steroids.
Sudden withdrawal of steroid medication, which is a secondary cause	Sudden decrease in circulating corticosteroids because adrenals are suppressed during steroid therapy. This is why you have to wean off steroids to allow sufficient time for the adrenals to kick back in.

Source: Created by the author from References 1 and 4.

Factoid

When first described in 1855 by Dr. Thomas Addison, adrenal insufficiency was most frequently associated with tuberculosis (TB),[35] but that is no longer true with the development of antibiotics for the treatment of TB.

Signs and symptoms and why?

Signs and symptoms	Why?
Asthenia (weakness); fatigue	Caused by fluid and electrolyte imbalances.
Fluid volume deficit	Sodium and water are excreted; hypovolemia.
Salt cravings	Sodium loss.
Orthostatic hypotension is common; vertigo, syncope	Fluid loss from vascular space; inability for vessels to constrict and a decreased peripheral resistance (normal compensatory mechanism).
Hyperkalemia: Muscle twitching, weakness, and flaccid paralysis; arrhythmias	Sodium and water are lost, potassium is retained.
Sodium imbalances	If water is lost, the client will be hypernatremic. If sodium is lost, the client will be hyponatremic. If sodium and water are lost equally, there will be no change in serum sodium. So who knows?
Decreased bowel sounds; GI upset	Hyperkalemia.
Muscle weakness, fatigue, muscle wasting, muscle ache	Decreased glucocorticoid causes decreased ability to maintain contractions; problems with fat, protein, and carbohydrate metabolism.
Hyperpigmentation: especially in skin creases, elbows, nipples, and pressure points; bronze skin; gums and mucous membranes become bluish black	Increased levels of ACTH. ACTH is very similar to the melanocyte-stimulating hormone.

(Continued)

Signs and symptoms	Why?
Increased risk of infection	Any time your steroids are messed up, you are at risk for infection. Infection is a stressor.
Hypoglycemia	Steroids are decreased, so blood sugar drops because of an inability to carry out gluconeogenesis.
Very little axillary and pubic hair (mainly in women)	Decreased sex hormones.
Inability to handle emotional or physical stress	Decreased glucocorticoids, which helps the body deal with stress.

Source: Created by the author from References 2 and 4.

Testing, testing, testing

- Serum cortisol levels: <10 mcg/dL low plasma cortisol in the morning.
- Urine tests show decreased corticosteroid concentrations.
- ACTH stimulation test: after a baseline serum cortisol level is established, the patient is given synthetic ACTH. No increase in serum cortisol level indicates adrenal insufficiency.
- Serum sodium is decreased because of excretion.
- Serum potassium is increased because of retention.
- Blood glucose is decreased because not enough steroids cause blood glucose to go down.
- Serum ACTH is increased because the pituitary secretes ACTH when adrenocortical secretions are low.
- CT and MRI of head detects pituitary tumors.
- EKG detects rhythm changes caused by hypovolemia and hyperkalemia.
- CBC: neutropenia (low white blood cell count); anytime steroids are not in balance, the immune system is altered.
- Hematocrit and eosinophils are elevated because blood is hemoconcentrated owing to fluid loss.
- CT may show adrenal atrophy. If the adrenals aren't working,

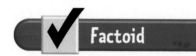

Factoid

Addisonian crisis is characterized by hypotension, weak, rapid pulse, rapid respirations with air hunger, pallor, and profound weakness, and can be precipitated by any physiologic or psychological stressor.

Interventions and why?

When the shocky patient is received in the emergency department, and the medical alert identification declares adrenal cortical insufficiency (Addisonian crisis), the immediate priority is to quickly restore circulating volume:

- Position the patient supine with legs elevated to drain peripheral blood into systemic circulation.
- Initiate venous access with a large-gauge catheter, simultaneously filling lab tubes for stat biochemistries (glucose, electrolytes) and CBC.

- Initiate cardiac monitoring and have crash cart/defibrillator available, being alert to arrhythmias associated with hyperkalemia.
- Administer prescribed hydrocortisone sodium succinate (Solu-Cortef) as soon as possible because without first giving steroids, IVF replacement is futile.

Clinical alert

Hydrocortisone sodium succinate is the only hydrocortisone preparation that can be given by the IV route.[12]

- Administer D5NS while monitoring blood pressure at frequent intervals (NIBP).
- Administer prescribed glucose as indicated. (The route of administration and amount vary according to serum glucose levels.)

While the patient's condition is being stabilized following immediate resolution of shock, hypoglycemia, and hyperkalemia, the Addison's patient will need:

- Bed rest: Provide assistance for all ADLs, avoiding any unnecessary activity or stress.
- I&O and daily weight to monitor fluid status.
- Initiate oral intake of fluids and foods (high-sodium, low-potassium) as soon as tolerated.
- Administer prescribed Florinef (mineralocorticoid replacement) as prescribed.
- Administer prescribed Prednisone (corticosteroid replacement) as prescribed.

Once the patient's condition and vital signs have stabilized, activity can be gradually resumed:

- Monitor three-step blood pressure: lying, sitting, standing.
- Instruct the patient to change positions slowly to avoid orthostatic hypotension.
- Evaluate degree of muscle weakness during short "in-room" trials (ie, bed to chair, or bed to restroom).
- Assist and/or monitor ambulation until patient is deemed "safe" for independent activity based on tolerance and muscle strength.
- Notify the physician of dramatic weight gain or loss and fluctuations in blood pressure so that Florinef dosage can be altered according to patient needs.

Case in point

A nursing student with Addison's disease always had to go to the emergency department on test days! He would wake up the morning of the test to find that he had lost 5 to 7 lb overnight and his Accu-Chek would reveal hypoglycemia!

- Restore fluid volume and blood circulation by administering IV fluid.
- IV (Solu-Cortef), then oral (cortisone) cortisol replacement, and oral aldosterone replacement (Florinef). Oral cortisone is administered to

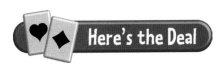

Giving IV fluids alone (in the absence of corticosteroids causing shock) will not restore circulating volume, because the patient is lacking sodium to hold the resuscitation fluid in the vascular compartment.

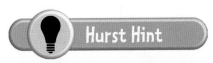

Because the patient with Addison's disease has adrenal cortical insufficiency, you have to "ADD-some" steroids!

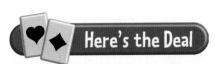

If your patient has lost 6 lb overnight, obviously the dose of Florinef (aldosterone) is insufficient and the doctor must be notified for adjustment of the Florinef dose. If your patient has gained 6 lb overnight, obviously he or she has too much aldosterone (retaining too much sodium and water) and you would hold the morning dose of Florinef and call the doctor!

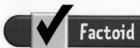

Factoid

When steroids are prescribed for patients, they are never the exact same dose every single day. The dose is always changing according to changing levels of stress!

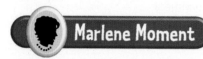

Marlene Moment

I don't know about you, but every morning when I wake up, I don't have a clue what new emergency or stressor is going to hit me right between the eyes! It's just a good thing my adrenal glands are alive and well, and can adapt to my changing levels of stress every day!

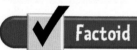

Factoid

More stress (illness, physical or emotional trauma) = need for increased dose of steroids!

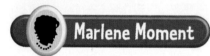

Marlene Moment

Nursing exams can be hazardous to your health! Even if you don't have Addison's disease!

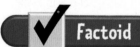

Factoid

Patients with Addison's disease learn how to manipulate their Florinef based on daily weight. Since aldosterone cause sodium and water to be retained, a weight gain would be an indicator to reduce or hold the morning dose of Florinef, whereas a significant weight loss would be an indicator to increase the morning dose!

replicate the normal secretion (two-thirds in the morning and one-third in the afternoon).

- Avoid all physical and psychological stress (exposure to extreme temperatures, exertion, emotional stress). Monitor for early signs of infection.
- Monitor for hypotension (thirst assessment, blood pressures in the lying, sitting, and standing positions).

PATIENT TEACHING For Addison's patient, or the Cushing's patient after surgical excision of the glands or radiation to destroy the glands, the patient taking lifelong steroid replacement therapy will be taught to:

- Wear medical alert bracelet or medallion and carry identification about the need for corticosteroids if found confused or unconscious.
- Curtail physical activity during hot, humid weather and increase intake of extra sodium and water to replace insensible loss.
- Vomiting and diarrhea can be very serious because of GI fluid loss, requiring replacement of sodium and water. Medical attention is needed if the condition does not resolve quickly.
- Consume a well-balanced diet (and between meal snacks) that are high protein and high carbohydrate with ample sodium.
- Adjust prescribed corticosteroid medication according to weight gain or loss, with increased dosages during times of stress.
- Evaluate lifestyle and hobbies to replace competitive, strenuous activities with leisurely enjoyable (low-stress) events (ie, attending a concert versus playing basketball).
- Call 911 or have someone drive you to the nearest emergency department if you are hypotensive, weak, or confused.
- Keep regularly scheduled follow-up visits with health care provider, being sure to stay current with recommended immunizations.
- Stay away from crowds, especially during flu and cold season.

Patient Teaching in a Nutshell

- Provide written and verbal instructions of replacement medication regimen.
- Adjust medication dosage and salt intake during episodes of stress.
- Provide instructions on how and when to use emergency kit (single-injection syringe of corticosteroids).
- Wear a medical alert bracelet and carry information on the need for corticosteroids.
- Weigh daily to monitor fluid status.
- Notify all health care providers of disease.
- Consume a high-carbohydrate, high-protein diet with adequate sodium.

What can harm my patient and why?

- Acute adrenal (Addisonian) crisis: severe sudden drop in blood pressure; nausea and vomiting; very high temperature; cyanosis

- Life-threatening arrhythmia because of hyperkalemia
- Hypovolemia and shock if severe fluid loss occurs
- Infection: immune system is impaired any time steroids are out of balance
- Adverse effects of steroid therapy
- Hypoglycemia

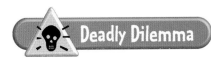

✚ Cushing's disease/Cushing's syndrome

What is it?

In general, think of Cushing's as a disease in which there are too many steroids present. The major steroids the body produces are glucocorticoids, mineralocorticoids, and sex hormones (also called androgens). The major steroid that the client with Cushing's has too much of are glucocorticoids, but you can have too much aldosterone and sex hormones as well.

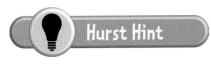

Causes and why?

Let's differentiate between Cushing's syndrome and Cushing's disease first. Many times the terms are used interchangeably, but this is incorrect. Let me re-emphasize, when someone is receiving steroids as a drug, this is referred to as *exogenous* steroids. In other words, the steroids came from **outside** of the body. At some time, you may see the statement, "The client is producing too much glucocorticoid **endogenously**." This means the client is producing too much glucocorticoid from within his or her own body. Remember, the adrenal cortex is responsible for producing steroids.

Basically, with each type of Cushing's you have too many steroids. The client either has an ACTH excess (coming from the pituitary) or a cortisol excess. As a result of the ACTH excess, the adrenal cortex is hyperstimulated and produces too many steroids. The client whose problem started with the adrenal gland itself overproduces steroids. Some clients are GIVEN steroids as a drug, and the steroid builds up in their blood. Other clients make too many of their own steroids. Either way, the client has TOO MANY STEROIDS!

Here's the difference between Cushing's syndrome and Cushing's disease:

- *Cushing's syndrome* is any condition in which there is a high level of glucocorticoids. This may be seen in a client who is receiving steroids as a medication (exogenous form of steroid) for problems such as asthma, COPD, autoimmune disorders, organ transplants, cancer (used with chemotherapy), or allergic responses. Cushing's syndrome is more common than Cushing's disease.
- *Cushing's disease* is a condition in which the **body** produces excess ACTH. Lots of diseases may cause this, such as any malfunction of the pituitary like a pituitary tumor, bilateral adrenal hyperplasia, malignancies, and adrenal adenoma or carcinoma.

Even though we differentiated between the terms *Cushing's syndrome* and *Cushing's disease*, we will just be using the term Cushing's from now on.

Signs and symptoms and why?

The signs and symptoms of Cushing's depend on how long and how much steroid the patient has been exposed to, if there is androgen excess or not, and if there are tumors secreting cortisol (steroids). As always, every patient is different. Some patients have all the symptoms listed below and some could have a few of the symptoms listed below.

Now let's get specific and look at how each steroid affects the body when there is an excess.

Glucocorticoids have four major effects:

1. Influence mood

2. Alter defense mechanisms

3. Cause protein breakdown, altered fat metabolism, and altered distribution of fat

4. Inhibit insulin

When you think of Cushing's, you probably think of the client having a moon face because of fluid retention and fat deposition, buffalo hump, skinny arms and legs, and a large abdomen.

Signs and symptoms	Why
Glucocorticoids	
Mood changes: depression, euphoria, irritability, and excess energy, which can lead to insomnia	Steroids play a part in neurotransmission, which can lead to mental changes. Steroids give you energy.
Skinny arms and legs	Muscle wasting and protein breakdown. Muscles are mainly made of protein.
Thin skin	Fibroblasts are inhibited, which leads to a loss of collagen and connective tissue. This leads to thin skin and poor wound healing. Little or no scar formation results.
Muscle weakness	Protein breakdown.
Poor wound healing	Lack of protein slows wound healing. Protein is needed to help wounds heal.
Bruising	Capillary weakness owing to protein loss (capillaries have a lot of protein), which leads to bleeding and ecchymosis. When capillaries are weak, they leak fluid out into the tissue, which produces ankle edema.
Ketonuria	When the body breaks down fat something called a KETONE is produced. Ketones are acids and cause the body to be more acidic, which naturally puts the client at risk for metabolic acidosis.
Buffalo hump: excess deposition of fat across the top of the back and shoulders	Altered fat metabolism and improper distribution of fat.
Truncal obesity: deposition of fat in the trunk	Altered fat metabolism and improper distribution of fat.

(Continued)

Signs and symptoms	Why
Pink/purple stretch marks on the breasts, abdomen, and thighs	Protein collagen fibers in subcutaneous tissue are diminished owing to protein breakdown, resulting in development of stria where they have been torn apart.
Risk for infection	Excess steroids in the blood decrease the body's ability to make as many lymphocytes and antibodies needed to fight infection. This also affects the body's ability to show signs and symptoms of inflammation.
Hyperglycemia	Glucocorticoids inhibit insulin. If insulin is inhibited, glucose won't move into the cell and the client becomes hyperglycemic. This is *why* you must perform frequent blood sugar checks on clients who receive steroids as part of their medical care. Also, glucocorticoids promote hepatic gluconeogenesis.
Glycosuria	Kidneys lower excess blood sugar by excreting it through the urine.
Osteoporosis	Steroids cause calcium excretion through the GI tract. The body works to replace the **blood** calcium (which has been lost through the GI tract) by pulling extra calcium from the bone into the blood. Why does this happen? Because your body wants your serum (blood) calcium to remain normal. When the body starts pulling the calcium from the bone to put it in the blood, then brittle bones result. Yes, the calcium level in the blood went up, but we have a client who IS STILL MAKING too many steroids. This process just repeats itself—which makes the bones more and more brittle and weak.
Peptic ulcer	Steroids cause increased gastric secretions, which eat away at the gastric mucosa.

Mineralocorticoids

Fluid volume excess	Fluid retention of sodium and water.
Hypertension	Fluid retention of sodium and water.
Hypokalemia	Sodium retention and potassium excretion.
Sodium imbalances	Retention of sodium and water; retention of more sodium than water can cause **hypernatremia;** or retention of sodium and water can be equal, causing a normal level of sodium. When answering test questions, think hypernatremia first when dealing with sodium.
Muscle weakness	Hypokalemia.

Androgens (sex hormones)

Voice deepening (female)	Adrenal androgen stimulation.
Beard growth (hirsutism) (female)	Adrenal androgen stimulation.
Menstrual irregularities (female)	Hormones are out of balance.
Thinning hair (female)	Adrenal androgen stimulation.
Ruddy complexion (same as facial plethora) (female)	Adrenal androgen stimulation.
Decreased libido (female and male); impotency (male only)	Decreased testosterone production; yes, females have testosterone too.

Source: Created by the author from References 2, 4, and 6.

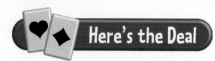

Here's the Deal

A client who receives heavy-duty steroid therapy in the hospital may develop steroid psychosis. Conversely, a client who receives a steroid injection at the doctor's office may just simply develop insomnia and irritability.

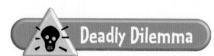

Deadly Dilemma

Excess steroids can cause immuno-suppression and infection. Things that do not make most people sick can make clients who take steroid therapy very, very ill!

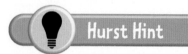

Hurst Hint

Both men and women may have a decreased sex drive (libido). When there are high levels of adrenal steroids, this interferes with the ability of the pituitary gland to secrete LH and FSH and for the testes to make testosterone, resulting in testicular atrophy and feminization such as gynecomastia.

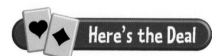

Here's the Deal

In pediatric clients, suspect Cushing's if there is increased obesity in the presence of delayed height on the growth chart.

Testing, testing, testing

- Serum cortisol level: In Cushing's, there are more steroids present in the blood in the morning and lesser amounts in the afternoon.
- Serum ACTH: This determines the origin of the problem (pituitary or adrenal gland).
- Dexamethasone suppression test: This determines the etiology of the problem.
- Midnight serum cortisol level: increased.
- 24-hour urine: increased levels of steroids.
- Serum sodium: increased (Mineralocorticoids cause sodium retention).
- Serum potassium: decreased (Mineralocorticoids cause potassium excretion).
- Serum glucose: Elevated (Steroids make blood glucose go up).

INTERVENTIONS AND WHY?

The treatment plan is based on the underlying cause of adrenal cortical excess:

- Iatrogenic Cushing's syndrome involves gradually reducing the dosage of prescribed glucocorticoids to the lowest possible dose for control of inflammatory symptoms. Doubling the dose and giving the double dose on alternating days may result in sustained remission of cushingoid symptoms.
- Treatment of choice for adrenal hyperplasia is surgery. If bilateral adrenalectomy is performed, the patient will require lifelong cortisol replacement.
- Treatment of choice for secondary Cushing's syndrome with an ACTH-secreting tumor of the pituitary gland is a transsphenoidal hypophysectomy. This procedure is generally successful, but with the surgical cure production of ACTH dramatically drops, requiring cortisol replacement therapy for one to two years in most patients and lifelong replacement in some patients.
- Radiation to the pituitary gland can be given over a six-week period in patients for recurrent cushingoid symptoms following a transsphenoidal hypophysectomy.
- Intensive critical care involves administration of oxygen, continuous monitoring of the electrocardiogram, pulse oximetry, and arterial blood pressure (preferably by radial arterial line).
- Swan-Ganz catheter insertion provides multiple lumen access with capability for hemodynamic monitoring, while simultaneously obtaining blood for frequent sampling of cortisol levels.
- Maintain NPO status while awaiting feasibility of adrenalectomy.
- Oral medications (if tolerated) to control the production of excess cortisol, such as ketoconazole, mitotane, aminoglutethimide, and metyrapone.

Oral medications are used when the patient must be stabilized before attempting surgery or because of persistently high serum cortisol levels resulting from surgery or radiation failure. Cortisol inhibitors can provide short-term relief of symptoms while awaiting full radiation effect or long-term relief of cushingoid symptoms owing to inoperable tumors. Selective agents may even accomplish "chemical adrenalectomy" by destruction of the gland. Drawbacks of the inhibitors of steroid biosynthesis (Table 10-8) include nephrotoxicity, neurotoxicity, and hepatotoxicity.

Table 10-8 Adrenal suppressant agents and nursing implications

Name and classification of steroid inhibitor	Action	Nursing implications
Metyrapone (Metopirone): Used also in cortisol stimulation test to drop serum cortisol levels quickly to test the negative feedback mechanism of the pituitary gland in producing ACTH. Effective as a single agent.	Potent blocker of a single enzyme (11 beta-hydroxylase) involved in cortisol production to halt synthesis of adrenocortical hormones.	• Monitor for remission of cushingoid symptoms and salivary cortisol levels for effectiveness. • Monitor blood pressure and heart rate at regular intervals, being alert for hypotension, which may forewarn of Addison crisis. • Monitor daily weight and I&O, being alert for rapid weight loss and increased urinary output, which can precede shock because of an aggressive lowering of serum cortisol.
Mitotane (Lysodren): This chlorophenothane analogue of the insecticide DDT is an adrenolytic antineoplastic agent, which makes it the drug of choice for adrenocortical malignancy. Effective as a single agent.	Blocks multiple enzymatic reactions to control high serum cortisol. Also induces degeneration of the mitochondrial tissue and selectively destroys adrenocortical tissue to produce chemical adrenalectomy.	• Administer prescribed antiemetic 30 minutes before dosing. • Monitor and record behavioral and neurologic signs throughout therapy. • Monitor hydration status if patient is experiencing nausea, vomiting, or diarrhea. • Monitor decreasing serum cortisol levels and increasing serum cholesterol.

(Continued)

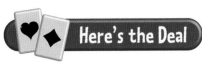

Deadly Dilemma

Hypertensive crisis, fluid volume overload, and heart failure require quick action. When the patient is too critical to tolerate oral cortisol suppressants, etomidate (imidazole derivative) is a nonopioid anesthetic that can be given IV for rapid action.

Here's the Deal

The intended use of etomidate is for inducing and maintaining surgical anesthesia, but it's major side effect, adrenal cortical suppression is "just what the doctor ordered" for the Cushing's patient in adrenal crisis because etomidate is the only cortisol suppressant that can be given IV. Obviously this drug is for short-term use, only until an adrenalectomy can be safely performed.[36]

Table 10-8 Adrenal suppressant agents and nursing implications *(Continued)*

Name and classification of steroid inhibitor	Action	Nursing implications
Aminoglutethimide (Cytadren): antiadrenal hormone, antineoplastic. Generally must be given in combination with other agents for effective treatment of hypercortisolism.	Blocks conversion of cholesterol to delta-5-pregnenolone in the adrenal cortex (multiple enzymatic reactions) to halt synthesis of adrenal steroids.	• Caution against alcohol use because effects of the drug are potentiated. • Drug must be taken exactly on schedule and doctor is to be notified if a dose is delayed or missed. • Can cause agranulocytosis and thrombocytopenia. Monitor for sore throat or signs of infection and easy bruising or bleeding (gums, nose, or stools for melena).
Ketoconazole: antifungal agent. Can be used alone or in conjunction with other agents to reduce serum cortisol. Best tolerated and is effective as monotherapy in about 70% of patients.	Potent inhibitor of the cytochrome P-450 enzyme system (multiple enzymes) to block production of cortisol.	• Requires gastric acidity for absorption. Patients with achlorhydria must take tablet dissolved in hydrochloric acid with full glass of water through a straw. • Nausea is transient and can be reduced by giving tablet with meals. • Monitor for increased ALT and AST. • Monitor WBC, platelet count, and hemoglobin, which may decrease.
Etomidate: Anesthetic/sedative used for rapid induction of anesthesia.[37] An adverse effect of the drug is adrenal cortical suppression, making it the only parenteral agent available for unpublished treatment of hypercortisolism. For short-term use only!	Blocks multiple enzymatic reactions to control high serum cortisol.	• Monitor level of sedation, airway, and breathing. • Administer oxygen as prescribed with continuous pulse oximetry. • Monitor for hypotension with continuous NIBP or radial arterial line. • Be prepared to treat hypotension with vasopressors as indicated.

Source: Created by the author from References 12, 38, and 40.

Hurst Hint

Drug therapy with single or multiple enzyme–blocking agents to inhibit synthesis of cortisol (see Table 10-8) are prescribed according to patient need. These patients are monitored closely for nephrotoxicity, neurotoxicity, and hepatotoxicity, and with the onset of Addison's disease.

PATIENT TEACHING Patient teaching for Cushing's syndrome is based on the prescribed treatment plan. If the patient is not a candidate for surgery or radiation to the gland, or if the iatrogenic condition cannot be remedied by gradually withdrawing corticosteroids, the patient will be taught to:

- Take antidiabetic medications and/or insulin as prescribed and monitor blood glucose (Accu-Chek) as indicated.

- Take antihypertensive medications as directed; adhere to a low-sodium diet; and self-monitor blood pressure on a routine basis.

- Routinely inspect skin (especially feet and legs), with attention to even minor cuts or abrasions that could become infected.

- Adhere to a diet low in sodium, calories, and carbohydrates, establishing a routine time for meals, evenly spacing calories throughout the day.

- Wear medic alert identification and carry a list of medications with you.

- Be alert to mood swings and the effect that they have on interpersonal interactions.

- Keep regularly scheduled follow-up visits with one's health care provider.

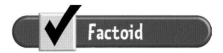

Factoid

ACTH is produced by the anterior pituitary to stimulate the adrenal cortex to produce adrenocortical hormones.

For Addison's disease or for the Cushing's patient following surgical excision of the glands or radiation to destroy the glands, the patient taking lifelong steroid replacement therapy will be taught to:

- Wear medical alert bracelet or medallion and carry identification about the need for corticosteroids if found confused or unconscious.
- Curtail physical activity during hot, humid weather and increase intake of extra sodium and water to replace insensible loss.
- Vomiting and diarrhea can be very serious because of GI fluid loss, requiring replacement of sodium and water. Medical attention is needed if the condition does not resolve quickly.
- Consume a well-balanced diet (and between meal snacks) that are high protein, high carbohydrate, and with ample sodium.
- Adjust prescribed corticosteroid medication according to weight gain or loss with increased dosages during times of stress.
- Evaluate lifestyle and hobbies to replace competitive, strenuous activities with leisurely enjoyable (low stress) events (ie, attending a concert versus playing basketball).
- Call 911 or have someone drive you to the nearest emergency department if you are hypotensive, weak, or confused.
- Keep regularly scheduled follow-up visits with health care provider, being sure to stay current with recommended immunizations.
- Stay away from crowds, especially during flu and cold season.

What can harm my patient and why?

- Peptic ulcer disease occurs because stress hormones increase gastric acid.

- Diabetes occurs because glucocorticoids raise the blood sugar and inhibit secretion of insulin.

- Hypertension occurs because of hyperaldosteronism because of increased sodium and water retention.[1]
- Heart failure is caused by increased afterload owing to systemic hypertension and increased preload caused by retention of sodium and water expanding the vascular space.
- Dysrhythmias, tetany, and acid–base imbalance are caused by excessive loss of potassium.

When Cushing's syndrome is caused by a rapidly growing adrenal tumor, and acute signs and symptoms with potentially fatal complications (adrenal crisis) can occur rapidly leading to:

- FVE leading to pulmonary edema caused by retention of sodium and water (too much aldosterone).
- Hypokalemia, leading to cardiac arrhythmias caused by potassium loss (too much aldosterone).
- Hypertensive crisis and heart failure in response to excessive preload and afterload.

Cutting edge

Advances in the technology of radiosurgery are no longer "point and shoot," but offer real-time imaging in conjunction with CT scan and MRI imaging. Currently available are the advanced Gamma Knife (Perfe-Xion unit) and the CyberKnife (with 1200+ beams), which have been touted as very effective for eradication of pituitary adenomas when given in a single high-dose treatment. Combining radiation with cortisol-inhibiting agents while awaiting full benefits of radiation treatment can help patients feel better while they are getting better.[39]

✚ Pheochromocytoma

Let's get the normal stuff straight!

The adrenal gland is composed of an outer portion (the cortex) that secretes steroids (glucocorticoids, mineralocorticoids, androgens, and estrogens) and the inner portion (the medulla) that secretes catecholamines (epinephrine and norepinephrine), which are neurotransmitters. Most of the norepinephrine from the adrenal gland is converted into epinephrine. Catecholamines are the stress hormones that enable fight or flight by increased CNS stimulation or inhibition (depending on the alpha or beta adrenergic receptor site), which results in:

- A sharp rise in blood pressure and heart rate
- Constriction of renal, visceral, and integumentary blood vessels
- Bronchial smooth muscle relaxation (getting more air into the lungs)
- Skeletal muscle vasodilation (getting more blood flow needed for flight)

What is it?

Pheochromocytoma is a tumor (usually benign) of the adrenal medulla that results in intermittent boluses of epinephrine being secreted and

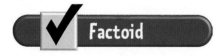
Factoid

Sometimes a little tumor can cause big problems, even when it is not malignant (Fig. 10-9)!

released into circulation. These tumors can occur outside of the adrenal gland, and when they do up to 10% to 15% of them can be malignant.

Causes and why?

The tumor is derived from chromaffin cells (stained with chromium salts) of the adrenal medulla caused by genetic predisposition and gene mutation. Pheochromocytomas are also associated with other syndromes: Von Hippel-Lindau disease, multiple endocrine neoplasia type 2, and neurofibromatosis type 1.[40]

Testing, testing, testing

Diagnosis of pheochromocytoma is verified by testing of urine and plasma for catecholamines, which break down into the catabolites metanephrines and vanillylmandelic acid (VMA).

- 24-hour urine for catecholamines and VMA will reveal higher than normal levels of both.
- Plasma catecholamines (blood is drawn with the patient at rest): Normal values <60 pg/mL for epinephrine and 120 to 680 pg/mL for norepinephrine.
- Clonidine (Catapres) suppression test can differentiate pheochromocytoma from essential hypertension, but is rarely used when diagnostic imaging is available.
- When catecholamine levels of blood and urine are elevated twice normal, imaging studies are indicated (US, CT, MRI) for detection of a suprarenal mass.

Clinical alert

A patient history of acute alcohol or clonidine withdrawal or cocaine abuse can cause false-positive testing for pheochromocytoma because these conditions also produce increased catecholamine catabolites in plasma and urine.

- I^{123}-MIBG (radioactive scintography) can be useful if imaging is negative.

  Genetic testing to identify gene mutation is indicated for patient and family members with high-risk syndromes (Von Hippel-Lindau disease, multiple endocrine neoplasia type 2, and neurofibromatosis type 1) to determine carrier states and for early detection and early intervention before symptoms arise.

Signs and symptoms and why?

During attacks of excess secretion of catecholamines the patient has sudden onset of the following signs and symptoms that resolve slowly:

- **Hypertension**
- **Headache** (severe "explosive" quality)
- **Hyperhidrosis** (profuse perspiration)
- **Hypermetabolism**

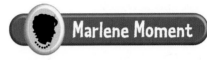

No vanilla ice cream while you are doing your VMA 24-hour urine collection. Vanilla can cause a false-positive! Everything with vanilla is a no-no!

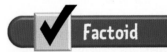

Best results are obtained if the 24-hour urine catch is started during or immediately after a hypertensive episode when increased levels of catecholamines are in circulation.[41]

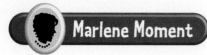

Marlene Moment

When is a nose bleed (epistaxis) a good thing? When your blood pressure is 310/180!!

Sometimes your nose can be a "popoff" valve to lower the pressure! Had you rather have a stroke or a bloody nose? Give me the bloody nose any day, even if it ruins my new dress!

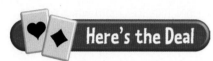

Here's the Deal

Recovery is characterized by return of normal blood pressure in approximately two-thirds of patients, but some may require continued antihypertensive therapy. Prolonged follow-up is recommended: 6 weeks, 6 months and then yearly for 10 years.

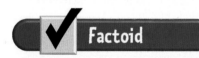

Factoid

Management of the hypertensive crisis and preventing cardiovascular complications is priority:

- Bed rest in a Semi-Fowler's position (cool, quiet room with dim, indirect lighting).
- Nasal oxygen as prescribed (especially important if chest pain is experienced).
- Initiate nitroglycerin infusion as prescribed.
- A concurrent nitroprusside (Nipride) infusion may be added to control blood pressure.
- Administer prescribed beta blockers (eg, metoprolol) to decrease heart rate, blood pressure, and anxiety level.

(Continued)

- **Hyperglycemia**
- Palpitations and chest pain
- Nausea and vomiting because of severe pain
- Blurring of vision
- Tinnitus
- Shortness of breath
- Polyuria
- Diarrhea
- Tremulousness and anxiousness[8,9]

The first five (bold) "Hs" are sufficient for making a clinical diagnosis,[42] which can be confirmed with diagnostic testing. Episodes may subside spontaneously and recur, or a severe episode can result in hypertensive or cardiac emergencies.

What can harm my patient and why?

Hypertension causes changes to vessel walls, increases afterload and strain on the heart, and can cause characteristic fundal changes (nicking). Acute complications include:

- Development of ectopic Cushing's syndrome with rapid progression of symptoms because of hyperplasia of the adrenal gland
- Hypertensive crisis triggered by excessive circulating catecholamines
- Stroke (cerebral venous thrombosis) caused by procoagulant substances secreted by tumor cells[43]
- Acute myocardial infarction and arrhythmias in response to excessive oxygen demand of the myocardial tissues and incompatible hypermetabolic needs
- Renal-induced diabetes insipidus (DI)

Interventions and why?

The only cure for pheochromocytoma is removal, but surgery must be delayed until stabilization of cardiovascular status and attainment of normotension is achieved. This may require a minimum of two weeks of alpha and beta blockage for optimal preoperative preparation.[7,48] Combinations of the following agents may be prescribed with frequent monitoring of blood pressure, heart rate, and volume status during the preoperative period:

- Antihypertensive of choice: Phenoxybenzamine (Dibenzyline), an alpha-adrenergic blocker to relax smooth muscles of vessel walls
- Beta blocker: Metoprolol (Lopressor, Toprol XL) to block sympathetic stimulation
- Calcium channel blocker: Diltiazem (Cardizem) to improve cardiac blood flow and treat arrhythmias

Intraoperative preparation is equally important for the reason that surgery is dangerous because massive release of catecholamines can occur during surgical manipulation or excision.

- Intraoperative monitoring for cardiac arrhythmias is imperative with immediate access to emergency medications in the event of hypertensive crisis.
- Continuous blood pressure via arterial line is indicated throughout surgery and recovery.
- Continuous hemodynamic monitoring per Swan-Ganz (pulmonary artery) catheter keeps a close record of fluid status.

PATIENT TEACHING

- Take all medications exactly as prescribed and return for all scheduled visits for blood pressure monitoring, weight, and physical examination.
- Caution the patient to arise slowly from a supine position and sit briefly before standing when taking Dibenzyline because orthostatic hypotension can occur.
- For collecting 24-hour urine: Place signs above the bed and in the restroom to save all urine until the time posted, and all additional urine (every drop) for the next 24 hours, keeping the last voiding that occurs during the time frame.
- Urine for the 24-hour specimen must be kept cold, in light-resistant jugs provided by the lab that have an acidifying agent added.
- Two to three days before collecting the 24-hour urine specimen, all ingested stimulants and vanilla (coffee, tea, cola, cocoa, chocolates) must be avoided, as well as bananas and citrus fruits because these alter the test results.
- Activities to avoid during the 24-hour urine specimen collection period are smoking and physical activity, which cause a false elevation of catecholamine levels in the urine.

Cutting edge

A recent study identified the superiority of a new tracer: F-18fluoro-L-dihydroxyphenylalanine positron emission tomography (^{18}F-DOPA PET). PET scans using this tracer picked up adrenal catecholamine-secreting tumors better than all other diagnostics! Outperforming (123) I-MIBG, CT, and MRI, the PET scan using this newest tracer (18) F-DOPA identified tumors that others missed![45]

PRACTICE QUESTIONS

1. What data from the nursing history would be the most likely contributing factor for the development of neuropathy and retinopathy in a Type 2 diabetic?

   A. A routine practice of running two miles each day

   B. Occasional episodes of not eating because of transient nausea

   C. A routine practice of drinking four beers daily (meals and bedtime)

   D. Occasionally forgetting to take prescribed oral hypoglycemic agent

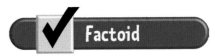

Factoid

- Incremental oral dosing of diltiazem (Cardizem) by mouth, starting at a low dose and increasing to the maximum dose as indicated to improve myocardial blood flow and prevent arrhythmias through calcium channel blockade.
- Continuous blood pressure monitoring (NIBP or radial artery line).
- Swan-Ganz line for hemodynamic monitoring during fluid repletion.

After the acute hypertensive crisis, monitor for damage to organs:

- Monitor I&O and daily weight.
- Monitor serum creatinine and BUN.
- Auscultate lung sounds bilaterally and posteriorly.
- Monitor activity tolerance. Compare blood pressure, heart rate, and respirations before and after activity and have the patient rate his or her degree of fatigue.
- Auscultate bowel sounds in all four quadrants at regular intervals.

Surgery will be delayed for 10 to 14 days until BP and heart rate normalize.

- Phenoxybenzamine (Dibenzyline), an alpha blocker, is prescribed for hypertension related to pheochromocytoma.
- Monitor for orthostatic hypotension and record three-step blood pressures.
- Monitor for reflex tachycardia associated with phenoxybenzamine.

2. While assessing a diabetic patient with known peripheral neuropathy, palpation of a thick darkened callous on the toe elicits pain. Which next intervention by the nurse is the priority?

A. Document the presence, location, and degree of peripheral neuropathy.

B. Notify the physician of assessment findings, relevant labs, and vital signs.

C. Place the patient on bed rest with the foot elevated and notify the doctor.

D. Have the patient rate the pain (scale of 1–10) and administer PRN analgesia.

E. Hang the leg in a dependent position and notify the doctor of intermittent claudication.

3. It is learned during report that a Type 1 diabetic patient who receives NPH insulin 40 Units AM and PM experienced the Somogyi effect during the previous shift. Which treatment plan will help to alleviate these phenomena?

A. Awaken the patient at 3 AM for a snack.

B. Include a protein serving with the bedtime snack.

C. Arrange to serve the patient's breakfast early (5–6 AM).

D. Administer the regular evening dose of NPH insulin at 10 PM.

4. A Type 2 diabetic has an 1800 calorie ADA diet with orders for AC and HS Accu-Chek. What is the next nursing implementation indicated when the bedtime glucose level is 180 mg/dL?

A. Notify the doctor of the blood glucose level.

B. Notify the lab to recheck the blood glucose level.

C. Withhold the bedtime snack (approx 15 g).

D. Administer the bedtime snack (100 calories) as prescribed.

5. For which of the following diabetic patients could the nurse safely omit the bedtime snack?

A. A Type 1 diabetic who has hypoglycemia unawareness

B. A Type 2 diabetic with bedtime blood glucose of 140 mg/dL

C. A Type 2 diabetic whose diabetes is controlled by diet and exercise alone

D. A Type 1 diabetic who received NPH insulin at supper time

6. Which would be inappropriate when planning care for the patient with hypothyroidism?

A. Employ meticulous hygiene.

B. Restrict animal fats in the diet.

C. Give instructions in simple concrete terms.

D. Exercise caution when applying external heat.

7. What is the priority for the patient experiencing hyperparathyroidism crisis?

   A. Support for airway and breathing

   B. Continuous cardiac monitoring for arrhythmias

   C. Diagnostics and imaging studies to find the cause

   D. Hurried preparations for emergency parathyroidectomy

8. Following simple sinus surgery, which postoperative assessment would be of greatest concern to the nurse at the time for outpatient discharge?

   A. The three-hour urine output is 660 mL of clear, pale urine.

   B. Complaint of a frontal headache (rated 4 on a scale of 1–10)

   C. Mustache dressing is soiled with a small amount of bright red blood.

   D. Blood pressure is 10 mm Hg lower than baseline and heart rate is increased 10%.

9. Which patient instruction is *least* important when the patient is scheduled for a vanillylmandelic (VMA) test?

   A. Eliminate sweets and pastries for 48 hours prior to the test.

   B. The 24-hour urine specimen requires starting with an empty bladder.

   C. Limit physical activity and smoking until the test is completed.

   D. Avoid all commercially prepared foods for 24 hours prior to testing.

10. A thin Caucasian patient with dark pigmented skin and gums whose clinical symptoms include muscle weakness, weight loss, and hypotension is undergoing diagnostic testing. If all of the following tests are ordered, which one would the nurse question for this patient?

    A. Serum electrolytes

    B. Fasting blood glucose

    C. Blood and urine cortisol levels

    D. ACTH stimulation test using metyrapone

    E. ACTH stimulation test using cosyntropin

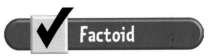

Factoid

The vanillylmandelic is a diagnostic test to evaluate the presence of catecholamines in the urine, which is associated with pheochromocytoma.

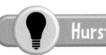

Hurst Hint

Don't ever try to answer a question like this without first asking yourself, "What's wrong with my patient?" You have to know what's wrong before you know what tests are indicated. If the question had been about nursing care for this patient, you have to know what's wrong with your patient before you can select an implementation answer. So when you see assessments in the question, you must always ask yourself, "What's wrong with my patient?" and formulate an answer before you ever even look at possible answers!

Hurst Hint

Before you consider any of these patients, you must ask yourself, "What's wrong with my patient?" before even looking at the four choices given! Your patient is immunosuppressed because of cortisol excess, so you are looking for a roommate who is NOT infected, or has a low potential for being infectious.

References

1. Porth CM. *Pathophysiology: Concepts of Altered Health States.* 7th ed. Philadelphia: Lippincott Williams & Wilkins; 2007.

2. Muretta JM, Mastick CC. How insulin regulates glucose transport in adipocytes. *Vitamins Hormones* 80(10):245–286, 2009.

3. National Diabetes Information Clearinghouse (NDIC). Available at http://diabetes.niddk.nih.gov/dm/pubs/hypoglycemia/#cause. Accessed July 14, 2009.

4. American Diabetes Association. PreDiabetes. Available at http://www.diabetes.org/pre-diabetes.jsp. Accessed July 10, 2009.

5. Hurst M. Endocrine. *Hurst Review's NCLEX-RN Review*. New York: McGraw-Hill Medical; 2008.

6. Beers MH, ed. *The Merck Manual of Medical Information. Diabetes.* Whitestation, NJ: Merck Research Laboratories; 2003.

7. Pagana KD, Pagana TJ. *Mosby's Diagnostic and Laboratory Test Reference.* 6th ed. St. Louis: Mosby; 2003.

8. National Center for Chronic Disease Prevention and Health Promotion. (2009). Diabetes public health information. Available at http://www.cdc.gov/diabetes/faq/prediabetes.htm. Accessed June 10, 2009.

9. Wonnacott K. Update on regulatory issues in pancreatic islet transplantation. *Am J Therapeut 12*(6):600–604, 2005.

10. Kamarzaman Z, Turner C, Clark F. How low can you go: A case presentation on a patient with diabetic ketoacidosis. *Resuscitation,* 2009. [Epub before print] Available at http://www.sciencedirect.com.lib-proxy.uams.edu/science?_ob=ArticleURL&_udi=B6T19-4-WGT650-6&_user=1496715&_rdoc=1&_fmt=&_orig=search&_sort=d&_docanchor=&view=c&_acct=C000053083&_version=1&_urlVersion=0&_userid=1496715&md5=b7e162614b3907d306aeff4b60e2e4d7. Accessed June 10, 2009.

11. Smeltzer SC, Bare BG, Hinkle JL, Cheever KH. *Brunner & Suddarth's Textbook of Medical-Surgical Nursing.* 11th ed. Philadelphia: Lippincott Williams & Wilkins: 2008.

12. Watts SA, Anselmo J. Nutrition for diabetes—all in a day's work. *Nursing2006 36*(6):46–48, 2006.

13. Kruger DF. Integrating innovative tools into the management of Type 2 diabetes to improve patient self-management. *J Am Acad Nurse Pract 20*(1):17–21, 2008.

14. Spollett GR. Diabetic neuropathies: Diagnosis and treatment. *Nurs Clin North Am 41*(4):697–717, 2006.

15. Kumareswaran K, Evans ML, Hovorka R. Artificial pancreas: An emerging approach to treat Type 1 diabetes. *Exp Rev Med Dev 6*(4):401–410, 2009.

16. Scemons D. Diabetic medications? *Nursing2007 20*(6):45–49, 2007.

17. Boyle ME. Optimizing the treatment of Type 2 diabetes using current and future insulin technologies. *MedSurg Nurs 17*(6):383–390, 2008.

18. Childs B. Complications and comorbidities. *AJN (Suppl) 107*(6):S5–S9, 2007.

19. Nathan DM, Buse JB, Davidson MB, et al. Management of hyperglycaemia in type 2 diabetes mellitus: A consensus algorithm for the initiation and adjustment of therapy. Update regarding the thiazolidinediones. *Diabetologia 51*(1):8–11, 2008.

20. Comerford KC, Labus D, eds. *Nursing 2010 Drug Handbook.* Philadelphia: Lippincott Williams & Wilkins; 2010.

21. Sheen AJ. Rosiglitazone: To be or not to be? *Diabetologia* 52:1448–1450, 2009.

22. Levine A, Brennan AP. Rethinking sliding-scale insulin. *AJN* 107(10):74–79, 2007.

23. Bentley J, Foster A. Multidisciplinary management of the diabetic foot ulcer. *Wound Care* 12(12):S6–S12, 2007.

24. Zgonis T, Stapleton JJ, Girard-Powell VA, Hagino RT. Surgical management of diabetic foot infections and amputations. *AORN J* 87 (5):935–947, 2008.

25. George-Gay B, Chernecky CC. *Clinical Medical Surgical Nursing: A Decision Making Reference.* Philadelphia: Saunders; 2002.

26. Flack S, Apelqvist J, Keith M, Trueman P, Williams D. An economic evaluation of VAC therapy compared with wound dressings in the treatment of diabetic foot ulcers. *J Wound Care* 17(2):71–78, 2008.

27. Saeed BO. Syndrome of inappropriate antidiuretic hormone secretion. *So Med J* 102(4):341–342, 2009.

28. Bowman AM. Promoting safe exercise and foot care. *Can Nurse* 104(2):23–27, 2008.

29. Sieggreen MY. Step up care for diabetic foot. *Nurs Mgmt* 37(6):25–31, 2006.

30. Evans-Molina C, Vestermark GL, Mirmira RG. Development of insulin-producing cells from primitive biologic precursors. *Curr Opin Organ Transpl* 14(1):56–63, 2009.

31. Chang CH, Liao JJ, Chuang CH, Lee CT. Recurrent hyponatremia after traumatic brain injury. *Am J Med Sci* 335(5):390–393, 2008.

32. Mount DB. The brain in hyponatremia: Both culprit and victim. *Semin Nephrol* 29(3):196–215, 2009.

33. Maggiore U, Picetti E, Antonucci E, et al. The relation between the incidence of hypernatremia and mortality in patients with severe traumatic brain injury. *Crit Care* 13(4):R110, 2009.

34. Bach-Huynh TG, Nayak B, Loh J, et al. Timing of levothyroxine administration affects serum thyrotropin concentration. *J Clin Endocrin Metab* [Epub ahead of print]. Available at http://jcem.endo-journals.org.libproxy.uams.edu/cgi/content/abstract/jc.2009-0860v1. Accessed July 26, 2009.

35. Addison T. On the Constitutional and Local Effects of the Disease of the Supra-renal Capsules. [HTML reprint]. London: Samuel Highley, 1855. Available at http://www.wehner.org/addison/x1.htm. Accessed July 30, 2009.

36. Dabbagh AA. Etomidate infusion in the critical care setting for suppressing the acute phase of Cushing's syndrome. *Anesthes Analges* 108(1):238–239, 2009.

37. Baird CRW, Hay AW, McKeown DW, Ray DC. Rapid sequence induction in the emergency department: Induction of drug and outcome of patients admitted to the intensive care unit. *Emerg Med J* 26(8):576–579, 2009.

38. Tombol Z, Szabo PM, Liko I, Racz K. Steroid biosynthesis inhibitors in the therapy of hypercortisolism: Theory and practice. *Curr Med Chem* 15(26):2734–2747, 2008.

39. Lunsford L, Dade LD. Letter to the editor: Stereotactic radiosurgery with the CyberKnife for pituitary adenomas. *J Kor Neurosurg Soc* 45(6):405–406, 2009.

40. Pasini B, Stratakis CA. SDH mutations in tumorigenesis and inherited endocrine tumours: Lesson from the phaeochromocytoma-paraganglioma syndromes. *J Int Med* 266(1):19–42, 2009.

41. Cook LK. Pheochromocytoma. *Am J Nurs* 109(2):50–53, 2009.

42. Bravo E, Tagle R. Pheochromocytomas: State-of-the-art and future prospects. *Endocrine Rev* 24(4):539–553, 2003.

43. Stella P, Bignotti G, Zerbi S, et al. Concurrent pheochromocytoma, diabetes insipidus and cerebral venous thrombosis—a possible unique pathophysiological mechanism. *Nephrol Dial Transplant* 15(5):717–718, 2000.

44. Wong C, Yu R. Preoperative preparation for pheochromocytoma resection: Physician survey and clinical practice. *Exp Clin Endocrinol Diab* [Epub ahead of print]. Available at http://www.ncbi.nlm.nih.gov/pubmed/19609840?ordinalpos=12&itool=EntrezSystem2.PEntrez.Pubmed.Pubmed_ResultsPanel.Pubmed_DefaultReportPanel.Pubmed_RVDocSum. Accessed July 30, 2009.

45. Fiebrich HB, Brouwers AH, Kersterns MN et al. 18F-DOPA PET is superior to conventional imaging with 123I-metaiodobenzylguanidine scintigraphy, CT, and MRI in localizing tumors causing catecholamine excess. *J Clin Endocrinol Metab* [EPub ahead of print]. Available at http://www.ncbi.nlm.nih.gov/pubmed/19622618?ordinalpos=1&itool=EntrezSystem2.PEntrez.Pubmed.Pubmed_ResultsPanel.Pubmed_DefaultReportPanel.Pubmed_RVDocSum.

CHAPTER

11 Sensorineural Dysfunction

OBJECTIVES

In this chapter you will review:

- The pathophysiology associated with selected eye and ear disorders.
- How sensorineural dysfunction affects patient safety.
- Primary prevention that helps maintain the highest level of wellness.
- Treatment modalities and nursing care to promote maximum sensorineural function.
- Pharmacology and technology that improve quality of life and minimizes sensorineural loss.
- The effects of age, lifestyle, genetics, and environmental factors on sensorineural wellness.
- Patient teaching to promote self-care and safety in the patient with impaired sensorineural function.

DISORDERS OF THE EYE

Let's get the normal stuff straight!

See Figure 11-1.

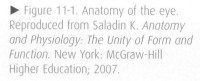

► Figure 11-1. Anatomy of the eye. Reproduced from Saladin K. *Anatomy and Physiology: The Unity of Form and Function.* New York: McGraw-Hill Higher Education; 2007.

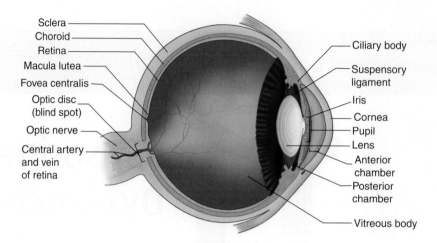

The eye (optic globe) consists of three layers, each of which also has multiple layers:

- The outer layer consists of the white fibrous sclera, the transparent, avascular cornea, the middle stromal layer, and the innermost endothelial layer.

- The middle layer (called the uveal tract) contains the iris, pupil, and ciliary body, as well as the vascular membrane called the choroid coat.

- The innermost neural layer is called the retina. Its photoreceptors receive transmissions of light and send impulses through the optic nerve to the brain.[1]

The middle of the eye is filled with clear, jelly-like substances (aqueous and vitreous humors) that allow light entering the pupil to be transmitted to the retina.

- The vitreous humor contained within a delicate membrane fills the eyeball behind the lens.

- The vitreous chamber extends from behind the lens to the retina.

- The aqueous humor occupies the anterior space between the lens and the cornea.

The eyelids cover the exposed surface of the eye to shut out light and protect it from injury and irritation.

- Mucus membranes line the eyelids to lubricate and keep the eyes moist.

- Tears bathe the eyes to reduce friction of the lids and hydrate.

- Irritants and injury cause increased tears to flush away the irritant.

The cornea contains no blood vessels, but is nourished by the scleral vessels, aqueous humor, which fills the anterior chamber, and tears. However, sensory neurons are abundant in the cornea! The three layers of the cornea are the:

- Thin outermost epithelial covering
- Stromal layer in the middle, separated from the epithelium by Bowman's membrane, which is an antimicrobial barrier
- The innermost endothelial layer, which is in direct contact with the aqueous humor of the anterior chamber[1]

Eyesight is valuable for:

- Entertainment
- Physical safety
- Work
- Educational pursuits
- Hobbies
- Communication
- Nonverbal expression (eg, eye contact)

Eyesight can be affected by:

- Trauma
- Cataracts
- Glaucoma
- Retinal detachment
- Macular degeneration

✚ Trauma of the eye

What is it?

Eye trauma is injury to any portion of the eye, and is described according to the type, extent, and depth of the wound.

Types of eye trauma:
- A **closed globe injury** is one in which the wound does not penetrate a full thickness into the wall of the eye (sclera and cornea).
- **Penetrating injuries** are characterized by an entrance wound and/or an intraocular foreign body (Fig. 11-2). Notice that the pupil is no longer round because the iris has been cut.

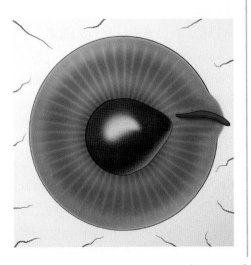

◀ Figure 11-2. Penetrating injury to the eye.

(Continued)

Hurst Hint

Tears or cuts of the eye can vary in depth. They are painful because the epithelial layer of the cornea has an abundance of sensory neurons.[1,2]

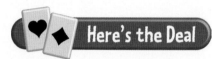

Here's the Deal

Penetrating injuries, perforating injuries, and corneal abrasions are usually accidental and related to work or recreational activities. These injuries are preventable with the proper use of safety precautions, such as goggles or glasses. Examples of accidents leading to eye trauma include:

- An ATV passenger gets hit in the eye with a tree limb.
- Sandblasting could drive a sliver of rock into the eye.
- A metal shard can enter the unprotected eye from using a grinding wheel or anything where metal strikes metal.
- A woman applying mascara gets bumped on the elbow, causing the brush to scrape across the eye, and resulting in a corneal abrasion.

- **Perforating injuries** (eg, BB or pellet) can have entrance *and* exit wounds. (The object enters one location and exits another.) This could leave a hole that oozes aqueous or vitreous humor.
- **Blunt impact** is direct physical trauma to the eye resulting in any of the following:
  - Bleeding into surrounding soft tissue (black eye)
  - Hyphema: bleeding *inside* the eye (in the anterior chamber)
  - Torn iris
  - Dislocated lens
  - Corneal abrasion
  - Tears or cuts
  - Vitreous hemorrhage (in the posterior chamber)
- **Foreign bodies:** "trash" or debris (eg, sandblasting)
- **Exposure to harmful chemicals:** sprays, splashes, or spills of any chemical substance
- **Nonpenetrating:** no entrance and exit wound

✚ Chemical injuries

What causes it and why?

Chemical injury occurs when an irritating substance gets into the eye (eg, splashing) from deliberate or accidental means. Serious chemical injuries are most often caused by acid and alkali burns, ranging from mild irritation to severe injury. The extent of the injury depends on the agent involved and the duration of exposure.[3] Carelessness and/or distraction in any environment (work or home) can lead to accidents. For example, wiping sweat from around the eyes while cleaning with muriatic acid solutions can cause chemical injury to the eye.

When the eye is exposed to acid:

- The acid immediately coagulates with proteins and the burning **stops** because coagulated proteins create a superficial barrier.[4,5]
- Toilet bowl cleaners (strong acids) can be accidentally squirted into the face while squeezing the bottle with the spout directed toward the face.

When the eye is exposed to alkali:

- Alkalis **continue** to be active.
- Collagenase is released from corneal epithelium adding to the destructive action of the alkali.
- Alkalis rapidly penetrate[6] the anterior chamber and can perforate the eye through liquefactive necrosis.[7]
- Drain cleaners (lye, a strong alkali) can lead to blindness

Knowing the agent responsible for the chemical injury helps with decision making and determination of prognosis.

Chemical injuries are graded 1 to 4 in terms of severity and prognosis:
- Grade 1 is the least injury and grade 4 describes the most severe injury.
- Grade 1 fully recovers with no visual loss while grade 4 has permanent damage with very likely severe visual loss.[6]

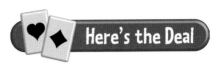

Here's the Deal

- An acid burn with a grade 3 haziness with less than half of the cornea involved should get *better* on the third or fourth day.
- An alkali burn with grade 3 haziness would be expected to be considerably *worse* on the third or fourth day owing to necrosis and ischemia.[6] Remember the alkali continues to be active, causing more damage than acids.

Signs and symptoms and why?

Direct Trauma Depending upon the type and extent of injury, the patient may experience a variety of symptoms.	Bleeding from the penetrating injury into the anterior segment of the eye (called hyphema) may color the front of the eye a red or rusty color or can obscure transmission of light past the pupil Hemorrhagic chemosis (swelling of the conjunctival tissue) Pain and a sensation of "something in the eye" Increased sensitivity to light (photophobia) Tearing (lacrimation) Redness and swelling of the eye and eyelid Blurring or dimming of vision.[7,8]
Chemical Injury The chemical irritant produces pain and burning that is immediate and extreme, causing reflex closure of the eyelids. This worsens the damage because the closed lid keeps the chemical in contact with the eye	Blurred vision Excessive tearing (lacrimation) Photophobia Red eye caused by hyperemia in mild to moderate burns (but can be white in severe burns because of ischemia of conjunctival vessels) Swollen eyelids A severe chemical burn will produce corneal swelling and opacification (white rather than clear) looking like "dead eyes"
Foreign Body Small, sharp, rapidly moving foreign bodies (eg, metal shards) can penetrate the eye so quickly that the signs and symptoms may not be immediately obvious	• Redness • Irritation • Tearing • Pain • Itching • Drainage

Testing, testing, testing

- An initial direct inspection in the emergency room can be accomplished with a hand held ophthalmoscope (Fig. 11-3), which has plus and minus numbers on the lenses that can be rotated for near focus (cornea) and more distant focus (retina).

▶ Figure 11-3. Physician using oph-thalmoscope. National Eye Institute, National Institutes of Health.

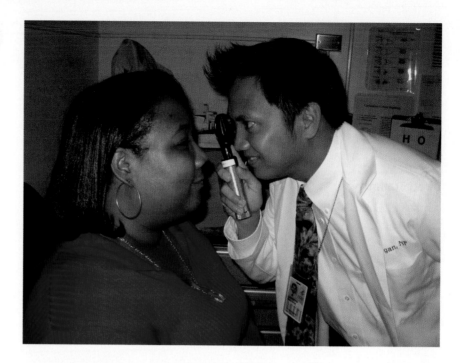

- The ophthalmologist uses a directed beam of high-intensity light and slit lens (biomicroscopy) or indirect ophthalmoscopy to view the damage from an eye injury (Fig. 11-4).[8]

▶ Figure 11-4. A slit-lamp being used to view the interior of the eye. National Eye Institute, National Institutes of Health.

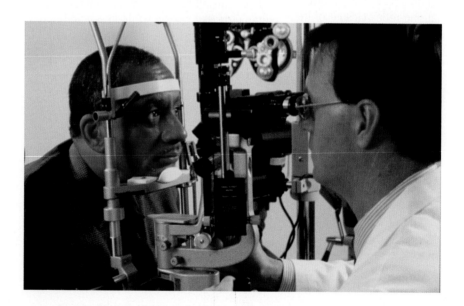

- A topical anesthetic drop facilitates examination of the eye with the slit-lamp (Fig. 11-5).[9]

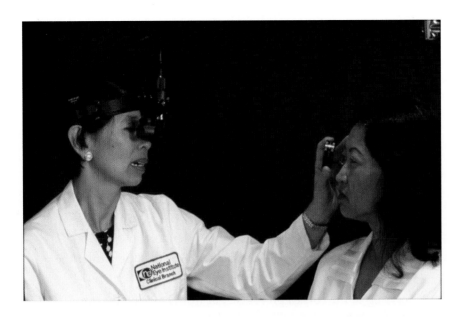

◄ Figure 11-5. Indirect ophthalmo-scope. National Eye Institute, National Institutes of Health.

- Additional imaging studies may be indicated:
  - CT (computed tomography) or US (ultrasound) can be used to localize a foreign body and determine its size and composition.
  - MRI (magnet resonance imaging) is NOT used because the foreign body has a high probability of being metal, and movement of the foreign body toward the magnet would cause further intraocular damage.

What can harm my patient and why?

DIRECT PHYSICAL TRAUMA

- Infection, especially if the object causing the injury is:
  - Contaminated with organisms in soil
  - Contains vegetative matter (eg, grass or leaf fragment)
  - Composed of metal (iron, copper, or steel)[2,4]
- Severe infections can lead to permanent loss of vision and possibly loss of the affected eye.[10]
- Any trauma to the eye can lead to vision loss because normally transparent structures become cloudy, no longer allowing penetration of light:
  - Traumatic cataracts
  - Scarring of the cornea[11]
- Trauma with intraocular bleeding and rupture of the optic globe can lead to increased intraocular pressure.
- Retinal detachment.
- Enucleation if the globe is irreparably damaged.
- Sympathetic ophthalmia (affects the uninjured eye) causing blindness.[2,4]

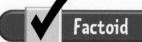

A scar on the cornea is like a curtain on the window! Light cannot enter!

- Glaucoma can also occur later in life if trauma or scarring has damaged (and narrowed) the drainage angle of the eye.[6]
- Do not attempt to remove a foreign object from the eye. This can cause further damage.
- Topical anesthetic drops containing preservatives can cause added damage if allergy occurs, but can be toxic to the retina if there is a penetrating injury.[12]
- Tetanus.
- Vomiting increases ICP.

CHEMICAL TRAUMA

- The longer the chemical is in contact with the eye, the greater the damage.
  - Scarring of the cornea prevents light from entering the eye.
  - Erosion and perforation of the eye damage internal structures.
  - Permanent blindness is always a risk.
- Alkali injuries are especially bad because they penetrate the eye more deeply than acids.[4,5]
- Prolonged (greater than the normal 30 minutes or 2 L) or repetitive irrigation following exposure to hydrofluoric acid may increase corneal ulceration and worsen the outcome.[5]

Interventions and why?

When the patient with eye injury presents in the emergency department, an immediate evaluation of the damage (or potential damage) directs the plan of action. Eyelids are never forced apart and topical preservative-free anesthetics are used to reduce the pain of eye opening.

- Chemical injury always involves flushing until the pH of the eye is normal, with close collaboration with an ophthalmologist.
- While irrigation is underway, gather information about the agent and check the pH of the eye at intervals, continuing irrigation until the pH is normal.
- An ophthalmology consult is initiated for emergency surgery (penetrating or perforating foreign injury, intraocular hemorrhage, dislocated lens, rupture of the orbit or retinal involvement),[12] or specialized intervention is required if vision loss is threatened.
- When there is damage and scarring of the cornea that leaves thick, rough surfaces or opacities, phototherapeutic keratectomy can be performed to improve functional vision.[4]
- Vitrectomy may be required to remove debris or blood causing opacity of the vitreous, which interferes with light projected to the retina (Fig. 11-6).

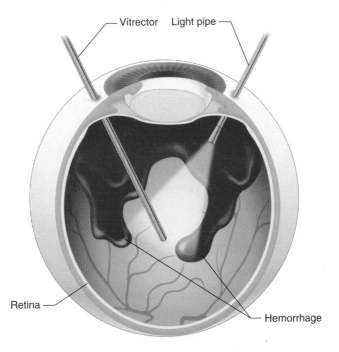

Vitrector   Light pipe

Retina

Hemorrhage

◀ Figure 11-6. Vitrectomy for intraocular hemorrhage.

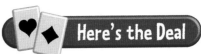

Here's the Deal

Vitrectomy can be performed as an outpatient procedure, and is indicated for many conditions such as diabetic retinopathy (Fig. 11-7), in conjunction with other surgeries (ie, macular hole repair) or procedures in which vitreous must be removed to accommodate a gas or silicone oil bubble into the vitreous for retinal compression.

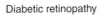

Diabetic retinopathy

Retina

Vitreous

Abnormal blood
vessels

Microaneurisms

Exudate

Hemorrhages

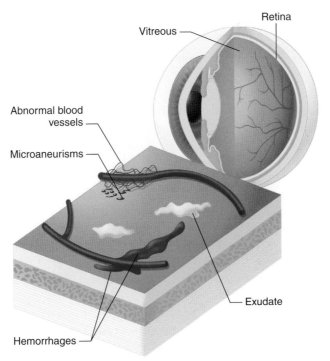

◀ Figure 11-7. Diabetic retinopathy.

- PRN administration of an antiemetic is considered because pain and psychosocial response can trigger nausea.

✚ Trauma

After examination and intervention by the ophthalmologist, the nursing care may include:

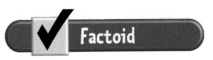

Factoid

Foreign bodies are surgically removed as soon as possible when necessary.

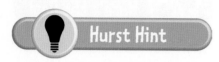

- Bed rest with the head elevated to decrease intraocular pressure.
- Administer prescribed IV antibiotics if the cornea or globe has been perforated.
- Administer tetanus booster (prophylaxis) for contaminated *penetrating* injuries if it has been more than five years since immunization.[4,10]
- Topical antibiotic ointment and pressure patch to immobilize the eyeball may be prescribed for a corneal epithelial defect.[4,8]
- The use of an eye patch is controversial because it may contribute to infection. If the physician orders a patch, be sure to monitor the patient's eye for signs of infection.

✚ Foreign bodies

- The priority is to prevent further injury.
- Do not attempt to remove an embedded foreign object from the eye because this can cause further damage.
- Immediately stabilize a visible penetrating foreign body.
- Make no attempt to remove a foreign body.
- Protect the object from any pressure or from moving.
- Protect the eye with a metal shield if available or a stiff paper cup (Fig. 11-8).
- Close and cover the unaffected eye to prevent contralateral movement of the affected eyeball.

▶ Figure 11-8. First aid to stabilize foreign body.

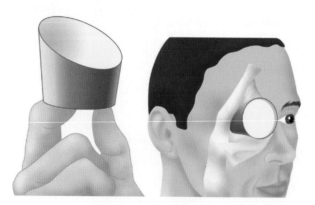

Nonpenetrating foreign bodies (trash, small nonembedded debris) can be removed with irrigation and eye movements or the gentle touch of a sterile applicator. The general practitioner never attempts:

- Removal of anything embedded
- Cleaning an injured eye (which could accidentally clean away an iris or a lens)
- Padding an injured eye (because intraocular pressure can increase, causing herniation)
- Putting creams or any medication containing preservatives into the eye[12]

CHEMICAL BURNS (ACIDS OR ALKALIS)

- The priority is to prevent further damage.
- Flush first, examine later!
- Hold eyes open and flush, flush, flush! Solutions and techniques vary according to availability and protocols.
- Severe eye pain can cause involuntary spasm of the eyelids, so irrigation can be very difficult if the eyelid is tightly closed because of pain.[3] Ophthalmic numbing drops can be administered to provide pain relief and aid in irrigation.
- Topical ophthalmic drops to relieve pain (eg, oxybuprocaine, tetracaine, or proparacaine 0.5%) may be prescribed to enable thorough, prolonged irrigation.[5]
- Prehospital irrigation: Dilute the chemical immediately with copious amounts of tap water or normal saline if available.
- Hospital irrigation can be accomplished at an eye wash station to deliver 0.4 gallons/minute for a minimum of 15 minutes (Fig. 11-9).

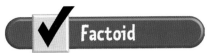

The cornea is the most sensitive tissue in the body, having **five** times more sensory neurons than the finger tips.

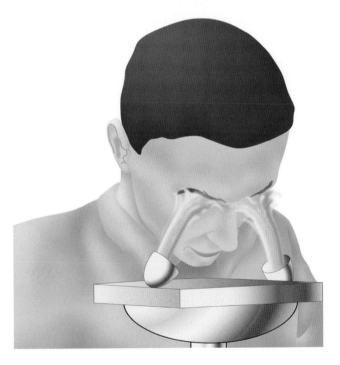

◄ Figure 11-9. Eye wash station.

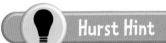

Suspect hydrofluoric acid exposure if the chemical agent is reported to be a rust remover, leather tanning fluid, high-octane gasoline, or glass/enamel etching material.[5]

- Continuous sterile IV solution (NS or Ringer's) using a drip set. Leave the roller clamp wide open while directing the flow of solution from the nasal corner outward (away from the lacrimal duct).
- If the clinical picture and patient history suggests corneal abrasion, a light source and fluorescein drops (a dye that will make scratches and cuts visible under the light) can be diagnostic.[2,4,8]
- The Morgan lens (a polymethylmethacrylate scleral lens with an attached perfusion tube)[5] fits over the eye and separates the lid from the cornea for patient comfort during prolonged irrigation.[3]

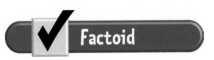

Hydrofluoric acid is the only acid that doesn't follow the rule. It is a weak acid but can penetrate the cell membrane as it becomes nonionized![6]

Hurst Hint

Nothing should delay irrigation! Not even for 20 seconds! If you can check eye pH while the irrigation is being set up, do it! But don't delay irrigation to assess whether it is an acid or an alkali because both require irrigation asap!

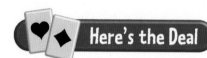

Here's the Deal

The critical first response to these two eye injuries (foreign bodies and chemical burns) means the difference between preserving vision and permanent blindness!

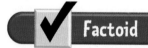

Factoid

Vomiting can increase intraocular pressure in the eye-injured patient, and is to be prevented if possible.

Factoid

Cycloplegic drops produce cycloplegia! This means that the medication paralyzes the ciliary muscle of the eye at the periphery of the iris.

- Warm solution for eye irrigation is more comfortable than cold, but the speed of initiating eye wash is a greater priority than comfort!
- Eye wash is not delayed for removal of contacts unless it can be accomplished quickly. Contacts must however be removed at some point because they hold the irritant in contact with the cornea, but removal is more easily accomplished after a few minutes of irrigation.[3]
- Evert upper eyelid and retract lower lid for irrigation to thoroughly remove the chemical.[3]
- Knowing the agent responsible for the chemical injury helps with decision making.
  - For example, you don't have to worry about flushing the eye too long after alkali exposure. Flushing may need to be continued for up to two hours (with breaks to allow the patient to rest, and to test the pH to see if it has returned to normal).
  - Prolonged (greater than the normal 30 minutes or 2 L) or repetitive irrigation following exposure to hydrofluoric acid may increase corneal ulceration and worsen the outcome.[5]
- Check pH of the eye (pH paper to the inferior fornix) at 30-minute intervals and continue irrigation until the pH is normal (7.0–7.3).
- Some physicians order testing of the pH 30 minutes after irrigation is discontinued in case of slowly dissolving particles in the conjunctiva.[5]

CHEMICAL INJURY   Measures to promote re-epithelization, healing, and comfort following chemical injury, grafting, or surgical intervention:

- Administer sterile lubricating agents (preservative free to decrease chance of allergic reaction).
- Apply topical antibiotic ointment (erythromycin or tetracycline) as ordered.
- Patch the affected eye (as prescribed), insuring that the lid is fully closed.
- Assess the pain level (scale of 1–10) and administer prescribed analgesia PRN.
- Topical corticosteroid (prednisolone or dexamethasone ophthalmic drops) may be prescribed to reduce the inflammatory response.[5]
- Instill cycloplegic ophthalmic drops as prescribed for pain relief and to prevent the complication of iris adhesion to the cornea or lens.[5]
- Tetanus status is assessed, and a booster is given if necessary.
- Photographs are indicated if the injury is a result of assault or a workplace accident and are helpful in documenting injuries. (Police are also involved for assault cases.)[12]

PATIENT TEACHING   To prevent eye injuries from trauma and infection, the patient wearing contact lenses should be taught to:

- Remove contact lenses at the very onset of discomfort!
- Use meticulous hygiene and care when inserting and removing contacts.
- Use daily wear disposable lenses rather than extended wear when vacationing or visiting high-altitude areas.

Extended-wear contacts (even those with high oxygen permeability) decrease oxygenation of the cornea, and high altitudes with "thinner air" even further decrease oxygen delivery to the cornea. Continuous extended wear eliminates recovery time of the cornea, which can cause contact lens–induced hypoxia and increased risk for infection.[8]

PATIENT TEACHING   Patient teaching to prevent eye injuries includes instructions to:

- Wear eye protection (polycarbonate glasses with side shields or goggles) whenever there is any risk of eye trauma.
- Avoid low-hanging branches when operating sports vehicles.
- Check the direction of spray nozzles before activating the spray to avoid accidental spray in the face.
- Read instructions and follow precautions when using tools and chemicals.
- Be alert to others who have potentially dangerous articles, such as scissors, pencils, darts, pellet guns, and projectiles, and stay out of harm's way.
- Buckle up! Penetrating eye injuries have decreased as a result of legislated compulsory vehicular seatbelt usage.[12]

Patient teaching to prevent or minimize damage from chemical exposure includes instructions to:

- Use goggles to protect swimmers from the chemical effects of chlorinated water.[7]
- Eye protection must be always worn when using potentially hazardous chemicals, especially acids and alkalis.
- Never rub an eye that burns and hurts from exposure to a chemical agent (whether it is hairspray or lye) because this spreads the irritant around the eye.
- Flush, flush, flush with running tap water immediately and then have the eye examined by a professional.

As a rule, the patient and family are always anxious when vision is threatened, and it is important to communicate optimistic yet realistic prognosis and expected outcomes of interventions.

Cutting edge

All's well that ends well! Periorbital cellulitis occurring 3 days after a fall from an ATV called for surgical exploration of the affected eye with no foreign body visualized. Ultrasound following surgery revealed the foreign body with characteristics of wood, removal of which was accomplished percutaneously with the guidance of sonography. No visual loss or impairment of any kind was noted at the 6-month follow-up.[13]

✛ Retinal detachment

Let's get the normal stuff straight!

The retina contains the neurosensory layer that transmits impulses to the optic nerve, so any damage, displacement, or ischemia of the retina equals loss of vision!

The retina is the innermost layer of the eye and is composed of a blanket of nerve fibers on the inside continuous with the vitreous and an outer pigmented layer (Fig. 11-10) nestled against the fine layer of capillaries in the choroid layer.

▶ Figure 11-10. Layers of the retina.

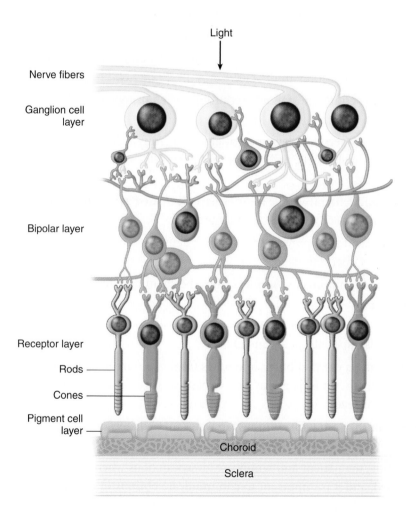

The receptor layer of the retina contains the photoreceptor cells of the rods and cones:

• Rods are responsible for low light, noncolor (black and white), night vision, and peripheral vision.

• Cones are responsible for perception of color, fine details, and central vision.

• The macula is a small central "yellow spot" in the retina (surrounded by, but containing no blood vessels) that is totally made up of densely packed cones (Fig. 11-11).

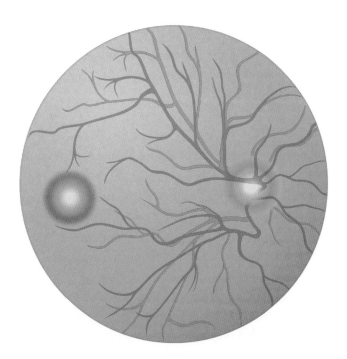

◀ Figure 11-11. Macula devoid of blood vessels.

- The only blood supply for the fovea centralis (in the center of the macula) comes from the capillaries in the choroids layer, which is attached to the pigmented layer of the retina.
- The optic nerve (cranial nerve #2) connects the eye to the brain. The optic nerve carries the impulses formed by the retina to the brain, where neural impulses are interpreted as images.
- The vitreous adheres to the macula, the optic disc, and around the edges of the retina.

The retina and optic nerve receive blood supply from the renal artery, which enters with the optic nerve at the center of the optic disc (via the optic papilla) and the choroid (Fig. 11-12).

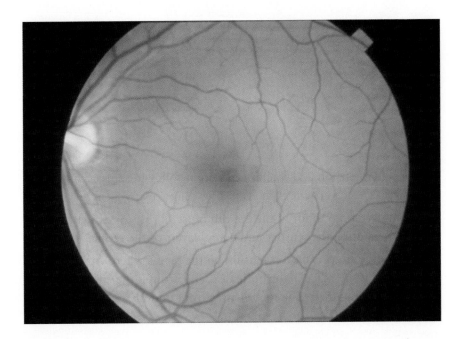

◀ Figure 11-12. Normal retina (vessels arising from optic disc). National Eye Institute, National Institutes of Health.

What is it?

The underlying support tissue of the retina separates from the pigmented layer, pulling the photoreceptor cells away from their major blood supply (the choroid).[1]

Causes and why?

Retinal detachment can be caused by the 4 Ts: trauma, tension, traction, and tumors!

- The impact of blunt trauma to the head can lead to immediate detachment or detachment that becomes apparent at a later time.

- Infection from penetrating trauma or chronic inflammation of the eye (uveitis) can lead to exudates, which can separate retinal layers.

- Perforating trauma can produce a rent or tear, causing a hole in the retina, allowing vitreous to leak out behind the retina, and separating the thin retinal surface from underlying tissue. This type of detachment is called *rhegmatogenous retinal detachment* because it only occurs when there is a hole in the retina (Fig. 11-13).

◄ Figure 11-13. Detached retina.

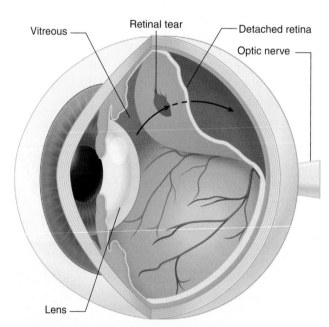

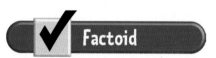

Factoid

Rhegmatogenous (REG-mah-toe-GIN-us) is actually two words: *rhegma* is a Greek word meaning a rip, rent, or tear producing a hole; and *genous* meaning originating from or the origin of.[14]

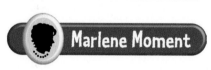

Marlene Moment

Rhegma? That's Greek to me! You didn't know that you would have to learn a foreign language when you applied to nursing school, did you? Now that you know it means "hole" there are all kinds of ways to use this word! (A black rhegma, a donut rhema,: lots of possibilities!) Isn't learning new words fun?

- Intraocular tension and traction can occur following surgery inside the eye. (This can occur even years after cataract surgery.)[1]

- A fluid-secreting tumor in the eye can cause fibrosis or exudates to form, separating the sensory and neural layers of the retina.

- Thick vitreous gel can exert tension on the places where vitreous is attached (at the macula, the optic disc, and around the edges of the retina), causing the retina to pull away from underlying tissue at these sites.

- Highly nearsighted (myopic) people have larger than normal, elongated eyeballs, which puts tension on the periphery of the retina, and can lead to lattice (criss-cross pattern) degeneration from having the retina stretched too thinly, and causing detachment (Fig. 11-14).

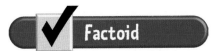
◄ Figure 11-14. Myopic (nearsighted) eyeball.

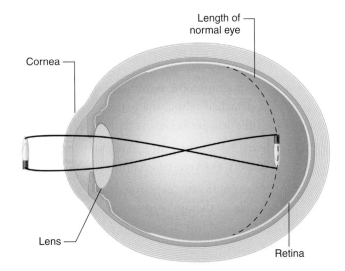

Length of normal eye

Cornea

Lens

Retina

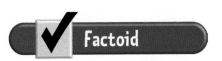
Factoid

Pilocarpine, a drug used to treat glaucoma, can also increase the risk for retinal detachment because it constricts the pupil, which causes pulling (traction) on the retina.

Testing, testing, testing

The eye must first be dilated in order to visually inspect for a retinal tear or retinal detachment:

- Ophthalmoscopy (direct or indirect; see Figs. 11-3 and 11-5)
- Slit-lamp examination (see Fig. 11-4)
- Ultrasound imaging
- Fluorescein angiography (photography of the retinal vessels using dye)

Other standard eye tests of visual ability to evaluate the intactness of the retina are:

- The refraction test determines the ability of the eye to focus light on the retina.
- Color perception (made possible by the photoreceptor cells of the cones) in the neural layer of the retina and the optic nerve
- The reflex response of pupils checks the ability of the ciliary bodies on either side of the iris to open and close the pupil in response to light and accommodation.

Electroretinography is used to record electrical currents in response to visual stimuli.

Signs and symptoms and why?

- Bright flashing spots of light (like sparks) caused by vitreous gel pulling on the retina
- Sudden increase in floaters (spots or "cobwebs" on the visual field) caused by condensations in the vitreous gel
- A dark curtain or shadow (like a shade being pulled down) progressing across the visual field

Factoid

Because there are no pain fibers in the retina, retinal pathology is painless.

What can harm my patient and why?

Once the retina begins to detach, the tendency is for detachment to continue until the entire retina is involved! No retina means no vision! If the detachment is not treated promptly total permanent blindness can occur. If the area of detachment involves the macula, surgical repair can restore peripheral vision. Central vision may be lost permanently.

Interventions and why?

As soon as ophthalmoscopic examination by the physician confirms a diagnosis of detached retina, the patient is prepared for surgery to close and seal the hole/tear in the retina and/or reattach the retina.

- Hold patients NPO when they have symptoms of retinal detachment because surgery needs to be accomplished as soon as possible.
- Reinforce the physician's explanations of the scleral buckle, diathermy, cryotherapy, laser therapy, or pneumatic retinopexy.
- Establish IV access and ensure that necessary labs and consent forms are on the chart.
- Provide factual reassurance about the success rate of repairing and/or reattaching the retina.

Eye Surgery: General Postoperative Care

Following eye surgery, the primary nursing interventions are directed toward supportive care and patient education.
- Maintain prescribed patient position.
- Ensure access to the patient call bell.
- Provide assistance with hygienic care and ADLs.
- Administer non-narcotic, mild PO analgesia as prescribed.

▶ Figure 11-15. Pneumatic Retinopexy. Postprocedural head down position floats the bubble toward the retina.

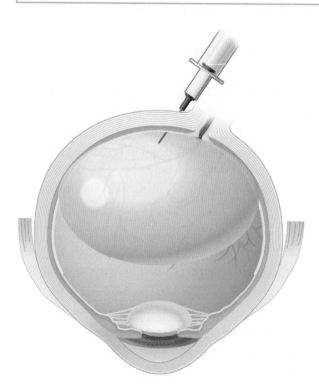

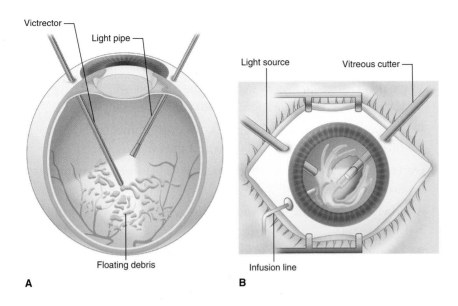

Victrector
Light pipe
Floating debris
A

Light source
Vitreous cutter
Infusion line
B

◀ Figure 11-16. Pars plana vitrectomy (A) and surgeon's view (B).

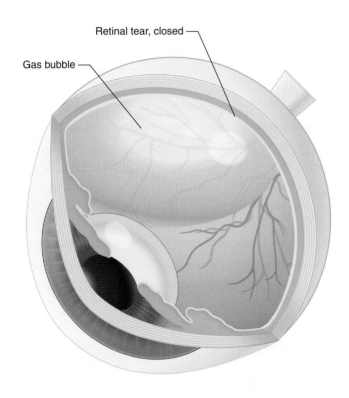

Retinal tear, closed
Gas bubble

◀ Figure 11-17. Pneumatic retinopexy.

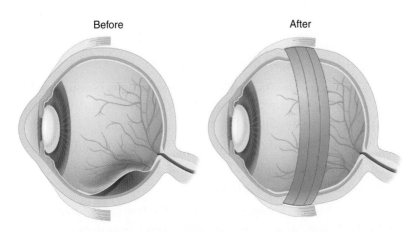

Before

After

◀ Figure 11-18. Scleral buckle for retinal detachment.

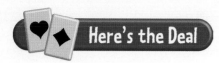

Here's the Deal

Depending on the location of the retinal detachment, the patient is required to maintain a position that will direct the injected bubble toward the detached area to press against the retina, pushing it back into place. The patient could be required to maintain a face-down position (or lie on the side with one cheek against the surface, depending on the area of the detached segment) for one to three weeks for the majority of each day (16–22 hours/day).

When dealing with retinal tears or retinal detachment, the longer the delay, the poorer the prognosis for return of vision. Depending on the characteristics of the retinal disorder, the following interventions may be indicated (Fig. 11-15):

- Pars plana vitrectomy to remove vitreous that is pulling against the retina, or building up behind the retina, having leaked out through a torn place causing detachment. Vitrectomy is also used in conjunction with pneumatic retinopexy when some vitreous must be removed to accommodate injection of the gas bubble (Fig. 11-16).
- Pneumatic retinopexy involves injection of a gas bubble, which will rise and apply internal pressure to push a torn place in the retina against the wall, sealing the tear (Fig. 11-17).
- Laser (photocoagulation) or cryosurgery (freezing) to bond the retinal tear to the eye wall, sealing the tear (Fig. 11-18).
- Scleral buckle with placement of a flexible band around the center of the eye to counterbalance the force pulling the retina out of place, sometimes also requiring a vitrectomy.

Prognosis is good following the above interventions if the macula is not involved.

PATIENT TEACHING   Following retinal intervention (vitrectomy, laser surgery, cryotherapy, diathermy, pneumatic retinopexy, or scleral buckle):

- Keep the head elevated at all times after scleral buckling.
- Vision may change after scleral buckling (the band pressing inward changes the shape of the eyeball); therefore, a follow-up vision exam is needed.
- Report double vision or strabismus (cross eyes) immediately after scleral buckle because the band can affect the eye muscles.
- Don't strain with lifting or bowel movements because this can increase intraocular pressure (IOP).
- Avoid vigorous exercise until your doctor gives the "okay" (usually 3–4 weeks).
- Report eye pain, redness, exudates, or hazy vision of the affected eye because of the risk for infection and cataract formation after invasive eye surgery
- Teach proper handwashing technique prior to instilling postop eye drops.
- Teach proper (no touch) technique of instilling eye drops into the lower conjunctival sac rather than onto the eyeball.
- Investigate various commercial positioning aids to maintain the prescribed position while promoting comfort and utility in activities of daily living.

Cutting edge

After only 30 minutes of on-site training in the use of bedside ultrasound, emergency physicians were able to diagnose retinal detachment with a high level of sensitivity and specificity. This study in Los Angeles, CA concludes that bedside ultrasound can be a valuable assessment tool for the nonophthalmologist physician in identifying retinal detachment.[15] There are additional advantages of bedside ultrasound:

- Bedside ultrasound is a safer and more comfortable diagnostic modality than a dilated eye exam following trauma, especially in the presence of hyphema.
- A complication of the medication Atropine (used to dilate the eye) is acute glaucoma.[16]

✚ Cataracts

As the population ages, cataracts continue to be an increasing health issue.[17]

Let's get the normal stuff straight!

The crystalline lens is structurally biconvex (curving outward on both sides) and is located directly behind the iris. It is suspended place by ligaments attached to the ciliary body.

- The lens is composed mainly of water-soluble protein fibers.
- Having no blood supply and a very low oxygen demand, the lens is nourished by the aqueous humor.
- The three layers of the lens consist of a thin transparent membrane (the capsule) that surrounds the soft cortex, with a firm nucleus in the center.

- The ciliary muscles control accommodation of the lens to ensure that light is focused on the macula for clear vision (Fig. 11-19).

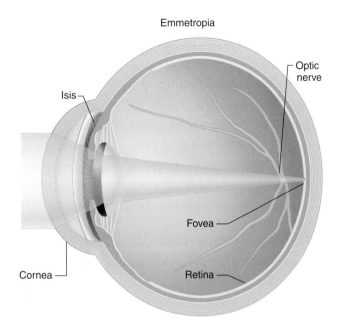

Emmetropia

Optic nerve

Isis

Fovea

Cornea

Retina

◀ Figure 11-19. Emmetropia of crystalline lens.

- The lenses change shape to become more or less spherical in response to the action of ciliary muscles.
- As the lens changes shape, the refractive power changes rapidly (in the presence of emmetropia) for near and distant vision (accommodation).
- As light enters via the cornea, it is focused by the lens onto the retina where the photoreceptor cells in the sensory layer send impulses to the neural layer for transmission to the optic nerve and interpretation by the brain as images.

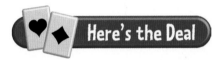

Here's the Deal

Emmetropia describes the visual ability to focus distant objects sharply on the retina without the need of corrective lenses.

What is it?

Cataracts are a progressive condition characterized by cloudy opacity of the lens that reduces light transmission to the retina and diminishes visual acuity.

- Opacity can develop anterior or posterior in any part of the lens: the capsule, the cortex, or the nucleus.
- Gradually the opacity increases in density and involves a greater area of the lens.
- Cataracts are the leading cause of blindness worldwide, affecting almost half of the population except in the most developed countries.[18]

Causes and why?

Cataracts are commonly associated with aging, but also may be precipitated by trauma, metabolic or genetic disorders, poor nutrition, ultraviolet irradiation, or various kinds of oxidative stress.

- Aging causes loss of flexibility/elasticity and increasing density of the lens because of clumping of alpha proteins.
- Injury associated with eye trauma or eye surgery can lead to intraocular inflammatory changes affecting the lens.

- Congenital cataracts (commonly seen with Down's syndrome) result from a genetic defect.
- Metabolic disorders (renal disease, metabolic syndrome with hyperlipidemia, diabetes) that increase systemic oxidative stress and decrease the efficiency of repair mechanisms of the lens.
- The damaging effect of prolonged exposure to UV rays is most risky at high altitudes or reflecting off water or snow.[8]
- Poor nutrition (lack of antioxidants), dehydration, or obesity (decreased percentage of body water) has a direct effect on the aqueous humor and health the lens.
- Certain medications (prolonged high-dose corticosteroids), chemicals (especially alkali), heavy metals (copper, iron, gold, silver, or mercury) and cigarette smoking and alcohol consumption have a toxic effect on the lens.[4,17]

Testing, testing, testing

Cataracts are easy to diagnose because they are clearly visible and alter visual acuity!

- Direct ophthalmoscopy (see Fig. 11-3) reveals opacity of the lens.
- Visual acuity testing is accomplished with use of the Snellen chart (Fig. 11-20).

▶ Figure 11-20. Snellen chart tests visual acuity.

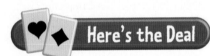

Here's the Deal

The Snellen chart (used to test distant vision) is composed of progressively smaller rows of letters, and the patient is asked to read the smallest letters that he or she can see from the usual distance of 20 feet. If the patient can read the 20/20 line, he or she is said to have normal vision. Each eye is tested separately. If a patient can only see the largest letter (the big E) clearly, he or she had 20/200 vision (legally blind), which means that this person sees at 200 feet what the person with normal vision can see at 20 feet. If the person cannot even see the first large letter at 20 feet, he or she keeps moving forward (to perhaps 10 feet away) until the largest letter can be identified. This visual acuity (at 10 feet) would be graded as 10/200.

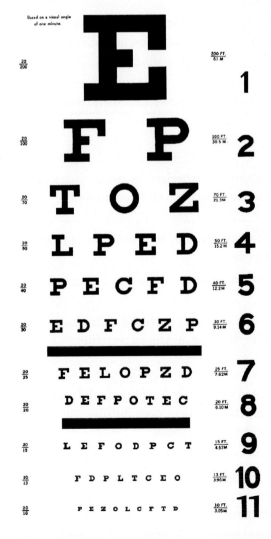

- Color perception is tested by using the Ishihara polychromatic plates, which are bound together as a booklet containing dots of primary colors making different patterns and shapes hidden against backgrounds of secondary colors. Patients with poor central vision cannot find the hidden pictures.[4]

Signs and symptoms and why?

Cataracts don't just happen overnight! Very gradually the patient will begin to notice hazy vision and a subtle change in color perception.

- Vision is described as cloudy, blurry, fuzzy, or dim (Fig. 11-21).

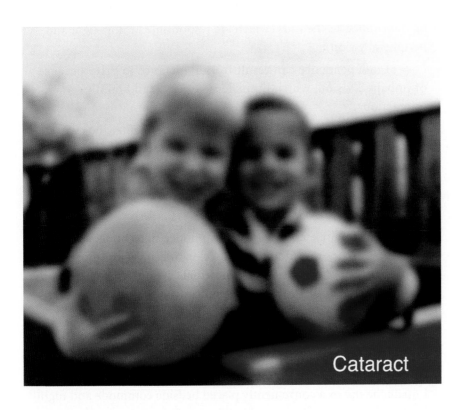

◀ Figure 11-21. How things might appear through eyes with cataract. National Eye Institute, National Institutes of Health.

- Double vision may be present in a single eye.
- There is difficulty in reading and brighter lights are required.
- Increasingly near vision is obscured and reading glasses are needed.
- Patient history reveals frequent prescription changes for eyeglasses or contacts.
- Color perception is altered, usually reported as a dulling or yellowing of color.
- Night vision is poor because light cannot be focused onto the rods, which are responsible for night vision.
- Eyes become very sensitive to light and to glares from headlights at night.
- The patient complains of eyestrain and blinks often to clear the visual field.

What can harm my patient and why?

Impaired vision caused by a cataract can interfere with all aspects of daily living:

- There is an increased risk of falls, especially when getting up at night to go to the restroom.
- There is an increased incidence of fractured hip caused by decreased visual acuity (ie, missing the bottom step or failing to see objects in the pathway).[19]
- Reduced quality of life, especially for those >65 years of age which includes limited opportunities for social interaction with resultant lack of social support and feelings of isolation.
- Driving becomes unsafe, especially at night, because light rays cannot be transmitted to the rods (which are responsible for low-light and peripheral vision).
- Loss of independence can result from reluctance to drive because of impaired vision, which limits leisure, work, and family interactions.

When both lenses are totally opaque (no light can enter the eye), the patient will be blind without cataract surgery and lens replacement.

Interventions and why?

The home health nurse may be the first to notice signs of decreasing vision, such as stains on clothing or the "clown-face" syndrome from inappropriately applied make-up.[20] Immediate action taken in the home for any visual impairment of elderly people involves safety issues first, followed by an evaluation for diagnosis:

- Eliminate potential threats to the patient's safety, such as loose throw rugs, electrical cords, and clutter or obstructions to a pathway (eg, a foot stool).[22]
- Initiate the use of a conveniently placed bedside commode and night-lights in bedroom, hallway, and bathroom areas.
- Place assistive devices close at hand and have the patient touch them to verify their location.
- Initiating a consult and/or appointment for a comprehensive eye exam by an ophthalmologist for evaluation of age-related vision loss (which could be cataracts or macular degeneration).

Preparation for cataract surgery (which is usually accomplished on an outpatient basis) involves:

- A thorough health history, including medications (especially anticoagulant therapy) and allergies (especially to local anesthetics and antibiotics).

Factoid

Age-related macular degeneration (ARMD) is the most prevalent cause of vision loss in the 69+ age group.[21]

Here's the Deal

Both cataracts and ARMD have similar symptoms—seeing dull colors, needing more light for close work, and blurry vision—but when the blurred vision is in the center of the visual field, macular involvement is suspected! Unlike cataracts, ARMD cannot be cured with surgery; however, the progression can be slowed with laser or transthermal laser photocoagulation and medications such as Macugen (pegaptanib) and Lucentis (ranibizumab), as well as eye protection against UV rays and increasing intake of antioxidants.[20,22] The patient with ARMD is given an Amsler grid to check vision every day for progressing visual dysfunction. The doctor is to be notified if the straight lines appear wavy or crooked and/or appear closer or more distant (Fig. 11-22).[5,20,22]

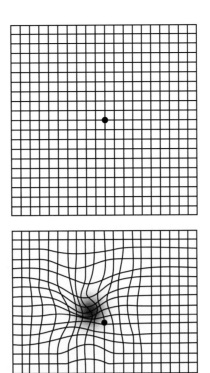

◀ Figure 11-22. Normal Amsler grid (top) and distorted view (bottom). National Eye Institute, National Institutes of Health.

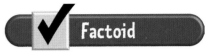

Factoid

With the use of smaller incisions, phacoemulsification (fak-o-e-mul-sih-fih-KA-shun) with suction and fold up plastic intraocular lens placed into the posterior membranous capsule, many patients are allowed to continue anticoagulant therapy without significantly increasing risk of bleeding.[20]

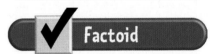

Factoid

Diopters are units to measure refractive error. A negative number represents nearsightedness (myopia) and a positive number represents farsightedness (hyperopia). A second number (positive or negative) reflects the amount of astigmatism (abnormal curve of the cornea), and lastly, presbyopia has to be considered if magnification is needed for clear vision at near distances (bifocals).

- Evaluation of family support system for assistance postoperatively.

- Getting the right lens! Biometric measures (diopters) of the axial length of the eye, the cornea, and the front of the optic disc are taken and keratometry measures the cornea at its tallest peak and flattest area for determining the most accurate power of lens to implant for best vision.[17]

In preparation for outpatient surgery the patient will need:

- To remain NPO for 12 hours before the procedure.

- Instillation of prescribed ophthalmic drops to dilate the eye according to surgeon preference. For example, two drops each of cyclopentolate hydrochloride 1% and phenylephrine hydrochloride 2.5% given 10 minutes apart.[23]

- Additional preoperative drops may include one drop each of ketorolac tromethamine 0.5% or nepafenac 0.1% (NSAID/anti-inflammatory) and gatifloxacin 0.3% or moxifloxacin 0.5% (anti-infective).

- Someone to drive the patient home and help with postop care.

- Verbal information outlining prescribed therapy postoperatively and the importance of adherence to written guidelines.

Once cataracts become symptomatic and significantly alter vision, surgery is the treatment of choice and can be accomplished by several techniques:

- Intracapsular cataract extraction removes the entire lens and the incision is closed with sutures. This old method is currently only used if the cataract is displaced or dislocated.

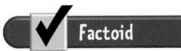

Factoid

Having the patient keep his or her eye closed after instilling the eye drop, and holding pressure for up to five minutes on the inner canthus of the affected eye will enhance uptake of the medication by tissues of the eye and minimize systemic absorption.[24]

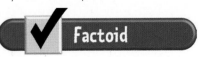

Factoid

Many elderly patients requiring cataract surgery live alone and are unable to perform postop self-care activities.[20]

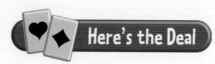

Hypopyon is a term that means "accumulation of white blood cells in the anterior chamber of the eye."[14]

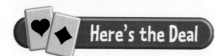

Implanted intraocular lenses (IOLs) are not for everybody! Diabetics with retinopathy, recurrent uveitis, neovascular glaucoma, or rubeosis iridis are not candidates for IOLs. Because IOLs don't have the capacity to change shape for accommodation, patients may still require reading glasses for close vision or prescription lens for distant vision. Contacts are another option if the patient can be successfully taught to insert, remove, and clean them (Fig. 11-23).[4]

▶ Figure 11-23. Intraocular lens implant.

- Extracapsular cataract extraction has a smaller incision to remove the anterior capsule, the lens nucleus, and cortex. The posterior capsule of the lens is retained to anchor an intraocular lens.

- Phacoemulsification can be accomplished with an ultrasonic device or with laser to break up the nucleus and cortex of the lens for removal by suction, leaving the posterior capsule intact. A phaco needle has the ability to cut and suction simultaneously to break up and evacuate the cataract.

- New silicone, foldable lens can be inserted during cataract surgery through the same tiny "phaco" hole, giving rise to fewer complications.[4]

Even though the surgery is accomplished on an outpatient basis, the patient is seen the next day to check for any iatrogenic complications, such as may occur with toxic anterior segment syndrome.

- This syndrome is caused by foreign material introduced into the eye that results in an inflammatory response, which is quickly symptomatic and may cause permanent damage to the anterior segment structures.

- The patient could react to the coating on the implantable lens or toxins remaining on surgical instruments from cleaning agents or from irrigating solutions or ophthalmic drops.

- Signs of toxic anterior segment syndrome (blurred vision, a red eye, hypopyon, and painless corneal edema) will occur within the first 24 hours.[23]

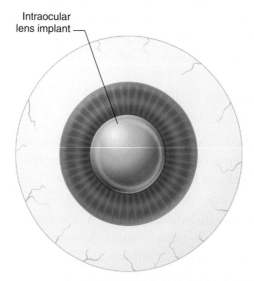

Intraocular lens implant

PATIENT TEACHING Prevention and early detection of cataracts is the focus for patient teaching:

- Have a comprehensive, dilated eye exam every two years or more often if the patient is at high risk for developing cataracts (ie, diabetic patients need a yearly eye exam).

- Persons with refractive errors need to have a visual acuity exam yearly.

- Don't wait for your regularly scheduled exam if your vision suddenly changes or you develop other symptoms!

Topics for postop teaching after phacoemulsification with intraocular lens implantation:

- Safely administer prescribed eye drops and observe the importance of handwashing.
- Protect the affected eye during sleep by faithfully wearing the plastic eye shield.
- Keep your plastic eye shield clean by washing it with soap and water.
- Observe for signs of infection daily, and be alert to excessive redness (erythema), swelling (edema), or "stickiness" when opening the lid.[17]

Cutting edge

Management of inflammation following intraocular surgery traditionally depends upon patient compliance with multiple eye drops taken as often as four times daily. A new strategy to offset poor patient compliance and variable corneal absorption tested by a group of ophthalmologists shows very promising results. Dexamethasone 0.1 mL (4 mg/mL) was injected through the paracentesis site into the anterior chamber at the end of cataract surgery. There were significantly fewer patient reports of ocular inflammation (redness, pain, sensation of something in the eye, lacrimation, and photophobia) on the first postoperative day by the nonglaucoma patients as well as improved subjective reports of recovery.[25]

✛ Glaucoma

Glaucoma is known as the "silent thief"[26] because by the time the person seeks treatment for this insidious, progressive eye disorder, the optic nerve may already be irreparably damaged.

Let's get the normal stuff straight!

The eye has an anterior and a posterior chamber, each of which has a well-defined boundary:

- The anterior chamber of the eye is enclosed by the cornea in front and the iris and middle part of the lens in the back.
- The posterior chamber is a narrow space behind the iris in front of the suspensory ligament of the lens and the ciliary processes.

There is normally a constant balance of the production of aqueous humor and the corresponding reabsorption and outflow of aqueous humor.

- The ciliary body maintains a constant production of aqueous humor to nourish the lens and cornea.
- Aqueous flows from the posterior chamber (where it is manufactured) over the lens and through the pupil into the anterior chamber.
- Once in the anterior chamber, aqueous flows over the anterior surface of the iris and filters through the trabecular meshwork.
- The trabecular meshwork containing spaces of Fontana (like a sieve) drains aqueous from the anterior chamber into the canal of Schlemm.

- The canal of Schlemm lies at the angle where the iris and the cornea meet between the anterior surface of the iris and the sclera (Fig. 11-24).

▶ Figure 11-24. Cross-section anterior and posterior chambers.

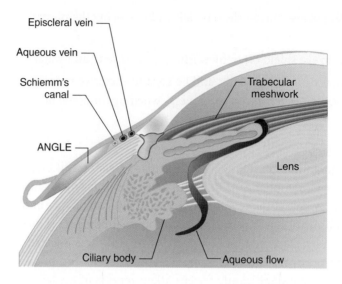

- The canal of Schlemm is a tiny thin-walled vein that goes all the way around the circumference of the iris.
- The endothelial membrane of the vein/canal of Schlemm is very porous and allows passage of large molecules.
- Some aqueous humor is reabsorbed in the trabecular meshwork with the remainder exiting via trabecular and uveoscleral outflow (Fig. 11-25).

▶ Figure 11-25. Inflow and outflow of aqueous humor.

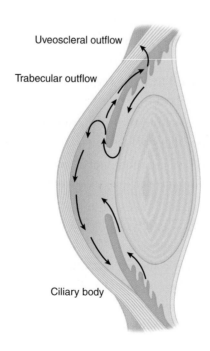

What is it?

Glaucoma affects >60 million people worldwide and is a leading cause of blindness in the United States.[1] Glaucoma is an optic neuropathy associated with increasing intraocular pressure (IOP) in most patients (80%–85%),[27] and is characterized by vision loss. Glaucoma disorders include primary angle-closure glaucoma, primary open-angle glaucoma, and secondary glaucoma.[1,18,26,27]

Causes and why?

Glaucoma is related to a variety of conditions that impede the flow of aqueous humor through the canal of Schlemm or an imbalance of the following factors:

- The rate of production and secretion of aqueous humor by the ciliary body
- Resistance to flow of aqueous from the posterior chamber to the anterior chamber
- Resistance to drainage through the trabecular meshwork into the canal of Schlemm

There are various risk factors for various types of glaucoma, each of which has differing presentations and causations (Table 11-1).

Table 11-1 Comparison of types of glaucoma

Primary open-angle glaucoma	Primary angle-closure glaucoma	Secondary glaucoma
Frequency:	Frequency:	Frequency:
Most common type of glaucoma	Not common, except in high-risk populations	Variable
Cause:	Cause:	Causes include:
Slow, insidious onset caused by a structural abnormality within the trabecular meshwork, resulting in decreased outflow of aqueous humor	Sudden obstruction of the angle of the anterior chamber by the peripheral iris. Can be acute (a medical emergency), subacute, or chronic	• Inflammatory conditions of the eye with edema closing off the canal of Schlemm • Intraocular tumors that obstruct the outflow of aqueous humor • Trauma with intraocular hemorrhage that obstructs the canal of Schlemm • Trauma in the form of corneal edema and scarring can obstruct the outflow of aqueous humor
Populations at highest risk: • African American and Hispanic populations because of genetic predisposition • Middle-aged and elderly people, because aging enlarges and pushes the lens forward	Populations at highest risk: • The East Asian population (Japanese and Chinese from Singapore and Hong Kong) comprise 87% of cases[28] because of an inherited anatomical defect resulting in a shallow anterior chamber[1]	

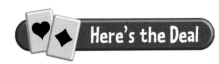

Here's the Deal

I have no problem understanding the cause of open-angle glaucoma and you won't either if you think about a stopped up sink with a leaky faucet! The water (aqueous) just keeps coming, but it cannot get out because the drain is clogged! The globe is closed, fluid builds up and applies pressure to the optic nerve. Got it?

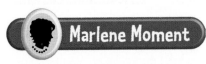

Marlene Moment

Angle-closure is just as simple! Imagine having soaked in the tub, and now the water won't drain out. You find that the drain is open, but a wash cloth was sucked over the drain and is blocking water from draining. With angle-closure the drain is functioning properly, but a portion of the peripheral iris is over the drain, blocking outflow. Remove the wash cloth and water drains out just fine! Likewise, open up a portion of the iris (iridotomy) and aqueous flows out normally because there is no problem with the drain.

(Continued)

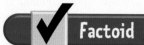

Factoid

If a medication causes the pupil to dilate, it can lead to acute glaucoma.[16]

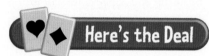

Here's the Deal

Mydriatics (drugs that dilate the pupil) cause the iris to bunch up around the periphery and increase the risk of closing off the drain! If the outflow of aqueous humor is blocked, intraocular pressure can build up quickly in patients at risk for angle-closure glaucoma.[1,16]

Table 11-1. Comparison of types of glaucoma (*Continued*)

Primary open-angle glaucoma	Primary angle-closure glaucoma	Secondary glaucoma
• Pre-existing elevated IOP exaggerates the response to additional aqueous humor • Family history (first-degree relative with glaucoma) • Nearsightedness (myopia), because excessive axial elongation is associated with flattening of the cornea[29] • Diabetes or hypertension because of peripheral vessel spasm	• Elderly persons, because the lens enlarges with aging, pushing the iris forward • Female gender • Farsightedness, because hyperopic persons have smaller anterior chambers with more narrow angles	Medications implicated in development of secondary angle-closure glaucoma are: • Glucocorticoids • Adrenergic agonists • Cholinergics • Sulfa-containing preparations • SSRIs • Tricyclic antidepressants • Anticoagulants • Histamine blockers

Source: Created by the author from References 1 and 27.

Testing, testing, testing

- Gonioscopy evaluates the drainage angle of the eye with a three-mirrored gonio lens (placed over the eye) to determine if the angle is open, narrowed, or closed, and to rule out any other conditions that could increase intraocular pressure (Fig. 11-26).

► Figure 11-26. Gonioscopy checks angle.

Goldmann three mirror goniolenses

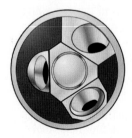 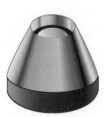

Front view   Back view

- Tonometry to measure the intraocular pressure. The normal range is 10 to 21 mm Hg.
- Biomicroscopy using the slit-lamp to examine the cornea, pupil, and anterior chamber
- Ophthalmoscopy to examine the optic nerve and optic disc for edema, damage, and structural damage

Signs and symptoms and why?

The patient with acute primary angle-closure glaucoma will have identifiable symptoms:

- Ipsilateral (severe headache on the same side as the affected eye) headache.
- Nausea and vomiting
- Painful red eye
- Semidilated, fixed, or nonreactive pupil
- Injected sclera
- Seeing halos around lights and blurred vision
- Photophobia (increased sensitivity to light)[27,30]

The patient with open-angle glaucoma doesn't feel any symptoms, not even noticing the loss of peripheral vision because of compensation by turning the head to the side. However, the patient may report sensitivity to light, and these signs may be seen:

- A hazy, edematous cornea
- One eye slightly larger than the other
- Increased lacrimation without discharge[26]

What can harm my patient and why?

The weakest point in the sclera is where the optic nerve exits the eye and this is where pressure becomes localized to compress blood supply and nerve cells, leading to:

- Optic nerve damage caused by multiple microinfarctions
- Permanent irreversible blindness because of damage to optic nerve fibers

Vision loss has a harmful impact in all areas of life: loss of employment and social interactions, emotional (depression because of loss of independence), and physical (increased fall risk).[31]

Interventions and why?

Acute primary angle-closure glaucoma is a medical emergency requiring immediate reduction in intraocular pressure! Prepare the patient for surgery and postop care:

- Explain the purpose of incisional or laser iridectomy or iridotomy, which creates an opening allowing aqueous to drain (reducing IOP).
- Administer the prescribed ophthalmic drops postprocedure to reduce inflammation and/or pain (Table 11-2).

Multiple topical medications (eye drops) may be prescribed in the initial management of primary open-angle glaucoma, which may create a financial hardship, and patients may be embarrassed to admit that they cannot afford the medications upon discharge from the hospital or clinic.

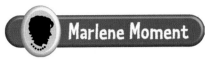

Marlene Moment

Everybody knows how a "brain freeze" feels (ie, eating ice cream fast). The headache with acute primary angle-closure glaucoma feels just like this, only worse!

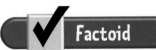

Factoid

Almost four million persons are estimated to develop bilateral blindness by 2010, and most of them will be of Asian descent.[30]

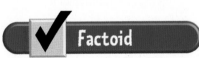

Factoid

Blindness can occur in acute angle-closure glaucoma if intraocular pressure (which can be as high as 40–80 mm Hg)[27] remains elevated for 24 to 48 hours.[32]

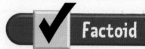

Factoid

Pharmacotherapy can stop the progression of glaucoma, but cannot restore sight. There is no cure for glaucoma, which can lead to blindness if untreated.

- Investigate the patient's financial ability to purchase needed medications and discuss the availability of patient assistance programs. Application forms can be printed from the hospital or clinic computer and given to needy patients.
- Teach the importance of pharmacotherapy as drops are being given, tell what they are used for, and mention the normalcy of transient local side effects.

Table 11-2   Pharmacology in a nutshell: Ophthalmic drugs/drops

Drug classification and name	Mechanism of action	Local and systemic side effects
Prostaglandin analogues are usually the first-line drugs: • Xalatan (latanoprost) • Lumigan (bimatoprost) • Travatan (travoprost)	Relax the ciliary muscle or alter the surrounding tissue to increase outflow of aqueous humor.	Local effects of redness and stinging. Low incidence of adverse effects: • The iris may darken in color. • Eyelashes grow and get thicker.
Beta-adrenergic blocking agents: Topical drops: • OptiPranolol (metipranolol) • Betoptic (betaxolol) • Betimol (timolol hemihydrate) • Timoptic (timolol) • Betagan (levobunolol)	Blocks receptors in ciliary epithelium to reduce the production of aqueous humor.	Causes minimal transient eye discomfort, but when absorbed systemically produces: • Bradycardia • Hypotension • Fatigue • Depression • Impotence • Exacerbation of COPD and asthma

Clinical alert

Have the patient keep the eye closed and be sure to hold fingertip pressure on the inner canthus (punctual occlusion) near the bridge of the nose for up to 5 minutes after each eye drop to minimize systemic absorption.[24]

Alpha$_2$-adrenergic agonists: • Iopidine: (apraclonidine) • Alphagan P (brimonidine)	Decreases production of aqueous humor and increases outflow (exact mechanism unknown).	Common adverse effects: • Dry nasal passageways • Dry mouth Less common adverse effects: • Allergic reactions • Redness of conjunctiva • Visual disturbances
Carbonic anhydrase inhibitors used only as adjunct therapy and only if the patient is NOT allergic to sulfa: Azopt (brinzolamide) Trusopt (dorzolamide)	Reduces production of aqueous humor by blocking an enzyme necessary for transport of sodium and water into the ciliary body.	Local discomfort after instilling the eye drop: • Stinging • Burning • Irritation The patient may experience a transient bitter taste that subsides quickly.

(Continued)

Table 11-2 Pharmacology in a nutshell: Ophthalmic drugs/drops (*Continued*)

Drug classification and name	Mechanism of action	Local and systemic side effects
Cholinergic agonists (miotic agents): • Isopto Carpine, Pilocar (pilocarpine) • Isopto Carbachol (carbachol)	Constricts the pupil, and the resultant pull on ciliary muscles opens up the trabecular meshwork that surrounds the canal of Schlemm.	Visual effects of miotics are: • Nearsightedness • Poor night vision • Blurred vision • Increased lacrimation

Systemic carbonic anhydrase inhibitors (ie, Diamox) are not commonly used because of the risk of potentially fatal aplastic and hemolytic anemic.
Source: Created by the author from References 24 and 30.

It is imperative that glaucoma be detected before injury to the optic nerve occurs, and the only way to accomplish this goal is with comprehensive dilated eye exams on a regular basis. The American Academy of Ophthalmology recommends the following timetable for persons with risk factors:

- Age 40 to 54: comprehensive exam at intervals of one to three years
- Age 55 to 64: comprehensive exam at intervals of every one to two years
- Age 65 and older: comprehensive evaluations every 6 to 12 months

With no added risk factors, the general population should have comprehensive eye examinations every two to four years (age 40–54), every one to three years (age 55–64), and every one to two years for persons 65 years and older.

When a patient is seen with acute primary closed-angle glaucoma, surgery is the primary option to quickly reduce the intraocular pressure:

- Iridectomy (either laser or incisional) to create an opening for the aqueous humor to drain.
- Prophylactic iridectomy is performed on the unaffected eye as well if an anatomic abnormality is the cause of the present emergency. The defect is usually bilateral and surgery can prevent a similar later occurrence.

Primary open-angle glaucoma is initially managed with topical medications to slow progression of the disease and control intraocular pressure in an attempt to preserve vision.

- The treatment plan includes pharmacotherapy primarily administered as eye drops.
- Topical pharmacotherapy works by reducing the production of aqueous humor, increasing outflow of aqueous humor, or a combination of both.

When pharmacotherapy fails because of nonadherence to the daily schedule of eye drops, poor response to medications, or intolerance to the drugs, invasive measures are indicated:

- Laser trabeculoplasty (either argon or selective laser): Both burn small tracts in the meshwork to enhance drainage. Postop inflammation and soreness is managed with NSAID drops.

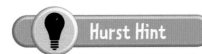
Hurst Hint

Miotics and mydriatics: Here's how to remember which classification of drug constricts and which dilates:
- MI**o**TIC = constricts the pupil (all capital letters, except the little bitty constricted **o** in the center. Remember that the pupil is in the center, round and tiny.)
- My**D**riatics = **D** means **D**ilate!

- Incisional trabeculectomy is indicated when medications and laser surgery have been ineffective in restoring unobstructed aqueous flow and relieving intraocular pressure. A small amount of trabecular tissue is excised to create a drainage pathway, and an antimetabolite such as mitomycin (Mutamycin) or fluorouracil (Adrucil) may be administered to keep scar tissue from forming and re-occluding the surgically created drainage tract.

- Deep sclerotomy is a last resort to "unclog the pipes" and restore drainage! This procedure tunnels through the sclera into the trabecular meshwork to let aqueous humor drain into a reservoir between the inner and outer layers of the sclera and drain into the blood stream.

- Finally, laser cryoablation may be required when all else fails to destroy the ciliary body so that the manufacture of aqueous humor is halted permanently.

There is a high rate of nonadherence to pharmacotherapy because of many factors:

- Many eye drops sting, burn, and cause local irritation.

- Some patients are forgetful rather than noncompliant, but the results (or lack of results) are the same.

- Some patients experience financial hardship because many of the prescribed agents are very expensive.

- Systemic side effects (especially those with beta-adrenergic blocking agents) make using prescribed drops intolerable.

- Many patients do not fully understand the consequences of glaucoma and don't believe that eye drops are really important because they don't improve vision or increase eye comfort.[24,30]

Nursing has the greatest impact on patient compliance through establishing trusting relationships for giving information to replace false beliefs, and patient teaching about glaucoma and the importance of compliance with prescribed treatment plans.

PATIENT TEACHING

- Do not take any over-the-counter OTC medications without first consulting your doctor or nurse practitioner.

- Consult your doctor or nurse practitioner for a list of "safe" medications for commonly occurring complaints (eg, seasonal hay fever or insect bites or stings).

- Seek immediate medical attention for a painful red eye accompanied by GI symptoms.

- Do not stop taking any prescribed topical medications! Let your doctor know about any local or systemic side effects that may occur.

- Report all medications being taken upon hospitalization because glaucoma medications must be continued throughout any hospital stay.

- Report all medications to each of your doctors at every visit as well as with every emergency department or outpatient visit because drug to drug reactions and interactions can occur with topical medications (eye drops).

- Patient assistance programs are available for help paying for prescriptions when you are experiencing financial hardship. Pharmaceutical web sites have applications that can be submitted with physician prescription and offer free medications or medications at a reduced cost. The American Health Assistance Foundation web site shows multiple resources when prescriptions coverage is lacking: http://www.ahaf.org/glaucoma/resource/Financial_Assistance.htm.

Because there is risk for infection deep in the eye following trabeculectomy or trabeculoplasty, the patient is taught:

- Meticulous eye care: Employ diligent handwashing before using eye drops or touching the eye.
- Keep the eye dry: Avoid pools, hot tubs, lakes, etc for at least one month.
- Showering is permitted being careful to keep soap and water away from the eye.
- Women are cautioned to avoid eye makeup for at least one month.
- Wear eye protection as a shield against trauma and debris, and sun glasses to reduce the discomfort of light sensitivity.
- Tape the shield over the eye while sleeping (up to several months postop).[26]

Cutting edge

A news release in 2008 announced that biomedical engineers have devised a contact lens that can continuously measure IOP and administer drops!![24,33] Researchers across the globe are now testing not only the accuracy of the IOP obtained in research labs and with patient volunteers, but also the uptake of glaucoma medications, which have been loaded onto soft disposable contact lens. Current findings show good correlations with results obtained with traditional methods.[34–36]

This innovation opens the door for advanced diagnosis and treatment of glaucoma.

DISORDERS OF THE EAR

Hearing loss can be categorized as conductive, sensorineural, or mixed.

✚ Conductive hearing loss

Something no bigger than a pea (lodged in the auditory canal) can lead to conductive hearing loss!

Let's get the normal stuff straight!

The paired organs of hearing that capture, transmit, and amplify sound consist of external and middle ear structures (Fig. 11-27). (Note that the inner ear is reviewed in the Ménière disease section.)

▶ Figure 11-27. Anatomy of the ear. Reproduced from Saladin K. *Anatomy and Physiology: The Unity of Form and Function.* New York: McGraw-Hill Higher Education; 2007.

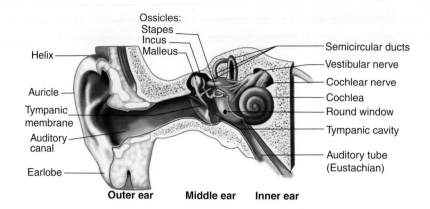

- The pinna (also called the auricle) is the external ear that is visible.
- The pinna is funnel shaped to direct sound into the auditory canal, which is a narrow tube about 1¼ inches long that forms a closed resonator (Fig. 11-28).

▶ Figure 11-28. Sound energy collected by the pinna.

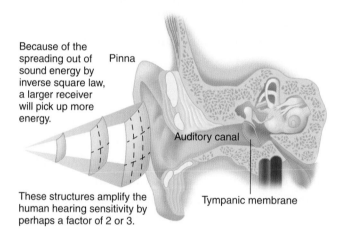

Because of the spreading out of sound energy by inverse square law, a larger receiver will pick up more energy.

Pinna

Auditory canal

These structures amplify the human hearing sensitivity by perhaps a factor of 2 or 3.

Tympanic membrane

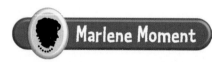

Does this mean that having big ears makes you hear better? It must be true, because when Little Red Riding Hood commented on the wolf's big ears, she said, "The better to hear you with!" (Please be advised that this may not be a scientific principle; otherwise, people with big noses should be able to "smell" better).

- The opening inside the auditory canal is called the *auditory canal meatus*.
- Cerumen, secreted by glands lining the auditory canal, has antimicrobial properties to protect the ear against infections and water repellant effects to excessive moisture, which could make the canal more susceptible to the growth of organisms.
- The auditory canal is also lined with tiny hairs and sebaceous glands.
- Excess cerumen and shed cells work their way out, moving toward the auditory meatus and new wax is laid down.[1,4]
- Waves of sound energy create vibrations within the auditory canal, which are transmitted to the middle ear by the thin, resilient, pearl gray tympanic membrane at the distal end of the auditory canal.
- The tympanic membrane vibrates in response to compressed sound energy coming down the auditory canal and pushes against the malleus (the first of the three tiny bones in the middle ear).

The primary function of the middle ear is to transfer sound energy from air waves to the fluid–membrane waves within the cochlea of the inner ear.

- The middle ear is bordered by the tympanic membrane on one side and the oval window on the other side.
- Structures of the middle ear consist of three uniquely shaped ossicles and the eustachian tube, which is continuous with the nasopharynx.
- The three tiny bones in the middle ear are called ossicles: the malleus (shaped like a hammer), the incus (shaped like an anvil), and the stapes (shaped like a stirrup) (see Fig. 11-27).
- The handle of the hammer (malleus) is attached to the tympanic membrane and receives sound waves from the external ear.
- Waves of sound energy are transmitted through the ossicles similar to the domino effect. One moves and transmits energy to the next.
- The base of the stirrup (stapes) occupies the oval window of the tympanum, which is the membrane-lined, air-filled bony cavity that houses the ossicles (see Fig. 11-27).
- There are muscles around the tiny ossicles in the middle ear that protect the inner ear against harmfully loud noises. The muscles contract in response to loud sounds, thereby reducing the transmission of sound to the inner ear. This is called the *acoustic reflex*.

The inner ear consists of three fluid-filled semicircular canals and the cochlea (because it looks like a snail), which converts the waves produced by sound energy into nerve impulses that are transmitted via the vestibulocochlear nerve (also known as the auditory or acoustic nerve) to the brain.[1,2]

What is it?

Conductive hearing loss occurs with mechanical problems of the external auditory canal or the middle ear and can affect patients across the life span. A number of conditions can obstruct sound waves from being transmitted from the external auditory canal and onward through the middle ear:

- Impacted cerumen is a condition wherein excessive brown wax builds up and becomes lodged in the auditory canal, usually only occurring in one ear.
- Foreign bodies can be anything small enough to get stuck in the auditory canal: a bean or pea, pebbles or beads. Insects can also crawl into the ear and become lodged.
- A perforated tympanic membrane (TM) happens when a hole or a tear occurs in the membrane that separates the middle ear from the external ear.
- Otitis externa (external otitis) is inflammation and/or infection of the external ear.
- Otitis media is inflammation and/or infection of the middle ear.

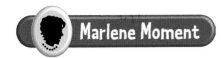

Marlene Moment

Medical terminology is more than just prefixes and suffixes, and it is learned gradually as you progress through clinical courses. Just make sure when you are talking about the little bones of the middle ear, they are Ossicles, not icicles! (You don't want people to laugh at you.) And don't be telling anybody that you have a pain in your "psychotic" nerve either. (Now, that's funny! I know I would have to laugh!)

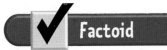

Factoid

Conductive hearing loss means that sound waves do not reach the inner ear because they are interrupted in either the external or middle ear.[32]

- Serous otitis media is a collection of fluid in the middle ear compartment that can be acute or chronic.
- Otosclerosis is a progressive form of low-frequency conductive hearing loss (more common in women) that involves inability of the stapes to carry sound waves forward through the oval window and may progress to the "mixed" variety that is a combination of conductive and sensorineural hearing loss.

What causes it and why?

The causes of conductive hearing loss are as varied as the factors that obstruct sound waves in the external ear.

Cause	Why?
Excess wax	Ceruminous glands produce excess wax, either because of overactivity of normally occurring glands, or an excessive number of glands, each producing a normal amount of wax, a tendency that is usually inherited.
Foreign body	Obstruction of the ear canal blocks sound waves. It can be caused when children, who are naturally curious, put things into their ears, or it can occur accidentally.
Perforated tympanic membrane	This can occur from trauma owing to a foreign object in the external canal, from the pressure of a direct blow to the external ear, or in conjunction with chronic otitis media because suppuration (pus formation) in the middle ear applies pressure against the TM. Any sudden change in pressure against the membrane can cause perforation: diving underwater, flying in an airplane, or being near an explosion.
Trauma and excoriations from scratching inside the external canal (external otitis) with a foreign object (ie, bobby pin/hair pin) or chemicals (eg, hair spray, perfume, or hair dye)	Inflammatory changes can occur, causing local edema that closes out sound waves.
External otitis	Causative organisms implicated in external otitis are *Staphylococcus aureus*, *Pseudomonas*, and *Aspergillus*. Water in the ear canal (which is warm and wet) after swimming provides a media for the growth of these organisms.

(Continued)

Cause	Why?
Serous otitis media	This results from any condition (edema owing to nasal allergy, upper respiratory infection, or an airplane flight) that blocks the eustachian tube, creating negative pressure in the middle ear, which then draws a fluid transudate out of the middle ear epithelium.
Otosclerosis	This is a hereditary condition caused by new, abnormal growth of spongy bone around the oval window resulting in a stiff, fixated stapes that is unable to vibrate in response to sound waves sent through the air in the middle chamber of the ear.[4]
Presbycusis	Age-related hearing loss is the slow loss of hearing that occurs as people get older. The hearing loss is most marked at higher frequencies

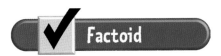

Factoid

If the foreign object that perforated the ear drum goes into the middle ear, the chain of ossicles could be dislocated, fractured, or pushed into the inner ear, causing even more problems!

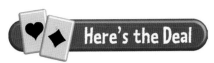

Here's the Deal

Infectious processes affecting the middle ear usually ascend the eustachian tube from the nasopharynx.

Testing, testing, testing

A hand-held otoscope (Fig. 11-29) provides effective means for visual inspection of the auditory canal, providing positive diagnosis for:

- Buildup of cerumen
- Foreign body
- Excoriations, inflammation, or infection
- Increased middle ear pressure (bulging of the ear drum)
- Perforation of the tympanic membrane

◀ Figure 11-29. Otoscope.

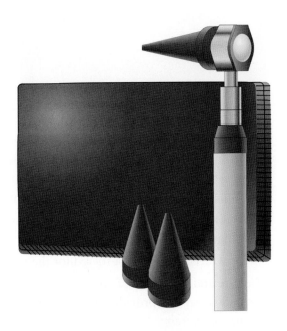

The Weber and Rinne test uses the tuning fork to differentiate between conductive and neurosensory hearing loss (Fig. 11-30).[37]

▶ Figure 11-30. Tuning fork.

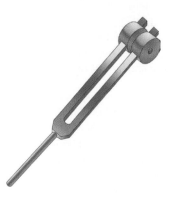

- Rinne test: The vibrating tuning fork is pressed to the mastoid bone (behind the ear) to conduct the vibration through the bone to the cochlea. When the patient can no longer hear the sound of the tuning fork, it is moved to the external ear canal of the same ear to see if the patient can hear better by sound or by bone (Fig. 11-31).

▶ Figure 11-31. Renne tuning fork test.

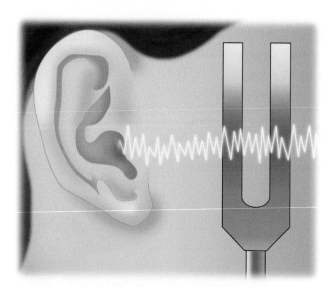

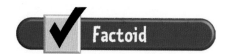

Factoid

Hearing will be better when sound waves are conducted by bone when the patient has otosclerosis.

- Weber test: The vibrating tuning fork is first placed on top of the head or against the center of the forehead. Normally the sound is heard in both ears simultaneously. When the sound is stronger in one ear than the other, conductive impairment may be present.[37]
- An audiogram hearing test can determine whether a person is hard of hearing and which ear has the problem.
- WBC with "diff" may be ordered for the patient with otitis media.
- Culture and sensitivity of any drainage or exudates from the external or middle ear will provide needed information for prescribed pharmacotherapy.

- A tympanogram measures the response of the middle ear muscle reflex to sound and measures compliance of the tympanic membrane (which can be absent or abnormal in sensorineural hearing loss).[38]

Signs and symptoms and why?

All of the conditions that interrupt conduction of sound energy to the middle ear are characterized by various degrees of hearing loss (conducted by air) in the affected ear. Additional signs and symptoms that accompany hearing loss are:

- Impacted cerumen: Feeling of fullness in the affected ear, possibly accompanied by a dull earache
- Obstruction by foreign body: Pain (may be severe), fullness in the affected ear, and auditory perception of noise if an insect is alive and moving inside the canal
- External otitis: Painful, reddened auditory canal with local edema. Visible clusters of white particles indicate infection in the canal.
- Otitis media: Pain (may be severe) with possible tenderness over the mastoid area (mastoiditis), red, inflamed or bulging ear drum with fever and elevated WBC.[32]
- Serous otitis media: Pain (may be severe) and a dull, bulging ear drum, afebrile.
- Perforated eardrum: Sudden severe pain initially and suppuration (formation of pus) occurring 24 to 48 hours later if the contamination occurred at the time of injury.[2]
- Otosclerosis: The patient cannot hear low frequencies and tinnitus may or may not be present.

What can harm my patient and why?

Sometimes the patient can cause additional harm with attempts at self-treatment, such as trying to remove a foreign body or ear wax and perforating an eardrum or worse.

- The complications of chronic otitis media or untreated acute otitis media are: perforation of the tympanic membrane because of fluid pressure or cholesteatoma, meningitis owing to spread of infection to nearby meninges, osteomyelitis of the skull caused by the spread of infection throughout the temporal bone, and facial paralysis because of secondary injury to the third cranial nerve.[1,2,32]
- Without early intervention, tympanic perforations can cause mixed or sensorineural hearing loss resulting from chronic inflammation.[39]

Define time

Cholesteatoma is a tumor growing in a confined place (eg, in the middle ear), creating a draining hole or pocket in the eardrum.[2]

- Without early intervention otosclerosis can result in mixed hearing loss.

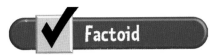

The measurement of hearing is classified according to the level of audible decibels (dB). The normal hearing threshold is 0 dB. Hard of hearing (20–25 dB) represents 10 times greater sound pressure to be heard.[1]

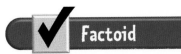

Pain with pressing downward on the tragus is a sure sign of external otitis.[32]

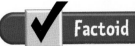

The tragus is that small firm projection in front of the external opening to the ear canal (adjacent to the cheek bone).

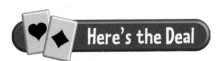

If the perforated tympanic membrane occurred during a fall while water skiing, lake water in the middle ear sets the stage for infection.

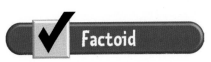

"Mixed" hearing loss involves conductive hearing loss that occurs in conjunction with sensorineural hearing loss, which is usually permanent.[1,2,4,32]

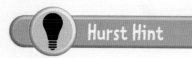

Interventions and why?

If the foreign body is not organic material (eg, bean, pea, bug) that will swell after contact with water, ear irrigation may be prescribed, providing that the ear drum is intact. If irrigation is for removal of hard, dry cerumen, an ear solvent may be instilled first to soften the cerumen.

- Warm the irrigating solution so the patient does not develop nystagmus.

Define time

Nystagmus is a term that describes involuntary movement of the eyeballs: rapid side-to-side oscillations.[40]

- Pull the adult up and back to straighten the auditory canal.
- Direct the flow against the canal rather than directly applying the force of the solution to the ear drum.
- Place an emesis basin under the chin and ear to collect the returning solution.
- Obtain specimens for culture and sensitivity for any drainage or purulent secretions from the auditory canal.
- Administer prescribed optic drops (analgesics and or antibiotics), possibly via a wick inserted into the canal by the doctor if drops cannot penetrate because of edema.

For painful, inflammatory, or infectious conditions of the external or middle ear:

- Administer NSAIDs or other prescribed analgesics PRN.
- Administer oral or parenteral antibiotics as prescribed.
- Instruct patients in the proper insertion and maintenance of a hearing aid and/or the availability of listening devices such as the "pocket talker."

PATIENT TEACHING   Impacted cerumen tends to recur in the same ear and patients need to know how to care for their ears:

- Don't stick anything smaller than your finger in your ear: No cotton buds (Q-tip), because this will just pack the wax (plus cotton fibers) against the tympanic membrane (which could also cause a perforation).
- Cerumen-softening agents (drops instilled into the affected ear) may prevent buildup and aid in movement of wax to the auditory meatus to prevent obstruction of the auditory canal.
- Soap and water on a cloth is sufficient for ear hygiene. Never use cotton swabs that push debris farther down, packing it against the eardrum.
- Use disposable ear plugs (one time use) and clean hearing aid devices that go into the ear daily to prevent growth of organisms that could cause infection.
- Acetic acid (vinegar) and alcohol (equal parts of each) before and after swimming can prevent swimmer's ear.[2]

Patients with ear infections are taught to take all of the antibiotics as prescribed, (even when ear pain has subsided) to completely eradicate the infection.

PATIENT TEACHING FOR TYMPANOPLASTY, MIDDLE EAR, AND MASTOID SURGERY Following surgery for tympanoplasty or insertion of tubes in the ear from drainage, the patient is taught to:

- Keep the affected ear dry until such time as the doctor deems a perforation has healed, or until ventilation tubes have been removed. No swimming and no water sports!
- Shower with a cotton ball treated on the outside surface (to shed water) with petroleum-coated cotton ball in the external ear over the opening to the auditory canal. Do not turn your head with the affected ear directly under the shower head.
- Avoid strenuous sports and blowing behaviors (ie, blowing up beach ball, blowing candles out on a birthday cake, or lifting weights, which is strenuous, and blowing with hard breathing).
- Return to your doctor for follow-up to visualize the tympanic membrane to monitor healing and spontaneous repair.

In addition to the above teachings, following middle ear or mastoid surgery the patient is taught to:

- Avoid any middle ear pressure by sneezing or coughing with an open mouth.
- Nose blowing must be gentle with both nostrils open.
- Expect popping sensations and temporary hearing loss for several weeks.
- Keep the suture line behind the ear clean and dry.
- Small amounts of blood tinged clear yellow fluid are normal after surgery, but the doctor must be notified for purulent ear drainage.[4]

Postop stapedectomy, the patient must adhere to similar restrictions: No nose blowing, open the mouth if you feel a sneeze coming on, no heavy lifting, no water in the ear. In addition, the patient is not to fly in an airplane for six weeks, and even after six weeks is not to fly if sick with a cold, or not able to "pop" the ears by swallowing.

Cutting edge

A newly engineered artificial eardrum has been created from water-soluble chitosan (a substance derived from shrimp shells)[39] that is more effective than spontaneous healing of the eardrum or tympanoplasty using paper patches.

Treatment modalities are prescribed beginning with least invasive procedures first:

- Impacted cerumen that cannot be removed with irrigation is removed with a rounded tip "scoop" or an instrument with a loop on the end, taking care not to damage the tympanic membrane.
- Foreign bodies (beads, eraser tips, etc) are removed with irrigation or instrumentation.

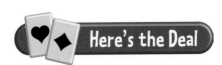

Here's the Deal

Following stapedectomy, the patient must be able to equalize pressure in the middle ear and swallowing should open the eustachian tube. Try swallowing right now! Go ahead, do it! Did you hear the click? What you just heard was the wet walls of the eustachian tube pulling away from each other to open. This should happen every time you swallow!

Irrigation is never used if the eardrum is perforated.

There are treatment options for a ruptured tympanic membrane:

- Wait for spontaneous healing to occur (usually two weeks), and monitor for a possible middle ear infection.
- Surgical tympanoplasty may be performed with use of novel tissue-engineered artificial eardrums fabricated from biomaterial (chitosan).

Infections of the ear can affect the external ear and auditory canal or the internal ear, and these infections may be categorized as acute, chronic, or serous.

- Broad-spectrum antibiotics are prescribed orally.
- Antibiotic otic drops are prescribed for drainage from the ear.
- Myringotomy or tympanotomy may be indicated to create an opening for serous or purulent fluid to drain from the middle ear.
- Ventilation tubes may be placed to equalize pressure in the middle ear when the eustachian tube is closed because of inflammation.
- Corticosteroids are prescribed for serous otitis media to decrease edema and inflammation.
- Cholesteatomas and mastoiditis require antibiotic therapy first, and then surgical intervention: tumor excision, tympanoplasty, ossiculoplasty, and mastoidectomy.

Otosclerosis (which affects one or both ears) is confirmed with audiometry with low-frequency hearing loss.

- Referrals for hearing aid (amplification) are the initial intervention.
- Treatment with sodium fluoride has shown some benefit on osteosclerotic growth,[41] but surgery provides the best option to restore hearing.
- Stapedectomy to remove the stapes and insert a tissue graft or a prosthesis for transmitting sound waves to the cochlea (Fig. 11-32).

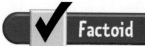

Only small perforations (less than half of the drum size) of the tympanic membrane can be expected to heal.[39]

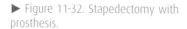
► Figure 11-32. Stapedectomy with prosthesis.

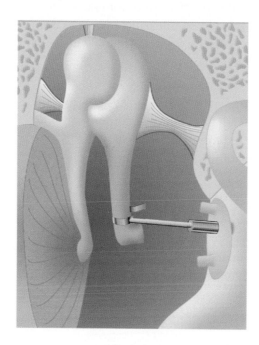

✦ Sensorineural hearing loss

Ménière's disease (a sensorineural hearing loss described by Dr. Prosper Ménière in 1861) involves irreversible damage and/or the death of nerve fibers.

✦ Ménière's disease

Almost 2½ million persons in the United States suffer from Ménière's disease, and about half of these have a family history of the disease.[4]

Ménière's (pronounced MEIN-jearz = rhymes with chairs) disease is an incurable inner ear disorder that not only causes hearing loss, but impairs balance as well. Ménière's disease usually occurs in only one ear, but a small portion of the population has bilateral disease.[4]

Let's get the normal stuff straight!

The structures of the inner ear consist of the cochlea (a coiled hollow tube) and the vestibule (central entrance way of the labyrinth):

* The vestibular system consists of sensory structures (saccule, utricle, and semicircular canals) comprising the organ of balance.
* The saccule (the smaller chamber of the membranous labyrinth) and the utricle (a small pouch in the membranous labyrinth) into which the semicircular canals empty are responsible for determining position sense.
* The looping, fluid-filled semicircular canals are responsible for balance.
* Electrolyte-containing fluid within the cochlea and the semicircular canals that bathe and nourish the sensory cells are maintained at a constant normal volume.
* The fluid-filled cochlea, which contains the organ of Corti, is the organ of hearing.
* Within the organ of Corti are specialized hair cells (cilia) that vibrate in response to different sound wave frequencies moving through the cochlear fluid.

What is it?

Ménière's disease (also called endolymphatic hydrops) is an incurable inner ear disorder that is usually unilateral. If another secondary illness coexists with Ménière's symptoms, the condition is called Ménière's syndrome.[38]

Causes and why?

Ménière's disease is caused by increased production of fluid within the labyrinth or a decrease in reabsorption of fluid, which may arise spontaneously with no exact known cause (idiopathic).[2]

* It is thought that there may be a membranous break that allows endolymph to mix with perilymphatic fluid, the combination of which causes erratic vestibular nerve firing that initiates an attack.[38]

- The syndrome is associated with autoimmune diseases such as lupus, rheumatoid arthritis, or hormonal problems such as thyroid disease.
- Increase in endolymph fluid, which causes the membranous labyrinth to dilate and balloon outward.

Testing, testing, testing

Several tests are performed to identify dysfunction within the inner ear:

Test	Clinical Significance
Auditory brain stem response (ABR)	Evaluates how the brain stem responds to specific sounds in order to differentiate sensory hearing loss from neural hearing loss.
Electronystagmogram (ENG)	ENG is a balance test that helps identify which ear is the problem.
Electrocochleography (ECOG)	This records the electrical activity of the inner ear in response to sound, and helps confirm the diagnosis of Ménière's disease. ECOG results are reported as an SP/AP (summating potentiation/alternating polarity) ratio, for which a ratio of 0.5 or greater is considered abnormal.[43]
caloric test	Performed to test the vestibular or balance system.
MRI	MRI is used to "rule out" a possible tumor that may be causing symptoms owing to pressure on the structures of the inner ear.
Audiometry testing	This may reveal sensory hearing loss in low frequencies.[44]

Signs and symptoms and why?

Incapacitating symptoms during an attack are described as:

- A feeling of fullness, pressure in the affected ear (using words like "plugged" or "stopped up").
- Rotational vertigo, described as a whirling or spinning sensation.
- Tinnitus (sounds heard are described as ringing, sea shell type roaring, or buzzing).
- Severe nausea and vomiting may accompany the rotational vertigo.

What can harm my patient and why?

The patient with Ménière's disease is literally living on a carnival ride, never knowing when someone is going to throw the switch, or how long the ride will last! The effects of the unpredictable and disabling symptoms can produce:

- Fear and apprehension because of never knowing when an attack may occur

- Fear of going out into public places and becoming a spectacle during an attack
- Loss of employment because of incapacitating attacks that can last from two to six hours (reported by patients), which are followed by headache and wobbly legs afterward[45]

Low-frequency hearing loss can progress to total, permanent, irreversible deafness, which has many negative psychosocial effects:

- Depression
- Low self-esteem
- Alteration in functional status[37]

Interventions and why?

Safety during an acute attack is the priority!

- Stabilize the head with pillows or sand bags to prevent movement, which will trigger nausea and severe vomiting.
- Stay with the anxious, fearful patient (who is probably holding onto the bedrail for dear life) and encourage him or her to take deep, slow breaths.
- Keep the patient NPO during the attack to prevent vomiting.
- To reduce sensations of vertigo and whirling, instruct the patient to be very still and to stare straight ahead with eyes fixed on an object taped to the ceiling or wall.
- Keep the bed in the low position, and the side rails up, and stay physically present during an attack.
- Administer sedation as prescribed (ie, valium IM or IV) for anxiety during the attack.
- Administer prescribed promethazine (Phenergan) as prescribed for nausea.
  Fluids and diet are offered when vertigo and nausea subside:
- Low-sodium diet with ample fluid.
- Administer thiazide diuretics (ie, HCTZ) as prescribed.
- Administer Antivert (meclizine) as prescribed for vestibular sedation.

PATIENT TEACHING   Living with Ménière's disease and coping with psychosocial issues involves knowing the patient and his or her unique needs and reinforcing available treatment options. Give assurance that he or she will feel "normal" between attacks, and that medications, diet, and lifestyle modifications can help:

- Take medications as prescribed.
- Drink 8 to 10 glasses of water daily.
- Keep sodium intake at 2000 mg/day (read labels for sodium content) and avoid obviously salty foods, with no added salt at the table.
- Include daily food sources of potassium in the diet when taking a thiazide diuretic.

• Avoid alcohol, smoking, and caffeinated beverages (Fig. 11-33).

▶ Figure 11-33. Ménière's disease: substances to avoid.

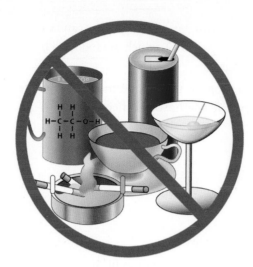

• Continue work, hobbies, and leisure activities, but have a safety plan in place in the event of an attack.
• Sleep with the radio tuned to static ("white" noise) to mask the annoying ringing in the ears.

To prevent sound induced sensorineural hearing loss:

• Wear ear protection when exposed to loud noises (gunshots, noisy machinery, rock concerts) and limit exposure time.
• Avoid or minimize exposure to ototoxic medications and substances (Table 11-3).

Betahistine (Serax) is a histamine precursor that is being prescribed abroad to reduce the frequency of attacks of vertigo; however, the drug is not FDA approved for uses in the United States.[46,47]

Conservative medical management of Ménière's disease is always the first plan:

• Reduction of fluid volume with a low-sodium diet (2000 mg/day) and Dyazide, a mild diuretic (hydrochlorothiazide and triamterene).
• Dexamethasone perfusion into the inner ear via a tiny ventilation tube has improved symptoms of ear pressure.[48]
• Chemical destruction of the inner ear with an ototoxic substance (eg, gentamycin or streptomycin) can be done to relieve symptoms when irreversible deafness in that ear makes trying to save the inner ear futile.

Surgical management may include the following procedures:

• Decompression of the endolymphatic sac by placing a drainage tube into the sac, creating a shunt to relieve pressure is the preferred initial surgical procedure.[42]
• Vestibular nerve section (lysis/cutting the nerve) relieves symptoms, but may cause permanent difficulty in maintaining balance.
• When hearing in the affected ear is functionally ineffective, a labyrinthectomy may be performed for removal of the vestibular canals and lysis of the vestibular nerve. This procedure relieves all symptoms, but leaves the patient permanently deaf.

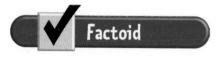

Factoid

Sensorineural hearing loss can be related to aging or can occur because of exposure to high decibel sound, prescribed ototoxic medications, and environmental ototoxics.

Define time

Presbycusis is progressive irreversible sensorineural hearing loss associated with aging (beginning in midlife), which is characterized by the inability to hear high-pitched tones as a result of inner ear changes.[4]

When ototoxic medications are prescribed (see Table 11-3), the nurse has a responsibility to monitor lab work reflecting renal function (BUN, creatinine) for indications that the patient is able to excrete the medication, and to caution the patient to report tinnitus immediately!

Table 11-3 *Hearing loss owing to drugs, substances, and environmental causes*

Ototoxic medications	Internal and external ototoxins
• Aminoglycoside antibiotics (especially high doses given IV)	• Alcohol
• Vancomycin, streptomycin, gentamycin: irreversible sensorineural hearing loss	• Arsenic
	• Heavy metals: gold, mercury, lead
• Metronidazole	• Toluene
• Diuretics: Lasix, Bumex, Edecrin	• Cyanide
• Quinine: Quinidex, Atabrine, Plaquenil, Chloroquine	• Styrene
	• Trichloroethylene
• Cisplatin and Nitrogen mustard (cancer chemotherapy drugs)	• Manganese
	• Benzene
• Aspirin (salicylate) reversible hearing loss when medicine is discontinued	• Ethyl benzene
	• Acetone
	• Pesticides
• NSAIDs and other analgesics	• Trimethyltin
	• Noise exposure: power equipment, gunfire, rock concerts, industrial noise

Cutting edge

Vertigo has been said to be the most disabling symptom of Ménière's disease, even more so than the hearing loss.

- Unilateral cases of Ménière's disease are becoming bilateral and recent advances in electrocochleography and MRI with intratympanic gadolinium-based contrast can predict disease progression.

- After initial conservative management American otolaryngologists, the next most commonly used therapy is a device manufactured by Medtronic, the Meniett™.

- Meniett™ is used by the patient for five minutes, three times daily. Low pressure pulsations reach the inner ear through a long-term ventilation tube placed in the tympanic membrane to reduce attacks of vertigo by stimulating endolymphatic flow.

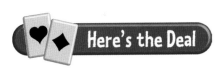

Here's the Deal

High-frequency hearing loss in the elderly (presbycusis) makes all consonants sound alike.[4] Hearing aids help, but nursing tips when conversing with the elderly are equally important:

- Always face the person directly with your face clearly visible when speaking.
- Do not shout, but speak slowly and distinctly with pauses.
- Have good lighting and turn off any competing noise source (ie, TV or music).
- Always validate that the person understands by having the message repeated.
- Utilize alternate forms of communication: written instructions, hand gestures and signals, sign language if appropriate.

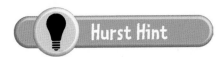

Hurst Hint

Decompression of the endolymphatic sac.

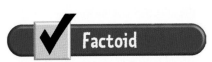

Factoid

If it says, "For decorative use only" on the bottom of the pitcher you bought in Mexico, the paint probably contains lead. Don't serve your orange juice in it!

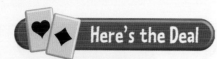

Here's the Deal

An entire family (except for the toddler) was getting sick and some family members developed tinnitus. After tests for lead were positive, the paint on a serving pitcher was identified as the source of the lead poisoning. The toddler was unaffected because his orange juice was poured directly into a "sippy" cup.

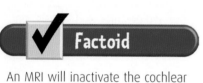

Factoid

An MRI will inactivate the cochlear implant! MRI is used when absolutely no other options are available for diagnosis.

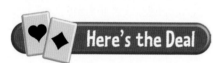

Here's the Deal

The cochlear implant bypasses the cochlea and sends the sound wave energy directly to the auditory nerve for transmission to the brain. The receiver is implanted in the temporal bone with an electrode placed in the inner ear. Auditory rehabilitation is accomplished with the help of an audiologist and a speech pathologist.

- Studies have shown remission of attacks for many patients and significant reduction of attacks in others.
- Cost of the device can be a major obstacle for patients who do not have insurance because the device is expensive. Critics say that there are complications from the tube, especially if it becomes plugged.[44]

An option for the totally deaf person is a cochlear implant (Fig. 11-34). Candidates are:

- Profoundly deaf in both ears
- Unable to recognize speech even with hearing aids
- Able to undergo general anesthesia
- Capable of receiving benefit from being able to hear

▶ Figure 11-34. Cochlear implant.

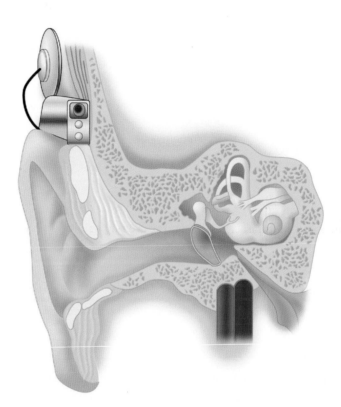

Hearing rehabilitation is required post–cochlear implant because the sounds are different and the brain must learn to interpret sounds. Adults who have already learned to speak have fewer problems adapting to the implant.[4]

PRACTICE QUESTIONS

1. Which intervention is the priority following a splash of cleaning fluid into the eye?

    A. Call 911 to get help on the way.

    B. Hold the eye lid open under running tap water.

C. Remove the contact lens from the affected eye.

D. Blink the affected eye rapidly to start the flow of tears.

2. A patient has the eye patch removed following successful surgical repair of a perforating injury from a BB gun. What can the nurse correctly assume when the patient reports being able to see her hair and scrub top, but not her face?

A. The injury damaged the macula.

B. There is edema of the optic disc.

C. This condition will resolve with healing.

D. Vitreous has leaked through the retinal hole.

3. A patient with "high risk for fall" activated the bed alarm, and the nurse responding to the alarm finds the patient on the floor in a pool of urine, having fallen from a standing position. While being assisted back to bed, the patient reports seeing bright flashing lights. Which next nursing interventions is the priority?

A. Darken the room.

B. Notify the doctor.

C. Obtain vital signs.

D. Apply a cool cloth to the patient's eyes.

4. Which of the following nursing measures is the priority when planning care for the preoperative cataract patient on the evening before surgery?

A. Administer cycloplegic drops every two hours.

B. Leave the night light and bathroom light burning.

C. Pull the side rails up and leave the bed in the low position.

D. Spend time to talk and listen for clues indicating preoperative anxiety.

5. An elderly patient is scheduled for impending outpatient phacoemulsification with insertion of a silicone intraocular lens. Which preoperative assessment must be reported to the physician immediately?

A. The sclera of the affected eye is red and injected.

B. The patient history reveals a coexisting diagnosis of glaucoma.

C. A stinging sensation is reported with drops to dilate the eye.

D. The systolic blood pressure is 10 mm Hg higher than baseline.

6. For which of the following patients might the nurse recommend earlier and/or more frequent than normal dilated ophthalmic exams with tonometry?

A. A Caucasian woman aged 55 whose aunt has glaucoma.

B. A 45-year-old Hispanic woman who has frequent headaches.

C. An African American man aged 45 with diabetes and hypertension.

D. An Italian accountant whose accounting job requires constant close work.

7. In addition to other musculoskeletal injuries, a young Japanese woman has suspected corneal abrasion of the right eye and possible retinal detachment secondary to deployment of the airbag upon impact during an MVA. Which order by the emergency physician should the nurse question?

A. Atropine 2%: two drops OD prior to slit-lamp exam.

B. Morphine 2 to 4 mg titrated IV PRN pain.

C. Instill proparacaine 0.5% (1) drop OD prior to examination.

D. Fluorescein ophthalmic drops (2) OD prior to direct ophthalmoscopy.

8. During irrigation of an ear for removal of impacted cerumen, the patient complains of nausea and both eyes begin side to side oscillations. The nurse's initial action is to stop irrigating the ear and

A. Raise the head of the bed.

B. Inspect the tympanic membrane.

C. Check the temperature of the water.

D. Notify the physician of the nystagmus.

9. Which statement by the nurse is accurate when responding to the patient's postoperative concern about the effectiveness of the newly performed stapedectomy?

A. "You can expect to hear out of both ears equally well."

B. "Your hearing will dramatically improve within weeks."

C. "The tinnitus you were experiencing will be totally corrected."

D. "The episodes of whirling vertigo should subside with healing."

10. Which of the following would be a next option when diet and oral medications have failed to reduce the disabling acute attacks of Ménière's disease?

A. Decompression of the endolymphatic sac.

B. Injection of gentamycin into the inner ear.

C. Scheduling the patient for a labyrinthectomy.

D. Insertion of a ventilation tube to equalize pressure.

References

1. Porth CM. *Pathophysiology: Concepts of Altered Health States.* 7th ed. Philadelphia: Lippincott Williams & Wilkins; 2007.

2. Beers MH, ed. *The Merck Manual of Medical Information. Diabetes.* Whitestation, NJ: Merck Research Laboratories; 2003.

3. Duffy B. Managing chemical eye injuries. *Emerg Nurs 16*(1):25–29, 2008.

4. Khodabukus R, Tallouzi M. Chemical eye injuries 1: Presentation, clinical features, treatment and prognosis. *Nursing Times 105*(22):28–29, 2009.

5. Ogg M. Eyewash stations in the OR. *AORN J 89*(5):912–913, 2009.

6. Khaw PT, Shah P, Elkington AR. ABC of eyes: Injury to the eye. *BM J 328*(7430):36–38, 2004.

7. Spector J, Fernandez WG. Chemical, thermal and biological ocular exposures. *Emerg Med Clin North Am* 26:125–136, 2008.

8. Smeltzer SC, Bare BG, Hinkle JL, Cheever KH. *Brunner & Suddarth's Textbook of Medical-Surgical Nursing*. 11th ed. Philadelphia: Lippincott Williams & Wilkins: 2008.

9. Watkinson S, Seewoodhary R. Common conditions and practical considerations in eye care. *Nurs Stand 21*(44):42–47, 2007.

10. Ellerton JA, Zuljan I, Agazzi G, Jeffrey JB. Eye problems in mountain and remote areas: Prevention and onsite treatment: Official recommendations of the International Commission for Mountain Emergency Medicine. *Wilderness Environ Med 20*(2):169–175, 2009.

11. Lee CH, Lee L, Kao LY, et al. Prognostic indicators of open globe injuries in children. *Am J Emerg Med 27*(5):530–535, 2009.

12. Linfield D, Das-Bhaumik R. Emergency department management of penetrating eye injuries. *Int Emerg Nurs* 17:155–160, 2009.

13. Close JK, Shiels WE, 2nd, Foster JA, Powell DA. Percutaneous ultrasound-guided intraorbital foreign body removal. *Ophthal Plast Reconstruct Surg 25*(4):335–337, 2009.

14. *Mosby's Medical Dictionary. Rhegmatogenous*. 9th ed. St. Louis: Elsevier; 2009.

15. Shinar Z, Chan L, Orlinsky M. Use of ocular ultrasound for the evaluation of retinal detachment. *J Emerg Med* [Epub ahead of print]. Available at http://www.ncbi.nlm.nih.gov/pubmed/19625159?ordinal pos=26&itool=EntrezSystem2.PEntrez.Pubmed.Pubmed_ResultsPanel.Pubmed_DefaultReportPanel.Pubmed_RVDocSum. Accessed August 12, 2009.

16. Budhram GG. Acute glaucoma after dilated eye exam in a patient with hyphema, retinal detachment and vitreous hemorrhage. *Acad Emerg Med 16*(1):87, 2009.

17. Seewoodhary R, Watkinson S. Treatment and management of ocular conditions in older people. *Nurs Stand 23*(25):48–55, 2009.

18. World Health Organization. *Causes of Blindness and Visual Impairment*. Available at http://www.who.int/blindness/causes/en. Accessed August 12, 2009.

19. Lockey J, Ul-Hassan M. Holistic approach to pre-operative assessment for cataract patients. *Br J Nurs 18*(5):323–327, 2009.

20. Young JS. Age related eye diseases. *Home Healthcare Nurse 26*(8): 464–471, 2008.

21. Spires RA. How you can help when older eyes fail. *RN 69*(2):38–43, 2006.

22. Whiteside MM, Wallhagen MI, Pettengill E. Sensory impairment in older adults: Part 2. Vision loss. *AJN 106*(11):52–61, 2006.

23. Mathys KC, Cohen KL, Bagnell CR. Identification of unknown intraocular material after cataract surgery: Evaluation of a potential cause of toxic anterior segment syndrome. *J Cataract Refract Surg 34*(3):465–469, 2008.

24. Sharts-Hopko NC, Glynn-Milley C. Primary open-angle glaucoma: Catching and treating the "sneak thief of sight." *AJN 109*(2):40–47, 2009.

25. Chang DTW, Herceg MC, Bilonick RA, et al. Intracameral dexamethasone reduces inflammation on the first postoperative day after cataract surgery in eyes with and without glaucoma. *Clin Ophthalmol 3*:345–355, 2009.

26. Halvorson P. The silent thief. *RN 68*(3):41–45, 2006.

27. Koch J, Sikes J. Getting the red out: Primary angle-closure glaucoma. *Nurs Pract 34*(5):6–9, 2009.

28. Yip II, Foster PJ. Ethnic differences in primary angle-closure glaucoma. *Curr Opin Ophthalmol 17*(2):175–180, 2006.

29. Gwiazda J. Treatment options for myopia. *Optom Vis Sci 86*(6): 624–628, 2009.

30. Kowing D, Kester E. Keeping an eye out for glaucoma. *Nurs Pract 32*(7):18–23, 2007.

31. Curtis C, Lo E, Ooi L, Bennett L, Long J. Factors affecting compliance with eye drop therapy for glaucoma in a multicultural outpatient setting. *Contemp Nurse 31*(2):121–128, 2009.

32. Smith D. Eye, ear, nose and throat health problems. In: Hogan MA, Hill K, eds. *Pathophysiology Reviews and Rationales.* Upper Saddle River, NJ: Prentice Hall; 2004.

33. UC Davis News Service. (2008). Press release: Smart contact lenses. Available at http://www.news.ucdavis.edu/search/news_detail.lasso?id=8722. Accessed August 22, 2009.

34. Liu YC, Huang JY, Wang IJ, et al. Intraocular pressure measurement with the noncontact tonometer through soft contact lenses. *J Glaucoma.* [Epub ahead of print]. Available at http://www.ncbi.nlm.nih.gov/pubmed/19593202?ordinalpos=1&itool=EntrezSystem2.PEntrez.Pubmed.Pubmed_ResultsPanel.Pubmed_DefaultReportPanel.Pubmed_RVDocSum. Accessed August 22, 2009.

35. Leonardi M, Pitchon EM, Bertsch A, et al. Wireless contact lens sensor for intraocular pressure monitoring: Assessment on enucleated pig eyes. *Acta Opthalmol 87*(4):433–437, 2009.

36. Shultz CL, Poling TR, Mint JO. A medical device/drug delivery system for treatment of glaucoma. *Clin Exp Optom 92*(4): 343–348, 2009.

37. Wallhagen MI, Pettengill E, Whiteside M. Sensory impairment in older adults. Part 1. Hearing loss. *AJN 106*(10):40–48, 2006.

38. Pullen RL. Spin control. *Nursing2006, 36*(5):48–51, 2006.

39. Kim JH, Choi SJ, Park J-S, et al. Tympanic membrane regeneration using a water-soluble chitosan patch. *Tissue Eng* [Epub ahead of print]. Available at http://www.liebertonline.com.libproxy.uams.edu/doi/abs/10.1089/ten.TEA.2009.0476. Accessed August 22, 2009.

40. Taber CW. Nystagmus. Venes D, ed. *Tabers Cyclopedia Medical Dictionary*. 20th ed. Philadelphia: F.A. Davis; 2007.

41. Naumann IC, Porcellini B, Fisch U. Otosclerosis: Incidence of positive findings on high-resolution computed tomography and their correlation to audiological test data. *Ann Otol, Rhinol Laryngol 114*(9): 709–716, 2005.

42. Kim HH, Weit RJ, Battista RA. Trends in the diagnosis and the management of Ménière's disease: Results of a survey. *Otolaryngol Head Neck Surg 132*(5):722–726, 2005.

43. Hain TC, Rudisill H. ECOG (Electrocochleography). Available at http://www.dizziness-and-balance.com/testing/ecog.html. Accessed August 23, 2009.

44. Nabi S, Parnes LS. Bilateral Ménière's disease. *Curr Opin Otolaryngol Head Neck Surg* [Epub ahead of print]. Available at http://www.ncbi.nlm.nih.gov/pubmed/19617826?ordinalpos=1&itool=EntrezSystem2.PEntrez.Pubmed.Pubmed_ResultsPanel.Pubmed_DefaultReportPanel.Pubmed_RVDocSum. Accessed August 24, 2009.

45. Ballentine J, Shiel WC, Jr. Ménière's disease. Available at http://www.medicinenet.com/Ménière_disease/article.htm. Accessed August 23, 2009.

46. Phillips JS, Prinsley PR. Ménière's disease. *Br J Clin Pharmacol 65*(4):470–471, 2009.

47. Teggi R, Bellini C, Fabiano B, Bussi M. Efficacy of low-level laser therapy in Ménière's disease: A pilot study of 10 patients. *Photomed Laser Surg 26*(4):349–353, 2008.

48. Silverstein H, Farrugia M, Van Ess M. Dexamethasone inner ear perfusion for subclinical endolymphatic hydrops. *Ear Nose Throat J 88*(2):778–785, 2009.

CHAPTER

12 Musculoskeletal Dysfunction

OBJECTIVES

In this chapter you will review:

- Common musculoskeletal disorders and the associated pathophysiology.
- Management of care for patients having acute and chronic musculoskeletal dysfunction.
- Safety precautions and rehabilitation needs.
- Medical and nursing interventions to promote attainment of maximum musculoskeletal function.
- Pharmacology and technology that improves quality of life and reduces threat to musculoskeletal activity when normal function is altered.
- The impact of age, lifestyle choices, genetics, and environmental factors that alter musculoskeletal integrity and function.
- Patient teaching to enhance self-care and promote safety when the patient has compromised musculoskeletal function.

MUSCULAR DYSFUNCTION

Problems with bones, joints, muscles, ligaments, and tendons can cause pain and loss of function. Pain and altered ability to function can result from seemingly simple musculoskeletal problems like contusions, strains, and sprains.

Let's get the normal stuff straight !

Joints are places where bones come together (articulate).

- Joints are freely moveable when the articulating surface is covered with cartilage and enclosed in a joint capsule.
- Joints are inherently weak and are susceptible to twisting, stretching, and becoming overloaded.[1]
- Ligaments strap muscles to the bone and provide mechanical and functional support.

Muscles supporting the cervical spine, elbows, and shoulders, the low back, knee, and ankle take most of the stress and strain of every-day living:

- Skeletal muscles are arranged in functional groups, with blood vessels and nerves enclosed in fascia lined compartments.
- Fascia that envelops muscles is comprised of dense connective tissue that provides flexibility and form to muscle tissue and serves the purpose of reducing friction between muscle groups.[2]
- As we age, we will experience decreased muscle mass and elasticity, which predispose muscles and muscle-tendon units to injury. Prevention measures include weight-bearing exercises and weight training.

What is it?

Soft tissue injuries involve muscles, tendons, or ligaments.[3] Let's get all these terms straight:

- A *contusion* is a bruise that appears as a discoloration underneath an intact skin surface.
- A *strain* is a tear of a muscle or muscle-tendon unit.
- A *sprain* is a tear of a ligament or tendon near a joint.
- There are degrees of muscle strain and muscle sprain: mild, moderate, or severe.

Causes and why?

- Unnatural movement or excessive pressure on joint can tear or rupture ligaments.
  - Being overweight (increasing the load on joints, ligaments, muscles, tendons).
  - When participating in sports, be sure to wear shoes specifically designed for the activity.

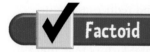

Factoid

Most soft tissue injuries occur because of excessive exercise or athletic activity in the presence of weak joints or ligaments and/or poor support.

- Inversion (turning inward) under pressure, which exceeds structural limitations, is the most common cause of a sprained ankle.[1]

Testing, testing, testing

- X-ray is used to rule out fracture[4] with severe strains and/or sprains.
- MRI can very effectively identify soft tissue damage for diagnosis of meniscal tears.
- Direct visualization with arthroscopy.

Signs and symptoms and why?

The patient with a muscle *strain* will have:

- Pain that increases with stretching of the muscle
- Local tenderness and stiffness of the muscle
- Soft tissue swelling

The patient with a *sprain* has symptoms that develop more rapidly and take longer to subside than a simple strain:

- Moderate to severe pain of the affected joint ligament or capsule.
- Rapid-onset edema with local discoloration and heat.
- Loss of function with various degrees of severity[5]
- A pulled *muscle* is a strain.
- A torn *ligament* is a sprain.

What can harm my patient and why?

Most soft tissue injuries heal with conservative measures, but acute injuries can become chronic with disability because of:

- Ligaments that become lax, offering poor support, because muscle contraction pulls the ends of healing fibers apart, causing healing in a lengthened position.
- Persistent pain, weakness, and instability of the joint,[6] because the tendon was not adequately healed before additional stresses were applied.

Interventions and why?

During the first 24 hours after injury, my patient with a soft tissue injury (sprain, strain, or contusion) needs R-I-C-E:[3]

- Rest: Get off the injured ankle! Don't use the injured wrist!
- Ice: Cold pack to either side of the injured area.
- Compression: Compression wrap to reduce edema and apply support.
- Elevate: Prop up the affected part with a pillow.

The nursing plan changes after 24 to 48 hours following soft tissue injury:
4 times a day
- Intermittent heat QID for 15 to 30 minutes.
- Avoid excessive exercise during the healing period to avoid re-injury and delayed recovery.

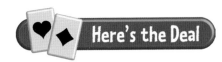

Here's the Deal

The anatomy involved determines whether the patient has a strain or a sprain.

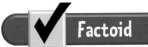

Factoid

Your patient may be a nurse! Nurses working in nursing homes have three times more lost work days owing to strains and sprains, and four times more lost work days owing to back injury when compared with the national average.[7]

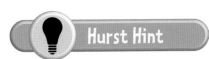

Hurst Hint

Remember that when wrapping an elastic compression bandage, begin distally and progress proximally, maintaining snug but not tight compression.[4]

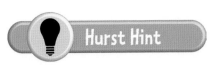

Hurst Hint

Perform a neurovascular check before and after application of compression bandages, splints, or braces to ensure adequate circulation.

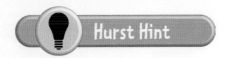

Hurst Hint

When applying an arm sling the strap should be adjusted and padded so that pressure is not applied to the neck.

● The patient may require a splint, sling, brace, or assistive device to promote rest of the injured part and provide support.

PATIENT TEACHING   Crutches, a quad cane, or a walker may be prescribed to avoid weight-bearing and protect the injured part while healing takes place.

● The assistive appliance is advanced forward with the injured part.

● When using crutches, do not bear weight on the axilla because of possible nerve damage (brachial nerve plexus).

● Take care to avoid re-injury by limiting movement and strain on soft tissues.

If splints and braces are removed for bathing and for sleeping:

● Use care with reapplication to avoid constriction or areas that rub.

● If wearing the appliance produces pain, loosen or remove the brace or splint and return to the clinician for re-evaluation.

PATIENT TEACHING   Patient teaching for prevention and/or re-injury:

● When running, watch the road for obstacles or irregular surfaces, curbs, etc.

● Wear appropriate footwear that is in good condition with a proper fit.

● Avoid athletic sports and activities for which you are not well conditioned.

● Use an ankle support brace if prone to ankle pain, twisting, or if previous sprains have occurred.[8]

Cutting edge

Technology allows measurement of pressure within a compartment of the upper or lower extremities. One such hand held device made by Stryker (Stryker Solid-State Transducer Intra Compartment [STIC] Pressure Monitor System, Stryker Corp., Kalamazoo, MI)[9] is available for validating clinical assessments that indicate the onset of compartment syndrome. Normal tissue pressure in the muscle ranges from 0 to 14 mm Hg at rest. If the pressure reaches 40 to 60 mm Hg, blood flow to the tissue and nerves may be compromised.[2] Even with this technology, the clinical priority is still astute observations and frequent neurovascular checks in patients at risk for development of compartment syndrome (Fig. 12-1).

▶ Figure 12-1. Stryker intracompartment pressure monitor. **A**. Set-up. **B**. Use.

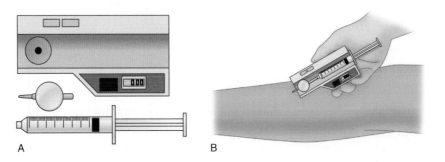

A   B

FRACTURES

Fractures can occur as a result of trauma or bone pathology.

Let's get the normal stuff straight !

The 206 bones in the body are classified according to their shape: long bones (arms/legs), short bones (wrists/ankles), flat bones (ribs, pelvis), and irregular bones (vertebra).

- The outer covering of bone is the fibrous periosteum, which contains nerves, blood vessels, and lymph network.
- The dense compact bone consists of mature osteocytes that rely on tiny canals through the irregular latticework of circular layers that provide pathways for blood vessels that nourish the bone cells.
- Bone cells require adequate blood supply for osteogenesis.
- Bone necrosis occurs when blood flow is absent, interrupted, or deficient.
- The medullary cavity in the shaft of the bone contains marrow (red and yellow).
- Long bones in adults contain fatty yellow marrow and red bone marrow is primarily found in flat bones.
- The vascular endosteum is the thin membrane that lines the marrow cavity of long bone.

What is it?

A fracture is a break in the continuity of a bone, which can be complete (all the way through the bone, with two distinct bone ends) or incomplete (partial break or splintering). Fractures are classified according to the location and characteristics of the break and whether the bone has penetrated the skin (open versus closed fracture). The characteristics of the damage provide definition to various types of fractures.

- Comminuted (bone is broken into numerous small pieces)
- Compressed (bones are squeezed together)
- Impacted (ends of bone are jammed together)
- Spiral (break shows evidence of being twisted)
- Greenstick (bone is not completely broken, rather is bent)
- Transverse (a complete break at a right angle to the long axis)[1,3,5]

Causes and why?

Fractures occur when the force (stress) placed on the bone exceeds the ability of the bone to absorb the shock.[1] Three categories of causations are listed:

- Sudden traumatic injuries: sudden direct blow, crushing or twisting.
- Stress or overuse injuries, such as occur in the feet of basketball players and shin splints in runners.

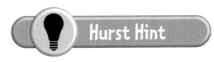

Hurst Hint

We want to keep joints moving (with support) because those familiar hazards of immobility include muscle atrophy, joint stiffness, and loss of proprioception (internal sense of where body parts are in relation to other parts).

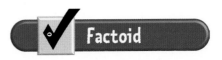

Factoid

The most commonly fractured bone is the tibia in the lower leg, the site of four compartments.

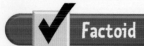

Factoid

Proton pump inhibitors are thought to increase the risk of hip fracture because of calcium malabsorption. Steroids can also increase risk for fracture because of increased excretion of calcium.[11]

• Bone pathology/conditions that weaken the integrity of the bone: infection, cysts, tumors, osteoporosis, or Paget's disease, and use of proton pump inhibitors or steroids.[1,3,5,10]

Testing, testing, testing

X-ray is the first diagnostic tool that is employed when a fracture is suspected. Other imaging can reveal features of the fracture as well as soft tissue injury surrounding the break.

• CT (computed tomography).
• MRI (magnetic resonance imaging).
• Bone scan with a radioactive substance can not only identify an obscure fracture, but any bone pathology that may have caused the fracture.

Signs and symptoms and why?

The patient who experiences a fracture of a bone initially has these signs and symptoms:

• Pain is continuous and increasing with movement, and muscle spasms occur soon after the fracture.
• Loss of function: Support to muscles is lost when the bone is broken. Pain is also a contributor to loss of function.
• Deformity: The limb or part may be crooked or abnormally rotated because of displacement from muscle spasm and edema.
• Shortening of the extremity: Muscle spasms pull bones out of alignment, and rather than end-to-end alignment, the bone fragments may be side by side.
• Crepitus: This is a grating or crackling sensation or sound associated with movement of bone fragment as they rub causing even more trauma to tissue, vessels, and nerves.
• Edema and discoloration: This may occur secondary to tissue trauma with injury.[5,11]

Interventions and why?

The fracture is splinted at the scene to prevent further tissue trauma because when bone fragments and ends are moved they can damage muscle tissue and nerves. After performing a baseline neurovascular assessment:

• Carefully splint the limb in a position of function with as little manipulation as possible.
• When the injured patient arrives at the emergency department wearing a C-collar, do not remove the neck brace or take the patient off the hard spine board until the radiologist has "cleared the C-spine." Removal of the C-collar in the presence of a neck fracture will most likely result in spasms of the neck muscles resulting in further injury to the patient.

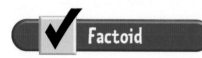

Factoid

A Thomas splint immobilizes and applies traction to overcome muscle spasms. It is most commonly used for femur fractures.

Musculoskeletal Dysfunction

When assisting the physician with application of a plaster cast:

- Perform a baseline neurovascular assessment. After application of splints, braces, or casts, frequent ongoing neurovascular assessments are needed.
- Elevate the extremity on a pillow, leaving the cast uncovered (open to air) to promote drying.
- Handle a wet cast with the palms of hands (never use fingertips, which could leave indentations).
- Protect the long leg or body (spica) cast around the groin area from excreta by taping clear plastic wrap over the outside of the cast prior to elimination.
- Following stabilization of a fracture, my patient needs to be monitored for potential complications. The nurse must constantly monitor the patient with a fracture for development of compartment syndrome:
  - The classic warning sign is intense pain not relieved with medication.[12]
  - The intensity of the pain is disproportionate to the injury.
  - Neurovascular check reveals a distal extremity that is pulseless, pale, painful, paresthesia, paralysis, cold to the touch, and nail beds that blanch with pressure and do not refill, or refill slower than the normal two seconds.
  - If palpation is possible, the muscle will be swollen and hard.
  - If circulation is compromised, relieve the pressure as quickly as possible! The cast may be bivalved (cut in down each side with a cast cutter) and loosened with a spreader between the two halves.

PATIENT TEACHING   Patient teaching when a cast has been applied:

- Do not place objects under the cast to scratch an itch because this can damage skin and increase the risk of infection.
- Blowing cool air under the cast is a safe option to manage an itch.[13]
- Do not rest a damp cast on a hard surface or sharp edges because indentations will become pressure places.
- Frequently observe the skin around the cast edges for irritation and keep the skin dry.
- Do not use a hair dryer to dry the cast. Use of a fan to circulate air is acceptable.
- Immediately report any unrelieved pain, burning, numbness, tingling, coldness, or discoloration of the casted limb.[13,15]

Be alert to signs of fat embolism or deep vein thrombosis (DVT), all of which are related to where the embolus lodges:

- Monitor LOC, mentation, and vital signs frequently: A cerebral emboli results in sudden loss of consciousness and a rapid spike in temperature reflecting hypothalamic response.[15]
- Monitor urinary output: The affected kidney will be compromised, or if the patient only has one functional kidney, renal failure can develop when the renal artery becomes occluded.[10]
- Administer nasal oxygen as indicated and notify the physician.

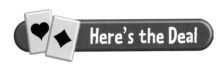

Reduce is a term used in orthopedics that means to bring the dislocation or fractures back into the correct position for proper healing. Traction can be applied with weights and pulley or manual traction applied as a slow, continuous pull to reduce a fracture.

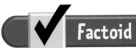

Drying time for fiberglass casts is minutes to hours, but for a plaster cast expect 24 to 72 hours for complete drying;[14] and the drying process of plaster produces heat.

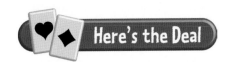

A thick plaster cast in a muggy environment can take up to three days to dry (cure) completely; during this time, precautions must be taken to avoid creating dents in the cast! A wet cast is grayish with a musty smell, and heat is generated and needs to escape as the wet cast dries. Don't cover a wet cast!

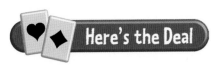

Indentations in a cast from being handled with fingertips, or propping the cast against a hard surface will cause pressure inside of the cast anywhere there is a dent. Pressure causes local ischemia and ulcer formation.[16]

604 MARLENE HURST ✚ Hurst Reviews: Medical-Surgical Nursing Review

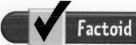

Factoid

Once a fracture is stabilized (not moving) the bone and surrounding tissue, pain should be minimal or totally relieved.

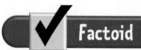

Hurst Hint

Cast cutters vibrate rather than cut the plaster and the patient cannot be cut; however, instruct the patient that it will feel very warm. Loosen the cast, leaving the two halves in place, or the top half can be removed, leaving the bottom in place as a splint.

Factoid

Monitor respiratory status: sudden shortness of breath, dyspnea, and low Spo_2, anxiety, and hemoptysis.

- Watch for petechiae that occur in strange places: conjunctiva of the eye, chest, neck, or axilla.
- Monitor Sao_2 and notify the physician for downward trends from the baseline reading.

Care of the patient in a spica (full body) cast:

- Positioning: Supine, prone (minimum of twice daily). Lateral side-lying position on uninjured side only. Pillows are required for support.
- Skin care: Apply protective plastic sheeting under the dry cast and over the edges when washing genitals to keep from wetting the cast. Dry well and remove plastic sheeting when bathing complete.
- Provide for elimination needs and toileting with small, flat fracture bedpan using plastic sheeting in and over the outside of the cast to prevent soiling. (Remove after cleaning.)
- Skin care: Inspect around edges frequently for signs of irritation or pressure.
- Monitor for physiologic cast syndrome: Decreased bowel sounds, abdominal distention, abdominal discomfort, and nausea and vomiting.
- Plan for muscle strengthening activities: Gluteal and quad setting, dorsiflex and plantar flex the feet. Teach patient how to pull up and reposition self with overbed trapeze bar.
- Plan for diversional activities according to patient interests. When prone, place mirror for watching TV. Stimulating mental activities and reading with pencil eraser to turn pages.
- Family involvement as indicated. Caregivers are taught basics of care for patient in a body cast: bathing, toileting, repositioning, and monitoring for complications.

When skeletal traction is used to reduce the fractured bone, orthopedic wires, pins, screws, or tongs affixed to the bone protrude through the skin surface and pulleys attached to weights to pull bone ends into alignment. External fixators are used to immobilize a bone when bone ends are aligned. The priority nursing concerns associated with pins, screws, tongs, and wires used with skeletal traction or external fixators are (Fig. 12-2):

▶ Figure 12-2. External fixator applied to a fractured radius.

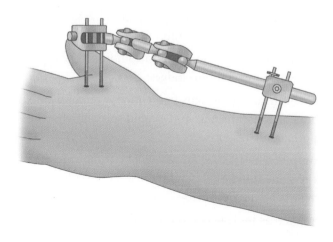

- Sterile technique pin care as prescribed: Common orders may be either saline or equal parts of hydrogen peroxide and normal saline (sterile of course), cleaning daily to TID.[13]

- Weights must hang freely at all times and the ropes must be in the grooves of the pulleys.

- Maintain proper alignment at all times, keeping the patient pulled up in the bed so that his or her feet are not touching the footboard and weights are not touching the floor (Fig. 12-3).

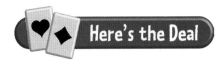

Here's the Deal

The patient who is immobilized because of a fracture could also develop a DVT, which could become dislodged from the lower extremity and lodged in the lung. So when your patient becomes symptomatic, the problem could be a fat embolus or a blood clot, both of which can be lethal, but remember that the fat embolus is not receptive to thrombolysis (see Chapter 4)! Treatment for fat embolism is supportive: oxygen and hydration to flush out fatty acids.[10]

◀ Figure 12-3. Skin traction. Left: Buck's traction. Below: Russell's traction. (Reproduced from *Hurst Student Handbook* Brookhaven, MS: Hurst Review Services; 2010:, p. 162).

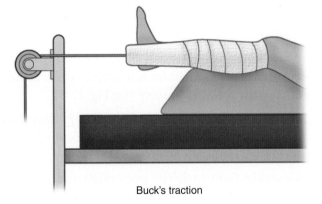

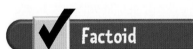
Buck's traction

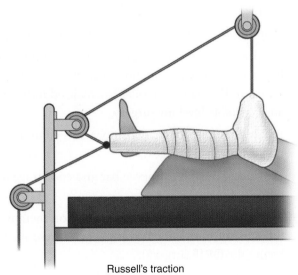
Russell's traction

Factoid

Advantages of the halo vest are that the patient is not confined to bed and can be up and about, getting on with life! A disadvantage is that if infection occurs it can quickly develop into osteomyelitis.

- Monitor for infection: Record temperature QID, and monitor pin sites often for purulent drainage (opaque, yellow, or green), redness, and localized heat at the site.

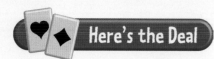

When toes are pointed straight up (toward the ceiling), that is neutral rotation. Toes slanting outward (laterally) is external rotation, and toe slanting inward toward the midline is internal rotation. Both internal and external rotation can cause dislocation of the fractured hip, leading to additional trauma at the site.

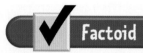

Skin traction exerts the mechanical "pull" directly on the skin! Can this cause a problem? Yes, especially for elderly people with thin, fragile (probably undernourished) skin.

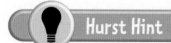

Use of the trapeze bar increases independence and reduces time on the call light for repositioning, but the secondary gain is even greater. Improved muscle mass and muscle strength of the upper torso, which will be needed postoperatively for ambulating with assistive devices such as walkers, crutches, and canes.

✚ Hip fractures: ORIF (open reduction with internal fixation)

Open reduction with internal fixation (ORIF) is a surgical procedure commonly used for a hip fracture, but internal fixation can be used with any fracture if indicated owing to the type and location of the break.

Many elderly patients who have sustained a fracture of the hip because of a fall have coexisting health problems (atrial fibrillation, heart failure, diabetes, hypertension, etc). They may also be taking anticoagulants. Management of comorbidities can delay surgery to repair the hip, but hopefully the patient can be stabilized within 12 to 24 hours, because further delay increases the risk for complications.

Preoperatively, my patient needs:

- Bed rest with immobilization to reduce further trauma.

- Maintain neutral rotation of the affected lower extremity with a trochanter roll wedged into position from the waist to below the knee.

- Each shift document that the trochanter roll is in place and that the leg is in neutral rotation.

- A firm mattress to provide for support (optimal for all orthopedic patients).

- Application of skin traction (Buck's extension) with weights as prescribed (usually 5–10 lb) for hip fracture while getting the patient nutritionally ready for surgery (see Fig. 12-3).

- Administer nutritional supplements to supplement high-protein, high-calorie diet with ample vitamin C, as prescribed for undernourished patients.

- Assess skin frequently (by inspection and palpation) and implement a plan for meticulous skin care any time skin traction is utilized.

- Monitor for pain and administration of analgesia as prescribed.

- For previously anticoagulated patients: Administer unfractionated heparin after discontinuation of warfarin home regime while awaiting return of INR (International Normalized Ratio/Prothombin Time) to an acceptable level for surgery.

- Provide a high-protein, high-fiber, and vitamin C diet while in skin traction awaiting surgery.

- Provide an overhead trapeze bar and encourage frequent repositioning.

- For patients who require anticoagulation therapy, prepare to discontinue use of unfractionated heparin as prescribed (usually hours before the ORIF surgery).

- High-top vented, canvas tennis shoes (or more expensive lamb's wool foot support) will prevent foot drop when a foot board cannot be utilized (because the frame for the Buck's extension traction takes up the entire footboard).

Postoperative care for the patient following ORIF, joint replacement, or total hip replacement:

- Monitor neurovascular status and compare with baseline findings to identify changes and deficits.
- Monitor for hemorrhage: Check vital signs, note character and amount of drainage in portable suction device (usually a JP drain with a bulb that must be compressed periodically). Excessive drainage is greater than 250 mL in the first 8 hours after surgery. Also report previously dark red drainage that becomes bright red.[5]
- Monitor for pain (have patient rate pain on a scale of 1–10) and administer analgesia as needed.
- Use TED compression hose and sequential compression devices (SCDs), as prescribed, removing for skin care and assessment at least 20 minutes twice daily.
- Monitor for development of DVT by being alert to any complaint of unilateral calf pain, local heat, erythema, or increase in the diameter of the calf.
- Supervise active exercise of the lower leg and ankle hourly to increase circulation.
- Administer prescribed prophylactic antibiotics as indicated and use aseptic technique for dressing changes and emptying portable drainage.
- Avoid positioning the patient on the operated side, or giving injections into the affected hip.
- Document the presence of abduction pillow and document use of same (Fig. 12-4).

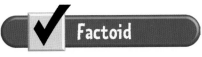

The abduction pillow maintains abduction of the hip (legs spread to the side), which forces the head of the femur into the acetabulum, preventing the head of the femur from dislocating.

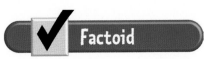

Patients having replacement joints are usually allowed to ambulate with a walker or crutches within 24 hours after surgery with specific weight-bearing limits prescribed by the surgeon.[5]

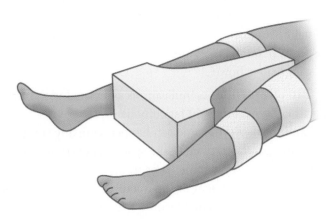

◀ Figure 12-4. Abduction pillow.

- Assist with ambulation using walker or crutches when surgeon deems appropriate.
- When the patient is out of bed and seated, the chair should be high and firm to avoid acute flexion of the hip.
- Warn the patient to avoid adduction to protect the affected hip from dislocation.

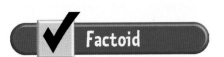

The two motions that encourage dislocation of a hip are flexion and adduction!

PATIENT TEACHING   Patient teaching following ORIF or hip replacement:

- Avoid sitting in low chairs or crossing the affected leg over the center of the body.

- When selecting a chair, the knees should always be lower than the hips.

- Do not sharply flex at the hip or rotate the foot inward or outward when dressing: putting on pants, stockings/socks, or shoes.

- Use a toilet rim extender to elevate the toilet seat.

- Keep the knees apart at all times and use a pillow between the legs when sleeping.

- Don't bend forward from the hip to pick up objects from the floor. Use a long pincer "grabber" with a hand held trigger instead.[5]

What can harm my patient and why?

Fractures don't heal as rapidly in adults as compared with children and adolescents because of a less vascular periosteum. The usual adult healing time of 10 to 18 weeks is influenced by a host of variables related to the general health of the individual and characteristics of the bone and the break. The normal bone-healing time for a child or adolescent ranges from 4 to 10 weeks, with faster healing occurring in the younger child.[1]

- Delayed union refers to healing of a fracture that does not occur at a normal rate but will eventually heal.

- Nonunion describes failure of bone ends to unite, which may require bone grafting.

- Signs of both delayed and nonunion are persistent discomfort and movement of bones (felt by patient inside the cast).

- Spica cast syndrome is a psychological and physiologic response to being confined within a full body cast characterized by ileus, abdominal discomfort, and nausea and vomiting. The worst-case scenario is pressure on the mesenteric artery and bowel ischemia, resulting in a gangrenous bowel.[5]

Two other serious complications associated with fractures are compartment syndrome and fat embolism.

Compression syndrome can happen with any condition that increases pressure within a limited tissue space: cellulitis or burns (edema fluid collects in the compartment) or trauma (bleeding within a compartment). With movement of the fractured limb, bone fragments can tear through vessels, causing bleeding within a compartment to produce compartment syndrome.

There are 46 such compartments in the body, and the majority of them (36) are in the upper and lower extremities. The four most common compartments that develop compression syndrome with resultant necrosis of tissue and nerves are the four chambers in the lower leg.[12]

- Compartment syndrome occurs because of limited space (such as occurs with snug fitting splints, braces, and casts) and increased pressure within the compartment, compressing blood vessels and nerves.[8]

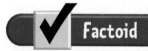

Blunt force is the most common cause of abdominal compartment syndrome, as occurs with pelvic fractures, but can also occur from ascites, abdominal obesity, cancer, pancreatitis, or even pregnancy![17]

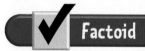

Fractures that are most commonly associated with fat emboli are those in the long bones (femur) and pelvis or any crushing injury.[11]

- Fat embolism occurs when continuity of the bone is interrupted, and fat globules released from the bone marrow enter the blood stream, forming emboli that especially like to go to the lungs.[11,14]

- The greatest danger period for developing a fat embolism is within the first 36 hours after a fracture.

- Petechiae develop in strange places: conjunctiva of the eye, chest, neck, or axilla.

AMPUTATIONS

Limb amputations occur frequently as a complication of other diseases.

Let's get the normal stuff straight!

Muscles and bones require adequate arterial blood flow:

- The femoral artery divides into the anterior and posterior arteries below the knee joint to perfuse the lower extremities.

- The subclavian artery divides into the brachial and axillary arteries, and further branches into the radial and ulnar arteries to provide blood flow to the upper extremities.

What is it?

Amputation is the process of severing (cutting) a limb away from the body. This drastic process is always a last resort, when all measures to promote healing or restore blood flow to a limb have failed. Amputations are performed at the most distal area that will heal and all attempts are made to preserve joints so that the patient will have a more normal gait and less disability.

Causes and why?

Any condition that produces ischemia to a limb can result in death of muscle and bone cells, necrosis and resultant gangrene, as well as traumatic injuries, which could compromise life and limb, necessitating amputation:

- Complication of casts: If it is applied too tightly to accommodate tissue swelling, or indentations that apply pressure to nerves and blood vessels, cutting off circulation

- Compartment syndrome, which is not relieved in a timely manner, producing tissue anoxia

- Vascular damage, as occurs in diabetes, in which distal blood flow is compromised

- Peripheral vascular disease (see Chapter 4 for more information about PVD)

- Arterial occlusion resulting from thromboembolism or fat embolism, which totally cuts off blood flow to a limb

- Poor wound healing because of vascular damage, decreased oxygen supply, and nutrients to support healing

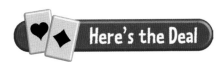

Here's the Deal

Petechiae are considered a hallmark sign of fat embolus![10] The strange reddish or purple pinpoint spots in the skin occur as a result of fat globules, either reaching the upper aorta and its more ventral tributaries occluding dermal capillaries, increasing capillary fragility, and causing local ischemia to the skin.[15]

Deadly Dilemma

Fat embolism happens most commonly in young men. Why? Because they are full of testosterone and they are risk takers!! Maybe you've known somebody who climbed up the 300 ft water tower with a can of spray paint to record the year of his high school graduation and his girlfriend's name! (Maybe you were the girlfriend!)

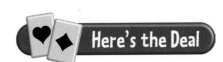

Here's the Deal

Complications related to patient noncompliance with cast instructions can be related to placing objects into the cast to scratch an itch or removing padding from the cast. Both of these actions can lead to trauma with resultant infection.[16]

- Catastrophic illnesses, such as bone cancer, or flesh-eating disease (necrotizing fasciitis caused by bacteria).
- Trauma: Crushing injuries that irreparably destroy tissues and traumatic amputations wherein the limb is severed at the time of injury

Testing, testing, testing

Any of the following tests may be indicated for the patient with PVD:

- Allen's test (to detect arterial insufficiency in the hand).
- Angiography (radiographic visualization of vessels using radiopaque dye) to identify arterial occlusions.[18]
- Ankle-brachial index (ABI) comparing systolic blood pressure with that of the affected extremity.
- CW (continuous wave) Doppler flow studies assess blood flow through vessels.
- X-rays can identify the presence or absence of foreign body, osteomyelitis, gas in soft tissues, and the spread of a disease process to adjacent bones/joints.[19]
- Duplex ultrasonography to measure velocity of blood flow[20]
- CT scan with contrast or MRI can diagnose deep abscess not clinically visible.

When amputation is anticipated, preoperative lab work commonly includes:
- CBC.
- Chemistry analysis (see Chapter 1).
- Blood type and cross-match with anticipatory units of PRBCs available for surgery.
- Culture and sensitivity of any lesions and wound drainage is performed to determine the infecting organism and the antibiotic of choice.

Signs and symptoms and why?

The patient may present with multiple injuries in addition to crushing limb injury with destruction of the entire vascular system, or a sudden traumatic amputation.

- Hypovolemic shock may be present, characterized by hypotension, tachycardia, cool clammy skin, and a sense of impending doom.
- Horror, dread, and anxiety are psychological responses to traumatic amputations, especially when the mangled, severed limb accompanies the patient to the hospital.
- Denial is commonplace when receiving the news that amputation is the recommended option.

More commonly the patient facing surgical amputation is diabetic with a pre-existing ulceration that becomes infected.

- Decreased or absent pedal pulses

- Visible, malodorous necrosis
- Black hard gangrenous lesions or toes (dry gangrene)

Soft tissue and bone involvement appears as deep craters with exposed tendon, joint capsule, or bone.

- Ulcers can be masked by overlying thick callous formation.
- Areas between fingers and toes may have thick dense hyperkeratotic tissue.
- Pain may not be present because of extensive peripheral neuropathy.
- If the patient has neuropathy and pain, a deep abscess or underlying infection is probable.[19]

The systemic response to infection of the extremity may include the presence of:

- Chills and fever
- Nausea and vomiting
- Malaise
- Hypotension and tachycardia
- Unexplained hyperglycemia (unrelated to diet, change in activity level, etc)

What can harm my patient and why?

When the immune-compromised diabetic patient presents with an infected limb, the patient may develop life-and-limb–threatening complications of:

- Sepsis with resultant metabolic instability and septic shock
- Necrotizing fasciitis
- Gas gangrene
- Ascending cellulitis
- Osteomyelitis
- Compartment syndrome[19]

What can harm my patient and why?

- Hemorrhage secondary to having severed major blood vessels.
- Infection from wound contamination following trauma.
- Phantom limb pain secondary to having severed peripheral nerves.
- Contractures of joints because of flexion deformity and protective positioning owing to pain and disuse.
- Pressure ulcers caused by poor fit or improper conditioning associated with the prosthesis.
- Psychosocial maladaptation may occur because of absent/ineffective crisis intervention at the time of trauma, or delayed/absent grief work.

Interventions and why?

The nurse caring for a patient with a traumatic amputation must act quickly to limit blood flow:

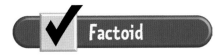

Factoid

Half the patients with limb-threatening necrotic ulcerations are physiologically incapable of mounting a normal immune response that is reflected in the clinical signs of infection.[19]

- Stay calm when initiating first aid because this will help calm the victim.

- Assess airway and respirations to see if there is a more acute problem, and then apply firm, direct pressure with layers of dry dressing over the residual limb.

- Apply pressure to the artery above the bleeding limb if direct pressure does not stop the bleeding.

- Keep reinforcing the soiled dressing with more layers of dry dressing material, but do not remove saturated dressings in effort to not dislodge clots that have formed.

- Apply elastic compression wrap or inflate blood pressure cuff above the amputation if direct pressure does not stop bleeding.

- Prepare to apply a tourniquet as a last resort if no other previous methods to halt hemorrhage have been effective.

- Take vital signs while collecting information about any health condition or medication that may contribute to free bleeding.

Immediate postoperative management focuses on patient needs of comfort and safety:

- Monitor postoperative vital signs frequently and assess the compression dressing for visible bleeding and intactness.

- Have a tourniquet readily visible and available at the bedside in the event of massive hemorrhage.

- Assess for pain frequently (rated 1–10) using nursing comfort measures and prescribed PRN medication as indicated.

- Elevate the residual limb (stump) on a pillow for the first 24 hours to reduce edema; thereafter, elevate the foot of the bed (for lower extremity amputations) to avoid flexion deformities.

- Provide psychological support and support the patient's grief process for his or her loss.

- Encourage expression of feelings regarding the loss and change in body image.

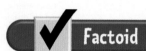

Peripheral Vascular Disease (PVD) accounts for the largest number of lower limb amputations, with the majority of amputees exceeding the age of 60.[21]

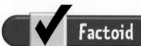

The compression dressing or (possibly a closed rigid plaster dressing) is used immediately after surgery to apply pressure and control bleeding. Later use of compression (elastic wrap over gauze dressing, compression limb sock) are used to control edema and for shaping the residual limb to fit into the prosthesis.

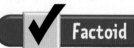

Getting amputees involved in self-care, and "normal" activities of daily living are important components of psychosocial adaptation.

To promote wound healing and prepare the residual limb for the permanent prosthesis:
- Assist with early mobilization: transfer from bed to chair, use of assistive devices for ambulation, upper body strengthening for use of crutches, and range of motion exercises.

- Change the dressing with sterile technique while drains are in place, and employ aseptic technique thereafter.

- Handle the residual limb carefully and gently during regular joint range of motion activity.

- Massage the stump gently with each dry dressing or limb sock application to increase circulation and reduce tenderness.

- If rigid and cast dressings are in place, monitor for compartment syndrome and signs of infection (elevated body temperature, unusual pain or odor, subjective complaints).

The nurse reinforces teaching outlined by members of the rehab team in preparation of use of a prosthesis:

- Residual limb shaping is accomplished with compression wraps and limb socks having incremental elastic pressure from distal to proximal. The goal of limb shaping is to achieve a tapered, cone-shaped stump that fits well into the prosthesis.

- Desensitize and toughen the stump by first pressing the healed stump into a soft pillow, then into a firm pillow, and then against a hard surface over a period of several days to weeks.

- To promote balance and joint mobility, move the residual limb in a normal gait pattern. (Swing the lower stump in rhythm with the other leg while crutch walking. Swing the upper residual arm in a normal pattern to the gait.)

- Instruct the patient to hold the residual limb in a flexed position when ambulating with crutches to avoid flexion deformities.

Cutting edge

- Because of vascular problems and trauma, the projected number of amputees by the year 2050 demands innovation to create a better, more user-friendly prosthesis than is currently available.

- Bioengineers at the University of Utah believe the answer lies in a novel osseointegrated intelligent design system for amputees wherein the implant into the bone creates an electric field at the bone interface, which decreases infection, enhances skeletal attachment and has a positive effect on bone remodeling.

- View the Seg3D CT program from the desk of Brad Isaacson, one of the researchers. You will be amazed: http://www.jove.com/index/Details.stp?ID=1237.[22]

- When a portion of lower limb has been amputated, the two greatest factors affecting optimal rehab and adaptation to a prosthesis are age and the level of the amputation.

- Obesity results in an increase in the frequency of requiring repairs or adjustments to the prosthesis.

- Psychological and cognitive factors (anxiety, depression, ability to learn, and attitude toward rehabilitation and life in general) impact the patient's autonomy in mobility.[21]

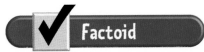

The multidisciplinary rehabilitation team includes the physician and vascular surgeon, the nursing team, a wound care nurse, an infectious disease specialist, physical therapists, the rehab engineer who designs the prosthesis, as well as a psychologist, and vocational and occupational therapists are all needed to accomplish the goal of getting the patient back into full participation in life, leisure, and work at the highest level of function.[19]

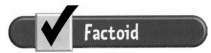

Amputees <65 years of age and those with the most distal level of amputation below the knee were predicted to adapt more successfully to mobility with a prosthesis.[21]

ACUTE LOW BACK PAIN

Let's get the normal stuff straight!

The spinal column consists of five cervical vertebra (C1-C5), 12 thoracic vertebra (T1-T12), four lumbar vertebra (L1-L4), and the sacral plexus

(L4-S5). The spinal cord passes through the cervical and thoracic verte-bra, ending at the first or second lumbar vertebra. Each vertebra has a flat spinal body with facets extending from each side and nerve roots for each vertebra passes through foramina in each facet to branch out as peripheral nerves, which innervate organ and body tissues.

- The spine has normal curvatures in the cervical and lumbar region that absorb shock from running and jumping.
- If the curvatures are abnormally flat (lordosis) or unnaturally curved (scoliosis), skeletal muscles in these areas are stretched or tightened, which can result in pain.
- Between each vertebra is a cartilaginous disk, which cushions the ver-tebral body and protects from damage during movement.
- With aging the vertebral disk narrows and the fluid within the disk diminishes.
- Compression injuries of the spine can damage the disk, causing cracks in the annulus (the fibrous covering of the disk), which allow disk material to bulge outward, putting pressure on nerve roots causing severe pain.
- Loss of calcium in the vertebral bodies can lead to compression frac-tures that impinge on nerve roots causing severe pain.
- The lumbar vertebra are the largest and thickest spinal bodies and carry the heaviest load in terms of keeping the body erect, lifting, and moving.
- Ligaments and tendons hold the vertebrae in place and attach the muscles to the spinal column.
- Abdominal and thoracic muscles give support to the spine during lift-ing activities.
- The cervical thoracic and lumbar muscles groups (cervical iliocostalis, thoracic multifidus, longissimus, semispinalis, spinalis and iliocostalis, and lumbar multifidus) are susceptible to overstretching and twisting injuries.[23]

Acute pain serves as a warning signal to alert the person to actual or impending tissue damage and is accompanied by these responses:

- Local musculoskeletal spasms and inadequately treated pain can pro-voke physiologic responses that alter circulation and tissue metabo-lism.
- Decreased mobility increased heart rate and decreased respirations to the point of breath-holding.
- Acute pain serves as an indicator for the need of professional help.

What is it?

Acute low back pain is short term and defines back problems and pain that subside spontaneously with or without treatment usually within 6 to 12 weeks, not persisting beyond three months.[23] Patients who do not improve with this time frame develop persistent (chronic) low back pain.

Low back pain is actually a symptom rather than a diagnosis, but when this common problem is acute it can usually be linked to a recent musculoskeletal event.

Causes and why?

Most commonly, acute back pain is caused by musculoskeletal strain or sprain associated with poor physical conditioning with weak supporting muscles of the back, having poor posture, or being overweight or tired.[3]

- Lifting activities (usually without help and using poor body mechanics)
- Trauma with sudden jolting or moving suddenly in unexpected ways
- Engaging in athletic events:

  Low back pain can be caused by a number of medical problems with referred pain to the back, such as urinary tract or kidney infection or conditions affecting the uterus, ovaries, or prostate. Other more serious problems can be implicated, such as:

- Malignancy
- Neurologic disease (ruptured or bulging disk)
- Cauda equina syndrome
- Disk degeneration
- Spinal stenosis
- Paget's disease

Testing, testing, testing

Usually low back pain is diagnosed based on patient symptoms, history of recent injury, and results of the physical exam. Diagnostic procedures that may be prescribed to rule out other causes of low back pain include:

- X-rays of the spine could reveal fractures, abnormal curvatures, degenerative changes, or osteoarthritis as well as indications of possible malignancy.[3,5]
- Bone scan and blood studies can reveal bone disease or tumors.
- MRI provides clear images of herniated disk, spinal stenosis, and cancer.[3]
- Electromyelogram (EMG) evaluates problems with the nerve root.

Signs and symptoms and why?

Pain is a subjective response that is usually accompanied by behavioral and psychological manifestations. The patient assessment may reveal:

- Pain usually related to a recent activity.
- Pain described as sharp, dull, deep, or aching.
- Pain that is usually constant and worsens in intensity at night.
- Deformity of the curvatures of the spine (lordosis or scoliosis).
- Very tender point areas noted on palpation.
- Impaired mobility: guarded movements, keeping the back still.

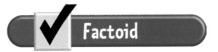

Factoid

At some time during their lives four out of five people will experience low back pain and only the common cold outranks low back pain as the most frequent reason for missed work.[3]

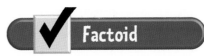

Factoid

Low back pain is costly! Yearly treatment costs exceed $80 billion; and insurance claims for disability because of low back pain are more than $8 billion yearly.[3]

- Straight leg raise produces pain in the low back.
- Spasm of the paravertebral muscles of the back (greatly increased tone)
- Restlessness, tension, anxiety, insomnia, and immobility owing to pain.

If there is spinal cord impingement or neurologic disease the patient may report:

- Pain radiating down the leg (sciatica or radiculopathy)
- Sudden bladder or bowel incontinence
- Foot drop
- Muscle atrophy
- Major muscle weakness

What can harm my patient and why?

Acute and chronic back pain is the leading cause of workers' compensation claims and has a significant impact on the quality of life:

- Disability because of the intensity of pain
- Loss of income because of disability
- Loss of social interactions, hobbies, and recreation because of pain
- Irritability, ineffective coping, feelings of worthlessness, and depression because of inability to work or play without pain

The mechanism of chronic low back pain differs as pain becomes chronic. The body's inflammatory response resolves and disappears, leaving soft tissue damage or spinal injury that continues to cause pain and mechanical problems. Therefore, nonsteroidal anti-inflammatory drugs (NSAIDs) are not helpful and side effects can be harmful.[23] Encourage the patient to stay active and moving. Bed rest is not indicated for acute low back pain.

Interventions and why?

Assess the precipitating event and the pain:

- Rate the pain on a scale of 1 to 10 and describe the onset, duration, quality, location, and radiation of pain.
- Describe functional impairment and impact of pain on activities of daily living, sleep, and rest.

Nursing care planning for relief of pain may include:

- Distraction
- Diaphragmatic breathing
- Relaxation to reduce muscle tension
- Guided imagery
- A firm mattress with pillows to maintain alignment and provide support
- Alternating periods of rest and activity

Implementation of prescribed therapies may involve:

- Application of heat or cold

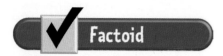

Factoid

The psychosocial strain of pain, depression, and disability places increased stress on relationships, and divorce is common.[23]

- Alternating heat and cold
- Stretching exercises
- Topical analgesic agents
- Massage therapy

When diversion and rest do not provide relief, pharmacologic intervention is necessary:

- Administer NSAIDs to decrease inflammation.
- Administer muscle relaxants as prescribed.
- Administer PRN analgesia that fits the level of pain the patient is reporting.

In order to reduce back strain and prevent re-injury, the patient should be taught to:

- Avoid factors that contribute to low back pain, such as stress, smoking, and heavy physical labor.
- Maintain good posture when sitting and standing.
- Sleep on a firm mattress with pillows under the waist and head when side-lying and under the knees when supine.
- Select chairs that allow feet to touch the floor with knees slightly bent and the low back against the back of the chair.
- Avoid sitting or standing for long periods of time without moving about and changing position.
- Exercise to strengthen muscles and achieve or maintain desirable weight.
- Use good body mechanics for proper lifting as well as activities of daily living and work.
- Save your back by using the stronger muscles of the arms and legs!
- Work smart. Push, pull, or roll rather than lift. Squat (keeping back straight) rather than bend. Use a sturdy footstool rather than lift over your head.

Reinforce back exercises prescribed by the physician or physical therapist. Pelvic tilt and abdominal curls to strengthen abdominal muscles. Knee-chest, hip, and quadriceps and sitting leg stretches.[3,5]

Cutting edge

A new study shows that an ounce of prevention more than accounts for cost of on-the-job back injuries! For nurses who work in residential care facilities, Park et al. (2009)[24] found that resident acuity and resident to staff ratio are variables associated with musculoskeletal back injury claims, but expenditures by the Ohio Bureau of Workers' Compensation for ergonomic equipment in nursing homes, resulting in fewer injuries and fewer insurance claims actually matched and balanced the cost of the new equipment, not even considering the unestimated benefit to the workers and the institutions.

► Figure 12-5. World Health Organization (WHO) pain relief ladder. http://www.who.int/cancer/palliative/painladder/en/

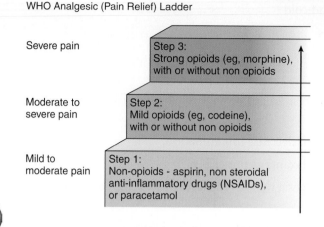

WHO Analgesic (Pain Relief) Ladder

Severe pain — Step 3: Strong opioids (eg, morphine), with or without non opioids

Moderate to severe pain — Step 2: Mild opioids (eg, codeine), with or without non opioids

Mild to moderate pain — Step 1: Non-opioids - aspirin, non steroidal anti-inflammatory drugs (NSAIDs), or paracetamol

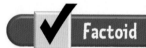

Factoid

Once acute low back pain becomes chronic, the treatment plan changes. Using the World Health Organization's (WHO) pain relief ladder, the patient's pain medication must fit the level of pain (Fig. 12-5).

Factoid

The WHO pain relief ladder was originally developed for cancer patients, but now it is being used for all types of pain.

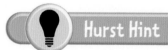

Hurst Hint

Never exceed a daily dose of 4000 mg of acetaminophen which is the maximum prescribed for healthy persons (aged 60 or below) with no organ damage or alcohol consumption.[23]

- Opioids are prescribed on daily basis (not PRN) for chronic low back pain.
- Referrals are made to pain clinics where patients with chronic low back pain are evaluated for a series of epidural steroid injections into the nerve root.
- Long acting medications are prescribed for patients needing 24-hour control (MS Contin, OxyContin, methadone, and Duragesic patches).

When pharmacologic therapy can no longer provide relief, surgery on the appropriate nerve root may be indicated.

PAGET'S DISEASE

What is it?

Paget's disease, also known as osteitis deformans, is a bone disease characterized by progressive bone remodeling, which causes bones to be larger and more vascular but structurally weaker because of increased bone turnover (rapid breakdown and rapid new bone formation), leading to skeletal deformities and fractures. It is the second most common bone disease in the older population following osteoporosis in frequency. Common sites of the disease are the vertebra, skull, pelvis, and weight-bearing bones of the femur and tibia. It is most common among people of European descent (see Fig. 12-6).

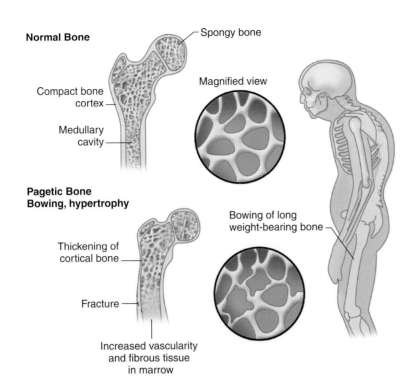

Normal Bone

Spongy bone

Compact bone cortex

Medullary cavity

Magnified view

**Pagetic Bone
Bowing, hypertrophy**

Thickening of cortical bone

Fracture

Increased vascularity and fibrous tissue in marrow

Bowing of long weight-bearing bone

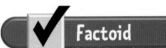
◄ Figure 12-6. Comparison of normal bone and Paget's disease.

Causes and why?

The cause of Paget's disease is unknown and most patients never know they have it. Patients are typically misdiagnosed with arthritis or skeletal changes owing to old age prior to a diagnosis of Paget's disease. There is evidence of family tendency, and up to 40% of patients with Paget's have a relative with the disorder. Possibly a viral infection contracted in childhood could cause a dormant skeletal infection that could later cause it.

Testing, testing, testing

Many times Paget's disease is discovered incidentally[25] after a fracture (ie, X-rays taken after a fracture show abnormal thickening of bone) or following a chest X-ray that reveals enlarged vertebra. Abnormal findings during X-ray or ultrasound screening tests for non-Paget complaints will prompt the health care provider to initiate these tests:

- Serum alkaline phosphatase (ALP), which will be elevated in the absence of renal or hepatic disease.
- Radionuclide bone scan (after initial ALP), which confirms a diagnosis after liver studies rule out any other disease.
- Lesser used biochemical tests: blood and urine N-telopeptide or C-telopeptide as well as specific tests for urinary hydroxyproline, pyridinoline, or deoxypyridinoline.

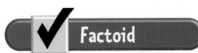

✔ Factoid

Alkaline phosphatase (ALP) is an indicator of bone "turnover" (breakdown and build up), which occurs at an accelerated rate in Paget's disease.

✔ Factoid

The bone scan uses a radionuclide material (Tc-99m), which emits gamma rays that are detected by a scintillator, which (using light patterns) provides realistic bone images. Light patterns are uniform in normal bone, but pagetic lesions (increased osteoblast and osteoclast activity) cause an increased uptake of the isotope. The concentrated spots of radionuclide are called "hot spots," which gives indication of the extent of Paget's disease throughout the body.[26]

Signs and symptoms and why?

Signs and symptoms	Why?
Severe, persistent pain worsened by weight-bearing activities	Bowing of legs causes mal-alignment of the hip, knee, and ankle joints, which cause arthritis, back, and joint pain; nerve compression causes pain
Cranial enlargement	Chronic bone inflammation; increased breaking down and rebuilding of bone in the area
Barrel-shaped chest	Chest and trunk flexes onto the legs to maintain balance
Asymmetric bowing of the tibia and femur	Chronic bone inflammation softens the bones causing them to bend
Kyphosis	Several vertebral fractures causing excess curvature of thoracic spine
Pathologic fractures	Diseased bones are highly vascular and structurally weak
Waddling gait	Bowed femurs and tibiae
Muscle weakness	Bone structural changes and deformity weaken surrounding muscles; hypercalcemia
Immobility	Abnormal bone formation impinging on the spine
Loss of height	Deformities of the femurs, tibias, and fibulas
Warmth and tenderness over affected areas	Increased bone vascularity
Paraplegia	Nerve compression from thickened bones
Blindness	Cranial nerve compression from thickened cranium
Hearing loss; tinnitus	Cranial nerve compression from thickened cranium; enlarged skull bones damage fragile inner-ear bones
Vertigo	Hearing loss and tinnitus; equilibrium off balance
Osteoarthritis	Bowing of legs causes mal-alignment of the hip, knee, and ankle joints, which cause arthritis; distortion of joints leads to osteoarthritis
Hypertension	Increased vascular demands owing to increased blood flow through the affected bones; hypercalcemia
Renal calculi	Hypercalcemia; dehydration
Hypercalcemia	Immobility; dehydration; bone breakdown causes increased calcium levels in the blood
Mental deterioration	Changes in shape of skull
Heart failure	Increased vascular bed and metabolic demands
Small, triangular appearing face	Cranium enlarges making face appear smaller
Headaches	Cranial nerve compression from thickened cranium
Bowel disturbances	Hypercalcemia
Fatigue, weakness, anorexia	Hypercalcemia

Very commonly the patient with Paget's disease complains of bone pain. Additionally the clinical picture includes:

- Warmth to touch over the bone lesion caused by increased blood flow.
- Painful hips and legs (if the bone lesions involve pelvis and femur).
- Neurologic symptoms: Paresthesia, weakness, and numbness if spinal vertebrae are impinging nerves.
- Elevated serum level of alkaline phosphatase (ALP) with no evidence of liver disease may be the only initial sign of Paget's disease if detected early.[25]

What can harm my patient and why?

Depending on how far advanced the disease has progressed before treatment to suppress disease activity; the patient may have already developed:

- Stress fractures because of large osteoclasts and pitting of bones
- Bowed limbs if long bones are affected
- Headaches and hearing loss if pagetic lesions involve the skull
- Physical disability owing to bone deformity
- Depression owing to decreased quality of life secondary to reduced independence, mobility, and constant pain[25]

Interventions and why?

- Calcitonin slows the rate of bone breakdown.
- Aspirin, acetaminophen, and NSAIDs reduce pain and inflammation.
- Heel lifts/walking aids make walking easier.
- Physical therapy improves mobility.
- Fractures are managed according to location.
- Hearing aids/sign language/lip reading facilitate communication with the hearing impaired.
- Surgery relieves pinched nerves; replaces arthritic joints; reduces pathologic fractures; and corrects secondary deformities

  When a patient is first diagnosed with Paget's disease, he or she may be hospitalized for a pathologic fracture having no additional symptoms other than those previously (and mistakenly) attributed to arthritis and other complaints associated with aging (hearing and visual impairments, dental complications).[25]

- Prepare for bone scan by administering prescribed PRN analgesia prior to scanning because lying for up to one hour on the hard scanning table will be very uncomfortable for the patient with pre-existing bone pain.
- Give information about the disease process, and collect information about siblings or other family members who should be tested for Paget's disease.

Prescribed doses of bisphosphate medication(s) will prevent the progression of Paget's disease and reduce incidence of future complications.[26]

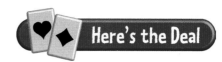

Here's the Deal

When an individual is diagnosed with Paget's disease, other siblings should be alerted immediately so that blood can be tested for elevated ALP levels because affected persons are asymptomatic in the early stages of the disease.

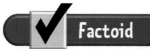

Factoid

The earlier that Paget's disease can be diagnosed and treated, the better response the patient will have to treatment, with decreased incidence of irreversible bone deformities and physical disability.

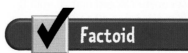

Factoid

Many of the same bisphosphonates are used in the treatment of osteoporosis, but the dosage and schedule varies. Boniva (ibandronate sodium) is the only bisphosphonate that is marketed solely for the treatment and prevention of postmenopausal osteoporosis and must be taken monthly (PO) or every three months (IV) for life.[32]

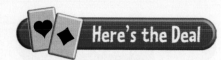

Here's the Deal

The patient with Paget's disease and the patient (female and male) with osteoporosis both have weak bones that are at risk for fracture and kyphosis, but the pathology is totally different.

- Calcium and vitamin D utilization and/or deficiency coupled with demineralization from lack of weight-bearing exercise is the root of the problem with *osteoporosis*, wherein the rate of new bone formation can't keep up with the rate of bone breakdown.

- In *Paget's disease* the rate of bone breakdown is accelerated, but so is the rate of new bone formation! Bone formation is increasingly rapid with larger than normal bone being produced but the bone formed has a disorganized structure with reduced mechanical strength (bigger but not better).

OSTEOPOROSIS

What is it?

Osteoporosis literally means porous bones. It is considered a metabolic bone disorder, which results in the loss of bone mass because of the rate of bone resorption exceeding the rate of bone formation. This decrease in bone density causes bones to become porous and brittle, which leads to easy bone fractures.

What causes it and why?

Causes	Why?
Inadequate calcium and vitamin D intake during young adulthood	Young adults drink caffeine drinks instead of milk, which has vitamins A and D as well as the calcium needed for bone growth and support
Rapid bone loss postmenopause	<ul><li>Low estrogen levels (hysterectomy)</li><li>Intake of caffeine and nicotine</li><li>Lack of weight-bearing exercises</li></ul>
Family history	Predisposes to low bone mass
Prolonged steroid therapy	Interferes with glucose utilization and causes breakdown of protein, which forms the matrix of the bone
Prolonged heparin therapy	Increases collagen breakdown
Osteogenesis imperfect	Imperfectly formed bones break easily
Immobility or disuse of bone	Bones need stress for bone maintenance
Medications: aluminum-containing antacids, corticosteroids, anticonvulsants, barbiturates	Affect the body's use and metabolism of calcium
Breastfeeding women	Bone density decreases during breast feeding but returns to normal after weaning
Age: As people age into their seventies and eighties, osteoporosis becomes a common disease[1]	Decrease in hormones and weight-bearing activity
Nutritional deficit: protein, calcium, vitamins C and D	Makes bones soft, thin, and brittle

(Continued)

Causes	Why?
Excessive intake of caffeine, nicotine, and alcohol	Worsen pre-existing osteoporosis; reduces bone remodeling
Bone tumors	Impair new bone formation
Diseases: Chronic kidney failure, liver disease, and hormonal disorders	Diseases cause hormone changes that affect bone density and bone loss
Rheumatoid arthritis	Causes generalized bone loss
Nutritional abnormalities: Anorexia nervosa, scurvy, lactose intolerance, malabsorption	Reduces nutrients needed for bone remodeling
Sudeck's atrophy: Localized in hands and feet with recurring attacks	Decreased circulation causes shrinkage of connective tissue and weakens bones
Sedentary lifestyle	Disuse of bones and muscles
Mild, prolonged negative calcium balance	Calcium needed for bone growth and support
Faulty protein metabolism	Caused by estrogen deficiency; leads to soft, thin, brittle bones
Declining gonadal adrenal function in males	Hormone changes affect bone density and loss

Testing, testing, testing

- Dual energy X-ray absorptiometry (DEXA): detects bone mass and decay
- Quantitative computed tomography (QCT): measures bone density
- X-rays: identifies suspected fractures
- Quantitative ultrasound (QUS): shows injured or diseased areas
- Blood tests: measures calcium, phosphorus, and alkaline levels; elevated parathyroid hormone
- Bone biopsy: shows thin, porous bone (Fig. 12-7)

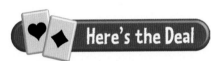

Here's the Deal

Osteoporosis can be prevented (which is more successful than treatment)[3] with lifestyle changes (less alcohol, less salt, stop smoking, regular weight-bearing exercise, increase vitamin D, and calcium intake),[28] but the only hope for patients with Paget's disease is early diagnosis with initiation of antiresorptive drugs to control the disease before deformity and disability occur.

◀ Figure 12-7. Osteoporosis. (Reproduced with permission from Hurst M. *Hurst Reviews: Pathophysiology Review.* New York: McGraw-Hill; 2008:398).

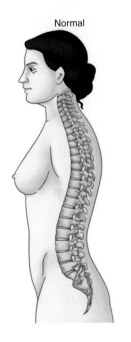

Normal

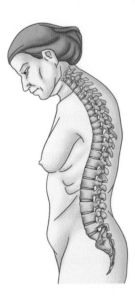

Signs and symptoms and why?

Signs and symptoms	Why?
Kyphosis of thoracic spine (called "dowager's hump")	Several vertebral fractures causing excess curvature of thoracic spine
Loss of height	Bones collapse or fracture
Fracture(s): back, hip, wrist	Weakened bones; hormonal imbalance; fractures heal slowly
Pain; tenderness	Can be sudden and associated with bending or lifting; back pain associated with vertebral collapse; worse when patient stands or walks; muscles may become tender
Immobility	Change in posture; pain; weakened muscles
Change in breathing pattern	Stooped posture; pain; weakened muscles
Deformity	Immobility because of pain; bone collapse or fracture
Decreased exercise tolerance	Pain; immobility
Markedly aged appearance	Body structure changes/deformity; pain
Muscle spasm	Muscle strain caused by weakened muscles; body structure changes/deformity

Source: Created by the author from References 1, 6, 10, 12, 13, and 15

Interventions and why?

- Physical therapy: slows bone loss
- Moderate weight-bearing exercises: slows bone loss
- Supportive devices (back brace, wrist splint): maintains function
- Surgery: hip replacement; open reduction and internal fixation for femur fractures
- Hormone replacement therapy (estrogen and progesterone): slows bone loss and prevents fractures
- Analgesics: relieves pain
- Local heat: relieves pain
- Calcium and vitamin D supplements: promotes normal bone metabolism
- Calcitonin (Calcimar): reduces bone resorption and slow loss of bone mass
- Bisphosphonates (etidronate [Didronel]): increases bone density and restores lost bone
- Fluoride (alendronate [Fosamax]): stimulates bone formation
- Diet rich in vitamin C, calcium, and protein: supports skeletal metabolism

- Smoking cessation
- Teriparatide (synthetic parathyroid hormone): builds bone and increases bone density
- Testosterone therapy for men: reduce osteoporosis
- AMG-162 (monoclonal antibody): inhibits bone resorption; in phase 3 clinical trials
- Vertebroplasty and kyphoplasty: repairs collapsed vertebra

The patient who has weak bones (either from Paget's disease or osteoporosis) teaching regarding lifestyle modifications for bone health:

- The diet should contain adequate amounts of calcium (1500 mg) and vitamin D (400–800 IU daily).
- Drink two 8-oz glasses of vitamin D–fortified milk. Exposure to the sun and/or supplements of calcium and vitamin D are recommended.[3]
- Increase the level of weight-bearing activity (walking daily, preferably outdoors without sunscreen).
- Avoid alcohol and cigarette smoking (first-hand or second-hand) and discuss risks and benefits of medications that reduce bone density (eg, corticosteroids, barbiturates, and anticonvulsants) with your doctor.[3]
- A safe home environment can be created with removal of scatter rugs, installation of hand rails, removal of clutter, and increased lighting.
- Indoor pets—which are wonderful for companionship and mental health—pose a risk of falls when underfoot. If pet adoption is not an option, contain the pet at night and be aware of the pet's whereabouts at all times, exercising caution.
- Take medications exactly as prescribed, notifying the health care provider of any complications.

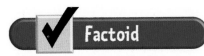

Factoid

Swimming is a great exercise, but it doesn't increase bone density! You don't bear weight on bones when you are swimming!

Depending on the progression of the disease when discovered, remission of early onset Paget's disease may be obtained with the administration of bisphosphonates. When the disease is advanced bisphosphonates are still used to arrest disease, but complications require additional interventional strategies:

- Fractures are managed with reduction and immobilization.
- Bowed limbs and instability require walking aids.
- Severe degenerative arthritis may require joint replacement.
- Hearing loss (Paget's lesions of the skull) is managed with hearing aids and learned techniques such as speech reading and interpreting body language.
- Weight management is important to reduce stress on weakened bones.

The mainstay of pharmacologic therapy for Paget's disease is the commonly used bisphosphonates. Additional drugs may be prescribed:

- Calcitonin given SQ or nasal administration (when bisphosphonates cannot be given) decreases breakdown of bone by reducing the number and activity of osteoclasts.[3]

- Plicamycin (Mithracin) a cytotoxic antibiotic is used for advanced Paget's disease with neurologic involvement when the patient is resistant to other pharmacologic approaches.[5]

Referrals are made to the rheumatologist or orthopedist as indicated.

Cutting edge

The first new Paget's drug of the decade is the newest bisphosphonate, zoledronic acid! When administered as a single intravenous infusion, it offers highly effective antiresorptive action and longer-lasting remission.[29] Even as much progress being made with drug-induced remission of Paget's disease of the bone, there is lesser progress with extramammary disease when the lesions appear on the nipple, areola, or around the genitals. Immunohistochemical staining of biopsy specimen is essential to accurate diagnosis of skin lesions and the treatment of choice is surgery. Frozen section–guided deep excision reduces the recurrence rate. Long-term follow-up is mandatory in these patients to identify and treat any subsequent recurrence or concurrent malignancy.[30]

PRACTICE QUESTIONS

1. Two days after a contusion to the thigh and a rotational injury to the knee, the patient in a knee brace from upper thigh to the mid-calf is complaining of pain. After having the patient rate the pain on a scale of 1 to 10, which next action is the priority?

   A. Elevate the leg on a pillow.

   B. Call the doctor to report the pain.

   C. Remove the brace and inspect the leg.

   D. Administer prescribed PRN medication.

2. Which nursing assessment is the priority following temporary external fixation of a tibial fracture when the nurse is monitoring the patient for complications?

   A. Patient complaint of pain

   B. Oral temperature of 100.2°F

   C. Alignment of the affected extremity

   D. Equal warmth of the lower extremities

3. The patient with a tibial fracture has a lower leg cast and the foot is edematous. After ascertaining that the foot is warm and pulses are palpable and the patient can wiggle all toes, which next action by the nurse is priority?

   A. Elevate the affected foot.

   B. Inspect for rough edges around the cast.

   C. Prick between the great toe and next toe to check sensation.

   D. Depress the nail bed on the great toe and watch for color return.

4. Your patient in a spica (body) cast has not had a bowel movement since the cast was applied four days ago, even though you have forced fluids and administered the prescribed Colace. The patient is complaining of abdominal pain rated 7 on a scale of 1 to 10. Which next action by the nurse is priority?

  A. Turn the patient to the prone position and manually check for fecal impaction.

  B. Elevate the head of the bed and place the patient on the bedpan with instructions to strain, using abdominal muscles.

  C. Slide the stethoscope underneath the top anterior rim of the cast (center of nipples) and auscultate bowel sounds.

  D. Administer prescribed PRN analgesia and reassess the patient in 30 minutes, notifying the physician if unrelieved.

5. A patient sustained two fractured femurs and a pelvic fracture is 24 hours postinjury and application of spica cast. Upon complaint of sudden sharp stabbing chest pain accompanied by sudden shortness of breath, which next nursing measure is indicated?

  A. Monitor vital signs, oxygen saturation, and chest sounds.

  B. Raise the head of the bed, apply oxygen, and call the doctor.

  C. Bivalve the cast from the axilla to the waist and loosen the upper portion of the cast.

  D. Turn the patient to the side opposite that of the pain and encourage deep breaths.

6. Workmen loading an overturned mower in which a partial amputation of the foot occurred, discover a portion of the shoe and present it to an industrial nurse on the scene, who finds three toes in the end of the shoe. Which first action (if any) should be taken regarding the severed toes that are discovered after the victim has been transported to the local hospital?

  A. Leave the toes in the shoe and transport both to the hospital.

  B. Gently remove toes from the shoe and submerge in ice water.

  C. Place the portion of shoe with toes in a watertight bag and apply ice.

  D. Place the shoe and toes in a labeled plastic bag for later burial if desired.

  E. Wrap each toe in sterile gauze, seal in a plastic bag, and submerge them in very cold water.

7. When the patient has low back pain, which of the following questions on initial patient interview is the priority?

  A. How long have you had this pain?

  B. Where (point to the area) are you hurting?

  C. What intervention or position relieves your pain?

  D. How would you rate your pain on a scale of 1 to 10?

8. A patient has a hip fracture, but comorbidities and malnutrition warrant delay of the ORIF; therefore, Buck's extension is prescribed with 5 lb of traction. When weights are near the floor, which plan is best for the patient and for optimal staff utilization when pulling the patient up in bed?

   A. Two nurses will use the turn sheet and after temporarily discontinuing the 5 lb weight, to pull her up in the bed with equal, even, and uniform manual power.

   B. Three nurses will pull together (one at the head, two on the sides) on the count of three and slide (rather than lift) her and the weights up in the bed.

   C. Two nurses, one on either side using the turn sheet, will pull her up in the bed, while a third nurse at the foot of the bed simultaneously brings up the weights.

   D. Four nurses, two on either side, will completely lift the patient up off the bed and place the patient at the head of the bed, letting the weights come up with the patient (rope over pulley).

9. A 65-year-old patient has ultrasound of the ovary to rule out a tumor, and the image reveals a grossly thickened and deformed pelvis. The physician confirms a diagnosis of Paget's disease with ALP. The results are more than twice the normal range. When planning care, which next diagnostic test should the nurse anticipate?

   A. Radiographic testing

   B. Radionuclide bone scan

   C. Urinary N-telopeptide or C-telopeptide

   D. Urinary hydroxyproline, pyridinoline, or deoxypyridinoline

10. Which discharge teaching is most important following outpatient infusion (IV) of the antiresorptive drug Reclast (zoledronic acid)?

    A. Notify the doctor immediately if flulike symptoms occur.

    B. Include good sources of dietary calcium in the diet each day.

    C. See your doctor immediately for loose teeth, bleeding, or receding gums.

    D. Report for follow-up laboratory evaluation of renal function (creatinine clearance).

References

1. Porth CM. *Pathophysiology: Concepts of Altered Health States.* 7th ed. Philadelphia: Lippincott Williams & Wilkins; 2007.

2. Salcido R, Scott J. Compartment syndrome: Wound care considerations. *Adv Skin Wound Care* 20(10):559–565, 2007.

3. Beers MH, ed. *The Merck Manual of Medical Information.* Whitestation, NJ: Merck Research Laboratories; 2003.

4. Laskowski-Jones L. First aid for sprains: Respond quickly to help the victim prevent complications and start healing. *Nursing 2006* *36*(8):48–49, 2006.

5. Smeltzer SC, Bare BG, Hinkle JL, Cheever KH. *Brunner & Suddarth's Textbook of Medical-Surgical Nursing.* 11th ed. Philadelphia: Lippincott Williams & Wilkins; 2008.

6. Gutierrez GM, Kaminski TW, Douex AT. Neuromuscular control and ankle instability. *PM & R: J Injury Func Rehab 1*(4):359–365, 2009.

7. Park RM, Bushnell PT, Bailer AJ, et al. Impact of publicly sponsored interventions on musculoskeletal injury claims in nursing homes. *Am J Ind 52*(9):683–697, 2009.

8. Altizer L. Compartment syndrome. *Orthop Nurs 23*(6):391–396, 2004.

9. Egol KA, Bazzi J, McLaurin TM, Tejwani NC. The effect of knee-spanning external fixation on compartment pressures in the leg. *J Orthop Trauma 22*(10):680–685, 2008.

10. Hurst M. *A Critical Thinking and Application NCLEX Review.* Brookhaven, MS: Hurst Review Services; 2008.

11. Sweeney J. What's a fat embolism? Clinical queries. *Nursing 2006* *36*(11):22, 2006.

12. Lynam L. Assessment of acute foot and ankle sprains. *Emerg Nurse 14*(4):24–33, 2006.

13. Fongiovanni MS, Bradley SL, Kelley DM. Orthopedic trauma: Critical care nursing issues. *Crit Care Nurs Q 28*(1):60–71, 2005.

14. Gore T, Lacey S. Bone up on fat embolism syndrome: Find out how to protect your patient from this potentially deadly complication. *Nursing 2005 35*(8):32hn1–32hn4, 2005.

15. Pullen RL. Clinical do's & don'ts: Applying a cast. *Nusing 2008 17*(4):12, 2008.

16. Carmichael KD, Groucher NR. Cast abscess: A case report. *Orthop Nurs 25*(2):137–139, 2006.

17. Comerford KC, Labus D, eds. *Nursing 2010 Drug Handbook.* Philadelphia: Lippincott Williams & Wilkins; 2010.

18. Puechal X, Fiessinger J-N. *Thromboangiitis obliterans* or Buerger's disease: Challenges for the Rheumatologist. *Rheumatology* 46:192–199, 2007.

19. Zgonis T, Stapleton JJ, Girard-Powell VA, Hagino RT. Surgical management of diabetic foot infections and amputations. *AORN J 87*(5):935–946, 2008.

20. Fraizer R, Forbes TL. Vascular images: Buerger's disease. *J Vasc Surg* 46:812, 2007.

21. Kelly M, Dowling M. Patient rehabilitation following lower limb amputation. *Nurs Standard 22*(49):35–39, 2008.

22. Isaacson BM, Stinstra JG, MacLeod RS, et al. Bioelectric analysis of osseointegrated intelligent design system for amputees. *J Vis Exp 15*(29):1–6, 2009.

23. D'Arcy Y. Treatment strategies for low back pain relief. *Nurse Pract* *31*(4):17–27, 2006.

24. Park RM, Bushnell PT, Bailer AJ, et al. Impact of publicly sponsored interventions on musculoskeletal injury claims in nursing homes. *Am J Indust Med 52*(9):683–697, 2009.

25. Sutcliffe A. Paget's disease 2: Exploring diagnosis, management and support strategies. *Nurs Times 105*(7):14–15, 2009.

26. Pagana KD, Pagana TJ. *Mosby's Diagnostic and Laboratory Test Reference.* 6th ed. St. Louis: Mosby; 2003.

27. Pountney D. Osteoporosis. *Nurs Older People 19*(3):19–21, 2007.

28. Abelson A. A review of Paget's disease of bone with a focus on the efficacy and safety of zoledronic acid 5 mg. *Curr Med Res Opin 24*(3):695–705, 2008.

29. Ekwueme KC, Zakhour HD, Parr NJ. Extramammary Paget's disease of the penis: A case report and review of the literature. *J Med Case Repts 3*(1):1752–1947, 2009.

30. Netzer G, Fuchs BD. Necrotizing fasciitis in a plaster-casted limb: Case report. *Am J Crit Care 18*(3):287–288, 2009.

31. Brush KA. Abdominal compartment syndrome: The pressure is on. *Nursing 2007 37*(7):37–40, 2007.

CHAPTER

13 Infectious Diseases

OBJECTIVES

In this chapter you will review:

- The responsible pathogens, signs, symptoms, and treatment of common infections encountered in med-surg nursing today. We will also cover a few uncommon sources of infection because you are likely to be tested on them:
  - Infectious diarrhea
  - STDs
  - West Nile virus
  - Legionnaires' disease
  - SARS
- Patient teaching.
- Isolation precautions for each type of infection.

INFECTIOUS DIARRHEA

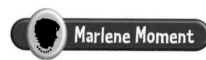

Remember to teach your patient not only the importance of hand hygiene, but also the *proper* way to wash his or her hands (Fig. 13-1).

What is it?

Diarrhea is the frequent passage of loose, watery stools. A person with diarrhea typically passes stool more than three times a day. People can have acute or chronic diarrhea. Acute diarrhea is a common problem that usually lasts one or two days and goes away on its own without special treatment. Diarrhea lasting more than two days may be caused by an underlying infection. More than 90% of cases of acute diarrhea are caused by infectious agents; these cases are often accompanied by vomiting, fever, and abdominal pain.

▶ Figure 13-1. Handwashing Sign. Good hand hygiene is crucial to avoid spreading infectious diarrhea! Graciously provided by the Centers for Disease Control and Prevention/ Minnesota Department of Health, R.N. Barr Library; Librarians Melissa Rethlefsen and Marie Jones.

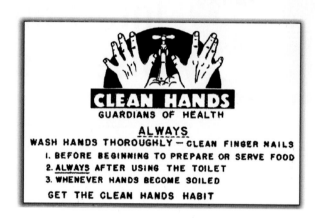

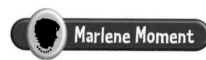

The GI system can be affected by your stress level. Many nursing students have their first episode of "explosive" diarrhea the night before their first unit exam or first day of clinical.

Causes and why?

Infectious diarrhea is transmitted by fecal-oral transmission or ingestion of food or water contaminated with pathogens from human or animal feces. The most common form of transmission is caused by an infected person with contaminated hands resulting from poor or absent hand hygiene after defecation. The infected person then handles foods, particularly uncooked foods, which are consumed by the public. Outbreaks are often seen at picnics, restaurants, and banquets where many people may prepare or handle the foods. Another form of contamination occurs when a person consumes foods, such as raw oysters and sushi, which are harvested in water contaminated with infected feces. Finally, a person may swallow water in a lake, hot tub, or other body of water that harbors pathogens. Diarrhea is a symptom of infection, but it may also be a symptom of many other diseases. Acute infection occurs when an ingested pathogen multiplies and overwhelms the person's gastrointestinal mucosa (gastric acid, digestive enzymes, mucus secretion, peristalsis, and suppressive resident flora) defenses. These infectious pathogens can be viral, bacterial, or parasitic (Table 13-1). Eating food that hasn't been properly stored (eg, not hot enough [140 ºF or above] or cold enough [40°F or below]) is one of the most common reasons for food-borne illness (Fig. 13-2).

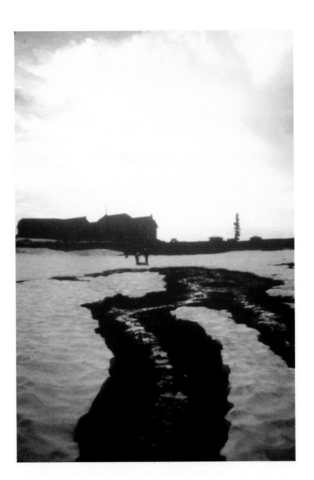

▶ Figure 13-2. Water contaminated with *E. coli*. Fluorescent dye placed in a toilet is shown spilling out of a sewer and contaminating the drinking water with *E. coli* at Crater Lake National Park, Oregon. Graciously provided by the Centers for Disease Control and Prevention, Mark Rosenberg.

Table 13-1   Summary of infectious diarrhea

Pathogen	Symptoms and why?	Testing	Interventions and why?	What can harm my patient?/ Patient teaching
Norovirus (Norwalk)	Incubation period of 24–48 hours. Characterized by acute onset of violent vomiting and diarrhea, abdominal cramps, nausea, and occasionally a low-grade fever.	Obtaining a good nursing history is important for the patient with diarrhea. Don't forget to ask about recent travel, vacations, attendance at a gathering where food has been served or antibiotic used. This will help expedite finding the cause.	Increase oral intake of fluids. May require IV fluids to replace lost electrolytes. Antibiotics for bacterial and parasitic infections. Diarrhea generally does not require special isolation precautions; however, if the patient is incontinent or diapered, "contact" isolation precautions should be instituted.	

(*Continued*)

Table 13-1   Summary of infectious diarrhea *(Continued)*

Pathogen	Symptoms and why?	Testing	Interventions and why?	What can harm my patient?/ Patient teaching
Rotavirus infection is rare in adults, but is very common in children and infants. Bacterial *Salmonella*	Incubation period 2 days. Characterized by vomiting and diarrhea, fever and abdominal cramps. Resolves in 3–8 days. Incubation 12–72 hours. Characterized by diarrhea, fever, and abdominal cramps. Resolves in 4–7 days.	Collecting a stool specimen can be tricky. Instruct your patient to defecate in a clean bedpan and use a tongue blade to transfer the sample to the laboratory collection container. You don't want the specimen to be obtained directly from the toilet, not because it is "dirty" but because it may have been recently cleaned with cleaners that "killed" what you are looking for. Last but not least, be sure to tell them to put the toilet paper in the toilet!	Standard isolation precautions are used on ALL patients, which means a barrier (usually gloves) should be worn if contact with blood or body fluids are anticipated. This applies to infectious diarrhea as a whole. Antidiarrheals may be used, but generally they are withheld until the GI tract has a chance to eliminate the invading pathogen. This applies to infectious diarrhea as a whole. Increase oral intake of fluids. May require IV fluids to replace lost electrolytes. Standard and isolation precautions. Most recover without treatment, as the bacteria are eliminated from the GI tract through diarrhea. Increase oral intake of fluids. May require IV fluids to replace lost electrolytes. Standard and isolation precautions.	
Bacterial *Shigella*	Incubation 1–2 days. Characterized by diarrhea, fever, and abdominal cramps. Diarrhea is often bloody. Resolves in 5–7 days.		Most recover without treatment as the pathogen is eliminated from the GI tract through diarrhea. Increase oral intake of fluids. May require IV fluids to replace lost electrolytes. May receive antibiotics depending on the severity of the infection.	
Campylobacter bacteria	Incubation 2–5 days. May have no symptoms or may have diarrhea, abdominal cramps, and fever. Diarrhea may be bloody. Nausea and vomiting resolve in 7 days.		Most recover without treatment. Increase oral intake of fluids. May require IV fluids to replace lost electrolytes. May receive antibiotics depending on the severity of the infection.	

(Continued)

Table 13-1   Summary of infectious diarrhea *(Continued)*

Pathogen	Symptoms and why?	Testing	Interventions and why?	What can harm my patient?/ Patient teaching
E. coli are normal bacteria for the colon and the most common cause of UTIs, but *E. coli* 0157:H7is a different strain of *E. coli* that produces deadly toxins.	Incubation 3–4 days. Begins slowly with mild abdominal pain and nonbloody diarrhea, but worsens over several days.		Increase oral intake of fluids. May require IV fluids to replace lost electrolytes. Use antibiotics to eradicate the pathogen from the GI tract.	HUS (hemolytic uremic syndrome) can occur 7 days after the first symptoms. Do not eat raw hamburger meat.
Bacterial *Clostridium difficile* (*C. diff*) is a bacterium that is related to the bacterium that causes tetanus and botulism.	Characterized by watery diarrhea, fever, loss of appetite, nausea, abdominal pain, tenderness.		Increase oral intake of fluids. May require IV fluids to replace lost electrolytes. Antibiotics. Standard and isolation precautions.	
Staphylococcus	Sudden onset. Characterized by nausea and vomiting, stomach cramping, and diarrhea.		Increase oral intake of fluids to replace lost electrolytes. May require IV fluids. May receive antibiotics depending on the severity of the infection. Standard and isolation precautions.	
Giardia parasite	Incubation 1–2 weeks. May have no symptoms, or diarrhea (often with foul-smelling, greasy stools), abdominal cramps, bloating, flatulence, fatigue, anorexia, and nausea. Resolves in 2–4 weeks.		Increase oral intake of fluids. May require IV fluids to replace lost electrolytes. May receive antibiotics. Standard and isolation precautions.	
Salmonella Reptiles, such as turtles, lizards, and snakes, are particularly likely to harbor *Salmonella*. Many chicks and young birds carry *Salmonella* in their feces and contamination can occur in the kitchen.	Foul-smelling diarrhea—may or may not be bloody.			Teaching: Surfaces and utensils that come in contact with raw poultry must be cleaned thoroughly. Poultry should be fully cooked prior to being eaten.

What Can Harm My Patient?

Complications may result from diarrhea of any etiology. The most serious result of acute diarrhea is dehydration and electrolyte loss (Na, K, Mg, Cl). Serious fluid volume deficit can develop rapidly in patients who have severe diarrhea or are very young, very old, or debilitated. Remember, the fluid in diarrhea is coming from the body and the vascular space is being depleted. HCO_3 loss can cause metabolic acidosis. Refer to the chapter on acid–base for a more thorough discussion. The patient who also has nausea and vomiting is at a higher risk of dehydration because of the inability to tolerate oral hydration. This information applies to all causes of infectious diarrhea.

PATIENT TEACHING   There is some debate over the use of sports drinks such as Gatorade® and PowerAde® for hydration in patients with acute diarrhea. The controversy centers around the value of the electrolytes verses the effects of the high sugar content in the sports drink. Although replenishing lost electrolytes in patients with diarrhea is important, the high sugar levels can make the diarrhea worse and last longer. Ultimately, the Centers for Disease Control (CDC) does not recommend the use of sports drinks in the treatment of these patients and recommends oral rehydration solutions such as Pedialyte® and Gastrolyte®.

CLOSTRIDIUM DIFFICILE   *C. difficile* is caused by a spore-forming bacillus. For this reason, alcohol hand cleaners are not as effective as soap, water, and friction.

Bacteria can be good, bad, or ugly! *C. difficile* is a bacteria found in the intestines of healthy and ill people. We all have "good" bacteria that help us digest food and ward off many "bad" bacteria. *C. difficile* is one of the bad guys that are usually kept at bay by the "good" guys. However, illness and/or antibiotics can reduce the number of "good" bacteria and allow the *C. diff* to overpopulate inside your intestine and colon. When this happens you may get an illness called *Clostridium difficile* colitis.

Although the antibiotic clindamycin (Cleocin) has been the most widely recognized as causing *C. difficile* colitis, many commonly prescribed antibiotics also cause *C. difficile* colitis. Examples of antibiotics that frequently cause *C. difficile* colitis include ampicillin, amoxicillin, and cephalosporins (eg, cephalexin [Keflex]) (Fig. 13-3).

▶ Figure 13-3. *Clostridium difficile* grown in a petri dish over 48 hours. Centers for Disease Control and Prevention, Gilda Jones.

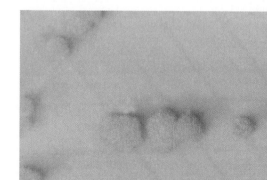

SEXUALLY TRANSMITTED DISEASES (STDs)

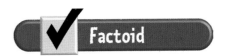

What is it?

A sexually transmitted disease (STD), also known as sexually transmitted infection (STI) or venereal disease (VD) is an illness that has a significant probability of transmission by means of sexual contact. Although in the past these illnesses have mostly been referred to as STDs or VD, in recent years the term *sexually transmitted infection* (STI) has been preferred, as it has a broader range of meaning. A person may be *infected*, and may potentially infect others, without showing signs of *disease*.

Causes and why?

Any person can become infected with an STD if there is unprotected (no condom) sexual contact with an infected partner. The greater the number of sex partners, the greater the risk of infection.

✛ Chlamydia

What is it?

Chlamydia is a bacterial infection, and is known as a "silent" disease because about three-fourths of infected women and about half of infected men have no symptoms. If symptoms do occur, they usually appear within one to three weeks after exposure.

In women, the bacteria initially infect the cervix and the urethra. Women who have symptoms might have an abnormal vaginal discharge or a burning sensation when urinating. When the infection spreads from the cervix to the fallopian tubes, some women still have no signs or symptoms; others have lower abdominal pain, low back pain, nausea, fever, pain during intercourse, or bleeding between menstrual periods. Chlamydial infection of the cervix can spread to the rectum.

Infants born to women with chlamydial cervicitis may develop chlamydial ophthalmia neonatorum and pneumonia.

Signs and symptoms and why?

Chlamydia is known as a "silent" disease because about three-fourths of infected women and about half of infected men have no symptoms. If symptoms do occur, they usually appear within one to three weeks after exposure. In women, the bacteria initially infect the cervix and the urethra. **Women** who have symptoms might have an abnormal vaginal discharge or a burning sensation when urinating. When the infection spreads from the cervix to the fallopian tubes, some women still have no signs or symptoms; others have lower abdominal pain, low back pain, nausea, fever, pain during intercourse, or bleeding between menstrual periods. Chlamydial infection of the cervix can spread to the rectum. **Men** with signs or symptoms might have a discharge from their penis or a burning sensation when urinating. Men might also have burning and itching around the opening of the penis. Pain and swelling in the testicles are uncommon.

What can harm my patient and why?

Chlamydia is known as a "silent" disease, and as a result can go untreated. Left untreated, this STI can progress and cause serious reproductive and other health problems. A common complication for women is pelvic inflammatory disease (PID), which can lead to chronic pelvic pain, infertility and ectopic pregnancy. An ectopic pregnancy is a potentially fatal complication. In addition, women who are infected with *Chlamydia* are up to five times more likely to become infected with HIV if exposed.

Testing, testing, testing

Laboratory tests can be performed on urine and as a culture from the cervix or penis. All sex partners should be tested and treated if infected. Testing for Chlamydia is routinely performed on all pregnant women during the antepartum period so that the infection can be identified and treated. Babies born to infected mothers can get infections in both their eyes and respiratory tract and is a leading cause of early infant conjunctivitis and pneumonia.

Interventions and why?

- Azithromycin 1 g orally ×1 **or** Doxycycline 100 mg orally twice daily orally × 7 days.
- Obtain a thorough patient history related to signs, symptoms, and sexual contacts.
- Obtain cultures as ordered.

✚ Gonorrhea

What is it?

- Gonorrhea is caused by the *Neisseria gonorrhoeae* bacterium.
- It infects the cervix, uterus, and fallopian tubes in women.
- It also infects the mouth, throat, eyes, urethra, and anus in women and men.

Signs and symptoms and why?

Some men with gonorrhea may have no symptoms at all. However, some men have signs or symptoms that appear two to five days after infection, although symptoms can take as long as 30 days to appear. Symptoms and signs include a burning sensation when urinating, or a white, yellow, or green discharge from the penis. Sometimes men with gonorrhea get painful or swollen testicles.

In women, the symptoms of gonorrhea are often mild, but most women who are infected have no symptoms. Even when a woman has symptoms, they can be so nonspecific as to be mistaken for a bladder or vaginal infection. The initial symptoms and signs in women include a painful or burning sensation when urinating, increased vaginal discharge, or vaginal bleeding between periods. Women with gonorrhea are at risk

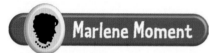

Factoid

Chlamydia is the most frequently reported bacterial sexually transmitted disease in the United States.

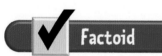

Marlene Moment

Now is not the time to be shy! You have to ask those "nosy," sometimes uncomfortable questions when obtaining a patient history from someone presenting with an STD. If sexual contacts are not identified and treated, then re-infection can occur and the sexual contact may go on to have long-term complications.

Factoid

State law mandates what infectious diseases have to be reported to the state. This not only provides important data for research, but also helps to protect the health of the public.

of developing serious complications from the infection, regardless of the presence or severity of symptoms.

The symptoms of rectal infection in both men and women may include discharge, anal itching, soreness, bleeding, or painful bowel movements. Rectal infection also may cause no symptoms. Infections in the throat may cause a sore throat, but usually cause no symptoms.

Testing, testing, testing

- Physical examination and patient history.
- Sexual contact information is collected so they may be treated also.
- Culture of cervix or penis discharge.

Interventions and why?

Ceftriaxone 125 mg IM ×1 *or* Cefixime 400 mg orally ×1.

What can harm my patient and why?

- Gonococcal and chlamydial ophthalmia neonatorum is a condition affecting a newborn's eyes. It occurs when they are contaminated during passage through the birth canal from a mother infected with either *Neisseria gonorrhea* or *Chlamydia trachomatis*. Eye drops containing erythromycin are typically used to prevent the condition. If left untreated it can cause blindness.
- An allergic reaction from the antibiotic may occur.
- Damage to reproductive organs may occur (Fig. 13-4).

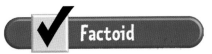

Factoid

During a patient interview, if your patient refers to a previous infection called the "clap," he or she is actually talking about gonorrhea. However, sometimes they use that term to refer to *any* sexually transmitted infection.

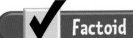

Factoid

The CDC has said the use of azithroycin ophthalmic solution (1%) is acceptable IF erythromycin ophthalmic ointment (0.5%) is n available.

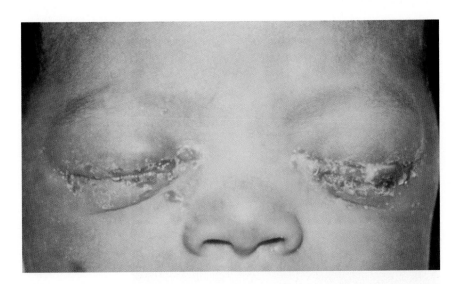

► Figure 13-4. Gonococcal ophthalmia in a newborn transmitted through the mother with a gonococcal infection. Centers for Disease Control and Prevention, J. Pledger.

PATIENT TEACHING

- Obtain prenatal care as soon as the patient realizes she is pregnant.
- Explain how STIs are transmitted.
- Describe the signs and symptoms of complications.
- Explain that the infection must be treated with medication.
- Explain that douches will not cure the infection.

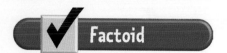

Factoid

Bacterium can be further described as "cocci" (cox-eye), rods, or spirochetes (spiro-keets). The syphilis bacterium is a spirochete.

✦ Syphilis

What is it?

Syphilis is caused by the *Treponema pallidum* bacterium and is called "the great imitator" because so many of the signs and symptoms are indistinguishable from those of other diseases. The patient may even be asymptomatic at first.

Signs and symptoms and why?

People infected with syphilis do not have any symptoms for years, yet remain at risk for late complications if they are not treated. Although transmission occurs from persons with sores who are in the primary or secondary stage, many of these sores are unrecognized. Thus, transmission may occur from persons who are unaware of their infection. All diseases have degrees of severity, and you may be taking care of a patient presenting with another complaint. Early diagnosis and treatment of the disease (at the earliest stage possible) is very important. This is why it's important to do a thorough nursing assessment.

PRIMARY STAGE The primary stage of syphilis is usually marked by the appearance of a single sore (called a chancre), but there may be multiple sores. The time between infection with syphilis and the start of the first symptom can range from 10 to 90 days. The chancre is usually firm, round, small, and painless. It appears at the spot where syphilis entered the body. The chancre lasts three to six weeks, and it heals without treatment. However, if adequate treatment is not administered, the infection will progress to the secondary stage (Fig. 13-5).

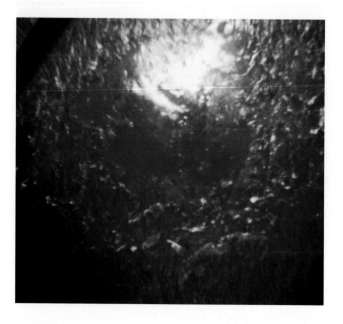

▶ Figure 13-5. A lesion (chancre) presenting during the primary stage of syphilis. Centers for Disease Control and Prevention, Dr. E. Dancewicz.

SECONDARY STAGE Skin rash and mucous membrane lesions characterize the secondary stage. This stage typically starts with the development of a rash on one or more areas of the body. The rash usually does not cause itching. Rashes associated with secondary syphilis can appear as the chancre is healing or several weeks after the chancre has healed. The characteristic rash of secondary syphilis may appear as rough, red, or reddish brown spots both on the palms of the hands and the bottoms of the feet. However, rashes with a different appearance may occur on other parts of the body, sometimes resembling rashes caused by other diseases. Sometimes rashes associated with secondary syphilis are so faint that they are not noticed. In addition to rashes, symptoms of secondary syphilis may include fever, swollen lymph glands, sore throat, patchy hair loss, headaches, weight loss, muscle aches, and fatigue. The signs and symptoms of secondary syphilis will resolve with or without treatment, but without treatment, the infection will progress to the latent and possibly late stages of disease (Figs. 13-6 and 13-7).

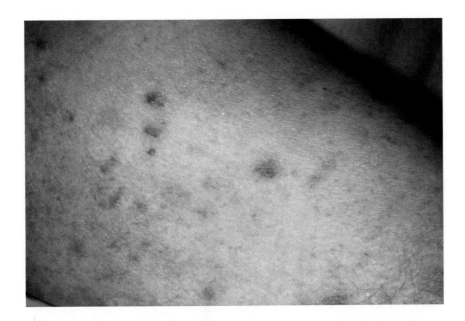

▶ Figure 13-6. A skin rash resulting from secondary stage of syphilis. Centers for Disease Control and Prevention.

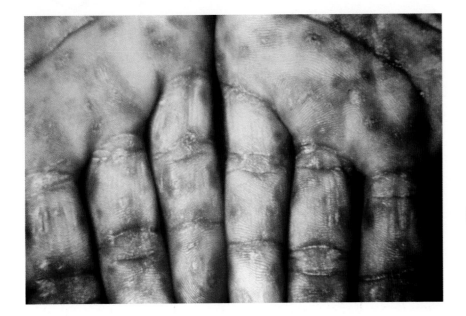

▶ Figure 13-7. Keratotic lesions on the palms caused by second-stage syphilis. Centers for Disease Control and Prevention.

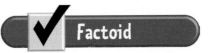

Factoid

Risk of transmission is about 30% from a *single* sexual encounter with a person with primary syphilis.

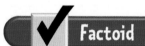
Factoid

One of the best-documented US cases of *unethical human medical experimentation* in the twentieth century was the *Tuskegee syphilis study*. The study researchers recruited a group of 600 black male *sharecroppers* in the rural area of *Tuskegee, Alabama*. Of these 600 men, 399 had the disease in the latent, asymptomatic stage. Two hundred and one men were uninfected control patients. The study was designed to measure the progression of untreated syphilis. Although the study lasted from 1942 until 1972, the infected men were not given any medications to treat the disease.

▶ Figure 13-8. *T. pallidum* spirochete, the causative agent of syphilis. Centers for Disease Control and Prevention, Bill Schwartz.

Factoid

When looking at a specimen (tissue or fluids) in the microscope, the pathologist looks for the syphilis spirochete, which has a worm-like, spiral-shaped form, and wiggles vigorously when viewed (Fig. 13-8).

LATE AND LATENT STAGES   The latent (hidden) stage of syphilis begins when primary and secondary symptoms disappear. Without treatment, the infected person will continue to have syphilis. Even though there are no signs or symptoms, infection remains in the body. This latent stage can last for years. The late stages of syphilis can develop in about 15% of people who have not been treated for syphilis, and can appear 10 to 20 years after infection was first acquired. In the late stages of syphilis, the disease may subsequently damage the internal organs, including the brain, nerves, eyes, heart, blood vessels, liver, bones, and joints. Signs and symptoms of the late stage of syphilis include difficulty coordinating muscle movements, paralysis, numbness, gradual blindness, and dementia. This damage may be serious enough to cause death.

Testing, testing, testing

- Physician examination and patient history.
- Sexual contact information is collected so that all potential contacts can be tested and treatment can be performed.
- Blood tests for VDRL and RPR.
- Microscopic exam of exudate from a chancre or lymph node aspirate.

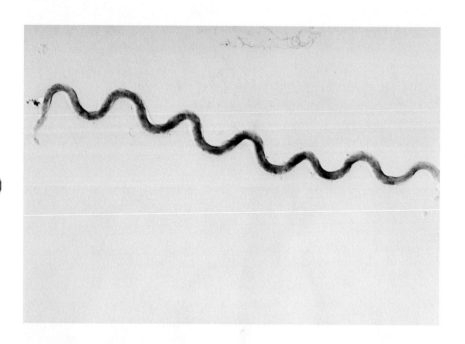

Interventions and why?

- Benzathine penicillin G 2.4 million units IM ×1.
- *Penicillin allergy:* Doxycycline 100 mg orally twice daily for 14 days.

✚ Genital herpes

What is it?

Genital herpes is caused by the herpes simplex viruses type 1 (HSV-1) or type 2 (HSV-2), although most genital herpes is caused by HSV-2. HSV-1 and HSV-2 can be found in and released from the sores that the viruses cause, but they also are released between outbreaks from skin that does not appear to have a sore. Generally, a person can only get HSV-2 infection during sexual contact with someone who has a genital HSV-2 infection. Transmission can occur from an infected partner who does not have a visible sore and may not know that he or she is infected.

HSV-1 can cause genital herpes, but it more commonly causes infections of the mouth and lips, so-called "fever blisters." HSV-1 infection of the genitals can be caused by oral-genital or genital-genital contact with a person who has HSV-1 infection. Genital HSV-1 outbreaks recur less regularly than genital HSV-2 outbreaks (Fig. 13-9).

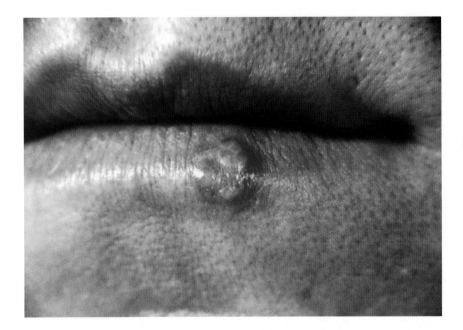

▶ Figure 13-9. Herpes simplex lesion caused by the (HSV1) pathogen. Centers for Disease Control and Prevention, Dr. C Herrmann.

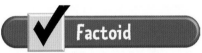

Fever blisters, chickenpox, and shingles are all caused by the HSV-1 infection.

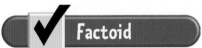

Type 1 infections usually occur from the waist up and type 2 infections usually occur from the waist down.

Signs and symptoms and why?

Many people infected with HSV-2 are not aware of their infection. However, if signs and symptoms occur during the first outbreak, they can be quite pronounced. Symptoms appear as blisters around the genitals and rectum that break and leave behind a painful sore. The first outbreak usually occurs within two weeks after the virus is transmitted, and the sores typically heal within two to four weeks. Other signs and symptoms during the primary episode may include a second crop of blisters, and flulike symptoms, including fever and swollen glands. However, many individuals with HSV-2 infection never have blisters, or they have very mild signs that they do not even notice or that they mistake for insect bites or another skin condition.

People diagnosed with a first episode of genital herpes can expect to have several (typically four or five) outbreaks (symptomatic recurrences) within a year. Over time these recurrences usually decrease in frequency. It is possible that a person becomes aware of the "first episode" years after the infection is acquired.

Testing, testing, testing

- Physician examination and patient history.
- Sexual contact information is collected so all sexual contacts can be identified, tested, and treated.
- Blood tests can identify the virus.
- Microscopic exam of exudate from a lesion.

Interventions and why?

Treatment of choice:

- First episode:
  - Acyclovir 400 mg 3× daily orally ×7–10 days
- Recurrent episodes:
  - Acyclovir 400 mg 3× daily orally ×5 days

PATIENT TEACHING

- Ensure patients and partners understand that safer sex practices should be used with daily therapy.
- Caution patients about touching the blisters and/or sores and then touching their eyes, as this can cause infection of the eye.

✚ Trichomoniasis

What is it?

- Trichomoniasis is caused by *Trichomonas vaginalis*, a single-celled protozoan parasite.
- The vagina is the most common site of infection in women.
- The urethra is the most common site of infection in men.
- The parasite is sexually transmitted through penis-to-vagina intercourse or vulva-to-vulva (the genital area outside the vagina) contact with an infected partner.
- Trichomoniasis does not affect the rectum.
- Women can acquire the disease from infected men or women, but men usually contract it only from infected women.

Signs and symptoms and why?

Most men with trichomoniasis do not have signs or symptoms; however, some men may temporarily have an irritation inside the penis, mild discharge, or slight burning after urination or ejaculation.

Some women have signs or symptoms of infection, which include a frothy, yellow-green vaginal discharge with a strong odor. The infection also may cause discomfort during intercourse and urination, as well as irritation and itching of the female genital area. In rare cases, lower abdominal pain can occur. Symptoms usually appear in women within 5 to 28 days of exposure.

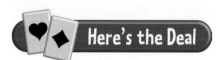

Factoid

The CDC recommends daily medication as part of a plan to reduce the risk of spreading genital herpes. Once-daily Valtrex is the only medication proved to reduce the risk of spreading genital herpes to a partner.

Here's the Deal

HSV-I and HSV-II are not curable. Once you contract it you have to live with it forever. The disease can be spread by sexual contact even when no outbreak is present.

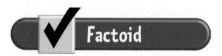

Factoid

Trichomoniasis is often referred to as "trick."

Testing, testing, testing

- Physical examination and patient history
- Culture of cervical scraping or penis discharge

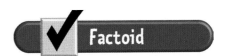

Cervical scraping is not as bad as it sounds. This is the same technique used to obtain a pap smear.

Interventions and why?

- Metronidazole (Flagyl) 2 g orally ×1

What can harm my patient and why?

The patient should be cautioned not to drink alcohol while taking Flagyl and for 48 hours following completion of therapy. This includes the use of preparations containing alcohol (perfume, OTC cough medicines), as these products and alcohol in conjunction with Flagyl can cause a disulfiram-like (Antabuse) reaction that causes vomiting.

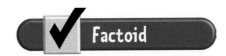

Pregnant women cannot take Flagyl.

✚ Genital warts

Let's get the normal stuff straight!

Most people with HPV do not develop symptoms or health problems. But sometimes, certain types of HPV can cause genital warts in men and women. Other HPV types can cause cervical cancer and other less common cancers, such as cancers of the vulva, vagina, anus, and penis. The types of HPV that can cause genital warts are not the same as the types that can cause cancer.

HPV types are often referred to as "low-risk" (genital wart–causing) or "high-risk" (cervical cancer–causing), based on whether they put a person at risk for cancer. In 90% of cases, the body's immune system clears the HPV infection naturally within two years. This is true of both high- and low-risk types.

What causes it?

- Human papillomavirus (HPV).
- It infects the skin and mucous membranes.
- There are more than 40 HPV types that can infect the genital areas of men and women.
- The skin of the penis, vulva (area outside the vagina), and anus, and the linings of the vagina, cervix, and rectum are affected.

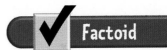

The HPV vaccine can prevent most cases of cervical cancer. The CDC recommends vaccination for females beginning at age 11 or 12. It can be started as early as age nine.

Signs and symptoms and why?

- Cauliflower-textured growths on the penis, vagina labia, or anal area

Testing, testing, testing

- Physical examination and patient history
- Culture of cervical scraping
- Many times, depending on the practitioner, the diagnosis can be made through clinical observation and assessment

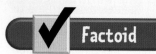

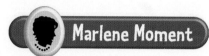

Granny said, "An ounce of prevention is worth a pound of cure!" Routine pap smears and the HPV vaccine can decrease number of women who develop cervical cancer. Each year 12,000 women are diagnosed with cervical cancer. In addition another 7,000+ develop cancers of the vulva, vagina, and anus.

Interventions and why?

There is no treatment for HPV infection; however, there are two vaccines available to help prevent certain types of HPV and some of the cancers linked to those types. They are Gardasil and Cervarix. These vaccines prevent the two types of HPV (HPV-16 and -18) that cause 70% of all cervical cancers. Gardasil also protects against the two types of HPV (HPV-6 and -11) that cause 90% of all genital warts.

What can harm my patient and why?

Certain types of HPV can lead to cervical cancer. In fact, we now know HPV is *the* cause of cervical cancer.

PATIENT TEACHING Patients often think that once they are diagnosed with an STD and treated, they cannot become infected again. Your patient should understand that if he or she resumes engaging in unprotected sexual activity the result can be in re-infection with the same or a new STD.

Birth control pills do not offer any protection from STDs.

WEST NILE VIRUS

What is it?

West Nile virus infection is a mosquito-borne infection. Arthropod-borne viruses (termed *arboviruses*) are viruses that are maintained in nature through a complex cycle of transmission between susceptible vertebrate hosts (birds) and blood-feeding arthropods (mosquitoes). The bird can become infected when an infected mosquito bites them to take a blood meal. The bird will host the virus for several days and usually becomes immune to the virus. An uninfected mosquito bites the infected bird and becomes infected, and the cycle goes on.

Although birds, particularly crows and jays, infected with West Nile virus can die or become ill, most infected birds do survive and continue to host the virus (Fig. 13-10).

▶ Figure 13-10. Mosquito. *Culex tarsalis* mosquito, the main vector responsible for West Nile virus in the Western United States. Centers for Disease Control and Prevention.

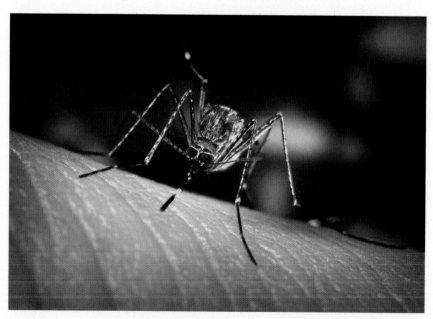

Causes and why?

West Nile virus is passed to humans when they are bitten by an infected mosquito. The cycle between birds and mosquitoes usually remains undetected until the virus escapes this cycle via a secondary host (people and animals) as the result of some ecologic change.

After the mosquito is infected and stores the virus in its salivary gland, it bites a human or animal and injects the virus where it can multiply and possibly cause illness.

Humans and domestic animals can develop clinical illness, but usually are incidental or "dead-end" hosts because they do not produce significant viremia (circulating virus), and thus do not contribute to the transmission cycle.

West Nile virus has been detected in dead birds of at least 300 species. There is no evidence that a person can get West Nile virus from handling live or dead infected birds.

Signs and symptoms and why?

SERIOUS SYMPTOMS IN A FEW PEOPLE About one in 150 people infected with WNV develop a severe illness, such as meningitis, encephalitis, or both. The severe symptoms can include high fever, headache, neck stiffness, stupor, disorientation, coma, tremors, convulsions, muscle weakness, vision loss, numbness, and paralysis.

These symptoms may last several weeks, and neurologic effects may be permanent.

MILDER SYMPTOMS IN SOME PEOPLE The body's recognition of the WNV as a foreign body accounts for the symptoms experienced. Up to 20% of the people who become infected have symptoms such as fever, headache, and body aches, nausea, vomiting, and sometimes swollen lymph glands or a skin rash on the chest, stomach, and back. Symptoms can last for as short as a few days, although even healthy people have become sick for several weeks.

NO SYMPTOMS IN MOST PEOPLE Approximately 80% of people (about four out of five) who are infected with WNV will not show any symptoms at all.

Testing, testing, testing

WNV infection can be suspected in a person based on clinical symptoms and patient history; however, laboratory testing is required for a confirmed diagnosis.

The most efficient diagnostic method is detection of IgM antibody to WNV in serum collected within 8 to 14 days of illness onset or CSF collected within 8 days of illness onset using the IgM antibody-capture, enzyme-linked immunosorbent assay (MAC-ELISA).

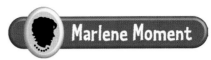

Marlene Moment

Increased dead birds in a geographic area may indicate increased infected mosquitoes flying around so keep your eyes as well as your feet on the ground.

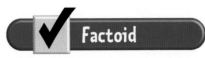

Factoid

People who have received a solid organ transplant may be at up to 40 times greater risk for developing severe WNV disease if bitten by an infected mosquito because the medications they take to inhibit rejection decreases their ability to fight off an infection.

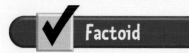

The American Academy of Pediatrics recommends that insect repellants containing no more than 10% DEET be used on children.

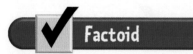

West Nile virus infection does not require special isolation precautions.

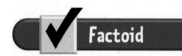

The bacteria got its name in 1976, when many people who went to a Philadelphia convention of the American Legion suffered from an outbreak of this disease.

Interventions and why?

No specific treatment is available. In severe cases treatment supportive care that often involves hospitalization, intravenous fluids, respiratory support, and prevention of secondary infections is provided.

PATIENT TEACHING   The easiest and best way to avoid WNV is to prevent mosquito bites.

When you are outdoors, use insect repellent containing DEET. Follow the directions on the package.

Many mosquitoes are most active at dusk and dawn. Be sure to use insect repellent and wear long sleeves and pants at these times or consider staying indoors during these hours. Make sure you have good screens on your windows and doors to keep mosquitoes out. Get rid of mosquito breeding sites by emptying standing water from flower pots, buckets, and barrels. Change the water in pet dishes and replace the water in bird baths weekly. Drill holes in tire swings so water drains out. Keep children's wading pools empty and on their sides when they aren't being used.

LEGIONNAIRES' DISEASE

What is it?

Legionnaires' disease is caused by the bacteria *Legionella*. The lungs are the most common site of infection. Legionella can be found in natural, freshwater environments, but they are present in insufficient numbers to cause disease. Potable (drinking) water systems, whirlpool spas, and cooling towers provide the three conditions needed for Legionella transmission—heat, stasis, and aerosolization. Therefore, these are common sources of outbreaks.

Causes and why?

People get Legionnaires' disease when they breathe in a mist or vapor (small droplets of water in the air) that has been contaminated with the bacteria. One example might be from breathing in the steam from a whirlpool spa that has not been properly cleaned and disinfected.

Outbreaks are defined as two or more people becoming ill in the same place at about the same time, such as patients in hospitals. Hospital buildings have complex water systems that can facilitate the conditions for growth of the bacteria in sufficient numbers to cause the disease. Many people in hospitals already have illnesses that also increase their risk for *Legionella* infection.

Other outbreaks have been linked to aerosol sources in the community, or with cruise ships and hotels, with the most likely sources being whirlpool spas, cooling towers (air conditioning units from large buildings), and water used for drinking and bathing. The bacteria are NOT spread from one person to another person.

Signs and symptoms and why?

Legionnaires' disease is a flulike syndrome with acute fever, chills, malaise, dyspnea, pleuritic pain, and hemoptysis, headache, or confusion. Nausea, loose stools or watery diarrhea, abdominal pain, and cough also frequently occur.

Testing, testing, testing

- Chest X-ray
- Staining of sputum
- Culture of sputum
- Urinary antigen assay

Interventions and why?

- Fluoroquinolone (Cipro) given IV or PO for two to three weeks.
- Legionnaires' disease does not require special isolation precautions.

PATIENT TEACHING   For patients on quinolones teach patients to:

- Limit intake of alkaline foods.
- Increase fluids to 3000 cc day to prevent crystalline formation in the kidneys.
- Avoid foods containing calcium and magnesium.
- Avoid exposure to UV rays.
- Do not take with theophylline.

SEVERE ACUTE RESPIRATORY SYNDROME

What is it?

Severe acute respiratory syndrome (SARS) is caused by a coronavirus, called SARS-associated coronavirus (SARS-CoV).

Signs and symptoms and why?

The illness usually begins with a high fever (measured temperature >100.4 °F [>38.0 °C]). The fever is sometimes associated with chills or other symptoms, including headache, a general feeling of discomfort, and body aches. Some people also experience mild respiratory symptoms at the outset. Diarrhea is seen in approximately 10% to 20% of patients. After two to seven days, SARS patients develop a dry, nonproductive cough that might be accompanied by or progress to hypoxia. In 10% to 20% of cases, patients require mechanical ventilation. Most patients develop pneumonia.

Testing, testing, testing

- Chest x-ray
- Swabs from the person's nose and throat for culture to test for the presence of the virus
- Blood test for SARS infection

Interventions and why?

- No antiviral treatment of proven value is available for SARS.
- O$_2$ delivery.
- May include mechanical ventilation.

SARS requires airborne, contact, and droplet isolation precautions. Isolation should be for the duration of the illness plus 10 days. An N95 (NIOSH-approved particulate filtering) or higher mask is required.

PRACTICE QUESTIONS

1. A nurse on a med-surg unit is caring for a patient who has been diagnosed with active tuberculosis and is placed in airborne isolation in a negative pressure room. The nurse knows that infections are spread through a process known as the *chain of infection*. Which best describes the chain of infection?

   A. Mode of transmission → Microorganism → Portal of entry → Host → Portal of exit

   B. Microorganism→ Mode of transmission → Portal of exit → Portal of entry → Host

   C. Microorganism → Portal of exit → Mode of transmission → Portal of entry → Host

   D. Portal of exit → Mode of transmission → Microorganism → Host portal of entry

2. A nurse on a med-surg unit is caring for a patient who is suspected of having a urinary tract infection. Which symptoms are indicative of a urinary tract infection? Select all that apply.

   A. Fever of 100.4°F

   B. Dysuria

   C. Hypotension

   D. Frequency

3. A patient is admitted to a hospital following an elective surgical procedure. Within 24 hours of admission, the patient develops a fever, cough, and chest pain. Which type of infection does the patient most likely have?

   A. Endemic infection

   B. Epidemic infection

   C. Community-acquired infection

   D. Hospital-acquired infection

4. A staff nurse is assigned to care for six patients during a 12-hour shift. Although the nurse is extremely busy, she knows that hand washing is a standard precaution used to prevent the spread of infection. When should the nurse's hands be washed? Select all that apply.

A. When visibly soiled

B. Before and after every patient contact

C. Before all dressing changes

D. After contact with objects near the patient

5. A nurse is caring for a patient with an intravenous line (IV). The nurse knows that IV lines are a major source of hospital-acquired infections because of their invasiveness. How often should the patient's IV line be changed?

A. Every 24 hours

B. Every 48 hours

C. Every 72 hours

D. Every 96 hours

6. A nurse is caring for a patient with a positive nasal swab for methicillin-resistant *staphylococcus aureus* (MRSA). Which precautions should the nurse take to prevent the spread of MRSA? Select all that apply.

A. Wear gloves and a gown when caring for the patient.

B. Wear a mask when caring for the patient.

C. Dedicate equipment, such as stethoscopes, to the patient.

D. Wash hands after removing contaminated personal protective equipment.

7. A nurse on a med-surg unit has been notified that a new patient is being admitted to the unit. The patient is a 24-year-old man with uncontrolled diabetes. Because only semiprivate rooms are available, which patient would be a suitable roommate for the new patient?

A. A 20-year-old woman with a broken femur

B. A 42-year-old man with MRSA

C. A 25-year-old man with pneumonia

D. A 50-year-old man who is HIV positive

8. A school nurse is reviewing the health records of enrolling kindergarteners. The nurse notices that several children have not received all of the immunizations necessary to attend school. The nurse knows that these children cannot attend school until they have been immunized against which vaccine preventable diseases? Select all that apply.

A. Tetanus

B. Tuberculosis

C. Diphtheria

D. Pertussis

9. A 19-year-old patient presents in a public health clinic complaining of fever, fatigue, nausea, and abdominal pain. While performing an initial assessment, a nurse notices a tattoo on the patient's leg. The patient reports that the tattoo is new and was done at home by a friend. The nurse is concerned that the patient may have an infection. Which infections should be suspected? Select all that apply.

A. Hepatitis A

B. Hepatitis B

C. Hepatitis C

D. HIV

10. A public health nurse is assessing a male patient who is complaining of painful urination, green discharge from the penis, and rectal itching. A psychosocial history reveals that the patient has had many sexual partners and seldom uses a condom. Based on this information, which sexually transmitted disease should the nurse suspect?

A. Syphilis

B. Gonorrhea

C. Trichomoniasis

D. Pediculosis

References

1. Centers for Disease Control and Prevention. *Sexually Transmitted Diseases.* Available at www.cdc.gov/std/.

2. Centers for Disease Control and Prevention. *Treatment Guidelines 2006. MMWR* 55(No. RR-11):1–94, 2006.

3. The Online Merck Manual of Diagnosis and Therapy. Available at www.merck.com/mmpe/index.html.

4. Camilleri M, Murray JA. Diarrhea and constipation. In: Fauci AS, Braunwald E, Kasper DL, et al., eds. *Harrison's Principles of Internal Medicine.* New York: McGraw-Hill; 2008.

5. Petersen LR, Marfin AA. West Nile Virus: A primer for the clinician [Review]. *Ann Int Med* 137:173–179, 2002.

6. Infectious Diseases Society of America/American Thoracic Society Consensus Guidelines on the Management of Community-Acquired Pneumonia in Adults. Mandell LA, et al. *IDSA/ATS Guidelines for CAP in Adults* 44(Suppl 2):S61, 2007.

7. Centers for Disease Control and Prevention. *Division of Vector-Borne Infectious Diseases.* Available at www.cdc.gov/ncidod/dvbid/westnile/index.htm. Accessed May 12, 2009.

8. Centers for Disease Control and Prevention. www.cdc.gov/ncidod/sars/.

9. http://www.cdc.gov/ncidod/dhqp/pdf/guidelines/Isolation2007.pdf.

10. http://phil.cdc.gov/phil.

14 Autoimmune and Rheumatic Disorders

OBJECTIVES

In this chapter you will review:

- The responsible pathogens, signs, symptoms, and treatment of common autoimmune and rheumatic disorders encountered in med-surg nursing today.

- You will also learn the associated signs, symptoms, and nursing care including patient teaching related to these disorders.

SYSTEMIC LUPUS ERYTHEMATOSUS (SLE)

What is it?

- Systemic lupus erythematosus (SLE) is a serious autoimmune disease. It can affect:
  - Connective tissue and joints
  - The cardiopulmonary system
  - The spleen
  - The neurologic system
  - The renal system
  - The pelvic organs
  - The hematologic system
  - The GI system
- Discoid lupus erythematosus (DLE) is a variant of SLE. It is also known as *chronic cutaneous lupus erythematosus*. It is characterized by a set of skin changes that can occur as part of lupus, with or without systemic involvement.
  - Skin rash (discoid rash) or lesions begin as skin rash plaques and progress to atrophic scars.
  - They cluster in light-exposed areas of the skin, such as the face, scalp, and ears.
  - Untreated, the lesions extend and develop central atrophy and scarring.
  - There may be widespread, scarring alopecia (hair loss).
  - Mucous membrane involvement may be prominent, especially in the mouth.

Causes and why?

- Normally our immune system produces proteins called *antibodies* that protect the body from foreign invaders.
- If the patient has an autoimmune disease, the immune system will make autoantibodies (*auto* means self and *anti* means against, as in *against self*) that destroy healthy tissue. These autoantibodies cause inflammation, pain, and damage in various parts of the body.
- About 70% to 90% of people who have lupus are young women in their late teens to thirties.
- Children (mostly girls) and adults can also be affected.
- Lupus may be mild or severe.

Signs and symptoms and why?

- Clinical findings vary greatly.
- SLE may develop abruptly with fever or insidiously over months or years with episodes of arthritis pain and malaise.

- SLE can manifest itself in almost all body systems. Joint and skin manifestations are the most common.

- Joint symptoms, ranging from intermittent arthralgias to acute polyarthritis, occur in about 90% of patients and may precede other manifestations by years.

- Skin symptoms include malar butterfly erythema (flat or raised rash) that generally appears on the face. This is known as a "butterfly rash" (Fig. 14-1).

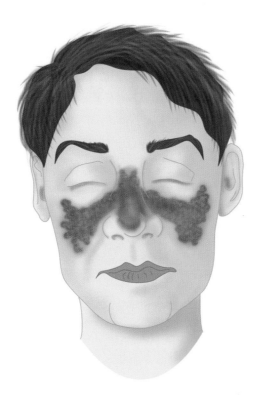

◀ Figure 14-1. Malar "butterfly" rash.

Malar erythema is redness over the cheeks of the face seen in SLE. Malar erythema is the formal name for a "butterfly rash."

Testing, testing, testing

The diagnosis of SLE is difficult and complicated. Establishing the diagnosis may require repeated evaluations over months or years.

As diagnostic criteria, at least four of the following are required to classify patients as having SLE according to the American College of Rheumatology:

- Malar rash

- Discoid rash (Fig. 14-2)

- Photosensitivity

- Oral ulcers

- Arthritis

- Serositis: Inflammation of the serous tissues of the body, the tissues lining the lungs (pleura), heart (pericardium), and the inner lining of the abdomen (peritoneum)

- Renal disorder
- Leucopenia
- Neurologic disorder
- Positive anti-DNA or anti-Smith antibody, or positive test for antibodies
- Antinuclear antibodies in high titers

▶ Figure 14-2. Discoid rash.

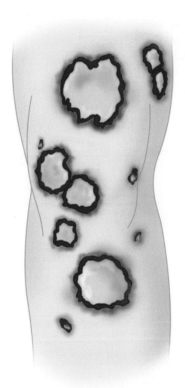

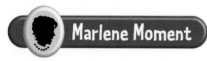
Hurst Hint

Photosensitivity is sometimes referred to as a sun allergy. It is an immune system reaction that is triggered by sunlight. Photosensitivity reactions may be characterized by an itchy rash eruption on patches of sun-exposed skin.

Marlene Moment

Photosensitivity doesn't mean crying while looking at old photos. Other tests to diagnoses SLE are blood and urine tests.

Signs and symptoms and why?

Side effects can be minimized by following the doctor's orders and keeping to the lowest dose possible. It is also important to avoid self-regulation of the dosage, either by adding more or stopping the medication without a schedule.

Corticosteroids must be gradually reduced so as to permit the adrenal glands to resume natural cortisol production. Eliminating doses too quickly can result in adrenal crisis (a life-threatening state caused by insufficient levels of cortisol).

Interventions and why?

To simplify therapy, SLE should be classified as mild (eg, fever, arthritis, pleurisy, pericarditis, headache, rash) or severe (eg, hemolytic anemia, thrombocytopenic purpura, massive pleural and pericardial involvement, significant renal damage, acute vasculitis of the extremities or GI tract, CNS involvement).

For mild SLE, little or no therapy may be needed. Symptoms are usually controlled with NSAIDs. For severe SLE, corticosteroids are the first-line therapy.

Medications used for treating SLE:

- Hydralazine (Apresoline)
- Procainamide (ProCair)
- Isoniazid (INH)

The diagnosis of SLE is very difficult and may take years. Treatments for SLE can be nothing or extremely complex combinations of drugs. The SLE course is usually chronic, relapsing, and unpredictable. Remissions may last for years. If the initial acute phase is controlled, even if very severe, the long-term prognosis is usually good.

RHEUMATOID ARTHRITIS

What is it?

Rheumatoid arthritis (RA) is an autoimmune inflammatory type of arthritis. Rheumatoid arthritis is the most common type of arthritis, which is triggered by the immune system (ie, autoimmune disease). The joints are primarily affected by rheumatoid arthritis, but organs may also be involved. The cause is unknown.

The incidence of RA is typically two to three times higher in women than men. Incidence studies from three populations show that incidence of RA in both women and men peaks in their sixties.

Signs and symptoms and why?

Pain, swelling, and redness in and around the joints are common manifestations. The inflammatory process primarily affects the lining of the joints (synovial membrane). The inflamed joint lining leads to erosions of the cartilage and bone and sometimes joint deformity, which is another visual symptom (Fig. 14-3).

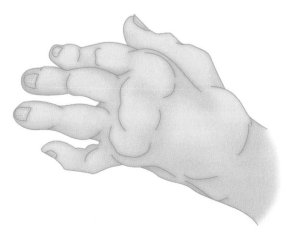

◀ Figure 14-3. Rheumatoid arthritis can lead to joint deformities.

Unlike the more common osteoarthritis (OA), RA is *not associated* with factors such as aging. It can affect any age.

Testing, testing, testing

- Physical exam of the joints
- Blood tests to detect:
  - Anemia, a deficiency of red blood cells.
  - Rheumatoid factor, an antibody often found in the blood of people with RA.
  - Elevated erythrocyte sedimentation rate (sed rate), an indicator of inflammatory process in the body and also an indicator of the severity of the disease.
  - C-reactive protein (CRP) is an additional test used to assess inflammation in the body. In some cases the sed rate will not be elevated, but the CRP will be or vice versa.
- X-rays are used to detect joint damage and see if the disease is progressing.

Table 14-1 shows the 1988 revised American College of Rheumatology criteria for classification of RA. *Four or more* of these criteria must be present to diagnose RA.

Table 14-1. 1988 revised American College of Rheumatology criteria for classification of RA

RA	Criteria
1	Morning stiffness >1 hour for >6 weeks
2	Swelling in three or more joints for >6 weeks
3	Swelling MCP or PIP in wrist >6 weeks
4	Symmetric joint swelling
5	Rheumatoid nodules
6	Serum rheumatoid factor
7	Hand X-ray changes—erosions or decalcification

The serum rheumatoid factor is a blood test to determine autoantibodies.

It is not uncommon for rheumatoid factor to be detected in healthy individuals. Approximately 1% to 2% of healthy people have detectable serum rheumatoid factor. And 10% to 20% of rheumatoid arthritis patients are NOT rheumatoid factor positive. Those rheumatoid arthritis patients who are rheumatoid factor positive are at greater risk for more aggressive disease.

MCP or PIP are anatomical joint sites in the hands and wrists. Swelling of the metacarpophalangeal (MCP) joints and proximal interphalangeal (PIP) joints are common in RA.

Some practitioners refer to the World Health Organization's International Classification of Functioning, Disability, and Heath (ICF) (Table 14-2). The ICF classification system focuses on human functioning and provides a unified, standard language and framework that captures how people with a health condition, like RA, function in their daily lives rather than focusing on their diagnosis or the presence or absence of disease.

Table 14-2. World Health Organization's International Classification of Functioning, Disability, and Heath (ICF)

Rheumatoid arthritis	Classification of function
Class I	No limitations
Class II	Adequate for normal activities despite joint discomfort of limitation of movement
Class III	Inadequate for most self-care and self-occupational activities
Class IV	Largely or wholly unable to manage self-care; restricted to bed or chair

People with RA have been reported to experience more losses in function than people without arthritis in every domain of human activity, including work, leisure, and social relations.

Interventions and why?

- There is no cure for RA, but new drugs are increasingly available to treat the disease.
- Exercise is known to reduce pain and disability.

Treatment of RA has traditionally followed the pyramid approach. That is, treatment starts with corticosteroids/nonsteroidal anti-inflammatory drugs, then progresses to disease-modifying antirheumatic drugs (DMARD) within three months of diagnosis.

FIBROMYALGIA

What is it?

Fibromyalgia is a syndrome predominantly characterized by widespread muscular pains and fatigue. The causes of fibromyalgia are unknown. Most people with fibromyalgia are women (female:male ratio, 7:1). However, men and children also can have the disorder.

Signs and symptoms and why?

- Fibromyalgia is characterized by widespread pain, abnormal pain processing, sleep disturbance, fatigue, and often psychological distress. People with fibromyalgia may also have other symptoms, such as:
  - Morning stiffness
  - Tingling or numbness in hands and feet

- Headaches, including migraines
- Irritable bowel syndrome
- Problems with thinking and memory (sometimes called "fibro fog")
- Painful menstrual periods and other pain syndromes

Testing, testing, testing

There are difficulties in diagnosing fibromyalgia, because its clinical picture can overlap other illnesses and there are no definitive diagnostic tests. Most people are diagnosed during middle age and prevalence increases with age.

The American College of Rheumatology criteria are used for clinical diagnosis classification. Diagnosis is based on the presence of two factors: widespread pain (at least three months' duration) and tenderness on 11 of 18 pressure points.

- Widespread pain
  - Pain is considered widespread when all of the following are present: pain in the left side of the body, pain in the right side of the body, pain above the waist, and pain below the waist. In addition, axial skeletal pain (cervical spine or anterior chest or thoracic spine or low back) must be present. In this definition, shoulder and buttock pain is considered as pain for each involved side. "Low back" pain is considered lower segment pain.
- Pain in tender point sites
  - Pain in 11 of 18 of the following tender point sites on digital palpation:
    - *Occiput:* Bilateral, at the suboccipital muscle insertions (where the neck muscles attach at the base of the skull)
    - *Low cervical:* Bilateral, at the anterior aspects of the intertransverse spaces at C5-C7 (front lower neck)
    - *Trapezius:* Bilateral, at the midpoint of the upper border (midway between the neck and shoulder)
    - *Supraspinatus:* Bilateral, at origins above the scapula spine near the medial border (muscle over the upper inner shoulder blade)
    - *Second rib:* Bilateral, at the second costochondral junctions, just lateral to the junctions on upper surfaces (edge of upper breast bone)
    - *Lateral epicondyle:* Bilateral, 2 cm distal to the epicondyles (2 cm below the side bone at the elbow)
    - *Gluteal:* Bilateral, in upper outer quadrants of buttocks in anterior fold of muscle (upper outer buttock)
    - *Greater trochanter:* Bilateral, posterior to the trochanteric prominence (hip bone)
    - *Knee:* Bilateral, at the medial fat pad proximal to the joint line (just above the knee on the inside)

Digital palpation should be performed with an approximate force of 4 kg (or about 10 lb). For a tender point to be considered "positive," the subject must state that the palpation was painful (Fig. 14-4).

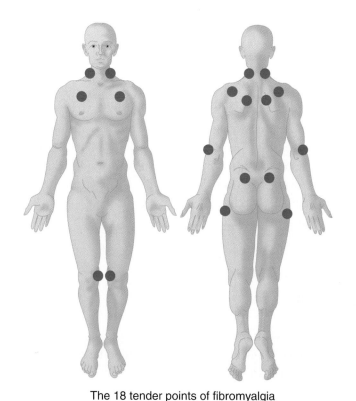

◀ Figure 14-4. Tender point sites of fibromyalgia.

The 18 tender points of fibromyalgia

For classification purposes, patients will be said to have fibromyalgia if both criteria are satisfied.

Fibromyalgia often occurs following a physical trauma, such as an acute illness or injury, which may act as a "trigger" in the development of the disorder.

Interventions and why?

- Because there is no known cure for FM, treatment focuses on relieving symptoms and improving function.

- A variety of prescription medications are often used to reduce pain levels and improve sleep. Lyrica is currently the most commonly used medication.

- Alternative therapies, such as massage, acupuncture, chiropractic, herbal supplements and yoga, can be effective tools in managing FM symptoms.

- Increasing rest, pacing activities, reducing stress, practicing relaxation, and improving nutrition can help minimize symptoms and improve quality of life.

Lyrica (pregabalin) was the first drug approved to treat fibromyalgia. Antiepileptic drugs, including Lyrica, increase the risk of suicidal thoughts or behavior.

PRACTICE QUESTIONS

1. The RN is planning care for the patient with mild systemic lupus erythematosus. Which of the following interventions is she likely to implement with this patient?

   A. Minimal or no interventions

   B. Corticosteroid therapy

   C. Isoniazid (INH) given on schedule

   D. Regimen of Apresoline

2. Systemic lupus erythematosus is a serious disease. Which of the following symptoms would typically be encountered when assessing the patient who has SLE?

   A. Involvement of many body systems

   B. One or two body systems affected

   C. Neurologic symptoms only

   D. Disorders of the skin only

3. The RN is reviewing the record for a patient with rheumatoid arthritis (RA). Which of the following blood tests is an indication of the severity of RA?

   A. Decreased RBC

   B. RA factor

   C. Increased sedimentation rate

   D. C-reactive protein

4. The nurse is teaching a patient about the diagnosis of rheumatoid arthritis (RA). Which of the following information should be included in the teaching plan?

   A. It is usually associated with aging.

   B. It is not usually associated with loss of function.

   C. It is more common in men.

   D. It causes erosions of cartilage and bone.

5. A 38-year-old patient has been diagnosed with fibromyalgia. Which of the following symptoms would be expected upon assessment of this patient?

   A. Pain in one or two sites

   B. Pain in many sites

   C. Constipation

   D. Joint stiffness lasting all day

6. A patient visits the wellness center to request information. She is concerned that she may have fibromyalgia. Which of the following information should be given to this patient?

　A. It usually has an onset in young adulthood.

　B. Is common in men.

　C. It follows some sort of "trigger."

　D. Its symptoms are unique.

7. The RN is performing an assessment of the skin on her assigned patient. Which of the following skin manifestations are characteristic of systemic lupus erythematosus?

　A. Rash on lower legs

　B. Butterfly rash on face

　C. Rash on upper back

　D. Itching intermittent rash

8. The RN is teaching a patient about corticosteroid therapy for the treatment of systemic lupus erythematosus. Which of the following information should be included in the teaching plan?

　A. The dose is typically increased rapidly.

　B. There is a universal prescribed regimen for corticosteroids.

　C. The dose will be reduced over time.

　D. The medications are usually discontinued without weaning.

9. A 40-year-old patient has been diagnosed with fibromyalgia. Which of the following interventions is appropriate for the patient?

　A. Eat a diet high in carbohydrates.

　B. Balance activity and rest.

　C. Take over-the-counter nonsteroidal anti-inflammatory medications for pain.

　D. Follow a daily intense exercise regimen.

10. The RN has been teaching the patient about the diagnosis of discoid lupus erythematosus (DLE). Which of the following patient comments indicates a lack of understanding?

　A. "I know that I can develop a rash on sun-exposed areas of the skin."

　B. "I know that scarring may occur."

　C. "The rash may look like plaques on my skin."

　D. "I am glad that I don't have to worry about hair loss."

References

1. Sacks JJ, Helmick CG, Langmaid G. Trends in deaths from systemic lupus erythematosus - United States, 1979-1998. *MMWR Weekly* 51(17), 371-374, 2002. Retrieved from http://www.cdc.gov/mmwr/preview/mmwrhtml/mm5117a3.htm.

2. LFA Response to CDC Report on "Trends In Deaths From Systemic Lupus Erythematosus, U.S., 1979-1998". Lupus Foundation of America, Inc. Retrieved from http://www.lupus.org/webmodules/webarticlesnet/templates/new_newsroomnews.aspx?articleid=1646&zoneid=59. Accessed on May 2, 2002.

3. http://www.cdc.gov/arthritis/index.htm.

4. World Health Organization. *International classification of functioning, disability and health: ICF.* Retrieved from http://books.google.com/books?id=pwb9ywSVKxwC&dq=World+Health+Organization's+International+Classification+of+Functioning,+Disability,+and+Health+(ICF).&printsec=frontcover&source=bn&hl=en&ei=6D4FS76TEoT_nAf5_THCw&sa=X&oi=book_result&ct=result&resnum=5&ved=0CBoQ6AEwBA#v=onepage&q=&f=false. Accessed in 2001.

5. Wolfe F, Smythe HA, et al. The American College of Rheumatology 1990 criteria for the classification of fibromyalgia. Report of the multicenter criteria committee. *Athritis Rheum 33*(2), 160-172, 1990

6. Branson BM, Handsfield HH, Lampe MA et al. Revised recommendations for HIV testing of adults, adolescents, and pregnant women in health-care settings. *MMWR Recomm Rep* 55(RR14), 1-17, 2006.

CHAPTER

15 Cellular Aberrations: Cancer

OBJECTIVES

In this chapter you will review:

- Risk factors for developing cancer.
- Carcinogens.
- The nurse's role in prevention.
- Patient care associated with radiation treatment.
- Patient care associated with chemotherapy treatment.
- Complications of treatment such as thrombocytopenia, neutropenia, and immuno-suppression; and related nursing care.
- Pain management and hospice.

Let's get the normal stuff straight first!

Carcinogenesis is accelerated cell division that results in malignancy (cancer). Cell division is also known as "mitosis." Normal cells reproduce according to an orderly set of events called the cell cycle during which all genetic material within the cell is duplicated and appropriately aligned to be received by the daughter cells.

The three kinds of special genes that stay on constant "red alert" to control healthy cell growth and replication are:

- Proto-oncogenes
- Tumor suppressor genes
- Apoptosis genes (the death genes) that program cellular death for the "duds."

What is it?

Cancer is a disease process that originates when the DNA of one abnormal cell undergoes genetic mutation, reproduces a clone cell, and rapidly proliferates without regard to the normal cellular growth–regulating signals. There is no part of the human body that is immune to cancer. Any cell in any tissue can develop malignant tumors (abnormal masses of cells). Once a malignancy develops, it can spread by metastasis to other parts of the body.

✚ The immune system and abnormal cells

A healthy immune system is able to "seek and destroy cancer cells".
T cells work as a team.

- T-cells are types of white blood cells that participate in the immune response.
- T-4 cells recognize foreign invaders and secrete cytokines. They alert the T-cells to start the cellular inflammatory response and B-cells to start producing antibodies.
- T-helper cells also secrete cytokines and activate other T-cells to "spread the word" producing a unified action against the foreign invader (also called the *humoral immune response.*)
- T-suppressor cells release lymphokines after the immune response has accomplished the goal.
- T-8 cells close down the immune response after the invading organism is destroyed.

✚ Environmental influences

Healthy behaviors reduce the risk for cancer by:

- Reducing exposure to carcinogens
- Increasing cellular health through healthy food choices

✛ Prevention

Primary and secondary prevention can stop cancer before it starts or catch it very early.

Primary prevention is the initial means for halting preventable cancer due to exposure to carcinogens.

Primary prevention behaviors (**lifestyle**) keep the person from developing cancer, which involves abstaining from or reducing exposure to known carcinogens such as tobacco or unprotected exposure to harmful sun rays and practicing a health-conscious lifestyle. Here are some examples of primary prevention.

* Eating healthy (small portions of red meat with generous servings of fruits, vegetables, and whole grains) can boost the immune system.
* Cruciferous vegetables (broccoli, cauliflower, and cabbage) contain high fiber and disease-fighting phytochemicals and are known to be associated with decreased incidence of prostate cancer.
* Nurses collaborate with organizations (American Heart & Lung Society, American Cancer Society, etc) to disseminate health information to the public, and to offer smoking cessation programs.
* Nurses are instrumental in talking with community groups and working with organizers to bring portable screening units to the workplace and to places in the community, accessible to the population.
* Risk reduction involves a commitment to dietary modifications, lifestyle changes, and preventive screenings with an annual health evaluation by a physician or nurse practitioner.
* Vitamin A foods (anything with color: squash, red bell pepper, carrots) and vitamin C can reduce the risk of cancer.
* High fiber diet increases gastric motility to move carcinogens through the intestine, reducing mucosal contact with carcinogens.

Screenings tests and other **secondary prevention** methods are indicated for early diagnosis and higher cure rate.

The goal of secondary prevention is **early detection** of cancer so the cancer can be removed in entirety or contained, thereby avoiding metastasis to other tissues. An example of secondary prevention is a routine yearly pap smear or colonoscopy **screenings**).

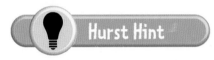

The phytochemicals in cruciferous vegetables inhibit cancerous tumor growth in the breast, endometrium, lung, colon, liver, and cervix.

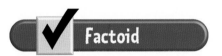

The American Dietetic Association refers to studies that link cruciferous veggies with protection against cancer!

✛ Examples of common screenings

* Monthly breast self exams (BSE) for females AND males (Fig. 15-1).
* Testicular exams for males.
* Males should begin BSE beginning at puberty.
* Females should begin BSE at menarche (onset of period).

- It is common to find "lumps" and "bumps" and a little breast enlargement *before* the onset of menses.
- The best time for BSE for females is *after* monthly menses to reduce discomfort. Many women experience sore breasts prior to and during their menstrual cycle. Some sources say to do the BSE between days 7 and 12 of the menstrual cycle. The most important thing is to make sure it is done consistently every month.

BSE

BSE is performed by palpating with an up and down motion over the entire breast while lying down. This helps the breast tissue spread evenly and as thin as possible over the chest wall.

- Postmenopausal females and males should perform the BSE on the same day of every month to promote consistency.
- Women greater than 40 years of age should have a yearly clinical breast exam (by a doctor or nurse practitioner) in addition to the BSE.
- It is recommended that women between the ages of 20 and 39 have a clinical breast (by a health care professional) exam every three years.

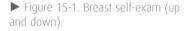

▶ Figure 15-1. Breast self-exam (up and down).

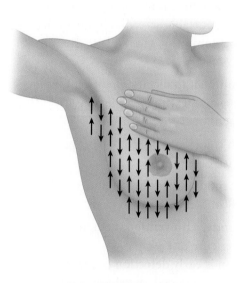

Breast Self-Examination
Examine up to the collarbone,
out to armpit, in to middle of chest,
and down to bottom of rib cage

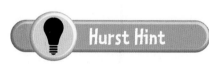

Hurst Hint

Don't forget the Tail of Spence when performing a breast exam! This is where 80% of breast cancers lurk.

- A baseline mammogram is recommended at age 35 to 40, and yearly after age 40 with two views of each breast.
- Prior to her mammogram appointment, the patient should be instructed not to use powder, deodorant, or lotion on the chest or axillary area because it could show up as a calcium deposit on the imaging study. If these products have been used, provide a warm cloth for removing them.

- A blood test called CA-125 (a protein biomarker), is a secondary prevention or screening. This test does not independently predict ovarian cancer. However, the CA-125 when utilized in conjunction with transvaginal ultrasound *can* detect ovarian cancer, the disadvantage to this particular secondary prevention option is that there are many false positives results that may result in unnecessary surgery.

  - In one clinical trial 570 women with abnormal results underwent a follow-up surgical procedure and 541 did NOT have cancer.

  - To date clinical trials have found no decrease in mortality rates from either the CA-125 or the transvaginal ultrasound as routine screening exams.

  - As a result the current recommendation *discourages* widespread use of these tests in the general population; however, data is still being collected from clinical trials.

- Women with a family history of breast cancer may elect to include genetic counseling and testing for the BRCA-1 and BRCA-2 genes. These mutated genes indicate an increased susceptibility to breast cancer.

- A yearly speculum *pelvic exam* (not pap smear) to visualize the cervix and a bimanual exam to palpate ovaries are recommended.

- A *pap smear* is only needed every two to three years, but since the *pelvic exam* is being performed yearly the specimen for pap-smear is usually collected at that time. Remember....yearly pelvic exam; pap smear every two to three.

- A colonoscopy is recommended for everyone (males and females) at age 50 and every 10 years after that if negative. For abnormal colonoscopy, follow-up is recommended more frequently.

- Males should perform a monthly self-testicular exam. Monthly is important because testicular cancers grow very fast.

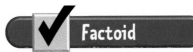

Ovarian cancer is deadly because initial symptoms are so insidious and vague. Many ovarian cancers are often in an advanced stage by the time they are diagnosed.

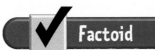

Testicular cancer affects young males (as young as 15 years old), so routine monthly testicular exams should start early!

Causes and why?

Healthy cells are transformed into cancerous cells (*initiation*) when a carcinogen (cancer causing substance) causes a mutation in the DNA. Some carcinogens are more prone to initiation than others; however, exposure to carcinogens is enhanced when other agents "team-up" to cause double trouble:

- Alcohol plus tobacco are co-carcinogenic, which means that in the presence of each other cancer can develop more rapidly.

- Tobacco is the number one cause of preventable cancer.

✚ Food choices

- Food choices are thought to be implicated in the development of cancer.

- Low fiber diet makes intestinal motility sluggish so carcinogens are retained in the intestinal mucosa for a longer period of time.

- Increased consumption of red meat and animal fat increases the risk of colon cancer (due to the iron and fat).
- Charbroiling meats using high heat creates higher levels of cancer-causing substances.
- Regular, frequent consumption of processed meats containing nitrites, nitrates, salt, and smoke residue increases colon and rectal contact with carcinogens.
- Prepared and packaged foods containing preservatives and additives also increase irritants in the colon.

✚ Aging

- The most important risk factor for developing cancer is aging. The older the individual, the greater the risk for cancer.
- Aging increases risk for cancer because the immune system ages too, becoming less able to destroy cancer cells.
- The immune system ages with the individual, becoming less responsive to abnormal cells that require removal.
- All immunosuppressed individuals are at higher risk because of a poor immune response.

✚ Chronic irritation

- Chronic irritation is known to increase cellular susceptibility to mutations.
- Smoking is an irritant to lung tissue.
- Chronic gastric reflux is an irritant to the esophagus.
- A mole that is constantly being rubbed by clothing or a belt causes irritation.
- Alcohol is an irritant to the upper GI tract especially the esophagus and stomach.
- Chronic inflammation causes irritation: Pelvic inflammatory disease leads to cancer of the uterus; ulcerative colitis leads to cancer of the colon.

✚ Environmental factors

- Exposure to X-rays (ionizing radiation)
- Exposure to chemical carcinogens (benzene, arsenic, methyl tertiary-butyl ether [MTBE], tetrachlorethylene, formaldehyde, lead, asbestos)
- Exposure to pollution (soot, tar and oils, diesel exhaust, cigarette smoke)

✚ Hereditary

- A genetic flaw in a cell can make it more susceptible to carcinogens.
- The two breast cancer genes (BRCA-1 and BRCA-2) also cause ovarian cancer.

✔ **Factoid**

Breast cancer occurs more frequently in women whose mother, grandmother, aunts, or sisters have had breast cancer.

- Some families have higher risk of developing certain cancers due to a single gene or due to several genes interacting together.
- Many cancers are related to a combination of multiple gene mutations plus environmental factors (multifactorial inheritance).

✚ Viral infections

- The human papillomavirus (HPV) causes cancer of the cervix (and venereal warts too).
- The hepatitis B virus (HBV) causes cancer of the liver.
- The Epstein-Barr virus causes Burkitt's lymphoma in Africa and nasal and pharyngeal cancers in China.

Testing, testing, testing

The blood tests, immunoassays for viruses, cytologic tests, tumor markers, and various imaging studies (US, CT, MRI) are listed with each of the specific types of cancers cited later in this chapter.

Signs and symptoms and why?

- The patient who has cancer may have a prolonged latent period in which no specific symptoms are apparent.
- Patient may be unaware of growing and spreading cancer. Once in the lymphatic system, it rapidly spreads (metastasizes).
- The American Cancer Society has identified seven warning signs of cancer which are often undetected.
  - **C**hange in bowel or bladder habits
  - **A** sore that does not heal
  - **U**nusual bleeding or discharge from any place
  - **T**hickening or lump in the breast or other parts of the body
  - **I**ndigestion (chronic) or difficulty in swallowing
  - **O**bvious changes in a wart or mole
  - **N**agging cough or hoarseness that is persistent

✚ External radiation

- When caring for a patient with cancer, many symptoms are related to adverse effects of the treatment. Symptoms of external radiation are generally limited to the exposure area.
- When one little area receives external radiation day after day in the same spot, that area can become really dry and may start to break down, causing local symptoms:
  - Erythema (local redness).
  - Shedding of the skin.
  - Altered taste, hair loss (alopecia), mouth sores (stomatitis) if radiation is directed toward the head as in treatment of a brain tumor.

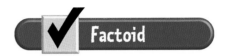

Factoid

The etiology is unclear, but African Americans have a higher incidence of cancer than do Caucasians.

- The side effects of external radiation (teletherapy or beam radiation) will always be confined to the area that is being irradiated.
  - Dry mouth occurs when salivary glands are within the site of radiation.
  - Alopecia (hair loss) occurs when the scalp is exposed to radiation.
- Systemic symptoms that can occur with external radiation therapy are:
  - Generalized fatigue is related to anemia (due to pancytopenia).
  - Pancytopenia (PAN-means everything), so all of the blood cells are decreases: RBCs, WBCs, platelets, everything!

What can harm my patient and why?

- One in four Americans will die as a result of cancer, making it the second leading cause of death.
- Harm to the patient can result from either:
  - The cancer itself
  - Adverse effects of treatment:
    - Radiation
    - Chemotherapy
    - Chemoradiotherapy (CRT)
    - Surgery
- Immunosuppression from treatment creates a high risk for infection.
- Pancytopenia causes:
  - Anemia due to decreased RBCs
  - Risk for infection due to decreased WBCs
  - Risk for bleeding due to decreased platelets
- Alterations in elimination (and change in body image) may result from surgically created fecal and urinary diversions (ostomies).
- Socioeconomic harm can occur due to staggering medical expenses coupled with loss of income and possible inability to obtain insurance or cancellation of existing policies.

Interventions and why?

The stage and grade of tumors (see Table 15-1 Staging and grading of tumors) are used when planning treatment options and estimating prognosis for of a wide variety of cancers.

- The stage of the tumor represents the size and extent of spread to nearby and distant tissues of the body.
- Staging becomes more complex with some cancers, especially in stages II and III where letters (A-B-C) are assigned to the stage (eg, IIA or IIIB) to more definitively describe the stage.
- Many different classifications are in place but the **TNM** system is most commonly used to describe:

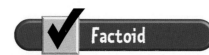

Factoid

Chemoradiotherapy is a combination of both chemotherapy and radiation used to improve local regional control and overall survival.

- **T** - extent of primary **tumor**
- **N** - absence or presence/extent of lymph **node** involvement
- **M** - absence or presence of distant **metastasis**

✛ Grading

- A process that may include various levels to describe the tumor or neoplasm.
- How abnormal the cells appear microscopically.
- How closely they resemble cells of the same tissue type (Refer to Table 15-1 for general descriptions of staging and grading.)
- Grading is different for different types of cancers.

Table 15-1 Staging and grading of tumors

Stage of the tumor	Grading of the tumor
Stage 0 • Precancerous (not considered true cancers by most oncologists). • Malignant cells are contained within ducts, lobules (in situ) only in the layer of cells where it began (no spread within the tissue, nodes or distant sites).	Grade X • Grade cannot be assessed. • Grade is undetermined.
Stage I Early cancer: present at the site of origin only (least extensive within tissue of origin).	Grade I • Resembles normal cells (well differentiated). • Grows and multiplies slowly. • Generally considered least aggressive.
Stage II (Localized) Cancer is limited to the organ in which it began with increased size and extensive growth without evidence of spread.	Grade II • Intermediate grade, growing and multiplying faster than normal. • Moderately differentiated (do not look like normal cells).
Stage III (Regional) Cancer has spread beyond the original (primary) site to nearby lymph nodes or organs and tissues.	Grade III • High grade (growing and spreading more rapidly than lower grade tumors). • Poorly differentiated (cells do not have mature structure or function).
Stage IV Cancer has spread from the primary site to distant organs or distant lymph nodes.	Grade IV • Undifferentiated or anaplastic (rapidly dividing with no resemblance to normal cell structure or function. • Generally more aggressive and less responsive to treatment.

Source: Created by the author from References 13, 14 and 24. National Cancer Institute web site: http://www.cancer.gov

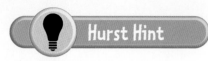

Hurst Hint

Poor skin prep prior to venipuncture leads to sepsis. According to research, scrubbing the area prior to venipuncture (back and forth rather than with a circular motion) with 2% chlorhexidine gluconate (FDA approved since 2000) and allowing to dry for 15 to 30 seconds decreases the bacterial count.

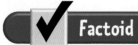

Factoid

PICC (peripherally inserted central catheters) at the antecubital area have a lower risk for infection than subclavian or jugular insertion sites. Subclavian and jugulars are in close proximity to the nose and mouth both having high bacterial counts.

✚ Infection prevention

General

The priority concerns for cancer patients with bone metastasis or those undergoing radiation or chemotherapy are risk for bleeding and risk for infection!

- Monitor WBC count and differential daily and report trends.
- Monitor and assist the easily fatigued patient to ensure meticulous personal hygiene.
- Instruct all personnel and visitors in careful hand hygiene before and after entering the patient's room.
- Screen visitors for those having recent or current infection or recent vaccination.
- Bottled purified water or fresh water in a single use disposable cup cannot sit at the bedside greater than 10 minutes once opened or having been poured.
- Monitor IV sites each shift for erythema, local heat, pain, or drainage.
- Re-site venipuncture sites at 48 to 72 hour intervals after thorough skin preparation.
- Change dressing to ventral venous catheter, PICC lines every 48 hours using strict aseptic technique.
- Change IV solutions and lines every 48 hours.
- Collaborate with physician for removal of indwelling catheters as soon as possible.

    When the WBC count is critically low (<1000 mm³):

- Collaborate with dietician to remove fresh fruit, fresh vegetables and salads, or coleslaw from the meal tray.
- Instruct all persons entering the room to thoroughly wash hands, wear mask, hair cover, and gown.
- Cut flowers in water and potted plants (soil) are not allowed in the patient room.
- Administer prescribed granulocyte colony-stimulating factor (G-CSF), granulocyte–macrophage colony-stimulating factor (GM-CSF), and/or prophylactic antibiotics.

    When the patient has thrombocytopenia (decreased platelets):

- Monitor lab results: platelet count, hemoglobin, and hematocrit.
- Plan care to minimize the number of venipunctures, such as drawing blood for labs while initiating IV therapy.
- Withhold any medication that may interfere with blood clotting.
- Monitor for bleeding: petechiae, bruising, free bleeding following venipuncture, bleeding from any orifice, or frank or occult blood in urine or stool.
- Observe bleeding precautions with use of electric razor, oral care with a soft toothbrush, and careful use (or avoidance) of dental floss.

- Encourage quiet, nonphysical activities (because of risk for injury).
- Hold pressure for five minutes after venipunctures and following removal of intravenous catheters.
- Avoid invasive procedures: rectal temperatures, suppositories, bladder catheterizations, enemas, IM injections.
- No IM injections if the platelet count is less than 100,000. This increases risk for bleeding.
- Administer blood and blood products (platelets) as ordered.

  When platelet count is critically low (<20,000 mm³) initiate rigorous safety measures:
- Bedrest with padded side rails helps to avoid trauma.
- Supervise activity when out of bed.
- Caution against straining or nose blowing.
- Administer prescribed platelet transfusions.
- In the presence of leukopenia (decreased WBC count) and/or immunosuppression, an infection can become deadly!
- Be alert to early signs of infection: cough, sputum changes, pain, local heat, exudates, discharge from any orifice, urinary frequency and burning, or malaise.

  After the initial diagnosis, the patient with cancer needs:
- A supportive, caring nurse who is optimistic and encouraging, to encourage the patient to view the diagnosis as any other chronic disease with exacerbations and remissions
- An unbiased sounding board to encourage expressions of feelings: anger, despair, sadness, and a wide range of other emotions
- A translator (ideally a well informed nurse) to communicate aspects of health care, such as treatment options and possible outcomes

+ Radiation therapy

- Interrupts the growth of malignant cells through use of ionizing radiation.
- Knowing the difference between internal and external is essential in order to create a safe, effective plan of care.
- When caring for a patient receiving internal or external radiation, the nurse exercises the appropriate precautions. (Refer to Table 15-2, Radiation therapy).
- **Brachytherapy (internal radiation)**—requires private room with restricted visitors
  - Sealed
  - Unsealed
- **Teletherapy (external beam radiation)**

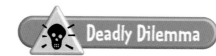

Deadly Dilemma

Even low grade fever in the immunosuppressed patient can be a cause for alarm! Immunocompromised patients generally do not demonstrate the normal response to infection.

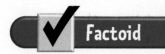

Factoid

Some radioactive implants emit radiation into the general environment and some do not.

Hurst Hint

For NCLEX if you can't remember which type emits radiation, in choosing your answer, assume they all do.

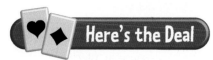

Here's the Deal

A nurse should never care for more than ONE internal radiation patient in any given shift.

Table 15-2   Radiation therapy

Radiation modality	Radioactivity
Internal radiation (brachytherapy): Sealed (solid) • Administered intercavitary or interstitial • May be temporary or permanent	• Solid radioactive material requires a delivery device such as wires, seeds, rods, needles, catheter or applicator into a cavity, or implanted into the tumor or nearby tissue. • Radioactivity is emitted from the body until removed (temporary) or until decay of radioactivity (permanent), leaving inert seeds that remain in the tumor. • Body fluids are not radioactive.
Internal radiation (brachytherapy): Unsealed • Administered orally or IV (example: radioactive iodine [I^{131}] for treatment of thyroid cancer) • May be injected into a body cavity	• Unsealed radiation causes the patient to emit radiation from their body and from body fluid. Body tissue acts like a shield but excreted body fluids are radioactive. • Patients are generally radioactive for 24 to 48 hours, after which radioactive precautions are discontinued. • The unsealed radioactive isotope is usually excreted from the body within 48 hours.
External radiation (Teletherapy) • Also called beam radiation	• A carefully focused beam of high energy rays is delivered by a machine outside of the body. • The higher the energy of the beam, the deeper the penetration. • Teletherapy can destroy nearby healthy tissue.

Source: Created by the author from Reference 9.

✛ Internal radiation

- Nurses caring for patients having internal radiation must wear a dosimeter badge that records the amount of radiation emitted in the environment, to monitor the exact amount of total radiation exposure that nurse receives.

- All patients having internal radiation will require a private room with restricted visitors.

- Restrict visitors less than 16 years of age and pregnant women.

- Known pregnant nurses (and nurses who could possibly be pregnant) are not allowed near the radiation source.

Marlene Moment

You cannot let somebody else wear your radiation badge because they left theirs at home!

- A radiation precaution sign is posted outside (usually on the door) with instructions to report to the nurse to verify instructions before visiting.
- The patient must avoid babies, small children, and pregnant women for 24 to 48 hours depending on the half life of the radioactive isotope.
- The patient should refrain from kissing anyone for 24 to 48 hours, because body fluids are radioactive.

✚ External radiation

- Use energy conservation techniques such as assisting with hygienic needs, bathing, and dressing.
- Exercise caution not to disturb the markings designating the area to be irradiated. Avoid using soaps, lotions, or other products to the area unless prescribed by the physician.
- Protect the fragile, inflamed skin at the site of irradiation during the time of treatment and for one year following external radiation. (See patient teaching about avoiding exposure of this skin to sun rays.)
- Monitor the irradiated skin area for changes in appearance and sensation.
- For systemic symptoms of weakness and fatigue enlist help for hygienic needs and activities of daily living.
- Arrange for home health nurse aide and housekeeping services during outpatient radiation therapy.
- Avoid sun exposure to the site of external radiation for 1 year following teletherapy.
- Avoid cologne, perfume, powder, lotions, or ointments at the site of external radiation.
- Protect fragile skin from coarse or rough clothing, straps or tight elastic on undergarments, extremes of temperature (hot or cold), soap, or any drying astringents.
- Treat thin, dry, erythematosus skin very gently (no rubbing or scratching) because of the danger of skin breakdown at the site.
- Check your mouth every day when radiation is applied to the head and neck.

✚ Radiation and exposure control

- Protecting oneself and others is a priority for planning care for a patient when radiation therapy is prescribed.
- Rotate nursing assignments daily so that one nurse is not overly exposed to radiation.
- Radiation exposure must be controlled to prevent health care professionals and visitors. Three methods used include:

  Time
  - Staff members wear badges.
  - The nurse must plan ahead to deliver organized and effective care at the bedside in a timely manner.

- Visitors are limited to 30 minutes per day of radiation exposure.

Distance

- Caution visitors to stay at least 6 ft away from source of radiation at all times.

Shielding

- Use a lead apron or portable shields between the patient and the staff member OR the patient and the visitor.

Chemotherapy

- Cancer chemotherapy (see Table 15-3) may be prescribed as a single drug or multiple drugs (combination chemotherapy) to attack the cancer cell in different phases of the cell cycle.
- Prescribed drugs are classified according to the specific phase of the cell cycle for which the agent is effective.
- Administer prescribed chemotherapy observing appropriate nursing precautions. (See Table 15-3, Chemotherapy classification, action, and precautions.)
- Chemotherapy is given in repeated doses over a prolonged period of time (usually scheduled every three to four weeks as outpatient therapy) to accomplish regression of the tumor.
- All of the cancer cells will not be killed by the chemotherapeutic agent, but enough of them are destroyed to enable the body's own healthy immune system to seek and destroy any remaining cancer cells.

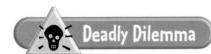

Always check WBC before administering any antineoplastic drug! Hold the drug if the white count is not at least 3000 mm³.

Table 15-3 Chemotherapy classification, action, and precautions

Site and/or general mechanism of action	Chemotherapy classification and commonly used drugs	Nursing precautions for adverse effects
Works on the S phase of cell cycle where nucleic acid is synthesized and chromosomes are replicated in readiness for cell mitosis. • Interferes with synthesis of DNA • Destroys cells that are actively reproducing by altering DNA structure or breaking molecular strands or the DNA molecule	Alkylating agents: • Bendamustine (Treanda) • Busulfan (Busulfex) • Carboplatin (Paraplatin) • Cisplatin (Platinol) • Cyclophosphamide (Lyophilized Cytoxan) • Dacarbazine (DTIC-Dome) • Ifosfamide (Ifex) • Melphalan (Alkeran) • Nitrogen mustard (Mustargen) • Oxaliplatin (Eloxatin) • Thiotepa (TESPA)	Clinical alert: • Follow facility policies for preparing and administering these IV agents • Absorbs through skin to be mutagenic, teratogenic, and carcinogenic General adverse effects: • Myelosuppression • Anaphylaxis • Hyperuricemia Patient safety precautions include: • Have epinephrine, glucocorticoids, and antihistamines on hand in the event of a hypersensitive reaction. • Administer prescribed antiemetic to reduce nausea. • Avoid all IM injections when platelets are less than 50,000/mm³.

(Continued)

Table 15-3 Chemotherapy classification, action, and precautions (*Continued*)

Site and/or general mechanism of action	Chemotherapy classification and commonly used drugs	Nursing precautions for adverse effects
Works on the S phase of cell cycle to interfere with synthesis of DNA and destroy cells that are actively reproducing, BCNU is not cell cycle specific; action is same as other alkylating agents but nitrosoureas cross the blood-brain barrier (necessary for treating brain cancers). Streptozocin is most active in the resting phase of the cell cycle.	Alkylating agents of the nitrosourea pharmacologic classification: • Carmustine (BCNU) • Lomustine (CCNU, CeeNU • Streptozocin (Zanosar)	Clinical alert: • Same as other alkylating agents, • Wear gloves when handling ANY form of BCNU. • Streptozocin is a vesicant: apply ice if it extravasates. General adverse effects: • Myelosuppression (delayed with BCNU, • Nephrotoxic • Hepatotoxic • Hyperuricemia Patient safety precautions: • Monitor uric acid level; can cause uric acid nephropathy. • Administer allopurinol and adequate hydration. • Administer transfusions as ordered for cumulative anemia.
Active late in the G$_2$ phase and in the M phase of cell cycle to prevent cell division and replication and to halt formation of the mitotic spindle. • Taxoids alter the microtubules to halt mitosis causing cell death.	Antimitotic drugs of the taxoid pharmacologic classification: • Docetaxel (Taxotere) • Paclitaxel (Taxol) • Paclitaxel protein-bound particles	Clinical alert: • Always wear gloves and follow agency policy when preparing and administering taxoids. • Label all waste CHEMOTHERAPY HAZARD.
• Vinca alkaloids (vinblastine, vincristine) work in metaphase to arrest mitosis and block cell division; disrupt assembly of microtubules to block spindle formation and prevent mitosis (vinorelbine).	Antimitotic drugs (vinca or plant alkaloids): • Vinblastine sulfate (VLB) • Vincristine sulfate (VCR) • Vindesine • Vinorelbine tartrate (Navelbine)	• For vesicants check the line prior to drug administration: free-flowing IVF with no puffiness or discomfort. • Have emergency equipment available in the event of cardiac arrest. • Immediately stop the infusion for complaint of pain or any signs of infiltration or red streaking, and follow vesicant protocols: docetaxel, paclitaxel, vinblastine, vincristine, and vinorelbine. General adverse effects: • Neurotoxicity • Myelosuppression • Hypersensitivity and/or anaphylaxis

(*Continued*)

Table 15-3   Chemotherapy classification, action, and precautions (*Continued*)

Site and/or general mechanism of action	Chemotherapy classification and commonly used drugs	Nursing precautions for adverse effects
		Patient safety precautions: • Administer pretreatment corticosteroids and antihistamines as prescribed to reduce reaction. • Tell patients to immediately report tingling, burning, or numbness. • Monitor vital signs closely during administration: may cause bradycardia and hypotension, dropping cardiac output.
Hydroxyurea may work in S phase to inhibit DNA synthesis. DNA synthesis doesn't happen without folic acid and folate: methotrexate binds to dihydrofolate reductase to block reduction of folic acid to tetrahydrofolate, a cofactor needed for purine, protein, and DNA synthesis. Pemetrexed (pronounced as peh-meh-TREX-ed) disturbs cell replication by inhibiting several folate-dependent enzymes involved in nucleotide synthesis. With combined chemotherapy, it inhibits growth of mesothelioma cell lines.	Pharmacologic class of antimetabolite (hydroxyurea) indicated for melanoma, resistant chronic myelocytic leukemia, head and neck cancers, and ovarian cancer that is inoperable or metastatic. • Hydroxyurea (Droxia, Hydrea) Antimetabolites of the pharmacologic classification folic acid/folate antagonist (indicated for acute lymphocytic leukemia, meningeal leukemia, Burkitt lymphoma, lymphosarcoma, osteosarcoma and head/neck cancers): • Methotrexate (amethopterin, MTX) • Methotrexate sodium (Methotrexate LPF, Rheumatrex, Trexall) • Pemetrexed (Alimta)	Clinical alert: Gloves must be worn when handling hydroxyurea capsules or the container. If powder is spilled from capsule, wipe up with damp towel and dispose of towel in a sealed plastic bag. Parenteral preparations of MTX are mutagenic, teratogenic, and carcinogenic: follow protocols for safe handling. General adverse effects: • Leukopenia, thrombocytopenia, anemia • Bone marrow suppression • Hyperuricemia and renal failure • Hepatotoxic (MTX) • CNS effects: seizure, neuropathy; intrathecal MTX may cause arachnoiditis within hours, leukoencephalopathy Patient safety precautions: • Monitor BUN, uric acid, liver enzymes, and creatinine. • Monitor CBC every two weeks (hydroxyurea can dramatically drop WBC in 24–48 hours) • Keep patient well hydrated and monitor urinary output. • Administer blood transfusions as indicated for anemia. • Give vitamin B_{12}, folic acid and corticosteroids before and during treatment with pemetrexed to reduce adverse effects and skin reactions.

(*Continued*)

Table 15-3 Chemotherapy classification, action, and precautions (*Continued*)

Site and/or general mechanism of action	Chemotherapy classification and commonly used drugs	Nursing precautions for adverse effects
Purine analogs work in the S phase to inhibit DNA and RNA synthesis. Fludarabine action is unknown, but after converting to its active metabolite it interferes with synthesis by inhibiting DNA enzymes.	Antimetabolites of the pharmacologic classification purine analogue (mercaptopurine indicated for acute lymphoblastic leukemia; fludarabine indicated for B-cell chronic lymphocytic leukemia unresponsive to standard alkylating drug regimen) • Mercaptopurine, 6-mercaptopurine, 6-MP (Purinethol)	Purine analog Clinical alert: Follow protocols for handling toxic drugs that are mutagenic, teratogenic, and carcinogenic. A diagnosis of ALL must be established before starting therapy with 6-MP. General adverse actions: • Leukopenia, thrombocytopenia, anemia due to bone marrow suppression • Hepatoxicity, jaundice, pancreatitis (6-MP), liver failure (fludarabine) • Hyperuricemia and renal failure • Thrombosis, stroke, transient ischemic attacks (fludarabine) • Severe and fatal neurotoxicity • Infection • Tumor lysis syndrome Patient safety implications: • Monitor WBC, RBC, platelet count, liver enzymes, bilirubin and uric acid. • No IMs if platelets are less than 50,000/mm^3. • Encourage 3 L fluid daily. • Watch for jaundice, clay-colored stools, and dark urine.
Works in cell phase S to interfere with DNA synthesis and (5-FU) resultant thymine deficiency that brings about irregular growth and cellular death	Pharmacologic classification of pyrimidine analog: 5-FU used for colon, rectal, breast, stomach, and pancreatic cancers. Topical application for actinic keratoses and superficial basal cell cancer; cytarabine used for acute nonlymphocytic leukemia, acute lymphocytic leukemia, meningeal leukemia, and lymphomatous meningitis. • Fluorouracil, 5-fluorouracil, 5-FU; (Carac, Efudex, Fluoroplex) • Capecitabine (Xeloda) is converted to active 5-FU • Cytarabine, ara-C, cytosine arabinoside; (Cytosar-U, DepoCyt, Tarabine PFS)	Pyrimidine analog Clinical alert: Intrathecal cytarabine is given with dexamethasone to help decrease symptoms of arachnoiditis which can be life threatening and physician must be present to observe for immediate toxic reactions. Use protocols for preparing and administering parenteral 5-FU which is mutagenic, teratogenic, and carcinogenic. Toxicity may be delayed 1–3 weeks.

(Continued)

Table 15-3 Chemotherapy classification, action, and precautions (*Continued*)

Site and/or general mechanism of action	Chemotherapy classification and commonly used drugs	Nursing precautions for adverse effects
Capecitabine (this is a hard one to pronounce: kap-ah-SEAT-ah-been) interferes with DNA synthesis to stop cell division, and also interferes with RNA processing and protein synthesis. Cytarabine (another hard one to pronounce: sye-TARE-a-been) inhibits DNA synthesis only.		General adverse actions: • Neurotoxicity • Leukopenia, anemia, thrombocytopenia, megaloblastosis, agranulocytosis (5-FU) • Hepatoxicity, jaundice • Pulmonary edema • Anaphylaxis Patient safety precautions • Monitor for toxic effects (bone marrow suppression and hepatic dysfunction). • Monitor lab reports for CBC, liver enzymes, BUN, and creatinine. • Implement bleeding precautions. • Tell the patient to report blurred vision or eye pain and watch for nystagmus, which may be the first sign of neurotoxicity (ara-C). • Notify the physician for diarrhea and stomatitis (signs of toxicity to 5-FU).
Pyrimidine nucleoside analogs cause hypomethylation of DNA and are toxic to abnormal hematopoietic bone marrow cells.	Pharmacologic classification of pyrimidine nucleoside analog: indicated for chronic myelocytic leukemia (azacitidine) • Azacitidine (Vidaza) • Gemcitabine (Gemzar)	Pyrimidine nucleoside analogs Clinical alert: Check liver function tests and creatinine before beginning therapy. Toxic reactions are nausea and vomiting (Gemzar). General adverse reaction: • Neutropenia • Leukopenia and febrile leukopenia • Thrombocytopenia • Anemia • Respiratory problems: atelectasis, dyspnea, rhonchi, pneumonia, wheezing Patient safety precautions: • Monitor CBC before each cycle and between times. • Initiate bleeding precautions. • Auscultate chest frequently. • Monitor lab results: CBC, BUN, creatinine, and liver enzymes. • Advise birth control (men and women) during therapy.

(*Continued*)

Table 15-3 Chemotherapy classification, action, and precautions (*Continued*)

Site and/or general mechanism of action	Chemotherapy classification and commonly used drugs	Nursing precautions for adverse effects
Active in S phase to inhibit DNA, DNA dependent RNA, and/or RNA synthesis. Mitomycin is similar to an alkylating drug, cross-linking strands of DNA altering cell growth, leading to cell death.	Antibiotic antineoplastics: • Bleomycin sulfate (Blenoxane) • Daunorubicin citrate liposomal (DaunoXome) • Daunorubicin hydrochloride (Cerubidine) • Doxorubicin hydrochloride (Adriamycin) • Doxorubicin hydrochloride liposomal (Doxil) • Epirubicin hydrochloride (Ellence) • Idarubicin hydrochloride (Idamycin PFS) • Mitomycin, mitomycin-C (Mutamycin)	Clinical alert: • Wear protective clothing: goggles, gown, gloves. • For vesicants: Check the line first for patency and any leak; remain at the bedside during the entire infusion, being alert to signs of extravasation. General adverse effects: • Myelosuppression • Anaphylaxis Patient safety precautions: • Be prepared to treat hypersensitive reactions (see alkylating agents). • Stop the infusion at the first sign of pain, burning, irritation, or infiltration; notify prescriber and follow vesicant protocols: daunorubicin (apply ice), doxorubicin, (ice), and epirubicin.
Interferes with hormone receptors in all phases of the cell cycle. • Aromatase inhibitors (AIs): In postmenopausal women inhibits the enzyme necessary for synthesis of estrogen (or inhibits conversion of androgens to estrogens), thereby blocking (estrogen receptor) ER-positive tumors from receiving estrogen needed for growth. • Estrogen and nitrogen mustard: action unknown, but the estrogen promotes uptake into prostate tissue. • Progestins inhibit hormone dependent tumors by inhibiting the pituitary and adrenal steroidal production. • Estrogen antagonists bind the estrogen receptors protein in breast cancer cells so they can't take up estrogen. • Nonsteroidal estrogen receptors: tamoxifen action unknown, but is selective estrogen modulator; toremifene competes with estrogen for binding sites in the tumor to block tumor growth by blocking estrogen.	Antineoplastics that alter hormone balance: Pharmacologic class of aromatase inhibitors (AIs) • Anastrozole (Arimidex) • Exemestane (Aromasin) • Letrozole (Femara) Pharmacologic class of estrogen and nitrogen mustard: • Estramustine (Emcyt) Pharmacologic class of progestin: • Megestrol acetate (Megace) Pharmacologic class of estrogen antagonist: • Fulvestrant (Faslodex) Pharmacologic class of nonsteroidal anti-estrogen: • Tamoxifen • Toremifene (Fareston)	Agents that alter hormone balance Clinical alert: • Contraindicated in pregnant or breast feeding women. • Decreasing estrogen increases osteoporosis risk. • Be alert to hepatotoxicity (nonsteroidal antiestrogens). General adverse effects: • Thromboembolytic disease (MI, stroke, PE) • Fluid retention • Electrolyte imbalance • Hot flashes and emotional instability (estrogen antagonists) Patient safety precautions: • Instruct patient to immediately report chest pain, leg pain, severe headache, shortness of breath, difficulty speaking, or one sided weakness. • Monitor weight and assess for peripheral edema. • Assess for fluid retention and signs of heart failure: auscultate lungs bilaterally. • Caution patients to avoid alcohol and tobacco use that can have an added adverse effect on decreasing bone density.

Table 15-3 *Chemotherapy classification, action, and precautions (Continued)*

Site and/or general mechanism of action	Chemotherapy classification and commonly used drugs	Nursing precautions for adverse effects
• Gonadotropin releasing hormone analogues work on the pituitary to decrease FSH and LH to sex hormones (estrogen in women and testosterone in men).	Pharmacologic class of gonadotropin-releasing hormone analogue: Goserelin acetate (Zoladex) Leuprolide (Lupron)	
• Nonsteroidal antiandrogen inhibits androgen uptake and keeps androgens from binding in the cell nucleus of target tissues.	Pharmacologic class: nonsteroidal anti-androgen • Flutamide (Eulexin)	Nonsteroidal antiandrogen Clinical alert: • Liver function tests are required at onset of therapy. • Repeat liver function tests at first sign of hepatic dysfunction. General adverse effects: • Hepatotoxic; can cause hepatic encephalopathy and liver failure • Leukopenia • Thrombocytopenia Patient safety precautions: • Immediately report dark urine, jaundice, nausea, vomiting, anorexia, or fatigue.
Miscellaneous antineoplastics: Podophyllotoxin derivatives inhibit the enzyme (topoisomerase II). • Prevents cells from entering mitosis. • Causes inability to repair breaks in the DNA strands leading to cell death. • Acts in late S phase or early G_2.	Miscellaneous antineoplastics: Pharmacologic classification of podophyllotoxin or podophyllotoxin derivative: • Etoposide (VP-16-213) (VePesid) • Etoposide phosphate (Etopophos) • Teniposide (Vumon)	Miscellaneous antineoplastics: Podophyllotoxin derivatives Clinical alert: Follow policies for administration: drugs are mutagenic, teratogenic, and carcinogenic! General adverse effects: • Anaphylaxis • Neurotoxic • Hepatotoxic • Myelosuppression Patient safety precautions: • Vesicant! Stop the infusion immediately upon burning or streaking. • Premedicate for nausea. • Have emergency medicines and equipment available in event of anaphylaxis. • Avoid IM injections when platelets are less than 50,000/mm³.
Monoclonal antibodies have different modes of action: • Some bind selectively to HER2 to inhibit tumor cells that overexpress HER2 (Herceptin).	Pharmacologic classification of monoclonal antibodies: • Bevacizumab (Avastin) • Cetuximab (Erbitux) • Panitumumab (Vectibix)	Monoclonal antibodies Clinical alert: Trastuzumab (Herceptin) is only for metastatic breast cancer whose tumor is HER2 positive.

Table 15-3 Chemotherapy classification, action, and precautions (*Continued*)

Site and/or general mechanism of action	Chemotherapy classification and commonly used drugs	Nursing precautions for adverse effects
• Inhibits vascular endothelial growth factor (Avastin). • Epidermal growth factor receptor antagonist (Erbitux). • Stops proliferation of cells and new blood vessel growth by inhibiting action between proteins and cell surface receptors (Vectibix). • Binds to an antigen (CD20) to mediate lysis of B lymphocytes (Rituxan).	• Rituximab (Rituxan) • Trastuzumab (Herceptin)	General adverse effects: • Cardiotoxicity • Neurotoxicity • Nephrotoxicity • Anaphylaxis • Myelosuppression Patient safety precautions • Baseline and ongoing cardiac assessment. • Have epinephrine and emergency resuscitation equipment available.
Proteosome inhibitors cause cells to die by inhibiting 26S proteosomes that regulate intracellular levels of certain proteins.	Pharmacologic classification of proteosome inhibitors are used for multiple myeloma (previously untreated or progressing) and mantle cell lymphoma progressive after at least one therapy: • Bortezomib (Velcade)	Proteosome inhibitors Clinical alert: Before initiating any cycle, platelet count should be 70 X 10^9/L or higher. General adverse reactions: • Neurotoxicity • Thrombocytopenia • GI effects: nausea, vomiting and diarrhea Patient safety precautions: • Make sure patient has order for antiemetic and antidiarrheal agent. • Monitor CBC during treatment, especially on day 2. • Monitor for burning, hyper or hypoesthesia, paresthesias, neurologic pain.
Leukemic cell growth is decreased through inhibition of a tyrosine kinase enzyme, (Sprycel and Gleevec) allowing bone marrow to resume production of normal cells (RBCs, WBCs, and platelets). Multiple tyrosine kinases are inhibited (Sutent) to halt tumor growth, pathologic growth of blood vessels, and metastatic progression of advanced renal cell carcinoma and GI stromal tumors that are intolerant to Gleevec.	Pharmacologic classification of protein-tyrosine kinase inhibitors are used to treat various types of leukemia with resistance, intolerance, or tolerance to prior therapy. • Dasatinib (Sprycel) • Imatinib mesylate (Gleevec) • Sunitinib malate (Sutent)	Protein-tyrosine kinase inhibitors Clinical alert: GI perforation with fatal hemorrhage has occurred. General adverse reactions: • Hemorrhage (cerebral and GI) • Hepatotoxicity Patient safety precautions: • Monitor hepatic function: bilirubin, AST, ALT, alkaline phosphatase. • Monitor for fluid retention: weight, blood pressure, edema.

(Continued)

Table 15-3 Chemotherapy classification, action, and precautions *(Continued)*

Site and/or general mechanism of action	Chemotherapy classification and commonly used drugs	Nursing precautions for adverse effects
Pharmacologic class kinase and multi-kinase inhibitors: Bind intracellular protein to stop the cell cycle and reduce tumor size Inhibit ErbB-driven tumor growth (Tykerb) • Decrease cell growth and formation of new vessels into the tumor by interacting with multiple kinases (Nexavar)	Pharmacologic class: kinase inhibitors (Torisel) for advanced renal cell carcinoma and as second line therapy (Tykerb) for metastatic breast cancer (with capecitabine) after prior therapy with taxane, anthracycline, and trastuzumab; chronic myelogenous leukemia (Philadelphia chromosome-positive) resistant or intolerant to Gleevec (Tasigna) • Lapatinib (Tykerb) • Nilotinib (Tasigna) • Temsirolimus (Torisel) Multi-kinase inhibitor used for advanced renal cell cancer and hepatocellular cancer: • Sorafenib (Nexavar)	Kinase and multi-kinase inhibitors Clinical alert: Left ventricular ejection fraction must be evaluated prior to therapy, and electrolytes (potassium and magnesium) must be within normal limits. General adverse reactions: • Prolongs QT interval • Reduces left ventricular ejection fraction • Neutropenia • Thrombocytopenia • Hemorrhage Patient safety precautions: • Monitor for pulmonary symptoms dyspnea and cough. • Monitor lab reports for anemia, neutropenia.
Inhibit DNA synthesis in leukemic cells, causing cell death	Pharmacologic class: DNA demethylation agent; indicated for T-cell acute lymphoblastic leukemia unresponsive to other treatment or relapse after treatment • Nelarabine (Arranon)	DNA demethylation agent: Clinical alert: Wear gloves and protective clothing when preparing drug; avoid skin contact. General adverse reactions: • Demyelination peripheral neuropathies • Neurotoxicity, seizures • Febrile neutropenia • Neutropenia, leukopenia, thrombocytopenia Patient safety precautions: • Monitor baseline and regular CBC. • Monitor for neurotoxic symptoms: confusion, somnolence, neuropathy. • Tell patient to immediately report numbness in hands or feet, weakness getting out of a chair or climbing stairs, tripping when walking. • Force fluids to prevent hyperuricemia from tumor lysis.
Interact with the enzyme topoisomerase I to break single strand DNA and bind to the DNA to prevent it from repairing itself	Pharmacologic classification of DNA topoisomerase inhibitors are indicated for first line therapy colorectal cancer (with 5-FU and leucovorin) or metastatic cancer of the colon or rectum that has recurred or progressed after treatment with 5-FU. Second line drug for metastatic cancer of cervix, ovary, and small cell lung cancer sensitive disease:	Topoisomerase inhibitors Clinical alert: Before initiating therapy the patient must have baseline neutrophil count in excess of 1500/mm³ and platelets greater than 100,000 mm³. General adverse effects: • Severe myelosuppression • Severe diarrhea (early or late in treatment)

Table 15-3 Chemotherapy classification, action, and precautions (*Continued*)

Site and/or general mechanism of action	Chemotherapy classification and commonly used drugs	Nursing precautions for adverse effects
	• Irinotecan hydrochloride (Camptosar) • Topotecan (Hycamtin)	Patient safety precautions: • Vesicant! Stop the infusion immediately upon burning or streaking. Flush site with sterile water and apply ice! • Administer colony stimulating factor for significant neutropenia.
Epidermal growth factor receptor inhibitor has an elective action on epidermal growth factor receptor 1 expressed on the surface of normal and cancer cells.	Pharmacologic class: epidermal growth factor receptor inhibitor used as first line therapy for pancreatic cancer when surgery is not an option, and advanced small cell lung cancer after failure of at least one chemotherapy regimen. • Erlotinib (Tarceva)	Epidermal growth factor receptor inhibitor Clinical alert: Use cautiously in pulmonary disease or liver impairment. General adverse reaction: • Pulmonary toxicity • Increases INR and PT • Increases risk for infection Patient safety precautions: • Teach patient to report new or worsened cough, shortness of breath, and fever immediately.
Stops cell reproduction by inhibiting formation of microtubules.	Microtubule inhibitor used alone for locally advanced breast cancer with capecitabine after failure of other chemotherapy drugs (taxane, anthracycline, or capecitabine). • Ixabepilone (Ixempra)	Microtubule inhibitor Clinical alert: Handle drug with care: wear gloves and avoid inhalation of vapors. General adverse reactions: • Neurotoxic • Hepatotoxic • Febrile neutropenia, leukopenia, anemia, thrombocytopenia • Hypersensitivity reaction Patient safety precautions: • Premedicate with H_1 and H_2 antagonists and corticosteroids. • Monitor liver function studies. • Teach patient to report fever, chills, cough, or burning pain on urination. • Instruct patient to report numbness and tingling of hands or feet.
Accumulates in leukemic cells to inhibit DNA synthesis which causes cell death.	Pharmacologic classification DNA demethylation agent, a prodrug of cytotoxic deoxyguanosine used for T-cell acute lymphoblastic leukemia and T-cell lymphoblastic lymphoma after relapse or unresponsiveness to at least two previous chemotherapy regimens: • Nelarabine (Arranon)	DNA demethylation agent Clinical alert: Wear gloves and protective clothing to avoid skin contact.

(*Continued*)

Table 15-3 Chemotherapy classification, action, and precautions (*Continued*)

Site and/or general mechanism of action	Chemotherapy classification and commonly used drugs	Nursing precautions for adverse effects
		General adverse reactions:
		• Neurotoxic: demyelination peripheral neuropathies
		• Febrile neutropenia, leukopenia, neutropenia, thrombocytopenia, anemia
		• Metabolic imbalance: hypo/hyperglycemia, hypocalcemia, hypomagnesemia, hypokalemia
		Patient safety precautions:
		• Tell patient to immediately report numbness or tingling in hands or feet and problems with gait and fine motor skills.
		• Monitor electrolytes and blood glucose.
		• Monitor WBC, platelet count, neutrophil count, RBC, hemoglobin, and hematocrit.
Enzyme destroys asparagines which is essential for protein synthesis in acute lymphocytic leukemia.	Pharmacologic class: *Escherichia coli*-derived enzyme • Asparaginase (Elspar)	E. coli derived enzyme: Clinical alert: Anaphylaxis may occur; skin test before 1st dose and repeat doses if greater than one week has lapsed. Negative skin test can still react; give tiny increments every ten minutes. till total dose is given. General adverse reactions: • Hemorrhagic pancreatitis • Renal failure • Hepatoxicity • DIC, hypofibrinogenemia • Anaphylaxis Patient safety precautions: • Have epinephrine, diphenhydramine, and IV corticosteroids in readiness for possible anaphylaxis. • Monitor amylase and lipase levels; stop drug if elevated. • Force fluids to reduce uric acid nephropathy from tumor lysis.
Modified K-asparaginase inactivates the amino acid asparagines to halt tumor growth. Leukemic cells cannot synthesize asparagines like normal cells and rely on the amino acid being available in the circulating blood volume.	Pharmacologic class: modified L-asparaginase used as part of a multidrug approach in treatment of acute lymphoblastic leukemia (ALL) . K-asparaginase works by depriving the tumor cells of the amino acid asparagines. • Pegaspargase (Oncaspar)	Modified L-asparaginase Clinical alert: Handle with extreme caution: gloves, protective clothing, avoid inhaling vapors, or contact with skin or mucus membranes.

(*Continued*)

Table 15-3 Chemotherapy classification, action, and precautions (*Continued*)

Site and/or general mechanism of action	Chemotherapy classification and commonly used drugs	Nursing precautions for adverse effects
		General adverse reactions: • Neurotoxicity: coma, seizures, status epilepticus • Hepatoxicity with liver failure • Acute pancreatitis • Anaphylaxis, sepsis, septic shock • Metabolic acidosis and hypoglycemia Patient safety precautions: • Have emergency drugs and equipment in readiness to treat anaphylaxis. • Monitor lipase and amylase to detect pancreatitis. • Monitor liver function studies. • Caution patients to report signs of infection immediately (fever, chills, malaise).
Anthracenedione is not believed to be specific to the cell cycle; reacts with DNA to kill cells.	Pharmacologic class: DNA-reactive agent; anthracenedione used as combination initial therapy for acute nonlymphocytic leukemia; given to reduce frequency of relapse in chronic progressive and progressive relapsing and worsening relapsing-remitting multiple sclerosis. Also used when prostate cancer does not respond to hormone therapy. • Mitoxantrone hydrochloride (Novantrone)	DNA-reactive agent; anthracenedione Clinical alert: Left ventricular ejection fraction must be evaluated prior to therapy. General adverse reactions: • Cardiotoxic: heart failure • Neurotoxic: seizures • Myelosuppression • Vesicant Patient safety precautions: • Avoid all IMs if platelet count is below 50,000/mm^3. • Stop the drug for any burning during infusion and instruct patient to report later burning at the site. • Caution patients to watch for signs of bleeding and infection.

Source: Created by the author from Reference 17.

• Administer prescribed antinausea medication prior to antineoplastic therapy as prescribed.
• Analgesics as prescribed.

✚ Pain control

Pain control is essential, and is treated without regard to risk for addiction. The WHO pain ladder is used to match the prescribed medication with the level of pain.

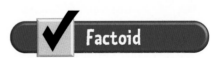

Factoid

The miscellaneous antineoplastics (see Table 15-3) are highly toxic and reserved for tumors which aren't responding to less toxic agents.

Hurst Hint

Tips for remembering notorious antimitotic vesicants:
VINS **E**AT VEINS
- VINS may **E**xtravasate and **E**at up the VEIN!
- Names of drugs that begin with "vin" (vincristine, vinblastine, vinorelbine)

AVOID T**AX**OID **AX**IDENTS
- Taxoid rhymes with **AVOID**, so you must avoid **AX**-i-dental t**AX**oid exposure.

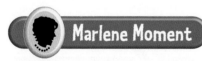

Here's the Deal

Remember, if a drug is carcinogenic, mutagenic, and teratogenic you certainly don't want any of it getting on your skin or splashing into your eyes. Take precautions!

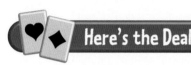

Hurst Hint

If you find a radioactive implant in the bed, worry **less** about the tumor not getting the prescribed amount of radiation and more about the nurse who is receiving radiation that has not been prescribed! Practice Question 4.

Marlene Moment

If you find a radioactive implant in the bed, don't take it to the nurses' desk and show everybody. NCLEX wants to be sure you can make safe choices by not irradiating yourself and your coworkers!

- Orally administered nonopioids (Tylenol and other NSAIDs, Cox-2 inhibitors) are used initially.
- Mild opioids (such as codeine) are the next step for mild to moderate pain.
- Strong opioids (such as morphine) are used on a regular basis for severe pain.
- Antidepressant and anticonvulsant (adjuvant) medications may be used with opioids when burning, tingling nerve pain is present due to radiation, surgery, or chemotherapy. An adjuvant is the "helper" to improve the effectiveness of another medication.
- Steroids are added for anti-inflammatory effect when the pain is due to pressure from edema.
- When oral medications or transdermal patches (Fentanyl) are ineffective, the parenteral route is utilized. Epidural catheters or venous access devices are placed for intravenous dosing.

What can harm my patient and why?

- Depression related to isolation and loneliness.
- Dislodgement of the implant. To prevent dislodgement:
  - Keep the patient on bedrest at all times to counter the effect of gravity allowing an implant into a cavity (uterus, vagina, or rectum) to fall out.
  - Low-fiber diet reduces intestinal peristalsis to decrease the incidence of an implant into an abdominal cavity from being expelled with a bowel movement.
  - Indwelling Foley catheter to keep the bladder decompressed because a distended bladder can apply pressure to an implant in the abdominal or pelvic cavity, causing displacement or dislodgement.
- Minimize staff members' exposure to radiation.
- Immunosuppression and infection.
- A common adverse effect of the antineoplastic medications is myelosuppression. If the white count is low, giving the medication will drop it even further. (Refer to patient teaching later in this section.)
- Use precautions when making patient assignments. The nurse taking care of the immunosuppressed patient shouldn't be assigned to a patient who has an infection. The nurse could transmit the infection to the immunosuppressed patient.
- The radiation dose and area of the body receiving the radiation are critical factors associated with toxicity. In adults significant production of blood cells and platelets (hematopoiesis) occurs in bone marrow of the sternum, ribs, and pelvis. Radiation to these areas can result in decreased bone marrow production of RBCs, WBCs, and platelets (myelosuppression).
- A rapidly growing cancer utilizes tremendous caloric expenditure at the expense of the patient's nutrition.

- Cachexia is the term that describes extreme wasting and malnutrition.
- Honor patient and family wishes regarding advanced directives. Provide information as needed.
- Administer nutritive supplements as tolerated (orally, enterally, or parenterally).
- Pad bony prominences, turn often, and provide meticulous skin care. Decubiti will not heal due to the extreme nutritional deficit.

Interventions and why?

The immunosuppressed patient needs instructions to avoid contracting infection, sustaining injury that could become easily infected, and for boosting the immune system.

- A private room is required with necessary equipment/supplies left in the room.
- Screen visitors for infection: use informative door sign to report to desk before entering patient room.
- Have patient wear mask if being transported through hospital corridors or while in waiting areas.
- Administer G-CSF (granulocyte colony stimulating factor) as prescribed.
- If WBC less than 2000 mm^3, implement infection control protocol.
- Take temperature orally at least once a day and report a temperature of 100.4°F.
- Avoid cuts or any break in the skin or mucus membranes by wearing protective gloves in high risk situations (using sharp tools or handwashing dishes).
- Stay away from crowds and persons having contagious illness (flu and colds).
- Avoid contact with children who have recently received immunizations.
- Protect lower extremities from injuries by wearing shoes and protective clothing when appropriate.
- Treat all cuts and abrasions immediately with running water and antibacterial soap and antibiotic ointment unless otherwise instructed by your doctor.
- Avoid direct contact with pets and other animals and under all circumstances avoid all direct contact with animal excreta, litter boxes, and bird cages.
- Do not eat raw foods or food that has not been properly refrigerated, including food that has been kept warm (buffet type restaurants) for long periods of time.
- Self administration of primary prophylaxis with G-CSF (granulocyte colony stimulating factor) if prescribed in conjunction with chemotherapy.

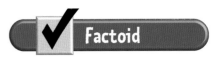

Factoid

External radiation is also called teletherapy or beam radiation. Side effects and toxic effects of teletherapy are dependent on location and dose.

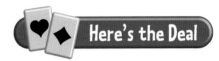

Here's the Deal

An infectious patient should never share a room with an immunosuppressed patient.

PATIENT TEACHING

- Instruct patients that a decreased energy level is a common side effect of radiation therapy. Reassure them it doesn't necessarily mean the cancer is getting worse.

- Encourage frequent gentle oral care to reduce the oral bacterial count and promote healing of any oral lesions. Meticulous oral care is a great strategy for reducing the risk for infection when the patient's immune system is in a weakened condition.

- Explain the rationale for radiation precautions when the patient has a radioactive implant, and provide diversion, encourage telephone contacts, etc to keep him/her from feeling unduly isolated.

- When the patient has a radioactive implant, family members must comply with a maximum time at the bedside (usually specified by the radiation safety officer from the X-ray department), use of shielding equipment, and special precautions if the implant becomes dislodged.

- Explain the family-centered concept of hospice with emphasis on palliative treatment and quality of life.

- Patients taking antineoplastic agents should be advised to watch for signs of infection and bleeding.

Cutting edge

The effectiveness of treatment prescribed for cancer (radiotherapy, chemotherapy, and surgery) is directly impacted by tumor hypoxia and resultant necrosis because the rapidly dividing cells "outgrow" the existing blood supply, causing hypoxic cells to be more resistant to the effects of radiation and many antineoplastic drugs. Laboratory studies are examining ways to circumvent tumor hypoxia by new technologies that enables measurement and monitoring of hypoxia in human tumors before and during the course of treatment. Hopefully these findings can pave the way for more therapeutic hypoxia-directed therapy for selectively targeting only the abnormal cells.

Antinausea medicines are used in combination with chemotherapy drugs to reduce nausea and as well as treatments for some causes of fatigue to help patients live a fairly normal life while receiving chemotherapy.

BREAST CANCER

The second most commonly diagnosed malignancy is breast cancer in females although males are also at a lesser risk.

Let's get the normal stuff straight!

Everybody has breast tissue (men and women), but the male breast isn't usually prominent because breast stimulating hormones remain at a low level.

- The adolescent breast consists of a very small amount of breast tissue and ducts which lie under the nipple and around the areola.

- Estrogen in females increases growth of breast tissue and male testosterone restricts the growth of breast tissue.

- Breasts consist of fat, connective tissue, and glandular tissue and are supported by Cooper's ligaments as well the fascia of the chest muscles.

- The breasts have an abundant supply of blood, nerves, and lymph nodes (Fig. 15-2).

◀ Figure 15-2. Anatomy of the female breast.

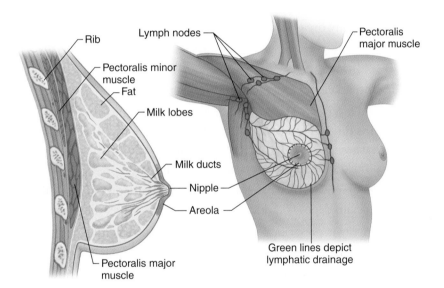

- Cooper's ligaments divide the breast into approximately 20 lobes of clustered glands interconnected by ducts within each lobe.

- Glandular alveoli are lined with secretory cells that produce milk under the proper hormonal influence.

- The nipple consists of four different tissue types: epithelial, glandular, erectile, and nervous and is surrounded by the darker smooth skin of the alveoli.

What is it?

Breast cancer is a malignancy that can originate in a milk duct, a lobule of breast tissue, or less commonly in surrounding fatty, fibrous connective (stromal) tissues. One in eight women (about 13%) in the United States will develop breast cancer as compared with 1% (1 in 1000) of men who are diagnosed with breast cancer.

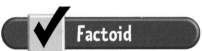

Anatomy of the male breast differs from that of the female in that ducts are present but with few (if any) lobules. Also men do not have the breast stimulating hormones necessary for growth and development of breast tissue.

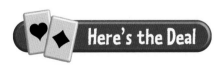

Nodules are more readily detected in the male breast because there is less tissue, but many men don't check their breasts because of the misconception that men don't develop breast cancer.

Causes and why?

Heredity is strongly implicated in the development of breast cancer (see "carcinogenesis" at the beginning of this chapter: BRCA-1 and BRCA-2). Other factors increasing the risk for breast cancer are:

- High estrogen levels

- Chronic liver disease or obesity (which can cause high estrogen levels)

- Exposure to radiation, which causes cell mutation

- Excessive alcohol consumption

- Klinefelter's syndrome and resulting gynecomastia

  - Klinefelter's syndrome is an inherited genetic syndrome wherein males carry an extra X chromosome (XXY instead of just the XY).

  - Gynecomastia (enlarged breast tissue) occurs in young males with the hormone surges of adolescence and in older men who experience changes in hormone balance. Gynecomastia can result in a growth under the nipple; however, even though gynecomastia can accompany breast cancer, it does not cause breast cancer.

Testing, testing, testing

- Tumor marker carcinoembryonic antigen (CA15-3).

- Her-2/neu status—Her-2/neu is a protein that appears in small amounts on the surface of normal breast cells, but some breast cancer cells have very large amounts of the protein (HER2/neu-positive) which makes the tumor grow and spread faster.

- Mammography can accurately detect cysts and pick up microcalcifications (tiny calcium deposits), which are indicators for further diagnostic testing.

- Chest X-ray is prescribed to detect metastasis to the lungs.

- Ultrasound is used when breast tissue is very dense making it difficult to palpate lumps, and can effectively distinguish a fluid filled cyst from a solid mass.

- MRI is used to evaluate suspicious breast lesions and can detect a mass in dense breast tissue. With newly diagnosed breast cancer diagnosis, further testing using MRI has detected cancer missed by mammogram in the opposite breast.

- PET (positron emission tomography) is used to check for metastasis when the location is unknown.

- Bone scan uses a low dose of radioactive material that is picked up by the bone and seen as "hot spots," which may or may not be cancer but require additional testing.

The treatment plan is based on staging and grading, patient characteristics (age, pre- or postmenopausal), and characteristics of the tumor.

+ Staging

- Imaging tests help to stage the disease.

- Staging of breast cancer is clear for Stage 0 (still contained inside the duct or lobule, not yet into breast tissue).

- Stage I (2 cm or less in size with no spread to lymph nodes).

- Stage 4 (distant metastasis), but Stage II and III have more definitive qualifiers with letters assigned (A-B-C).

   For more detailed breast cancer staging, go to the American Cancer Society website:

   http://www.cancer.org/docroot/CRI/content/CRI_2_4_3X_How_is_breast_cancer_staged_5.asp?sitearea=)

   Once an abnormality is found by imaging, a biopsy is performed to obtain a sample of cells from suspicious tissue to determine whether the breast lesion is benign or malignant. Biopsy can be accomplished by the following means to obtain cells for microscopic examination:

- Fine needle aspiration: A small needle is inserted into the breast lump, a cell sample is aspirated, and the needle is withdrawn.

- Core biopsy: A larger needle is used to remove actual breast tissue (not just a sample of cells) for microscopic examination.

- Ultrasound guided biopsy: Ultrasound guides the needle into the exact spot of the breast lesion so a sample can be obtained of the abnormal tissue.

- Stereotactic biopsy: Used when a breast lesion can be seen on mammogram, but can't be palpated. Once the exact coordinates of the lesion are obtained with digital mammography, the radiologist injects a local anesthetic to make a small nick for insertion of a needle into the lump and tissue samples are obtained.

- Open excisional biopsy: An incision is made and a lumpectomy is performed wherein the entire "lump" of abnormal breast tissue is removed. If there is healthy tissue all the way around the diseased tissue, the lumpectomy can be therapeutic/curative as well as diagnostic.

- Wire needle localization: Used when a lump can be visualized with imaging tests, but cannot be palpated. The wire is inserted into the lump using radiographic imaging and is left in place for the surgeon who, after making the incision, follows the wire to the tip for excision of the diseased tissue.

Signs and symptoms and why?

The signs and symptoms of breast cancer vary according to the size of the growth (nodule versus tumor) and involvement of lymph nodes:

- Painless lump in the breast, usually fixed and hard with an irregular border.

- Enlargement of axillary lymph nodes.

- Change in the uniformity of the breasts or nipple.

- Retraction or discharge from the nipple.

- Skin dimpling (orange peel appearance) or puckering of the breast tissue as the growing tumor pulls on breast tissue.

- Paget's disease of the breast presents as redness or scaling of the nipple or skin over the breasts.

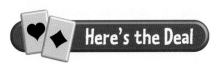

Here's the Deal

Abnormal lumps are more often found near or under the nipple or in chest tissue in men[5] and more commonly detected in the axilla (at the Tail of Spence) in women.

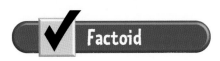

Factoid

Retraction of the tissue and skin dimpling are late signs giving evidence that earlier signs could have been missed, ignored, or denied.

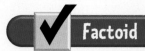

Paget's disease of the breast is Stage 0 (and totally curable) when only the nipple is involved.

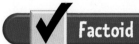

There is no cure for lymphedema so lifelong commitment is required for daily exercises, wearing compression garments/wraps, and using protective measures.[29]

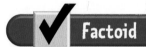

Many patients having a breast biopsy are more worried about the possible findings than the procedure itself.

What can harm my patient and why?

Ductal carcinoma in situ has a great cure rate when detected early as a calcification on mammogram, but when undiagnosed and untreated progresses from a microcalcification to invasive breast cancer with metastasis into surrounding tissue and to distant sites. Depending on the type and aggressiveness of the cancer, my patient may experience:

- Adverse effects related to the treatment (surgery, chemotherapy, radiation).
- Change in body image (females) due to mastectomy or orchiectomy (males).
- Lymphedema as a result of faulty lymphatic drainage, which can cause discomfort, impaired function, and long-term emotional distress.
- Hematoma (collection of blood in the tissue) and seroma (collection of serous fluid in the axilla) formation.
- Metastatic involvement of the bone (ribs, thoracic spine), lung, liver and brain.
- Complications such as lymphedema, seroma, and postoperative decreased range of motion are greatly increased following axillary lymph node dissection.

Interventions and why?

For outpatient biopsy:

- Review medications and have the patient discontinue any agent that will increase risk of bleeding.
- Instruct NPO according to the type and timing of the biopsy (could be several hours prior to the procedure or after midnight).
- Postprocedurally, monitor vital signs and inspect the dressing for bleeding.
- Discharge with instructions (see patient teaching to follow) when the patient is fully recovered from light to moderate sedation and local anesthesia, able to drink and retain liquids, ambulate, and void.
- Someone must be available to drive the patient home.
- The follow-up contact at 24 to 48 hours provides an opportunity for answering questions, investigating sources of concern, and reinforcing instructions.

Define time

Sentinel lymph node biopsy involves injecting a radioactive tracer and blue dye into and around the tumor before breast surgery (lumpectomy or mastectomy), allowing the dye to travel the same pathway as the malignant cells. This enables the surgeon to determine by the blue stain which of the nodes will most likely test positive for cancer.

- Even when breast reconstructive surgery is planned, the hospital stay is still very short, so priority patient needs for comfort, psychological adjustment, and self care management must be addressed urgently at a time when the patient is physically, emotionally, and psychologically stressed.

- Spend time with the patient specifically to talk about fears and concerns, coping strategies, and utilization of all available support systems. Provide contact information so that as issues arise, they can be discussed.

- Discuss Breast Cancer Network of Support (available at http://www.networkofstrength.org/support/#), with a 24/7 "YourShoes" toll free number that will be answered by a trained volunteer who is also a breast cancer survivor.

- Administer PRN analgesia as indicated.

- Monitor JP drainage (color and amount) and keep bulb decompressed.

- To reduce transient edema postoperatively, encourage the patient to make a fist on the affected side and/or squeeze a soft foam ball at intervals.

- Assist, remind, and encourage the patient to raise the affected arm above heart level while performing the prescribed exercises several times a day beginning on the second postoperative day. (See patient teaching to follow.)

- Reassure the patient that the blue dye being excreted in urine and stool with the radioisotope is generally not harmful because only a tracer dose was given before surgery.

- Monitor for hematoma formation (swelling, tightness, pain, bruising at the surgical site) and apply compression dressing (usually 12 hours) as prescribed by the surgeon.

- A large hematoma may require surgical evacuation, but small hematomas usually resolve in several weeks using warm compresses or a warm shower as advised by the doctor. Small seromas resolve spontaneously, but large collections of serous fluid can lead to infection.

- Monitor the axilla or under the breast incision for a seroma, which can develop after removal of a drain or if the drain is clogged. Look for: swelling, heaviness, discomfort, and fluid slosh with movement and notify the surgeon.

- Monitor the surgical dressing and encourage the patient to "look" as the dressing is changed. Describe the wound using positive terms to convey the normalcy of the surgical appearance.

- Encourage participation in care by having the patient hold the hypoallergenic tape, etc or to assist by helping to remove the existing dressing.

Administer adjuvant chemotherapy (usually after surgery and before radiation) as prescribed if indicated (ie, positive lymph nodes, tumors 1 cm or greater in size).

- Tamoxifen (plus an anthracycline) or aromatase inhibitor (AI) if the tumor is estrogen dependent.

- Paclitaxel (Taxol) plus a doxorubicin agent for breast cancer treatment failure or recurrence, and as adjuvant therapy for node positive breast cancer.

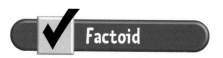

Normal drainage is bright red (sanguinous) immediately after surgery and gradually become serosanguinous (yellow clear serum mixed with blood), and last is serous (clear yellowish).

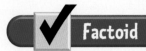

Factoid

Lymphedema can occur early (within the first three years after breast surgery) or late (three years or more after breast surgery) and is most commonly associated with lymph node dissection but can follow sentinel node biopsy, radiotherapy, or trauma to the area.

PATIENT TEACHING   Discharge teaching following a breast biopsy:

- Change the large band-aid dressing after 48 hours, but leave the Steri-Strips intact over the incision to maintain wound closure.
- Wear a well-fitted bra for comfort and support.
- Provide a foam inlay for the bra to reduce self-consciousness while awaiting breast prosthesis.
- For one week: avoid jarring or vigorous muscle activity that pulls chest muscles, moving the affected breast.

Discharge teaching following breast surgery with lymph node dissection:

- Use the demonstration/return demonstration method for teaching approved arm exercises on the affected side: wall climbing, over door pulley tug, hand behind head and swing elbow outward; brushing hair, etc.
- Monitor for signs of infection: redness, increased local heat, tenderness, malodorous drainage, and fever in excess of 100.4°F.
- Give information to the patient and significant other about breast cancer resources in the hospital, the community, and online breast cancer support services: social workers, psychologists, psychiatrists, breast cancer survivors, and support groups such as Reach to Recovery.
- Demonstrate how to empty a compress bulb suction drain (refer to detailed instructions Chapter 1) and discuss the expected amount of drainage, color, and indication for removal (< 30 mL) in 24 hours.
- Notify your doctor for persistent swelling (early or late) in the affected arm or anywhere near the site of surgery (neck, shoulder, breast, chest area), which may be preceded by a feeling of heaviness, burning, or numbness in the arm.

Lifelong care of the affected arm with lymphedema (or risk for lymphedema) will include attention to daily preventive behaviors. (Refer to Table 15-4.)

Table 15-4   Reducing risk and managing lymphedema in breast cancer survivors

Risk	Action
High risk for infection	• Remove all possible sources of infection by keeping the area clean, dry, and moisturized.
	• Keep nails clean with smooth, supple cuticles free of cracks.
	• Avoid portals for entry of microorganisms: don't cut cuticles (use oil instead and gently push them back), use electric razor for shaving axillary area (neck area for men).
	• Apply insect repellent to avoid skin excoriation from scratching itchy bites.
	• Inspect the area daily for changes in size, shape, texture, or firmness being alert to subjective changes (tight, heavy, sore).
	• Immediately treat any puncture wound, cut, or abrasion by washing area thoroughly with antibacterial soap and apply a topical antibiotic cream or ointment.
	• Notify the doctor immediately for redness, feverish skin, rash, pain, or fever greater than 100.4°F.

(Continued)

Table 15-4 Reducing risk and managing lymphedema in breast cancer survivors (*Continued*)

Risk	Action
High risk for injury	• Wear gloves for any activity that might result in injury: gardening, cleaning, and washing dishes (no knives in the sink!). • Use caution when cooking to avoid steam, splash burns, and use long oven mitts to protect the arm as well as the hand. • Avoid all injections in the affected arm: no shots, no IVs, no drawing blood samples. • Apply sunscreen to the area when outdoors to avoid local burn injury.
High risk for impaired lymph drainage	• Lie down and elevate the affected arm using pillows above heart level for 45 minutes several times daily (or as advised by your doctor). • While arm is elevated and supported above heart level (above), open and close the hand 15 to 25 times (or as advised by your doctor). • Plan for healthy meals and snacks plus regular light aerobic exercise (walking, swimming) daily or at least 3 times weekly to attain or maintain optimal weight. (Extra fat requires more blood vessels which equals more fluid coming into the area). • Elevate the affected arm or wear prescribed compression sleeve when traveling by air in a pressurized cabin.
Risk for muscle strain	• Wear prescribed compression garment during any strenuous activity. • Wash compression garment/sleeve in cool water, line dry, and replace every six months to ensure proper elasticity and compression. • Do not overuse of the affected arm. (Note: If you go to the point of fatigue, you've gone too far). • Don't use the affected arm to lift or carry heavy objects.
Risk for restriction of affected arm	• Don't allow anyone to take a blood pressure in the affected arm. • Bra (no underwire) should be well-fitted but not tight anywhere. • Select a prosthesis that is lightweight and soft. • Don't carry a handbag using the affected arm or a bag with a shoulder strap over the affected side. • Avoid tight fitting clothing (elastic sleeve, constricting arm opening, or sleeve bands). • Avoid tight rings or a watch band on the affected hand/arm. • Purchase a body pillow to help you remember not to sleep on the affected side.
Risk for excessive exposure to extremes of temperature (hot or cold)	• Avoid all prolonged exposure to excessive heat (hot tubs and saunas). • Do not use a heating pad on the affected arm because heat favors tissue edema (fluid build up). • Avoid immersion of the affected arm in water above 102°F. • Avoid extreme cold (wear coat, scarf, and gloves) because of rebound swelling with rewarming.
Risk for emotional distress related to chronicity of symptoms and disfigurement of lymphedematous arm	Explore and engage in coping strategies: • Find new hobbies and interests if previous ones exacerbate symptoms or increase risk for complications (eg, give up needle point in favor of china painting). • Integrate self care activities (ie, exercise and care of arm) into activities of daily living (getting ready for day or going to bed, placing frequently needed kitchen items on a higher shelf that requires reaching over the head using the affected arm). • Find a support group or online blog to communicate with other breast cancer survivors with lymphedema, share experience and tips for skills of applying compression bandages or sleeves, performing manual lymph drainage, etc.

Source: Created by the author from References 27-30.

Cutting edge

A new surgical procedure uses blue dye to differentiate lymph nodes draining the breast versus those draining the arm identified with a radioactive tracer. This procedure may open the door for reducing the incidence of lymphedema after sentinel node biopsy and axillary lymph node dissection. The lymphedema would be prevented by only excising the nodes that drain the breast and preserving the ones draining the arm.

Women at high risk for breast cancer may be candidates for chemoprevention using nonsteroidal antiestrogens (also called selective estrogen receptor modulators [SERMs]) such as tamoxifen or raloxifene or they may opt for prophylactic mastectomy followed by immediate breast reconstruction.

When breast cancer is noninvasive, surgery alone can be curative:

- Breast conservation can be accomplished by lumpectomy, wide excision, quadrantectomy, or segmental mastectomy.

- A total mastectomy may be required.

Define time

Neoadjuvant chemotherapy refers to the chemotherapy that is given prior to surgery to shrink large tumors, increasing potential for breast conservation (lumpectomy versus mastectomy) and also giving the oncologist an idea of how the tumor will respond to a particular agent.

If neoadjuvant chemo doesn't work *before* surgery, it probably won't work *after* surgery, so the oncologist should choose from other drugs if there was a poor response to the neoadjuvant administration.

When breast cancer is invasive, lymph nodes are removed for biopsy followed by combinations of chemotherapy and radiation as indicated:

- Taxol and Adriamycin.

- Estrogen receptor blocking agents (tamoxifen).

- Aromatase inhibitors have replaced tamoxifen for postmenopausal women.

- Estrogen synthesis inhibitors (Lupron and Zoladex).

- Trastuzumab and lapatinib are used with combination chemotherapy to increase survival benefits when the patients has HER2-positive disease (Table 15-3).

Often men present with advanced disease and because they are also likely to be HER-2 positive, the treatment is similar: adjuvant endocrine therapy and chemotherapy.

Metastatic breast cancer is incurable; however, a palliative effect and increased survival time can be obtained with anti-Her2/neu–directed therapies.

- Trastuzumab to suppress Her2/neu

- Lapatinib to suppress Her2/neu

- Bisphosphonate therapy for bone metastases

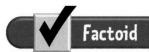

Factoid

Chemotherapy used for estrogen-dependent breast tumors will inhibit estrogen, but this also puts women into menopause.

CANCER OF THE CERVIX AND UTERUS

Let's get the normal stuff straight!

The good news is that cancer of the cervix and uterus can be 100% curable when detected early.

The uterus is a pear-shaped hollow organ that is located in the female pelvis behind the bladder and in front of the rectum. The cervix forms the narrow neck of the uterus (Fig. 15-13):

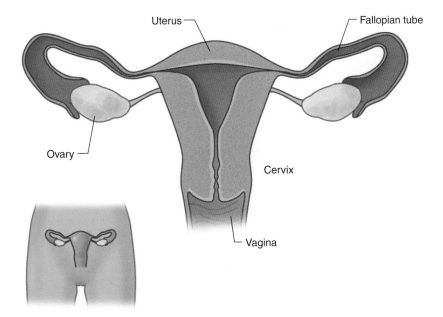

Uterus
Fallopian tube
Ovary
Cervix
Vagina

◀ Figure 15-3. Uterus and cervix.

- The lower part of the cervix (called the ectocervix) protrudes into the vagina and can be visualized after parting the vaginal walls with a speculum.
- The opening of the ectocervix is called the external os, the appearance of which varies according to the woman's age, parity, and hormonal status.
- The endocervical canal is the passageway from the external os upward into the uterine cavity.
- The normal cells that make up the cervix are squamous, glandular, and metaplastic epithelial cells.
- Squamous epithelial cells cover the outer surface of the cervix and line the vagina.
- Glandular cells that produce mucus line the inner canal (ectocervix) of the cervix.
- Squamous metaplastic cells originate from the zone where the inner (endocervix) and the outer (ectocervix) meet.

Squamous cells of the cervix are stacked in distinct layers (stratified):

- The top superficial layer of cells is under hormonal influence to shed continuously.

- The intermediate (parabasal) layer pushes up as cells mature to replace those that are shed.
- The basal (base) or reserve cell layer is from whence the above layers arise.

The uterus is normally anteriorly flexed over the bladder and is shaped like an upside-down pear, approximately three to four inches wide and two to three inches high (Fig. 15-4).

▶ Figure 15-4. Cross-section of normal uterus: anterior flexion over bladder.

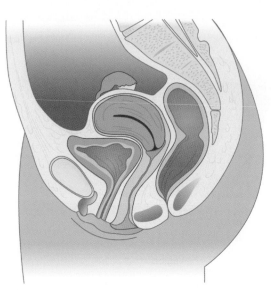

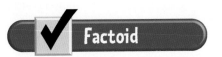

Factoid

Cancer that begins in the cervix is a different kind of cancer than that which begins in the uterus. Most uterine cancers begin in the endometrial tissue, but another different kind of cancer (sarcoma) can form in the uterine muscle tissue.

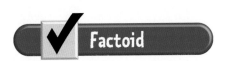

Factoid

A reserve cell (first identified at 20 weeks, gestation) arises from Müllerian epithelial cells for endocervical reserve cells and endocervical columnar cells. During early cervical development, these stem cells have the capacity to transform into both endocervical columnar and squamous-type epithelium in the endocervix.

Just like an army reservist who is on standby until needed, the reserve cell is a stem cell that helps repair normal wear and tear, only coming into "active duty" when conditions get really bad requiring reinforcement or replacement. The reserve cell arises from the base layer of the squamous epithelium and becomes *metaplastic,* which increases the likelihood of cancer developing, especially in the presence of the human papillomavirus (HPV).

- The body of the uterus is made up of muscle tissue; endometrial tissue lines the inside cavity.
- The endometrial lining sloughs off monthly under the influence of estrogen and progesterone and is excreted in menstrual fluid.
- The endometrium is replaced on a monthly basis by new tissue arising from the intermediate layer (decidua media) that pushes up from the base layer of the endometrium (decidua basalis).

What is it?

Cancer of the cervix originates at the squamous-columnar junction either in the cervical canal or at the opening of the cervix. Cervical cancers are staged according to their size and the depth of invasion into the stromal tissue of the cervix, whether the growth is only seen microscopically as opposed to gross lesions with ulcerations, and metastasis to nearby vagina, bladder, and rectum, or to distant organs through lymphatic flow or by way of the blood stream.

Causes and why?

The majority of cancers of the cervix (90%) are squamous cell (epidermoid) cancers and a very small percentage (10%) are adenocarcinomas. Cancer of the cervix is caused by changes to the reserve cells that may arise from any three types of cells (columnar, glandular, or epithelial) cells in the cervix.

Define time

Metaplasia is a term that means transformation of one type of tissue into another, an example of which could be cartilage turning into bone.

Risk factors for cervical cancer:

- Infection with human papillomavirus (HPV)

- Sex or pregnancy at a young age

- Repeated STDs (chronic irritation) causing dysplasia

When considering sex or pregnancy at a young age, the age of the person at the onset of menses is an important defining factor. For example, one girl may have commenced having a monthly period at age 12 and another may have only just started a period at age 16. If both of these girls were having sex or got pregnant at age 17, which one would be considered "youngest?" Who would be more *reproductively* mature? The one who has been having a menstrual cycle for the longer period of time!

Risk factors for uterine cancer:

- Endometrial hyperplasia (increase in the number of cells in the lining of the uterus).

Endometrial hyperplasia is not cancer, but it can turn into cancer, which is why they usually want to do a hysterectomy for treatment of this condition. Here's how it happens: When cells get old they are supposed to die and be replaced by new cells. Likewise, old endometrial cells don't do the apoptosis thing where they are programmed to die, and they just hang on, piling up cell on top of cell (which is not normal) and can become malignant. Endometrial hyperplasia causes heavy menstrual periods, bleeding between periods, and even postmenopausal bleeding.

- Greater than 50 years of age (the risk increases with aging)

- A positive family history of cervical cancer

- Late menopause and no pregnancy

- Obesity (resulting from increased production of estrogen in fatty tissue)

The length of time that a woman's body is exposed to the effects of estrogen has a direct relationship with the risk for cancer, so beginning menstruation at a young age and entering menopause at a late age increase exposure time. Women who take estrogen replacement to stop menopausal symptoms will have an increased risk for reproductive cancer unless they also take progesterone for the uteroprotective effect.

Testing, testing, testing

The pap smear is the most important screening test for diagnosis of cervical cancer. The timetable for pap smear screening and HPV testing takes the woman's age and onset of sexual activity into consideration.

- Pap smear testing should begin within three years of first becoming sexually active or by age 21 (whichever comes first).

- An annual pap smear is advised for women under age 30.

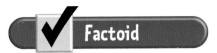

Factoid

HPV is the leading cause of cervical cancer worldwide.[35]

Factoid

Anybody who has struggled with infertility or has never ever been able to get pregnant always has a higher risk of reproductive type cancers. Never being pregnant means prolonged exposure to estrogen effects without a break during gestational periods.

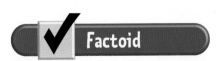

Factoid

It is incredibly rare for cervical cancer to develop in the under-25 age group.

- Women aged 30 to 65 should have a pap smear every two to three years if they have previously had three negative pap smears.

- Women aged 65 to 70 and above who are at low risk (few or no known risk factors), and have had three normal pap smears in the past 10 years should discuss the need for continuing routine screening with their doctor.

- Women who have had a hysterectomy, but still have their cervix, must still have routine pap smear screening.

- High-risk women or those who have had abnormal results on a pap smear require more frequent screening:

  - Women who have had a total hysterectomy for cancer or precancer

  - Women who have risk factors for cervical cancer: smoking, poor nutrition, STDs (especially HPV and chlamydia), HIV, or a positive family history

  - Women who have cervical dysplasia or atypical squamous cells with undetermined significance (ASC-US)

  Terms used for cytology findings with the pap smear:

- ASC-US = atypical (not completely normal) squamous cells with undetermined significance (meaning that they will continue to watch it closely with a repeat pap test in one year)

- CIN = cervical intraepithelial neoplasia (a new growth in a cervical epithelial cell)

- LSIL = low-grade squamous intraepithelial lesions are mild abnormalities caused by HPV; early changes in the size and shape of cells calls for a repeat pap test in four to six months.

- HSIL = high-grade squamous intraepithelial lesions show marked abnormalities in precancerous cells that have a high likelihood of progressing to invasive cancer which necessitates a prompt colposcopy.

- AIS = (endocervical) adenocarcinoma in situ shows precancerous cells in the glandular tissue.

The HPV DNA test is indicated for women over the age of 30 because the virus usually is self-limiting and goes away on its own with no intervention; however, if the pap test is slightly abnormal (atypical cells), this test can help determine if more testing or treatment is indicated.

The CA-125 blood test is used to rule out ovarian involvement, which may or may not be an indicator. The most definitive diagnostic tests obtain tissue for microscopic examination:

- A punch biopsy of the cervix and a colposcopy.

- Depending on the stage, a dilatation and curettage (D&C) may be performed with endometrial biopsy to detect uterine cancer.

  Tests to evaluate for metastasis include:

- Chest X-ray

- IVP

- Barium enema

- CT of the abdomen

- Liver and bone scans

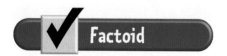

✓ Factoid

The FDA approved the first HPV genotyping assay in March 2009, and this test is now being used to monitor women aged 30 and older who are HPV positive having atypical squamous cervical cells, but who are currently negative for cytology.

✓ Factoid

Anytime a woman has an abnormal pap smear, the test will always be repeated.

Signs and symptoms and why?

Cancer of the cervix is often without symptoms when the cancer is pre-invasive, which is why the pap smear is such an important screening test. Once women are symptomatic, cervical cancer has already spread to surrounding tissues and lymph nodes. Painless vaginal bleeding is the classic sign of invasive cancer of the cervix. Other symptoms are:

- Watery, blood-tinged vaginal discharge.
- Leg pain that follows the sciatic nerve pathway.
- Flank pain and back pain with sciatic nerve pain owing to pressure.
  Major symptoms of uterine cancer:
- Postmenopausal bleeding is a classic sign.
- Watery, bloody, vaginal discharge.
- Low back or abdominal pain, pelvic pain.

What can harm my patient and why?

- Fistula formation and ostomies related to surgery.
- Major postoperative complications are hemorrhage and infection.
- Decreased libido secondary to loss of fertility.

Signs and symptoms and why?

Signs and symptoms related to chemotherapy and radiation include:

- Nausea, vomiting, anorexia
- Immunodeficiency and risk for infection
- Hematopoietic syndrome, myelosuppression
- Anemia and easy fatigability
- Neurotoxicity, hepatotoxicity, or cardiotoxicity depending on the agent

Interventions and why?

- **Cryotherapy** is a procedure used to freeze a premalignant cervical lesion.
- **Loop electrocautery excision procedure (LEEP)** is a procedure used for premalignant lesions of the cervix (LSIL, CIN I and II).
- If a **conization** is performed to preserve fertility in young women, the patient needs to know that frequent monitoring for recurrence is important.
- If cervical cancer is invasive (>1–3 mm) more extensive surgery is indicated (see postoperative care for hysterectomy).

Interventions and why?

Postoperative nursing care (total hysterectomy, bilateral salpingo-oophorectomy, and node sampling)

- Monitor vital signs and check for bleeding frequently.
- After removal of indwelling (Foley) catheter, check voiding and monitor for bladder distention.

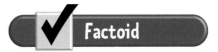

There is a 50% chance of a cancer diagnosis when postmenopausal bleeding occurs. Women must be taught that vaginal bleeding recurring after menopause must be reported to the doctor IMMEDIATELY!

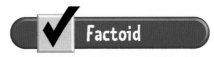

The greatest risk for hemorrhage is during the first 24 hours after abdominal hysterectomy.

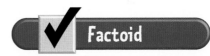

Women who have an abdominal hysterectomy are at greater risk for hemorrhage, but women who have a vaginal hysterectomy are at greater risk for infection.

- If unable to void within the next 8 hours, collaborate for an order to catheterize with a small French catheter (in and out) to prevent distention.

Interventions and why?

- Depending on the stage of lesion, treatment for cervical or uterine cancer involves surgical removal of diseased tissue. When cancer of the cervix is diagnosed in the early stage with a pap smear and the woman desires that fertility is preserved, a conization is performed through utilization of:
  - Electrosurgical excision
  - Laser ablation
  - Cryosurgery

Define time

Conization is removal of a cone-shaped wedge of the cervix. More radical surgery (hysterectomy) followed by radiation and chemotherapy is reserved for later stages of cervical cancer (<3 mm deep) and uterine cancer that has become invasive.

Define time

Pelvic exenteration is the most radical surgery in which the uterus and all of the pelvic organs are removed. This means that in addition to a radical hysterectomy, the patient may be left with a colostomy or an ileal conduit because the colon and bladder have also been removed.

- Intracavitary radiation may be indicated to prevent vaginal recurrence.
- Chemotherapy and estrogen inhibitors are indicated if tumor is estrogen dependent.

Clinical trials are constantly recruiting patients who have recurrence and poor response to the standard prescribed regimes. Many clinical trials offer hope for extended life while research progresses to find new drugs and/or new combinations of tested drugs.

What can harm my patient and why?

Prevent abdominal distention after pelvic surgery to avoid tension on the suture line, which could lead to wound dehiscence and evisceration.

Interventions and why?

- Semi-Fowler's position to promote drainage, but avoid high Fowler's position after pelvic surgery to reduce pelvic congestion of blood.
- Monitor dressings (abdominal and/or perineal for more radical surgery) and change PRN.
- Antiembolus stockings and pneumatic compression sleeves are used to prevent venostasis of the lower extremities.
- Assist with early ambulation to reduce risk for pneumonia, thrombophlebitis, and constipation.

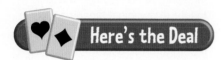

Here's the Deal

Total abdominal hysterectomy sounds like everything (total) will be removed; however, this term only means the total uterus and cervix. If the tubes and the ovaries are to be excised, the op-permit must include bilateral oophorectomy and bilateral salpingectomy.

✚ Infection prevention

Because of the risk for infection following surgery, the nursing care plan will include:

- Administration of prophylactic antibiotics as prescribed
- Monitoring for signs of infection
- Reporting of fever or foul vaginal discharge

Depending upon surgical staging and diagnosis of recurrent vaginal lesions or metastasis beyond the uterus, my patient may be receiving adjuvant external beam radiation (whole pelvis radiotherapy) or intracavitary radiation alone or with chemotherapy (see Table 15-1).

- Observe general radiation precautions and nursing precautions cited earlier in this chapter.
- Observe clinical alerts and patient safety precautions with prescribed chemotherapy used in combination with radiation and surgery.
- Platinum-based agents (cisplatin or combination cisplatin/fluorouracil) may be administered for invasive cervical cancer.
- Hormonal therapy (Progestin) or chemotherapy with two and three drug regimes (paclitaxel doxorubicin, cisplatin) may be administered according to the stage.

Refer to Table 15-3 for clinical alerts and patient safety precautions.

PATIENT TEACHING   For prevention or early detection of uterine/cervical cancer:

- Prophylactic vaccination to reduce risk of cervical cancer by preventing HPV infection (but this only works if not previously infected with the HPV subtypes covered by the vaccines).
- Menopausal women are to report any vaginal spotting or bleeding immediately!

Postoperative discharge instructions:

- Take showers rather than baths, because sitting submerged in a tub promotes ascending infection.
- Do not use douches or tampons and do not have sexual intercourse pending the followup exam by the doctor.
- Avoid activities that can cause bleeding: lifting heavy objects, climbing stairs, sexual intercourse, exercise, and driving. Your doctor will decide when these activities can be resumed safely.
- Expect a whitish vaginal discharge, but report color change (yellow) immediately.

Cutting edge

When cervical cancer is invasive and young women desire future childbearing, only the affected tissue of the cervix can be excised, using frozen section to check the margins of the incision. This procedure called a radical trachelectomy is an alternate to hysterectomy and is now being performed by robotics, which allows for better visualization and fine dissection. The pelvic lymph nodes are removed and uterine arteries are preserved. Closure of the cervix is accomplished with a cerclage, which uses a drawstring procedure.

TESTICULAR CANCER

Let's get the normal stuff straight!

The testes are two egg-shaped glands inside the scrotum whose function is to produce sperm and testosterone (male hormone).

- The testes are outside of the abdominal cavity to avoid exposure of the testicles to internal heat, which would decrease fertility.
- The scrotal sac has a layer of fascia and smooth muscle with a thin septum that provides a separate compartment for each testicle.

What is it?

Testicular cancer is a rare condition (1% of all male cancers) that is more prevalent in the white population and occurs in young males. It is the most commonly occurring cancer in the 20- to 30-year age group. Testicular cancer is a treatable condition with a good cure rate and when detected in the early stage can result in 100% cure. There are two types of testicular cancer: seminoma or nonseminoma, the more common being seminomas (40% of all testicular germ cell tumors).

Causes and why?

The exact causes are unknown; however, most testicular malignancies (90%) begin in germ cells (seminomas) and nonseminomas are choriocarcinomas, yolk sac tumors, embryonic cancers, and teratomas (neoplasms that contain different kinds of tissue—chorionic or embryonic or both), none of which is native to the testis. Increased risk testicular cancer is associated with:

- Undescended testes (even following surgical repair)
- Genetic syndromes (Down's and Klinefelter's)
- Abnormally developed testicles and infertility
- Family history of testicular cancer
- Infection with HIV and AIDS

Malignant cells grow within the testicle and replace normal parenchymal tissue.

- The disease spreads by lymph and vascular channels to lungs, bone, or liver.

Testing, testing, testing

- Tumor markers (radioimmunoassay studies) are sensitive blood tests that can indicate testicular cancer even before the solid tumor is palpable on physical exam:

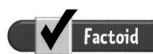

Men with certain occupations (eg, miners, oil field workers, utility workers) have a higher incidence of testicular tumors, but evidence is lacking to confirm chemical exposure as a direct cause.

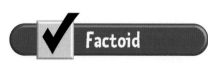

Metastasis of testicular cancer can occur even before a large mass is detected in the scrotum.

- Alpha-fetoprotein (AFP)
- Beta-human chorionic gonadotropin (BHCG)
- Lactate dehydrogenase (LDH)
- Ultrasound is used to determine whether the lesion is fluid filled (usually a cyst) or solid (usually a malignancy).
- Biopsy is accomplished with tissue obtained following inguinal (groin incision) orchiectomy (removal of the affected testicle). The inguinal approach (incision in the groin) is used to avoid cutting into the scrotum, which could cause the cancer to spread. If the man only has one testicle, a tissue sample may be obtained and checked for malignant cells prior to the orchiectomy.
- CT, X-rays, and liver function studies are used to assess for metastasis.
- If testicular cancer is confirmed by the pathologist, additional tests are performed to accomplish staging of the tumor, which will determine the best treatment approach:
  - Computed tomography (CT scan)
  - Lymphangiography (X-rays of the lymph system)
  - Bone scan
  - Chest X-ray

Signs and symptoms and why?

Depending on the size and metastasis of the malignancy, various signs and symptoms may occur:

- Painless lump or swelling of a testicle
- Testicular pain or scrotal discomfort
- Enlarged testicle with a difference in sensation
- Perception of heaviness in the scrotum
- Dull ache in the lower abdomen, back, or groin area
- Rapid collection of fluid in the scrotum

What can harm my patient and why?

Although low-stage disease approaches a 100% cure rate, liver, bone, brain, and lung metastasis are risks associated with higher stages. Effects of radiation and chemotherapy can be harmful and lead to long-term health issues.

- Infertility, depending on the type of treatment received
- Secondary leukemia with use of prolonged use of alkylating agents or radiation
- Decreased creatinine clearance by average of 15% (usually without further deterioration)
- Diminished hearing at the 4- to 8-kHz range (although normal conversational tones aren't affected)
- Increased cardiovascular morbidity (bleomycin, etoposide, and cisplatin)
- Pulmonary toxic effects (bleomycin)

Orchiectomy can lead to changes in body image. (Note: This effect is reduced if prosthesis is inserted at the time of surgery.)

Interventions and why?

The diagnosis of testicular cancer can be overwhelming for a young man, his family, and significant other. The initial diagnosis and the implications of the disease may impact the patient and family severely. The nurse is often present when the physician explains the condition and treatment options and possible outcomes. The initial patient priorities are:

- Offer compassionate holistic care that provides for physical, emotional, and spiritual needs.
- Reinforce information in lay terms and answer questions about the disease.
- Provide educational support and encouragement that the loss of a single testicle does not produce infertility, and a vast majority of treatment regimens can preserve fertility.
  Testicular cancer is treated according to:
- Stage
- Size of the tumor (bulky versus nonbulky)
- Involvement of retroperitoneal lymph nodes
- Metastasis to brain, liver, and/or bones

The T (tumor) N (nodes) M (metastasis) S (serum tumor markers) further helps to classify the stage (IA, IIA, IIB, IIC, IIIA, IIIB, and IIIC), but usually the stages are referred to as:

- Stage I: Confined to the testicle
- Stage II: Spread to retroperitoneal lymph nodes
- Stage III: Beyond lymph nodes to brain, liver, and/or bones

After inguinal radical orchiectomy and lymph node dissection, treatment options based on staging may utilize:

- Radiation alone to lymph nodes.
- Retroperitoneal lymph node dissection.
- Single-dose carboplatin.
- Combination chemotherapy with cisplatin (bulky Stage II seminomas).
- Single course of bleomycin, etoposide, and cisplatin (BEP) (Stage I non-seminoma).
- Multiple courses of BEP chemotherapy.
- Less commonly used chemo combinations are cisplatin plus vinblastine plus bleomycin or etoposide plus ifosfamide plus cisplatin.

In some instances after radical orchiectomy and lymph node dissection, patients with fewer than six positive nodes are followed with frequent checkups (as often as monthly), which include:

- Physical exam
- Chest X-ray

- Serum markers (alpha-fetoprotein, human chorionic gonadotropin, and lactate dehydrogenase)
- Chemotherapy for relapse

Thankfully, on initial evaluation and diagnosis of testicular cancer, the percentage of the population having metastasis is small (10%–15%), with most testicular cancers being highly responsive to treatment and curable. Because radiation and chemotherapy reduce sperm and sperm quality, men are offered an option for banking sperm before treatment.

Postoperative care:

- Monitor vital signs.
- Monitor dressings and drains.
- Administer prescribed analgesia.

Administer chemotherapy (usually on an outpatient basis) as prescribed:

- Cisplatin (Platinol), bleomycin (Blenoxane), and etoposide (VePesid).
- Etoposide (VePesid plus cisplatin [Platinol] (see Table 15-3 for patient safety precautions).
- Monitor vital signs during chemotherapy or radiation treatment as well as fluid balance because of the expected adverse effects: nausea, vomiting, and diarrhea.

PATIENT TEACHING

- If fertility is desired, inform the patient of options (such as sperm banking), which must be considered prior to chemotherapy.
- Perform a monthly testicular self-exam of the remaining testicle.
- Have a yearly clinical examination and physical.

Men who have had testicular cancer are at higher risk for developing cancer in the remaining testicle, making regular self-examination important (Fig. 15-5).

◀ Figure 15-5. Testicular self-exam.

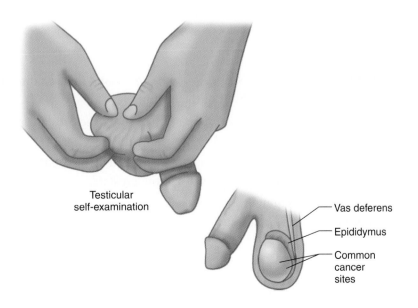

Testicular
self-examination

Vas deferens

Epididymus

Common
cancer
sites

- After a warm bath or shower, gently roll the testicle between the thumb and fingers, also palpating the cord leading upward from the top of the testicle.
- The testicle should feel smooth and firm. Notify your doctor immediately if any lump, swelling, hard nodule, or fluid is detected.

Cutting edge

The scrotal imaging modality of choice is high-resolution, real-time sonography, which is highly accurate and sensitive for identifying prepubescent scrotal lesions and differentiating fluid-filled lesions (cysts) from solid tumors in adults.

PROSTATE CANCER

The prostate cancer diagnosis was projected to be in excess of 192,000 men in 2009, with an expected 27,000 deaths from the disease (Fig. 15-6).

Let's get the normal stuff straight!

▶ Figure 15-6. The prostate gland.

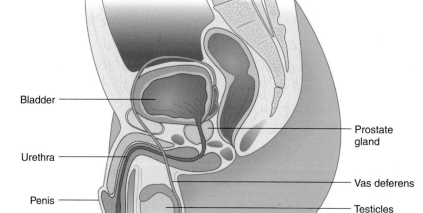

The prostate is a donut-shaped, walnut-sized gland that sits directly under the bladder and in front of the rectum.

- Two small glands (seminal vesicles) sit just above the prostate and secrete seminal fluid (semen).
- Nerves that control erectile function are located alongside the seminal glands and are attached to the sides of the prostate.
- The urethra emerging from the bladder goes directly through the prostate gland and continues through the urethral opening in the distal penis.
- Urinary sphincters are bands of muscle tissue at the base of the bladder and at the base of the prostate that prevent stored urine from leaking out.

- Sphincters relax during urination to allow urine to flow from the bladder through the urethra and out of the body.

What is it?

Other than skin cancers, prostate cancer is the most common cancer in America, which currently affects more than 2 million men, with new cases occurring at an alarming rate of one every 2.7 minutes and a death from prostate cancer every 19 minutes! Prostate cancer is most commonly a slow-growing malignancy that takes years to become detectable, and even longer to spread beyond the prostate. Only a small percentage of prostate cancers are of the more aggressive forms that grow more rapidly.

Causes and why?

Unregulated growth produces abnormal cells within the prostate tissue that outlive normal cells and rapidly multiply to create small tumors, 95% of which are adenomas. The incidence of prostate cancer increases with age: 65% of cases occur in men 65 years of age and older (Fig. 15-7).

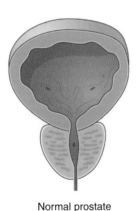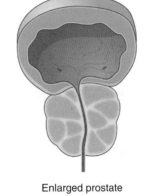

Normal prostate   Enlarged prostate

◀ Figure 15-7. Normal prostate and enlarged prostate.

Other risk factors include:
- Family history of a single first-degree relative with prostate cancer confers twice the risk of developing the disease, but having two first-degree relatives increases the risk fourfold.
- Race/ethnicity: African-American men are at highest risk.
- Increased dietary consumption of red meat and fatty foods.
- Excess body fat (especially around the middle) because of increased secretion of hormones and inflammatory mediators with increased cellular oxidation that contributes to development/progression of aggressive prostate cancer.
- Moderate and high occupational exposure to ammonium perfluorooctanoate (PFOA).

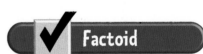

Factoid

When father, brother, or son (first-degree relatives) are diagnosed with prostate cancer at an early age (prior to age 60) the risk is even greater.

Testing, testing, testing

Screening tests and physical examination alerts the health care provider to a potential problem, but biopsy provides definitive confirmation of the diagnosis of prostate cancer.

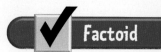

- Prostate specific antigen (PSA).
- Digital rectal exam (DRE) with palpation of the prostate for hard nodules.
- Transrectal fine needle aspiration for biopsy.
- Transrectal ultrasound (TRUS) guided biopsy.
- Endorectal MRI and MR spectroscopic imaging is used as an aid for staging prostate cancer.
- Alkaline phosphatase (increased levels with bone metastasis of the spine, sacrum or pelvis).
- Acid phosphatase (highest levels found in the prostate) used for diagnosis and staging of prostate cancer.

Signs and symptoms and why?

Signs and symptoms of prostate enlargement (which could be benign or malignant) detectable by men are changes in urinary and sexual function:

- Difficulty passing urine (hesitancy, small stream, urinary retention).
- Frequency of urination and nocturia with decreased voided volume accompanied by a sensation that the bladder has not completely emptied.
- A hard nodule is palpated on the digital rectal exam.
- Urinary retention and painful bladder distention occurs with large lesions.
- Hematuria and/or blood streaks in semen with painful ejaculation (later sign that may indicate cancer invasion into the bladder or urethra).

What can harm my patient and why?

Prostate cancer that begins as a malignancy contained within the prostate gland can progress to a systemic disease involving the seminal vesicles, lymph nodes, skeleton (sacrum, pelvis, and spine), and other distant organs. Aggressive prostate cancer that advances and metastasizes quickly is lethal.

Adverse effects of treatment can have a negative impact on the individual:

- Urinary dribbling and leaking owing to damage to the urinary sphincter at the base of the bladder caused by surgery or radiation
- Bowel problems caused by radiation damage of the nearby rectum
- Infertility (sterility) caused by loss of the prostate, which creates retrograde ejaculation
- Erectile dysfunction because of surgical damage to the pudendal nerve
- Hemorrhage (read more about this in interventions and why below)

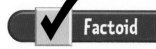

Interventions and why?

Small, primary tumors within the prostate detected at an early stage have cure rates of 90% or better with standard interventions such as surgery or radiation to remove or kill all cancerous cells in the prostate.

Unfortunately, at this stage the cancer produces few or no symptoms and can be difficult to detect. Treatment decisions are complicated because it is difficult to differentiate which prostate cancers will grow slowly and which small percentage will grow aggressively.

- Watchful waiting is indicated with advanced age or in patients with other comorbidities, in whom the treatment options would have a detrimental effect on quality of life.

- Transurethral resection of the prostate (TURP) does not effect a cure for cancer, but can offer the patient symptomatic relief of obstructed urine flow when curative surgery is not an option.

- Radical prostatectomy (via the suprapubic, retropubic, or perineal approach) is indicated when the cancer is localized to the prostate and a cure can be expected.

- When there is no lymph node involvement and acid phosphatase is normal with no evidence of metastasis, the surgeon will try to preserve the pudendal nerve.

- If a frozen section of pelvic lymph nodes reveals metastasis, radiation therapy is an option to control local symptoms.

- Androgen suppression therapy (AST), such as a luteinizing hormone–releasing hormone agonist (leuprolide or goserelin) and the anti-androgen flutamide.

When patients are not candidates for surgery and decline radiation, final treatment options are:

- Palliative treatment for metastatic or progressive prostate with estramustine phosphate (Emcyt), continuing as long as the response is favorable

- Recommending entry into existing clinical trials

In men with localized cancer of the prostate with no added additional illnesses, radical prostatectomy plus radiation therapy and six months of AST therapy offers improved survival rates even with high-risk disease.

Following transuethral (TURP) a three-way catheter will be in place for continuous irrigation to maintain patency and flush out clots:

- Tape the tube securely to avoid accidental trauma of the bulb pulling against the neck of the bladder and caution the patient not to pull on the tube.

- Monitor urinary output carefully, subtracting the amount of GU (genitourinary) irrigant from the total output to determine the actual amount of urine.

- Monitor for kinks or clots in the tubing that could obstruct the outflow of urine.

- Monitor for bladder distention, looking for a rounded swelling above the pubis. If urine flow is obstructed, the bladder will become distended, causing pressure to disrupt the incision (if any) or operative area. Even worse, acute renal failure (secondary to hydronephrosis) can occur if the urine flow is blocked.

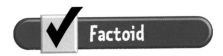

TURP is the most popular surgery today! Benign prostatic hypertrophy (BPH) obstructs urine flow.

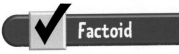

The payoff for radical prostatectomy (even when the pudendal nerve and capability for erection cannot be saved) is being cancer free! When nerve-sparing radical prostatectomy is possible phosphodiesterase-5 (PDE-5) inhibitors (sildenafil [Viagra], vardenafil [Levitra], and tadalafil [Cialis]) can be effective treatment for erectile dysfunction. PDE-5 inhibitors are also helpful after radiation therapy for localized prostate cancer.

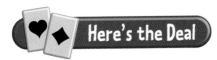

Researchers recently reported the benefit of postponing treatment while actively monitoring the cancer's progression, stating that the vast majority of older men who decline treatment will die of something other than prostate cancer.

- Monitor for hemorrhage through direct observation of increased viscosity of drainage with clots, vital signs, hematocrit, RBCs, and patient symptoms. Hemorrhage is the major complication of TUR or TURP.
- If hemorrhagic hypovolemic shock occurs, treatments described in Chapter 5 are implemented.

Venous bleeding (dark and less viscous) can be controlled with pressure by applying traction to the catheter, which pulls the bulb against the operative site for local compression. Arterial bleeding (bright red and viscous) requires surgical intervention. Either way, you are to notify the doctor promptly at the first sign of hemorrhage!

Never hand or manually irrigate a catheter after fresh surgery because the operative site is still too fragile!

The absorption of large volumes of bladder irrigation fluid during TURP can produce a complication known as transurethral resection syndrome, which is characterized by hyponatremia, hypovolemia, and hyperammonemia. Initial signs of hyponatremia are headache, confusion, and disorientation.

- Monitor electrolytes (be especially alert to hyponatremia).
General nursing care to prevent complications and promote healing:
- Monitor dressings (perineal, suprapubic, or low abdominal) and the surgical incision if present.
- Post perineal prostatectomy, avoid rectal thermometers, rectal tubes, or enemas, which could injure the prostatic fossa and cause bleeding.
- After the initial dressing has been removed by the surgeon, change dressings PRN using sterile technique.
- To prevent DVT continue SCDs or antiembolus stockings until the patient is fully ambulatory and ensure that the patient is well hydrated.
- Encourage early ambulation to reduce pain and improve circulation, but do not allow sitting, which encourages pelvic congestion of blood.
- Administer prescribed stool softeners (Colace) and provide prune juice to prevent straining.
- Assess pain on a scale of 1 to 10 and administer PRN analgesia as prescribed.
- Administer smooth muscle relaxants flavoxate (Urispas) or oxybutynin (Ditropan) as prescribed to relax bladder spasms PRN.
- Provide warm sitz baths or warm compresses to the pubis as needed to help relieve bladder spasms and promote healing of the surgical incision.

In addition to the above considerations for general nursing care, refer to priorities for nursing care (cited earlier in this chapter) when the patient is receiving radiation therapy or chemoradiation.

PATIENT TEACHING   Trim men are less likely to develop prostate cancer!
- A healthy lifestyle (nutrition and exercise) is an important preventive measure.
- Reduce intake of red meat, dairy products, and other high-fat foods.
Primary and secondary prevention modalities:

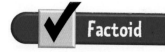

Factoid

Anything that causes the patient to strain increases venous pressure and will result in bleeding.

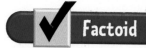

Factoid

The B&O (belladonna alkaloids and opium) suppository used to relax painful bladder spasms after TURP is one of only three medications to contain opium and is the only drug listed in the US Pharmacopeia that contains opium in suppository form.

- Annual prostate specific antigen (PSA) and digital rectal exam (DRE) after age 50 or sooner (by age 45) with high-risk factors.
- Chemoprevention (finasteride [Proscar]) to reduce the incidence of prostate cancer may produce undesired side effects such as erectile dysfunction, loss of libido, and gynecomastia.

Patient instructions related to self-care and monitoring:

- Watch for signs of infection (urinary tract or epididymitis) after prostate surgery and report immediately: chills, fever, urinary frequency, urgency, or pain or straining to void.
- Teach Kegel exercises to strengthen the pelvic floor muscles to reduce urinary dribbling.
- Avoid sitting for long periods of time (pelvic pressure) or lifting heavy objects (increased venous pressure), which predisposes to bleeding.
- Stay well hydrated by drinking plenty of fluids. Dehydration can predispose to the formation of clots, which could obstruct flow of urine.
- Avoid alcohol, coffee, tea (caffeinated beverages), or spicy foods that may cause bladder discomfort.
- When taking Lupron (leuprolide acetate), signs and symptoms will become worse! This results from "tumor flare" and usually disappears after about a week.
- When taking Eulexin (flutamide) be alert to signs of liver dysfunction (dark urine, yellowing of the skin, no appetite, fatigue) and notify the doctor immediately!

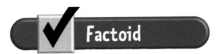

Factoid

In addition to inhibiting enlargement of the prostate gland and decreasing PSA levels, finasteride (Propecia) can make bald men grow hair and hairy women (polycystic ovary syndrome hirsutism) lose hair. Propecia is not indicated for male pattern hair loss (androgenic alopecia) in women.

Cutting edge

High serum levels of macrophage inhibitory cytokine (MIC-1) have been identified as a new biomarker for predicting progress and prognosis of prostate cancer. Poor cancer survival was found to be threefold higher with elevated levels of MIC-1, and pretreatment high levels were associated with an eightfold incidence of cancer death.

The newest treatment modality for relieving prostate obstruction resulting from BPH is to "zap" the gland with green light laser. Photoselective vaporization of the prostate (PVP) uses potassium-titanyl-phosphate (green light) laser for bloodless prostatectomy. PVP lessens the risk for absorption of GU irrigant solution because the laser produces effective superficial tissue coagulation, but unlikely complications have occurred. The first report of transurethral resection syndrome was thought to have occurred in conjunction with injury incurred with introduction of the laser cystoscope. Another incidence of transurethral resection syndrome associated with PVP thought to result from a perforated bladder, was again unlikely because PVP carries a low risk of penetration through the fibrous prostatic capsule. These events sparked the recommendation to utilize normal saline rather than sterile water for irrigation with PVP TURP.

LUNG CANCER

Lung cancer is the leading cause of cancer deaths (both sexes) in the United States. In 2009 an estimated 219,440 new cases of lung cancer were diagnosed and 159,390 lung cancer deaths occurred.

Let's get the normal stuff straight!

With each inhalation the billows effect of the lungs (made possible by the diaphragm and intercostal muscles) draw air into nasopharyngeal passageways through the trachea to the right and left mainstem bronchus. From there air follows an unobstructed pathway to smaller air passageways all the way to the alveolus where oxygen is extracted in exchange for carbon dioxide, which will be exhaled.

- The lungs are divided into lobes: three in the right lung and two in the left lung.
- The lungs are surrounded by a thin double-layered serous membrane called the pleura.
- A thin film of serous fluid separates the two layers of the pleura, allowing the layers to glide smoothly over each other as the lungs expand and contract with respirations.
- Lung compliance refers to the ease with which the lungs are able to inflate with the incoming volume of air.
- Lung compliance is decreased by stiff lungs, blockages of the bronchi or smaller airways, increased surface tension of the fluid film in the alveoli, or impaired flexibility of the rib cage.

What is it?

Lung cancer consists of small cell or non–small cell (most prevalent) malignancies that usually develop in the lining of the air passageways.

Causes and why?

The single greatest cause of lung cancer (80%) is smoke from tobacco because of all the carcinogens contained in the smoke and the constant irritation.

- In 2006 the Surgeon General reported that there is NO existing safe level of second-hand smoke.
- Other causations are attributed to environmental exposure to carcinogens (radon, asbestos, arsenic, chromium, nickel) and air pollution.
- Obstructive pulmonary disease with low forced expiratory volume increases risk for developing lung cancer.

Testing, testing, testing

Noninvasive testing is the initial approach to diagnosis after the physical exam identifies alterations in breath sounds, enlarged lymph nodes, or enlarged liver.

- Chest X-ray to identify tumors or masses or bone metastasis
- CT or spiral CT of the lungs to identify gross pathology
- MRI to more precisely visualize layers with greater contrast between soft tissues in the lung
- Sputum cytology for microscopic analysis of cells

Samples of tissue or fluid are obtained by a variety of means for analysis by a pathologist:

- Fine needle aspiration (transbronchial or transthoracic) to obtain lung tissue, lymph, or fluid for cytology
- Needle thoracentesis to obtain pleural fluid for cytology
- Thoracotomy to obtain lung tissue samples and lymph nodes for analysis
- Mediastinoscopy for intrathoracic visualization and to obtain tissue and lymph node samples for analysis

Staging of lung cancer is accomplished with CT/positron emission tomography, bone scans, and MRI of the brain.

Signs and symptoms and why?

Lung cancer in the early stages does not produce symptoms, and there are currently no screening tests (eg, mammogram for breast cancer). Once the patient develops symptoms the following signs and symptoms are reported:

- Persistent cough that worsens rather than subsides
- Dyspnea and shortness of breath
- Chest pain that is persistent and constant
- Pleuritic pain on inspiration
- Displacement of the trachea by a large tumor or pulling of tissue
- Hemoptysis (usually expectorated after a cough)
- Persistent and progressive hoarseness
- Constant fatigue with a low energy level, which may manifest as a change in endurance
- Unexplained weight loss, anorexia, cachexia

What can harm my patient and why?

Non–small cell lung cancers comprise 80% of all cases and these cancers grow very rapidly and by the time of diagnosis may have already metastasized to the liver, adrenal glands, bones, or brain. Prognosis is not good. Five-year survival is only 15%.

- Patients with advanced disease who defer active therapies have little time for making final preparations.
- Length of time (before death) after hospice enrollment averages 24 to 34 days.
- Brain metastasis is the most common occurrence in advanced lung cancer.
- A small number of patients (3%) experience sudden fatal hemoptysis.

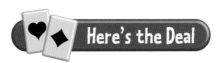

Here's the Deal

There are currently no recommended screening test for lung cancer, but results of the National Lung Screening Trial who accepted 50,000 patients for screening by the end of 2004. Low dose helical chest CT was compared with chest X-ray for asymptomatic patient aged 60 years or older with a history of 10 pack years smoking or more. The National Cancer Institute predicts that results of the study will be available before 2011.

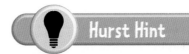

Hurst Hint

Sometimes the symptoms of lung cancer can be confused with those of TB, but remember that patients with TB also have night sweats, which are not present in lung cancer.

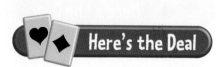

Here's the Deal

Respiratory depression (hypoventilation) is a rate that is less than 12/minute with a depth that does not adequately supply needs and results in increased concentration of carbon monoxide. This is not to be confused with hypopnea, which is decreased respirations that is expected when the patient receives sedation such as is given prior to a bronchoscopy.

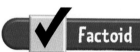

Factoid

Subcutaneous emphysema (also called crepitus) is air in the tissues under the skin covering the neck or chest wall that may appear as a smooth bulge, but when palpated makes a "Rice Krispy" crackling sensation as gas is moved about in the tissue.

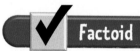

Factoid

Photodynamic therapy (PDT) involves administration of a photosensitizing agent with a specified distribution time allowing malignant cells to take up the agent followed by laser light activation, resulting in apoptosis (programmed cell death) of cancerous cells. PDT enables selective damage to be obtained because only the tumor tissues that rapidly absorbs the photosensitizing drug will be destroyed when light energy changes the drug into a reactive chemical compound.

Interventions and why?

During the diagnostic phase of lung cancer the nurse collects specimens and monitors recovery of patients who undergo invasive diagnostic procedures. Collection of sputum for cytology requires a sterile specimen in a sterile container:

• Collect an early morning specimen before the first meal of the day.

• Instruct the patient in the use of the sterile sputum container with lid.

• Instruct the patient to rinse his or her mouth with clear water to reduce the bacterial count.

• Emphasize that the patient's lips must not touch the lip of the container, which would contaminate the specimen.

Monitoring the patient following bronchoscopy:

• Keep the patient NPO until the gag reflex returns to prevent aspiration.

• Watch for complications, such as respiratory depression, hoarseness, dysphagia, or SQ emphysema.

• Notify the physician promptly upon detection of any of the preceding complications.

Treatment differs according to the two main types of lung cancer: non–small cell or small cell, further divided into adenocarcinomas, squamous cell, or large cell carcinoma.

• Surgery (lobectomy, pneumonectomy) remains the cornerstone of treatment for Stage I, II, and some Stage III depending on the location.

• Cisplatin is currently the drug of choice for adjuvant chemotherapy, but clinical trials are investigating others (see Cutting edge, this chapter).

• Photodynamic therapy is used for tumor regression in very early (Stage I) and symptomatic relief of very late non–small cell lung cancer.

• Second-line therapy uses docetaxel (gives estimated extended survival of two to three months) or pemetrexed (multitarget antifolate), which requires vitamin B_{12} and folic supplements and concurrent dexamethasone to reduce toxicity.

• Stage IIIB (T4-N3-M1^c) is treated with chemotherapy and radiation (with or without surgery) to achieve an average survival of 16 to 17 months.

The T-N-M classification system (tumor-nodes-metastasis) for Stage IIIB (T4-N3-M1^c) would mean that the tumor (T4) has invaded nearby tissue (mediastinum, esophagus, trachea, vertebra, etc.) and there is metastasis through the lymph nodes (N3) across the mediastinum, into the muscle and/or up the neck with distant metastasis (M1^c).

Older patients have the same survival rates as younger patients, but the incidence of toxicity to chemoradiotherapy is more severe. Palliative care relieves some of the distressing symptoms. Hopefully clinical trials currently in progress will translate into genomics that will target molecular markers for specifically tailored drug therapy to raise the current dismal survival rate and improve quality of life for persons having non–small cell lung cancer.

Nursing management of the lung cancer patient does much to relieve distressing symptoms and improve quality of life. Dyspnea is the most common complaint, affecting 65% of patients because the cancer occludes main airways and pneumonia and pleural effusions also compromise respirations.

- Administer oxygen therapy and monitor response.
- Administer prescribed adjuvant therapies of morphine plus benzodiazepines for anxiety.
- Stay physically present until anxiety subsides and breathing improves.
- Direct cool air vents toward the patient or use fans on low.
- Implement stress reduction measures and relaxation techniques.

Collaborate with the oncologist for screening and treatment for fatigue caused by anemia, pain, depression, or thyroid dysfunction. Other nursing measures to relieve fatigue are:

- Exercise! Patients who walk 10 to 12 minutes (or as tolerated) on a treadmill with nurse coaches can turn fatigue from a negative experience into a positive experience: a good fatigue with exercise as the cause (rather than the cancer).
- Distraction and relaxation during IV chemotherapy can consist of watching videos, listening to music with headphones, and unraveling challenging mental tasks such as solving mysteries or puzzles.
- Energy conservation and monitoring of response to activity, allowing rest periods as needed.
- Sleep measures such as manipulating the environment via temperature, noise, fresh linens, and hygiene (eg, bathing face and hands, oral care), back massage, and deep breathing relaxation techniques.

When the patient has a cough and hemoptysis, mouth care is indicated after each expectoration to reduce the metallic taste and breath odor. Other measures may be helpful to reduce the cough:

- Opioids to suppress the cough reflex and non-narcotic cough suppressants such as benzonatate.
- Administer prescribed steroids if pneumonitis is secondary to inflammation following radiation therapy.

Palliative radiation may be prescribed for pain reduction and PRN medications are given as needed:

- Combinations of NSAIDs, opioids, non-narcotic adjuvant medications, corticosteroids, and bisphosphonates.
- Evaluate the patient response, and watch the clock! Administer repeat doses regularly, before the pain can intensify.

Postoperative nursing care of the patient following lobectomy or pneumonectomy (Table 15-5) involves routine interventions such as obtaining vital signs and oxygen saturation levels; monitoring dressings, drains, or tubes; and positioning. (See Chapter 6 for additional nursing care post thoracotomy).

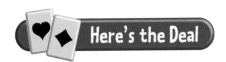

Here's the Deal

Intensive care monitoring is necessary following photodynamic therapy because of the possible need for emergency intubation and ventilation. Obviously the nursing priority would be monitoring for hemoptysis, bronchial hemorrhage, dyspnea from swelling of airways and secretions, and pleural effusion.

Table 15-5   Nursing interventions post-thoracotomy

Surgical procedure	Nursing interventions	Rationale
Lobectomy: A portion of the lung is surgically excised and chest tubes are placed in the pleural space for evacuation of drainage around the affected lung.	Position: • Surgical (affected) side up! • Elevate the head of the bed. • Change position from affected side to back at 2-hour intervals, leaving the head of the bed in a low Fowler's position. Maintain and monitor chest drainage system: • Note hourly drainage color and amount. • Report color change from pink to red or dark red to bright red immediately. • Report drainage of 100 mL/h or greater. Continuous cardiac monitoring as ordered: • Be alert to dysrhythmias. • Be alert to tachycardia greater than 100 beats/min and intervene per protocol or PRN orders. (See additional applicable interventions for thoracotomy).	• Lying on the affected side would compromise lung expansion and the remaining lung would fill up with fluid, resulting in pneumonia. • Change of position discourages fluid from accumulating in the lung. • Elevate the head of the bed to promote lung expansion. • Color change or increase in volume indicates fresh (new) or excessive bleeding. • Atrial dysrhythmias (atrial flutter and atrial fibrillation) are common following pneumonectomy. • Tachycardia is an indicator of hypoxia (especially when coupled with restlessness) or inadequate pain control.
Pneumonectomy: An entire lung is removed leaving a cavity previously occupied by the diseased lung. There are no chest tubes because there is no lung to drain.	Position: • Unaffected (nonsurgical) side up! • Avoid severe lateral positioning. • Elevate head of bed to 30 degrees when patient is oriented and stable. Note: There are no chest tubes (because there is no lung) and there is usually no water seal drainage. Escape of fluid by extravasation is desired because the resultant effusion eventually fills the empty space. (See additional applicable interventions for thoracotomy).	• Lying on the surgical side allows the only remaining lung to better expand. • Severe lateral positioning shifts the remaining lung into the empty cavity to create a mediastinal shift.
Thoracotomy: Surgical incision of the chest wall for above lung surgeries, open lung biopsy, or wedge resection in which only a small section of diseased lung tissue is removed.	Postoperative breathing exercises: • Deep breathe and cough every 1–2 hours during the first 24 hours. • Assist patient to sit upright and splint during cough. • Monitor all expectorated sputum for bleeding or signs of infection and report to surgeon. • Incentive spirometry for sustained maximum inhalation as prescribed. Monitor respiratory status: • Rate, depth, pattern • Breath sounds • Oxygen saturation • ABGs	• Breathing exercises and incentive spirometry help to prevent atelectasis by full inspiration and effective cough that raises secretions. • Upright position promotes lung expansion and splinting reduces discomfort of coughing. • Sputum changes indicate changes in pulmonary status. • Respiratory status may be compromised by ineffective airway clearance or hypoventilation secondary to pain or analgesic medications. • Vibration/percussion helps loosen secretions and gravity helps drain the lung.

(Continued)

Table 15-5 Nursing interventions post-thoracotomy (*Continued*)

Surgical procedure	Nursing interventions	Rationale
	Perform chest physiotherapy as prescribed • Avoid using percussion or vibration directly over the incisional area. • Stay in constant attendance to monitor patient tolerance to dependent position. Pain management: • Assist with repositioning or turn every 2 hours. • Use pillows to support upper limbs off of chest wall. • Supervise passive and active range of motion of shoulder and arm on the surgical side. • Administer prescribed PRN analgesics after determining location, character, quality, and rating on pain scale. • Monitor respirations frequently after administration of opioid analgesics giving reminders to deep breathe and cough. • Collaborate with surgeon for PCA pump if indicated.	• Patients with reduced ventilatory capacity may require immediate assistance during postural drainage if poorly tolerated. • Repositioning and maintaining proper alignment reduces muscle strain and fatigue. • Shoulder and arm exercises prevent painful stiffness and prevent frozen shoulder. • PRN analgesia is administered according to the patient's level of pain. • Opioids can depress respirations and lead to respiratory insufficiency. • Patient controlled analgesia allows self dosing at the onset of pain without waiting and affords better pain control within a safe, preset limit.

Source: Created by the author from References 9.

Define time

Wedge resection is named for the wedge-shaped section of tissue or mass that is removed. This procedure is commonly used for small areas of diseased tissue of the ovary or lung.

PATIENT TEACHING   Patient teaching is indicated for myelosuppression due to chemotherapy and/or radiation that is adjuvant to surgery:

• See previous teachings for immunosuppression.

• See previous teaching indicated with risk for anemia or bleeding.

• Teaching about community services available when fatigue necessitates help with personal hygiene and housekeeping needs.

• Teaching about the concept of inpatient and home care with hospice: options and advantages associated for self and family.

Cutting edge

Biotechnology applying the techniques of genetics and molecular biology (genomics) is becoming a consideration in targeted therapy for lung cancer.

• Clinical trials are underway using erlotinib plus bevacizumab (each having a different mechanism of action) as combination therapy.

• Other combination therapy for lung cancer in clinical trials is the anti-vascular endothelial growth factor receptor agents sunitinib and sorafenib (dual inhibitors: both previously approved in combination for other types of cancers).

- Researchers have found a DNA repair protein that may explain cisplatin resistance.

- Another tumor-suppressor gene involved with DNA synthesis and repair appears to be related to the effectiveness of gemcitabine chemotherapy.

These new findings are leading the way toward genetic blueprinting that may predict the patient's response to combinations of such agents in the future.

LARYNGEAL CANCER

The National Cancer Institute estimates that in 2009 there were 12,290 new cases of laryngeal cancer in the United States with an estimated 3660 deaths.

Let's get the normal stuff straight!

Structures of the upper airway (mouth, nose, oropharynx, larynx, trachea, and bronchus) are lined with mucus membranes, which warm and moisten the air entering the lungs. The purpose of the larynx (also called the voice box) is to protect the trachea and to produce sound. The larynx consists of three sections (Fig. 15-8):

▶ Figure 15-8. The larynx.

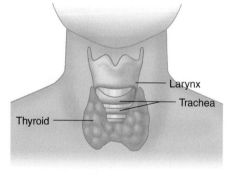

Larynx
Trachea
Thyroid

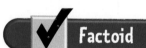

Audible voice is an echo of air forced through the throat, mouth, and nose.

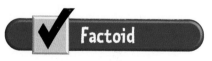

Vocal folds in the glottis vibrate, making sound as air moves against them.

- The glottis is the middle section that contains the vocal cords.
- The supraglottis is the area above the vocal cords.
- The subglottis is the area below the vocal cords that is continuous with the trachea.

The epiglottis is the "lid" that covers the larynx with swallowing to protect against aspiration.

The larynx branches into the trachea (also known as the windpipe) just below the cricoid cartilage (commonly called the Adam's apple).

- Cartilaginous rings (20 total) of the trachea hold the airway open.
- The trachea and the esophagus are two separate tubes—the anterior tube for air and the posterior tube for food.

- The trachea branches into the right and left mainstem bronchus, which comprises the air passageway into the right and left lungs.

What is it?

Cancer develops when malignant cells form in the squamous epithelium of the larynx. Laryngeal cancer can develop in any part of the larynx, but most often originates in the glottis, which contains the vocal cords.

Causes and why?

The majority of laryngeal cancers are caused by squamous cells that undergo change because of constant irritation from:

- Smoking and all other forms of tobacco use
- Excessive chronic alcohol use
- Concurrent tobacco and alcohol use (co-carcinogenic)
- Voice abuse, chronic laryngitis
- Inhaled industrial chemicals (sulfuric acid mist, nickel, asbestos fibers, paint fumes, cement dust, wood dust)
- Gastroesophageal reflux with chronic acid flow up into the esophagus

Testing, testing, testing

- An indirect laryngoscopy uses a local anesthetic spray to decrease gagging while a long-handled mirror is positioned to visualize the vocal cords.
- Direct laryngoscopic exam uses a laryngoscope with a light source to look deeper into the throat, focusing on areas that can't be seen with a mirror.
- A tissue sample may be obtained during the laryngoscopic exam for microscopic exam.
- X-rays, CT scan, or MRI may be performed for the purpose of staging to determine whether the cancer has spread to lymph nodes, the neck, or lungs.
- Positron emission tomography (PET) scanning may be used after treatment when recurrence of a laryngeal tumor is suspected.

Signs and symptoms and why?

There are no early signs and symptoms of laryngeal cancer. Once the patient becomes symptomatic, the cancer is well on its way:

- Hoarseness
- Difficulty swallowing
- Burning, such as when a patient swallows things that didn't used to burn the throat, but do burn now
- Persistent sore throat
- Swelling in the neck
- Loss of speech (indicates vocal cord involvement)

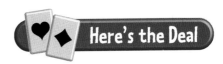

Here's the Deal

Swallowing causes backward motion of the tongue to push the epiglottis over the opening of the larynx, thereby preventing food or fluids from entering the trachea.

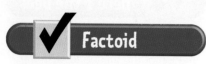

Factoid

The patient's ability to laugh, sing, speak, whistle, or suck through a straw will be lost when the larynx is removed.

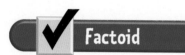

Factoid

Most malignant lesions of the larynx begin in the glottis and are squamous cell cancers.

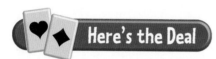

Here's the Deal

When malignant squamous cells of the larynx spread to the lungs, the cancer cells in the lungs are laryngeal cancer cells, not lung cancer. Treatment is still according to the primary cancer, which is laryngeal cancer.

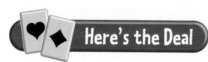

Here's the Deal

When the entire larynx is removed the patient will require a permanent tracheostomy or laryngectomy, in which the trachea is re-routed through the neck. This prevents aspiration because the epiglottis is responsible for covering the airway (trachea) during swallowing.

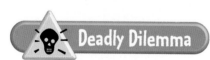

Deadly Dilemma

A pulsating trach is a sign of rupture of the innominate artery. Call the physician stat. This is a medical emergency.

- Mouth sores
- Bad breath (halitosis)
- Lump in the neck
- Color changes in the mouth or tongue (The patient may say that his or her dentures do not fit anymore.)
- Unilateral ear pain (The tumor is causing unilateral pressure.)

What can harm my patient and why?

Cancer of the larynx can have a major effect on eating, breathing, and speaking.

Alteration in nutrition occurs because of the effects of surgery and/or radiation therapy:

- Soreness and changes in smell and taste
- Difficulty swallowing (dysphagia)
- Dry mouth and decreased saliva as a result of irradiation of salivary glands
- Metastasis to the neck and lungs is common.

A number of post-treatment complications can significantly alter the quality of life:

- Development of esophageal strictures in the cervical region, which restrict the passage of food
- Development of a salivary leak and draining fistulas, leading to infection
- Dry mouth syndrome (no saliva), because of damage to the parotid glands

Postoperative "killer" complications can occur:

- Carotid artery rupture and hemorrhage because of the proximity of the carotids to the operative site, an accidental "nick" could occur.
- Rupture of the innominate artery with hemorrhage can also occur.
- Vocal cord paralysis is a possibility because of surgical trauma. If both cords are paralyzed, the larynx will go into a spasm and close off the airway.
- Respiratory distress caused by hypoxia, aspiration, airway obstruction, or tracheal edema.

Define time

A laryngectomy tube (inserted into the remnant of the larynx) is shorter and has a larger diameter than the tracheostomy tube, which is inserted in the trachea when the entire larynx has been removed. The tubes are a little different, but both hold the airway open and require the same care.

Interventions and why?

- When cancer of the larynx is confirmed by biopsy, the treatment may be either radiation or surgery (including laser excision) alone for small tumors in early stage disease (Stage I or II).

- Sometimes the decision is to use radiation alone based on the ability to salvage the voice, reserving surgery for treatment failure or recurrence.
- Radiation may be used prior to surgery to shrink the tumor or combined with chemotherapy for advanced laryngeal cancer.
- Cisplatin plus fluorouracil (5-FU) followed by radiation therapy.
- Radiation therapy administered concurrently with cisplatin.

Because of the proximity of the thyroid gland to the larynx, there is a high incidence of hypothyroidism after radiation therapy, so thyroid screening tests and possible hormone replacement therapy are in order.

When surgery is performed, one of four procedures may be done, depending on the stage and grade of the cancer:

- Partial laryngectomy is removal of the affected vocal cord, a portion of the larynx, and all of the tumor.
- Supraglottic laryngectomy is removal of the top part of the larynx—the glottis, the false cords, and the hyoid bone—or can be tailored to just the structure that is diseased, hopefully preserving the voice.
- Hemilaryngectomy is excision of one side of the larynx, which is split in the middle to remove one true cord and one false cord plus the tumor, leaving the person with a raspy voice.
- Total laryngectomy is removal of the vocal cords, the epiglottis and the thyroid cartilage, and two or three rings of the trachea.

Speech-language pathologists play an important role both before and after surgery. Voice and artificial voice options may include voice prostheses placed during surgery or at a later date, non-indwelling devices that are removed, cleaned, and replaced by the patient, or indwelling devices that stay in place until the need for replacement, which is performed by a medical professional.

- Battery-powered artificial larynx.
- Pneumatic (air-driven) device that directs tracheostomal air from a tube into the mouth to be expelled as speech. It uses the principle of the older method of belching air into the mouth to speak.
- Tracheoesophageal puncture uses a valve placed in the tracheal stoma to divert air into the esophagus and out of the mouth as the voice.

Even before the beginning the treatment plan, assessment of tobacco and alcohol use and psychologic readiness for coping with possible outcomes is fundamental. Input from the multidisciplinary team (oncologist, surgeon, nurse, speech therapist, nutritionist) is beneficial to support patient adaptation and an uneventful recovery.

- The patient is counseled and encouraged to quit smoking with referrals to resources known to be effective, such as American Heart Association "Fresh Start" program and toll free assistance at 1-877-44U-QUIT (1-877-448-7848).
- Pattern of daily alcohol intake is taken into consideration because of the risk for withdrawal syndrome (delirium tremens) during the treatment period.

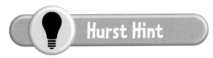

When the patient has a total laryngectomy, breathing takes place via the stoma.

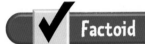

Voice prosthesis is actually a misnomer, because it does not actually generate sound, only the air needed to make sound possible.

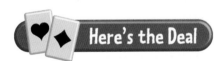

With a TEP valve in place, the patient takes a deep breath and covers the stoma (a hands-free option is also available); then the air goes through the one-way valve up the esophagus, where the pharyngoesophageal (PE) muscle vibrates to produce vocal sounds.

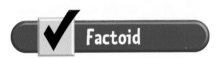

Patients who continue to smoke have shown lower responsiveness to radiation with shorter survival duration than patients who quit smoking in advance of treatment.

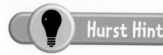

Hurst Hint

If the patient has a laptop, he or she is encouraged to bring it to the hospital to write notes and communicate with family members by e-mail. "Point to the picture" charts at the bedside can communicate needs, and a system can be established for yes and no. The peace sign (index and middle finger spread) looks like a Y for yes, and NO (two letters) can be signified by two blinks of the eye. Whatever is used should be practiced preoperatively and communicated in the nursing report.

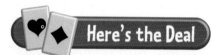

Here's the Deal

The remnant of the larynx or the trachea react to change in the quality of incoming air that is no longer being naturally warmed and moistened by the upper mucus membranes and mucus production is increased dramatically until the tracheobronchial mucosa adapts to this altered physiology.

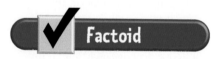

Factoid

Cold, dry air increases tracheobronchial mucous production.

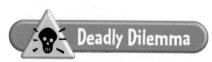

Deadly Dilemma

In the event of respiratory distress, do not leave the patient! Use the call button to get help.

- Preoperative evaluation and support of the speech therapist with input regarding aids to swallowing and speech.

- Alternate means for communication are established prior to surgery so the patient can make his or her needs known and communicate postoperatively.

- Options for treatment are explained by the surgeon and oncologist and reinforced by the nurse and speech therapist.

- The nutritionist evaluates preoperative nutritional status to plan for postoperative needs.

Ensuring a patent airway and protecting the suture line will be the initial priorities of care following a total laryngectomy.

- Postoperative positioning: Elevate head of bed 35° to 45° (mid-Fowler's) to reduce any edema close to the airway.

- Caution the patient not to try to talk (or use the artificial larynx) during the first days after surgery to avoid tongue movement, which could disturb the suture line.

- Provide alternate means for communication: small white board with marker or previously agreed upon signals or charts.

- Increase room temperature and humidity to offset thick mucus production that can potentially obstruct the airway.

- Maintain patency of the redirected airway (the laryngectomy tube or the tracheotomy tube) at all times.

- Gently and cautiously perform sterile tracheal suction PRN for mucus secretions.

- Clean the inner trach cannula (if one is present) every 8 hours per protocol.

- Exercise caution to maintain secure tracheostomy ties or manually hold the device in place when changing ties to prevent accidental dislodgement.

- Monitor respirations and pulse oximetry, being alert to early signs of hypoxia (restlessness and tachycardia).

- Be prepared for any respiratory emergency and ready to respond quickly if intubation or mechanical ventilation is necessary.

Suctioning tips:

- Suctioning depletes the patient's oxygen.

- Hyperoxygenate the patient before and after tracheal suctioning to prevent oxygen depletion.

- Avoid suctioning longer than 10 seconds.

- Remember to apply the suction on the way OUT.

- Have the patient deep breathe and cough, being prepared to wipe away secretions that are expelled through the tracheostomy.

- Initiate NG tube feedings to protect the fresh suture line. We want to protect the suture line from becoming disrupted by the muscle movement associated with swallowing.

Nursing measures to prevent complications (infection, hemorrhage) and promote healing:

- Clean about the stoma with sterile normal saline solutions and gauze squares.

- Provide frequent mouth care with a toothbrush and toothpaste to decrease bacterial count in the mouth and prevent associated infections. When bacteria build up in the mouth, they can travel to the patient's new trach site or go all the way down into the lungs to cause pneumonia.

- Monitor drains if any are present to prevent fluid from accumulating around the surgical site.

- Monitor the surgical site for bleeding, hematoma formation, and pulsation.

- Cover the trach with a bib for a filter effect (also patient preference for body image).

- Other treatments for laryngeal cancer include radiation and chemotherapy. (Review previously listed nursing priorities for radiation and chemotherapy.)

- Beam radiation is directed toward the neck; therefore, dietary and nutritional considerations are important because the salivary glands and taste buds will be affected.

- After a swallowing study determines that oral feedings can be safely started, the initial feedings will consist of thick liquids such as thick soups, pudding, and milkshakes.

- The nasogastric tube is left in place until nutritionally adequate oral feedings are well established.

- Even if the speech (and swallowing) specialist think it's ok to resume oral feedings, the nurse must stay with the patient during the first meal. The suction should be assembled and ready to use in case the patient has problems.

- When swallowing is well coordinated and less painful, collaborate with the dietician for soft bland foods moistened with sauces and gravies, because eating is difficult with a dry mouth.

- Monitor daily weight, intake and output, and 24-hour calorie count to determine the adequacy of oral intake.

- Nutrition is critical for healing, rebuilding healthy tissues, and regaining strength. If caloric intake is inadequate (calories and proteins) to prevent weight loss, a feeding tube may be placed into the stomach for nutritional supplements until the patient is able to swallow and/or regains interest in food.

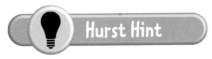

Hurst Hint

On NCLEX®, if you are asked to choose why the NG feeding is given, choose disruption of suture line. Always pick the "killer" answer. Painful swallowing won't kill your patient, but a disrupted suture line can cause many complications.

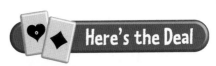

Here's the Deal

Any time your patient is NPO, he or she needs really good mouth care with a toothbrush and toothpaste (not with a lemon glycerin swab, which doesn't remove bacteria).

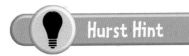

Hurst Hint

If NCLEX® presents this situation: "The patient's new tracheostomy is pulsating. Which action would you take? Call the doctor or check the vital signs?" Calling the doctor is the right answer. Although checking the vital signs is a good choice, it's not the best choice. This situation is a medical emergency; therefore, the doctor has to be notified immediately. In the real world, somebody would be calling the doctor for you while you're checking the vitals, but for the purposes of the test, NCLEX wants to know what YOUR priority is!

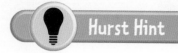

When selecting material for a tracheostomy bib, the priority is that air can move through the bib. Another consideration is that the material should not contain loose fibers (as can occur when cutting gauze squares), which can be inhaled into the airways.

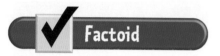

Commercial trach covers provide a protective filter. They also help some patients feel more secure about the appearance of having a trach.

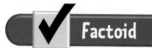

Soreness and changes in smell may cause anorexia, and the patient may not be interested in food.

PATIENT TEACHING   Teach the "Dos and Don'ts" when the patient has a tracheostomy or laryngectomy:

- Do not use powder (which can be inhaled into the lungs) around the trach.
- Use a humidifier to prevent drying and irritation of the membranes lining airways and to reduce viscosity of secretions for removal with coughing.
- Wear a tracheostomy cover (air comes in shielded bottom opening) when showering, and do not ever swim!
- Increase humidification in the home with a nebulizer or humidifier.
- Notify the health care provider for signs of infection at the operative site: redness, tenderness, or pus around the tracheostomy.
- Notify the health care provider for signs of lung infection: cough, fever, or coughing up purulent secretions.
- Stress the importance of handwashing before touching the stoma, or cleaning or removing crusts from the stoma.
- Have an emergency plan in place in the event of breathing difficulty or bleeding. Keep emergency phone numbers visible near the phone or on speed dial.

Cutting edge

Impressive results from a recent Taiwanese study (1999–2008) found that early laryngeal cancer (Tis, T1, T2 glottic cancer) using transoral CO_2 laser microsurgery not only preserved the larynx, but had a five-year survival rate of 97%, and almost half of the survivors demonstrated intelligible voice over the phone.

COLORECTAL CANCER

Colon cancer is listed as the third most commonly diagnosed cancer in both men and women in the United States, with 106,100 new cases reported in 2009. The staggering total of colorectal cancer deaths for this same period was 49,920.

Let's get the normal stuff straight!

The lower gastrointestinal tract is composed of the large intestine, the rectum, the anal canal, and the anus. The liquid contents of the small intestine, which comprises the middle GI tract, empties into the cecum, which forms the junction between the distal small bowel (the ileum) and the large intestine (Fig. 15-9).

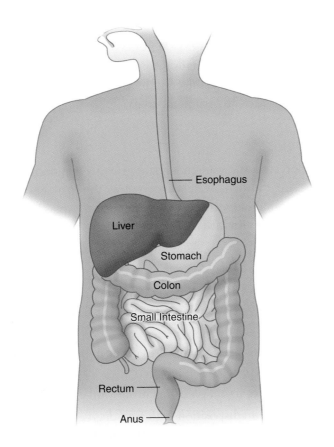

- Once liquid feces from the ileum enter the cecum, the ileocecal valve prevents backflow into the small intestine.
- The colon is divided into anatomic portions: ascending, transverse, descending, and sigmoid colon.
- The rectum extends from the sigmoid portion of the colon to the anus.
- Sphincter muscles of the anus prevent fecal incontinence.
  The innermost of the five layers of the intestine is the mucosal layer:
- Epithelial cells of the mucus membranes lining the intestine produce the mucus that protects and lubricates the inner surface of the bowel.
- There is a very fast turnover of epithelial cells in the mucosal layer (4–5 days).
- The layer of connective tissue underneath the mucus membrane contains vessels, nerves, and secretory glands.
- Two layers of muscle tissue (circular and longitudinal) contract to produce peristaltic motions, which move bowel contents forward.
- The peritoneum is a loosely attached, secretory membrane that covers the intestines.
- Serous fluid produced by the peritoneum makes the intestines slippery and reduces intra-abdominal friction with intestinal peristaltic movements.
- Ascites develops when peritoneal fluid accumulates.

- An apronlike filmy fold of protective mesentery containing blood vessels, lymph, and nerves is divided into the greater and lesser omentum.
- The mesentery functions to protect the intestines from cold and wall off any intestinal infection by adhering to the inflamed area to halt entry into the peritoneal cavity.

What is it?

Colorectal cancer are malignant growths that occur within the colon or rectum. Most colorectal cancers (two-thirds of all cases) occur low in the rectosigmoidal region and are adenocarcinomas beginning in secretory cells, which produce mucus or fluid.

Causes and why?

Most colorectal cancers begin as a polyp (a precancerous tissue growth), which undergoes changes over time. Risk factors for the development of colorectal cancer include:

- Increasing age (95% of cases occur in persons >50 years of age)
- Inflammatory bowel disease (Crohn's disease or ulcerative colitis) because of irritation from chronic inflammation
- Genetic predisposition with first-degree relatives who have colorectal cancer (the risk is increased threefold)
- Familial adenomatous polyposis (autosomal dominant) in which the person develops multiple polyps (adenomas) at an early age, making cancer of the colon commonplace by age 40 unless a total colectomy is performed.
- Constipation owing to retaining carcinogens in contact with the intestinal mucosal surface.
- Increased consumption of refined carbohydrates, high-fat diet, and red meats, especially those overcooked with high heat (fried and charbroiled). High dietary fat causes the liver to increase production of bile acids, which are converted to potential carcinogens by bacterial flora in the colon. Add high refined sugars to this picture and the bacterial flora responsible for this conversion goes to work overtime!

Testing, testing, testing

- Stool specimen for fecal occult blood
- Flexible sigmoidoscopic examination to visualize the sigmoid colon with a light source and obtain specimens for biopsy
- Colonoscopic exam to visualize the colon with a fiberoptic light source and obtain tissue samples for cytology
- Barium enema
- If both tests are prescribed, the colonoscopy should precede the barium enema because barium sulfate can cling to mucosal surfaces and folds, obscuring small polyps

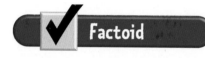

Factoid

Elderly patients and those with spinal cord injury are more likely to experience constipation secondary to decreased peristalsis and decreased innervation to the intestines.

Signs and symptoms and why?

Cancer of the colon does not produce symptoms for a long time, but the earliest noticeable sign is a change in bowel habits (constipation and/or diarrhea). Later signs include:

- Blood in the stool or rectal bleeding
  - Cancerous cells aren't well attached to each other, and the vessels supplying the tumors are fragile.
  - Trauma from the passage of stool causes microscopic bleeding that can be detected as occult blood in stool.
  - As the tumor grows it may invade a nearby blood vessel to cause massive bleeding, or the tumor itself could ulcerate and bleed.
- Anemia owing to chronic intermittent bleeding
- Vague abdominal pain
- Feeling of abdominal fullness
- Weight loss owing to caloric utilization by the growing cancer

If the growing tumor is large enough to obstruct the bowel, these signs and symptoms may be present:

- Nausea and vomiting, possibly with reverse peristalsis and foul-smelling fecal emesis
- Visible peristaltic waves across the abdomen in an effort to push impacted stool through the bowel
- Hyperactive, high-pitched tinkling bowel sounds auscultated above the bowel obstruction
- Hypoactive or absent bowel sounds auscultated below the bowel obstruction

What can harm my patient and why?

Colorectal cancer (men and women combined) is the second leading cause of all cancer deaths in the United States. Colorectal cancer can produce:

- Rectal hemorrhage caused by invasion of the tumor into local blood vessels
- Bowel obstruction caused by excessive growth of the tumor
- Perforation of the bowel and resultant sepsis caused by excessive internal pressure and/or poor wound healing
- Draining fistulas caused by leakage of bowel contents, which creates a tract (openings between the bowel and bladder or the outside skin)
- Metastasis to the liver (with jaundice and ascites), lung, or bone caused by invasion of the malignancy to nearby tissue and lymph nodes

Postoperative harm can present itself as any of these possible complications:

- Necrosis of ostomy stoma caused by poor blood supply
- Retraction of the stoma down into the wound
- Infection because of microbial contamination and wound dehiscence
- Malnutrition, fluid and electrolyte imbalance, and/or fatigue

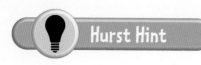

Hurst Hint

Ingestion of the hemoglobin contained in red meats can cause a false-positive result on stool for occult blood.

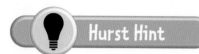

Hurst Hint

Bowel prep can be exhaustive and may cause severe dehydration in the elderly patient.

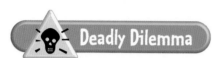

Deadly Dilemma

Retained barium can solidify and cause an intestinal obstruction!

Interventions and why?

Collect stool specimen for fecal occult blood (guaiac) or give patient supplies and instructions for home collection and return the Hemoccult specimen cards by mail:

- Refrain from eating red meat for three days before specimen collection.
- Don't mix urine with stool.
- Review the medication history for drugs that could cause rectal bleeding (anticoagulants, NSAIDs, aspirin), bleeding gums, or swallowed blood from recent dental procedures.
- Always wear gloves when collecting or handling a stool specimen! Normal stool contains many bacteria and fungi!
- The nurse may administer the prescribed bowel prep (or give written instructions to the patient for home bowel prep) prior to barium enema or endoscopic exams:
  - Have clear liquids for lunch and supper (no red Jell-O) the day before the test.
  - Administer the prescribed cathartic (magnesium citrate, X-prep, Dulcolax [bisacodyl] tablets), and Fleet enema.
  - Remain NPO after midnight.
- After the barium enema, it is important that the patient has a bowel movement, laxative, or enema to facilitate evacuation of the barium from the colon.

Nursing actions for bowel surgery:
- Liquid or low residue diet preoperatively to reduce bowel contents.
- Administration of bowel sterilizing antibiotic (such as neomycin).
- Hydration with prescribed IV and oral fluids (for unobstructed bowel).
- Hyperalimentation (TPN with lipid emulsions) may be prescribed if poorly nourished.
- Nasogastric tube (Salem sump, Miller-Abbott tube) to suction as prescribed for decompression of the stomach or bowel (if obstructed).
- Intake and output and daily weights to monitor nutritional status.
- Monitor abdominal and perineal dressings and drains (abdominoperineal resection).
- Relieve stress on the abdominal suture line by elevating the head of the bed 35 degrees and teaching the patient to splint the abdominal incision when deep breathing and coughing.
- Administer PRN analgesia as prescribed to enable patient to participate in postoperative activities (turning, coughing, leg exercises, etc).
- Assist the patient up on the bedside (first to dangle) and then to the chair on the first postoperative day, progressing to ambulation in the room as soon as possible after surgery.
- Assist and accompany the patient to ambulate in the hall (progressively increasing duration as tolerated).
- Monitor for return of bowel sounds, at which time the nasogastric tube may be discontinued.
- Encourage participation in ostomy care with the first dressing change (even before return of bowel sounds).
- Arrange for a meeting with an "ostomate" as indicated, and coordinate ostomy care with an enterostomal specialist.
- Teach ostomy care and colostomy irrigation if indicated.

The United Ostomy Association, which is available by phone (1-800-826-0826) or online (http://www.uoaa.org/) provides information and support for persons living with ostomies or continent diversions. Qualified members serve as "ostomates" to visit patients with newly created bladder or bowel diversions, offering encouragement, information, and support for returning to a normal, healthy, and active lifestyle.

PATIENT TEACHING   Early detection of colorectal cancer improves outcomes. Patient teaching should include the following means for primary and secondary prevention:

- Schedule a yearly digital rectal exam after age 40 as a part of the annual physical.
- At age 50 begin annual fecal occult blood testing.
- Schedule a flexible sigmoidoscopy every 5 years or a colonoscopic exam every 10 years or sooner if polyps are detected, or for high risk conditions.
- See your doctor immediately for any change in bowel habits or rectal bleeding!
- Increase dietary fiber by adding whole grains (cereals and breads), fruits, and vegetables.
- Increase protective micronutrients in the diet: vitamins A, C, and E.
- Eat less red meat, smaller portions of lean cuts, and bake, broil, or poach rather than frying or charbroiling.

Instructions regarding colostomy care and diet:

- Irrigate at the same time each day (preferably after a meal when peristalsis is increased) to promote regularity.
- Increase liquids to 2000 mL per day (minimum).
- Use prune or apple juice and increased fiber and fluids as needed for constipation.
- Select ostomy pouches and stoma covers (available with charcoal filters to deodorize gas) according to individual preferences and needs.
- When changing the ostomy appliance, wash peristomal skin gently using a soft cloth and mild soap, pat dry, and allow to air dry before reapplying the pouch.

Cutting edge

Clinical trials have shown that timing the administration of anticancer drugs to the patient's circadian rhythms has been linked to 50% greater effectiveness (in terms of antitumor activity) of anticancer drugs and a fivefold increase in patient tolerance to therapy (in terms of toxicity).

Colon cancer risk is reduced by removal of small polyps seen during routine colonoscopy and regularly scheduled follow-up in high risk patients.

The primary treatment for colorectal cancer is surgery which has a good cure rate if the tumor has not penetrated the wall of the bowel.

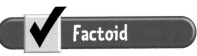

Do not take rectal temps on any patient who is thrombocytopenic, immunosuppressed, or post abdominoperineal resection! This is an absolute "NO-NO!"

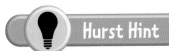

A gauze square can serve as a wick to keep drainage off the skin while drying.

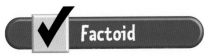

There are only two reasons for irrigating a colostomy: to establish regularity or to promote evacuation of hard stool.

Prognosis and treatment varies depending upon how far the cancer has advanced at the time of diagnosis.

The TMN staging system is recommended by the American Joint Commission on Cancer (AJCC) rather than older Dukes or the Modified Astler-Coller classification schema. The TNM system takes into consideration three factors:

- Penetration of the **T**umor through the muscularis (muscle layers of the intestine)
- The presence or absence of lymph **N**ode involvement (with a minimum of 12 nodes examined to verify absence)
- The presence or absence of distant **M**etastasis

Depending upon staging of the cancer, surgery (with or without temporary or permanent colostomy) could consist of:

- Bowel resection.
- Hemicolectomy.
- Total colectomy.
- Abdominoperineal resection radiation and/or chemotherapy are the cornerstones of treatment for colorectal cancer.

After excision of the primary tumor, adjuvant chemotherapy is indicated for Stage II, III, IV, and recurrent colorectal cancer:

- Adjuvant treatment with 5-FU is indicated with Stage II colon cancer (capecitabine has been established as an equivalent alternative to 5-FU and leucovorin).
- Adjuvant treatment with 5-FU/LV (leucovorin) is indicated for Stage III colon cancer after complete surgical resection of the primary tumor.
- Oxaliplatin (Eloxatin) plus 5-flourouracil and leucovorin (5-FU/LV) is the first line treatment of advanced colorectal cancer.

Follow-up monitoring using CEA levels alone to evaluate response to treatment is not recommended, and CEA immunoscintigraphy and positron emission tomography are being investigated as improved means for surveillance.

BLADDER CANCER

The National Cancer Institute estimates that 70,980 new cases of bladder cancer were diagnosed in 2009 with the most current US bladder cancer statistics at 14,330 deaths.

Let's get the normal stuff straight!

The bladder functions as a reservoir for urine, being attached to the kidneys by the right and left ureters (Fig. 15-10). The bladder is composed of four layers:

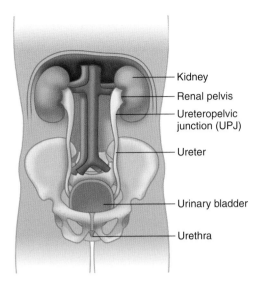

◀ Figure 15-10. Anatomy of the urinary system.

Kidney
Renal pelvis
Ureteropelvic junction (UPJ)
Ureter
Urinary bladder
Urethra

- The outer serosal layer is continuous with the peritoneum.
- The second layer of smooth muscle fibers make up the detrusor muscle which contracts when urinating to squeeze out urine.
- A third submucosal layer comprised of loose connective tissue surrounds the inner lining (interstitial layer) of the bladder.
- When the bladder is full, the muscles in the bladder wall contract to allow urination.
- Urine leaves the bladder through the urethra.

What is it?

Bladder cancer is more common in men than women and usually involves a superficial tumor that begins near the base of the bladder or in the neck of the bladder near the urethral opening. Bladder tumors most commonly begin in the inner lining of the bladder (transitional cell carcinomas), or as adenomas or squamous cell carcinomas. Transitional cells are named because of their changing appearance when the bladder is full or empty. These cells make their "transition" when the bladder is full by their capacity to stretch and to shrink when the bladder is empty.

Causes and why?

The single greatest risk factor for bladder cancer is smoking, because nicotine in the blood causes irritation of the lining of the bladder. Other sources of chronic irritation that increase the risk for developing bladder cancer are:

- Chronic urinary tract infections
- Recurrent bladder stones
- Indwelling urinary catheters

The majority (90%) of tumors begin in the epithelial cells lining the bladder when carcinogens excreted in the urine and stored in the bladder cause cellular mutations:

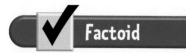

- Excessive intake of coffee, phenacetin, sodium, saccharin, sodium cyclamate
- Workplace chemicals that get into the blood by inhalation or absorption

Industrial exposure is implicated in the development of bladder cancer. The greatest risk for exposure is in chemical plants, rubber manufacturing and beauty shops. Painters, printers, textile workers, and truck drivers are also at risk.

- Chemotherapy with cyclophosphamide (Cytoxan)

Additional risk factors are related to age (> 40), gender (male), and race (Caucasians) as well as a personal family history of bladder cancer.

Testing, testing, testing

The cystoscopy is the most important diagnostic tool because the interior lining of the bladder can be directly observed and specimens can be taken for biopsy, which provides the most definitive diagnosis. Other diagnostic tools that can help to detect bladder cancers are:

- Urinalysis to check for blood in the urine
- Cytology to examine transitional cells shed in the urine
- CT of the bladder can detect a tumor
- Newer bladder tumor markers: nuclear matrix protein (NMP22 BladderChek), cytoskeletal proteins, telomerase (an enzyme put off by cancer cells), and adhesion molecules are the focus of clinical studies for early detection of bladder cancer in susceptible individuals. (See Cutting edge, bladder cancer.)

Signs and symptoms and why?

Painless intermittent gross or microscopic hematuria is the cardinal sign of bladder cancer! Additional signs/symptoms of bladder cancer are:

- Change in pattern of urinary elimination
- Dysuria
- Pelvic or back pain

What can harm my patient and why?

Bladder cancer metastasizes to the prostate gland, the rectum, ureters, and vagina. Deaths from bladder cancer are directly related to metastasis into adjacent organs as well as the periaortic lymph nodes that disseminate the cancer throughout the body.

Interventions and why?

Most bladder tumors are superficial, being confined to the bladder mucosa or submucosal layer with no muscle invasion, which allows these malignancies to be treated by transurethral resection (TUR) and fulguration. Follow-up cystoscopies are indicated because superficial malignancies tend to recur and progress in a small number of patients.

Fulguration (also called electrofulguration) is application of electrical current to destroy tissue. To prevent or postpone recurrence and/or progression, TUR may be followed by:

- Intravesicular administration (instilled directly into the bladder) of the bacillus Calmette-Guérin (BCG). BCG (immunotherapy) is particularly useful for transitional cell carcinoma in situ to prevent relapse.

- Intravesical therapy with thiotepa, mitomycin, doxorubicin, or bacillus Calmette-Guérin (BCG) is most often used in patients with multiple tumors or recurrent tumors or as a prophylactic measure in high-risk patients after transurethral resection.

  Intravesicular chemotherapy (directly into the bladder) avoids the systemic effects of cytotoxic drugs.

- Radical cystectomy may be indicated for invasive bladder cancer. This procedure in men requires removal of the bladder, the prostate, and the lower end of the ureters.

  In some cases cystectomy in the male can be accomplished by a nerve sparing surgical technique, but generally results in erectile dysfunction due to nerve damage.

  Radical cystectomy in women involves removal of the bladder, urethra, lower end of ureters, the uterus, fallopian tubes, and possibly ovaries as well as the front wall of the vagina.

- After removal of the bladder a procedure is necessary to divert urine. An older procedure is the ileal conduit (a non-continent urinary diversion):

  - A piece of the ileum is harvested to create a reservoir for urine.

  - The ileal segment is closed on one end and the ureters are attached.

  - The other end of the intestinal reservoir is brought out through the abdominal wall and a stoma is created.

  Advances in surgical technique have made more options available for urinary diversion that allow for continence, eliminating the need for external collection pouches to collect urine that drains continuously. Some procedures allow the patient to drain the internal reservoir with a small tube, and the most recent procedure creates a new bladder (orthotopic neobladder) that can be connected to the patient's urethra, provided that there is no urethral involvement.

- The orthotopic neobladder (a new bladder in the same place) is fashioned out of a segment of harvested bowel that is connected to the patient's own urethra allowing urination to take place by increasing intraabdominal pressure and bearing down efforts.

  Since nerves are cut the patient doesn't feel the sensation to void and must remember to urinate at regular intervals during the day.

- Indiana pouch or the Kock pouch (other variations are the Mainz reservoir) are internal reservoirs that are emptied by inserting a small tube into the stoma to empty urine, and must be periodically flushed (irrigated) to keep mucus flushed out.

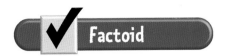

Factoid

BCG is a strain of the *Mycobacterium bovis* initially used to for TB prophylaxis.

Continent catheterizable urinary diversions and orthotopic neobladders have improved health related quality of life because patients have more control without hours spent in care of draining stomas, and the related skin complications.

Patients with metastatic bladder cancer can benefit from palliative radiation to improve symptoms, assist with cystoscopic procedure for intravesical administration of bacillus Calmette-Guèrin (BCG) or chemotherapy:

- Give preprocedural instructions: NPO not required. Set up table and prescribed antineoplastic agent, observing clinical protective precautions and using patient safety precautions. (See Table 15-3: methotrexate, 5-fluorouracil, vinblastine, doxorubicin, cisplatin, or docetaxel.)

- Have the patient void.

- Position the patient in stirrups and drape.

- Make the patient comfortable for the two hours that the agent must be retained in the bladder.

- Withhold fluids for two hours to avoid overdistention of the bladder.

- After voiding, force fluids to flush the agent from the bladder

- My patient will need interval cystoscopies to monitor for recurrence, and it is helpful to make phone contact as a reminder prior to the appointment.

- When bladder cancer is resistant to BCG, antineoplastic agents, or becomes invasive, radiation may be prescribed. (Review radiation precautions cited earlier in this chapter.)

- When urinary tract surgery is performed for recurrent or invasive bladder cancer, the priorities are maintaining urinary output, monitoring the patient, and checking incisions and dressings for signs of hemorrhage, infection, or complications.

- Monitor hourly urinary output after any urinary tract surgery!

- Increased fluid intake: 2000 to 3000 mL daily to flush out ileal conduit.

- Change the urinary ostomy appliance in the morning when urine output is lowest before the patient has anything to drink.

- The person with an ileal conduit has to drink a lot of fluids during waking hours to keep the conduit flushed out and the stoma drains urine continuously. Output is always lowest in the early morning because the patient has gone all night without drinking. If necessary, a gauze square can be placed in the stoma to absorb urine during skin care, but be sure to remove it!

- Never put anything in the urinary tract to clog it up! Renal failure can occur if urine flow is obstructed.

- Because the urine reservoir is made from a segment of intestine (mucus membrane), the urine will naturally contain mucus.

- With an ileal conduit, the patient's diseased bladder had to be removed and a portion of the small intestine was used to create a bladder. Ureters are attached to this portion of bowel tissue, which forms a pouch for collection of urine that will be diverted out through a stoma on the skin surface.

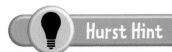

Hurst Hint

Always worry if the urinary output drops after urinary tract surgery!

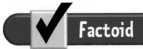

Factoid

Urine from any urinary diversion or neoileal conduit (a urinary diversion) will contain mucous because a piece of the intestine was used to create a new bladder (a pouch to collect urine), and healthy intestinal tissue will always continue to make mucus.

- Monitor and observe appearance of stomas, reporting dark mucosal coloration.

- A normal, healthy stoma should be beefy red, moist, and glistening. Nonviable stomas are bluish, purple, or black and dry.

- Report any hematuria after 48 hours, or previously clear urine that changes to become blood tinted after 48 hours.

- Empty continent urinary diversions (catheterization) regularly to prevent distention (and stress on suture lines) of the newly created internal pouch.

- Be alert to leaks in the external collection appliance and monitor peristomal skin for irritation.

- Report foulsmelling urine and obtain a specimen for culture and sensitivity as instructed.

PATIENT TEACHING   Care of urinary diversions, continent and noncontinent:

- Change pouch in the morning when urinary output is lowest (because the patient has not been drinking water during the night). Bending over several times can compress the conduit and help it to empty.

- Treat peristomal skin (pat dry or use cool blower rather than rub) very gently to avoid abrasions.

- Until a routine is developed, wear a watch with a beeper as a reminder to empty the orthotopic neobladder because loss of sensation can lead to overdistention and possible rupture.

- Mark your calendar for follow-up cystoscopies to monitor for recurrence to ensure a timely response.

Cutting edge

The results are in for a phase I clinical trial that administered 6 weekly treatments of intravesical docetaxel given to patients with recurrent bacillus Calmette-Guèrin (BCG)- resistant non–muscle-invasive bladder cancer. No other maintenance was given, and intensive long term follow-up (four years) found docetaxel to prevent recurrence in a select number of patients.

An FDA approved urine test with (nuclear matrix protein) NMP22 BladderChek (cost $20 per test) can be used for diagnosis of bladder cancer in high risk individuals.

Positive or negative results are available in 30 to 50 minutes without high laboratory cost or inconvenience. A Dallas, Texas study that screened asymptomatic, high risk individuals (based on age, smoking status, and occupation) using the NMP22 BladderChek detected a relatively small number of noninvasive bladder cancers verified by follow-up cystoscopy, although a some of those submitting to cystoscopy had normal bladder lining and others with normal NMP22 BladderChek developed later hematuria and small tumors.

Frequent dip-stick check in high risk persons for microscopic hematuria may continue to be used for bladder cancer screening tests.

STOMACH CANCER

There were 21,130 new cases of gastric cancer reported in 2009 with a total of 10,620 deaths during this reporting period. Historically Americans had fourfold increase in gastric cancer prior to 1930, but since then better food storage has reduced the intake of salted, smoked, and preserved foods and this improvement is speculated to be one reason for the current decline.

Let's get the normal stuff straight!

Everything entering the GI tract enters the mouth and passes through the esophagus to the stomach (Fig. 15-11).

▶Figure 15-11. Anatomy of the stomach.

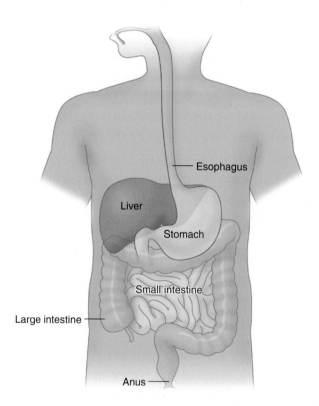

- The uppermost part of the stomach which connects to the esophagus is called the cardiac orifice because of its position near the heart.
- The stomach lies in the upper abdomen in front of the pancreas with the liver to its right, and the spleen and kidney to the left.
- The stomach has three layers: an outer serosal layer that is continuous with the peritoneum, a middle layer of muscle (muscularis), and the innermost mucosal layer.
- Stomach contents are churned by peristaltic contractions, mixed with hydrochloric acid and pepsin, and released into the small intestine.
- The gastric mucosal barrier (refer to Chapter 9) protects the stomach lining from autodigestion by the acid and pepsin.
- Gastric epithelial cells are tightly connected and covered by a water-resistant lipid layer that makes a barrier against acid.

- The fundus of the stomach is the rounded hump to the left of the cardiac orifice.
- The middle portion is the body of the stomach and the area emptying into the small intestine is the pylorus.
- Contractions of smooth muscle in the pylorus control the rate of gastric emptying.

What is it?

Gastric (stomach) cancer is a malignancy that begins in the mucosal layer lining the stomach and spreads through the other two layers as it grows. The majority of gastric cancers are adenocarcinomas (90%) of the intestinal type, which occur in the distal stomach and tend to become ulcerative.

Causes and why?

There are many identified risk factors for development of gastric cancer, but three top targets are age, diet, and stomach disease. Medical conditions that place the person at risk for developing gastric cancer include the following:

- *Helicobacter pylori* (*H. pylori*)
- Chronic gastritis (inflammation of the stomach) or atrophic gastritis that can occur after stomach surgery (Billroth II, a partial gastrectomy)
- Pernicious anemia and achlorhydria (not enough acid in the stomach)
- Intestinal metaplasia (normal gastric mucosal layer is replaced with cells that line the intestines)
- Familial adenomatous polyposis (FAP)
- Gastric polyps

  Other risk factors are related to diet, lifestyle, and family predisposition.
- Eating a diet high in salted, smoked foods and low in fruits and vegetables.

  The dietary carcinogenic factors implicated in gastric cancer are the N-nitros compounds and benzopyrenes in smoked and preserved foods.
- Eating foods that have not been prepared or stored properly
- Being older or male
- Smoking cigarettes
- Having a mother, father, sister, or brother who has had stomach cancer

  Partial gastrectomy (especially the Billroth II procedure) for benign causes may predispose the person to the development of gastric cancer; however, this risk factor is disputed.

Testing, testing, testing

When the patient has vague complaints that may be attributed to other conditions, initial lab tests may prescribed:

- Fecal hemoccult (looking for blood in the stool).
- CBC (will reveal decreased RBCs and anemia related to chronic blood loss form a gastric ulceration).

- Gastric analysis may reveal achlorhydria.

  Diagnosis of stomach cancer relies on tests that examine the stomach:
- X-ray (Upper GI using barium
- Endoscopic examinations: esophagogastroduodenoscopy (EGD) to visualize the lining of the stomach
- Biopsy of specimens obtained with EGD
- Cytology of gastric secretions (obtained by nasogastric tube aspiration)
- CT and ultrasonographic endoscopy used for staging of the tumor to delineate the spread of diagnosed gastric cancer

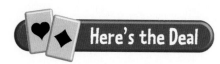

Here's the Deal

The gastric tumor occupies space, and the patient gets "full" very quickly because there is insufficient room in the stomach for normal sized portions.

Signs and symptoms and why?

Most stomach cancers are not symptomatic until much later in the course when bleeding gives evidence of ulceration. In the early stages of gastric cancer, patient's symptoms are often attributed to diet or aging, which delays treatment:

- Indigestion and vague epigastric discomfort
- Feeling of fullness after eating only a small portion of food
- Bloated feeling after eating
- Heartburn
- Mild nausea
- Loss of appetite

As gastric cancer progresses to more advanced stages, an abdominal mass may be present and more definite symptoms initiate health care intervention!

- Melena (dark tarry stools); blood in the stool
- Vomiting frank blood (hematemesis)
- Vomiting with coffee ground emesis
- Unexplained weight loss
- Stomach pain
- Dysphagia (difficult swallowing)
- Jaundice (metastasis to the liver)
- Ascites (free fluid in the peritoneal cavity)

What can harm my patient and why?

Complications of untreated cancer of the stomach:

- Hemorrhage due to perforation or tumor ulceration into an artery
- Cachexia (extreme malnutrition) due to malabsorption of nutrients and decreased ability to eat
- Anemia due to blood loss, malabsorption of vitamin B_{12}, and iron
- Hepatic failure and coma secondary to portal hypertension, because tumors occupy space within the liver

Complications secondary to gastrectomy, chemotherapy, and/or radiation:

- Dumping syndrome due to small stomach pouch remaining after debulking the tumor

   Surgical removal of the entire tumor is the only hope for cure of gastric cancer and this is only possible when the cancer is confined to the stomach. However, most stomach cancers are adenocarcinomas, which tend to recur in other places; so rather than performing a radical gastrectomy, as much of the tumor is removed as is possible, leaving a small pouch for food so the person can still eat.

- Vitamin B_{12} deficiency and pernicious anemia due to loss of intrinsic factor post gastrectomy

- Immunosuppression, anemia, and organ failure due to toxic effects of chemotherapy and/or radiation

Interventions and why?

The A-B-Cs guide nursing interventions when priority needs are threatened:

- Position the patient with ascites or anemia in semi-Fowler's position and administer PRN oxygen.

- In the event of hemorrhage, administer blood (whole blood or packed RBCs), blood products (cryoprecipitate, fresh or frozen plasma), and IV fluids to restore circulating blood volume.

- Monitor vital signs, respiratory, circulatory, and renal status closely and communicate findings to the primary care physician.

   For the patient who cannot eat:

- Administer prescribed TPN and fat emulsions observing protocols for care of central line and monitoring blood glucose levels.

- Administer IV hydrating solutions with multivitamin additives as prescribed.

   The patient with a gastric tumor (especially one near the pylorus) can become obstructed:

- Monitor for signs of gastric obstruction: abdominal distention, nausea, and vomiting, and stomach pain.

- Withhold food and fluids (NPO) upon recognition of above signs/symptoms.

- Insert NG tube and connect to intermittent suction as prescribed.

- Provide frequent oral care with hydration/wetting solutions and scrubbing teeth and tongue with foam toothettes/peroxide-based cleaner.

   In addition to the standard (see Chapter 1) postoperative considerations:

- Fowler's position to decrease stress on the suture line.

- Maintain securely anchored nasogastric tube to reduce movement or migration of the tube that could possibly interrupt the suture line.

- Maintain low intermittent nasogastric suction to prevent abdominal distention and nausea/vomiting, which would increase stress on the suture line.
- Monitor suction canister for change in color and amount of gastric fluid, and notify the surgeon for significant increase or decrease in gastric secretions.

A change of gastric secretions from dark red to bright red means fresh bleeding and increasing amounts indicates hemorrhage. If the secretions decrease significantly, the small pouch (possibly as small as 30 mL) could become distended and rupture at the incision site causing internal hemorrhage.

- Collect urine for Shilling's test when ordered to aid in diagnosis of pernicious anemia.
- Administer vitamin B_{12} injection as prescribed because the patient cannot absorb this vitamin orally.

PATIENT TEACHING For prevention and/or early detection of gastric cancer, teach high risk patients to:

- Avoid smoked, pickled, charred, preserved or highly salted foods, alcohol, and tobacco.
- Eradicate the bacterium *H. pylori* by taking prescribed medication for the appropriate length of time, followed by testing to ensure complete eradication.
- Be alert to vague GI symptoms (see "What's wrong with my patient") and report them immediately to initiate screening tests.

The patient with "dumping syndrome" needs help to maximize nutrition and to prevent distressing symptoms:

- Meals and snacks are to be consumed while in a semireclining position to allow gravity to help keep food in the stomach longer.
- Liquids are consumed between meals because more liquid contents empty faster.
- Avoid concentrated sweets and carbs because they empty from the stomach rapidly.

With postoperative loss of the intrinsic factor in the stomach, the patient cannot absorb oral vitamin B_{12}.

- Teach technique for IM injection using aseptic technique.
- Administer vitamin B_{12} injections weekly for 1 month and monthly thereafter.
- Notify your doctor if signs of anemia become apparent: fast heart beat, feeling cold, and being tired all the time.

Cutting edge

The field of endoscopy is advancing rapidly with many new therapeutics (such as chromoendoscopy, magnification endoscopy, and confocal laser endomicroscopy) but the most exciting advanced surgical procedures are

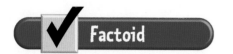

Shilling's test measures the urinary excretion of vitamin B_{12}.

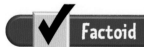

Vitamin B_{12} is essential for the manufacturing of mature red blood cells, without which the patient will quickly become anemic because of the relatively short lifespan of an erythrocyte (120 days).

endoscopic mucosal resection and endoscopic submucosal dissection because these are providing alternatives to the more radical gastric resection. And the best news is that select patients undergoing these procedures have 100% five-year survival rates.

Laparoscopic gastrectomy for removal of early gastric adenocarcinoma, commonly practiced in the east because of the higher incidence of gastric cancers, is infrequently used in the western world even though the less invasive benefits are proved and the procedure is deemed safe.

At the 2009 annual meeting of the American Society of Clinical Oncology, results of several clinical trials garnered much attention. The breast cancer drug, trastuzumab is responsible for the first increase in gastric cancer survival (26% reduction in death rate) when given for tumors showing high levels of the protein HER2. An added benefit for advanced gastric cancer patients in this phase III clinical trial is that trastuzumab added to standard agents for gastric cancer rather than being given in conjunction with an anthracycline (standard breast cancer protocol) had fewer cardiotoxic effects.

The treatment plan for gastric cancer depends on staging (depth of invasion, nodal involvement, and distant metastasis) but most commonly includes surgery in the form of a radical subtotal gastrectomy with or without chemotherapy and radiation.

The recent introduction of active "new-generation agents" is offering hope for better patient outcomes:

- Taxane based agents
- Irinotecan (CPT-11)
- Oxaliplatin
- Capecitabine

Docetaxel is one of several new-generation agents that are being combined with older agents for new-era chemotherapy:

- Docetaxel/cisplatin/5-fluorouracil (5-FU) (DCF) has shown promise in clinical trials.
- The "DCF" regimen (above) is being used in advanced gastric cancer in selected patients.

Radiation can offer relief of symptoms for the patient who has advanced gastric cancer with metastasis.

SKIN CANCERS

The American Cancer Society estimates that this year more than one million new skin cancer cases will be diagnosed in the United States and about 8000 people die each year from melanoma of the skin, the most deadly form of skin cancer.

Let's get the normal stuff straight!

The skin has three layers: the dermis, the epidermis, and the subcutis (subcutaneous tissue). The basement membrane divides the epidermis and the dermis from the subcutaneous tissue. Within the top layer of skin, the epidermis, there are also distinct layers:

- The deepest layer of the epidermis (stratum basale) is a single layer of basal cells from which all cells of the epidermis arise and change shape as they are pushed upward.
- Basal cells divide to form keratinocytes (squamous cells) that make a protein called keratin, which produces sulfur containing horny tissue (hair and nails).
- Melanocytes make brown pigment (melanin) to protect the skin from harmful ultraviolet (UV) rays.
- Melanocytes have fine cytoplasm-filled extensions that infiltrate the epithelial layer to pass pigment granules to the keratinocytes.
- The thickest outermost layer that is constantly shedding is the stratum corneum, which is made of stratified layers of dead keratinized cells.

What is it?

Skin cancer is a rapid unregulated growth of skin cells (basal cells, squamous cells, or melanocytes) that become malignant. Melanocytes are the cells that can develop into any one of the four types of melanoma (listed in order from most common to least common): superficial spreading, nodular, lentigo maligna, and acral lentiginous melanoma. Other skin nonmelanoma cancers develop from cells other than melanocytes. These nonmelanoma (basal cell and squamous cell) skin cancers are much more common and much less deadly since they rarely spread (nonmetastasizing). Basal cell cancers are of two primary types: nodular ulcerative and superficial, which is easy to confuse with other dermatologic conditions. Squamous cell cancers are also of two types: intraepidermal that remains in the original location or invasive, which can spread either slowly or rapidly with metastasis.

Causes and why?

Genetics and the immune system are implicated in skin cancers and melanomas, but solar radiation is more likely the major cause.

Basal cell, squamous cell, and melanoma all have one thing in common, sun exposure! Basal and squamous cell cancers are related to accumulated total ultraviolet rays (UVR) while melanoma is associated with intermittent intense UVR exposure.

- Years of unprotected sun exposure
- At least one incident of severe sunburn during childhood
  Risk factors for the development of melanoma are:
- Caucasian because light skin makes less melanin, which is a barrier to UV rays
- Youthful tanning bed exposure to UV rays
- Actinic keratosis (precancerous lesions) due to sun damage
- Genetics: family history of melanoma, red or blond hair and fair skin with blue, green, or gray eyes, and marked freckling on upper back.

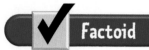

The squamous cell that becomes invasive may start as an itchy little rough place (actinic keratosis) and progress to a fast growing invasive cancer. Intraepidermal squamous cell cancers can be confined to the epidermis for years before changing into the slow growing or rapidly invasive type.

All squamous cell skin cancers should be immediately and completely removed as soon as they are detected because they are unpredictable: at any time a lesion may convert from a local epidermal lesion to the fast growing invasive type that penetrates the basement membrane, gaining access to blood vessels in the dermis which enables spread to distant sites.

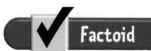

The bulk of lifetime sun exposure will occur during childhood, under age 18!

Testing, testing, testing

Diagnosis of skin cancer is confirmed with excisional biopsy with a 1-cm margin of normal tissue all around or incisional biopsy for larger lesions. Additional tests are needed for staging (determining the extent) of the disease:

- CBC
- Liver function studies
- CT scans (with or without contrast)

Signs and symptoms and why?

The patient may not notice an early stage lesion unless he/she practices regular self monitoring of the skin (see patient teaching to follow). The A-B-C-D descriptive system was devised in 1985 and a fifth sign (E) was recommended in 2004 to warn of dangerous lesions.

- **A** = asymmetry
- **B** = border irregularity
- **C** = color with uneven pigmentation
- **D** = diameter is greater than 6 mm (size of pencil eraser)
- **E** = evolving changes in a lesion over time (itching, bleeding, scales, tenderness, or any other noticeable changes in appearance)

The patient may present with a lesion that differs in size, shape, color that may be anywhere on the body. Refer to Table 15-6 for descriptive signs and symptoms of three types of malignant lesions.

CASE IN POINT   A woman seeking medical care for an enlarged lymph node in the groin area had no symptoms of any illness: no pelvic or urinary infection or anything amiss that could explain the enlarged lymph node. Upon biopsy of the enlarged node melanoma was discovered, but the primary lesion could not be found until a pelvic examination revealed the lesion hidden inside the left labia majoris.

Table 15-6   Characteristics of skin cancer lesions

Malignant melanoma	Basal cell cancer	Squamous cell cancer
Color: • Black or brown • Uniform blue-black color (nodular melanomas) • Dark pigment can be mottled with red (inflammation), white (scales), or blue (new growth)	Color: • Skin colored, pink (nodular ulcerative type basal cell) • Darkly pigmented in dark skinned persons (nodular ulcerative type) • Red scaly areas (superficial basal cell)	Color: • Red scaling lesion • In blacks the lesions are hyperpigmented (darker black)

(Continued)

Table 15-6   Characteristics of skin cancer lesions (*Continued*)

Malignant melanoma	Basal cell cancer	Squamous cell cancer
Shape or configuration: • Slightly raised edges (superficial spreading melanoma) • Dome shaped (nodular melanomas) • Flat (lentigo maligna melanoma)	Shape or configuration: • Small and smooth in early stages • Becomes nodular or nodulocystic as lesion grows • Over years, a dip or depression will occur in the center of the lesion with raised edges	Shape or configuration: • Slightly elevated lesion • Borders are irregular
Secondary changes: • May be red or inflamed and tender around the perimeter • Bleeding with rapid growth	Secondary changes: • Ulceration of the central area (nodular ulcerative type) • Ulcers are surrounded by the original shiny, waxy border • Raised nodular borders (superficial basal cell) • Telangiectasia (spidery little visible capillaries) develop around the base of the lesions	Secondary changes: • A beginning shallow chronic ulcer • Outward growth as the ulcer spreads to a larger surface area • Crusty exudates form over the ulcer • Borders become raised and red
Usual location: • Sun-exposed areas of elderly persons (primarily seen with lentigo maligna melanomas) • Palms of hands and soles of feet, nail beds, mucous membranes (rare acral lentiginous type only) • Nodular melanomas can occur anywhere • Most common male locations are head, neck, trunk, and arms • Most commonly occurs on female legs	Usual location: • Sun exposed areas of the body (head and neck) • Can occur on areas not exposed to sun	Usual location: • Sun exposed areas of persons with light skin and fair complexion • Non–sun-exposed areas in dark skinned persons • Most common locations are: nose, forehead, bottom lip, tops of ears, and dorsal surface of hands

Source: Created by the author from Reference 9.

What can harm my patient and why?

Many of the 8650 estimated melanoma deaths were related to metastasis to vital organs such as:

• Unresectable liver metastasis from melanoma of the eye
• Central nervous system involvement due to melanoma of the head or neck
• Lung metastasis from a melanoma on the back
• Lymphatic spread throughout the body from a melanoma on the vulva

Surgery for removal of large melanomas wherein a deep, wide band of tissue is removed and therapy that follows may result in:

• Obvious and visible disfigurement
• Numerous phases of reconstruction and skin grafting
• Adverse effects of radiation and chemotherapy (see Table 15-2 and Table 15-3)

Interventions and why?

Preparing the patient for excisional or incisional intervention, Mohs micrographic surgery, cryosurgery, electrosurgery after curettage or electrodessication, and/or radiation (see Table 15-7):

- Reinforce risks and benefits of the intervention (as explained by the physician).
- Monitor results of all diagnostic tests for evidence of metastasis.
- Monitor the patient for symptoms that could reflect metastasis: breath sounds, cough, dyspnea (lung), bone pain or pathologic fractures (bone), jaundice, abdominal pain, ascites, elevated liver enzymes (liver), changes in mentation, or LOC (brain).
- Provide nursing care based on the patient's symptoms.
- Provide emotional support through physical presence and therapeutic communications.

In addition to general postoperative care (see Chapter 1), the nursing plan will include:

- Management of pain due to surgical excision and grafting using diversion, protective positioning, and administration of prescribed analgesia
- Attention to anxiety and depression related to complications, metastasis, and disfigurement using therapeutic communications, collaboration with the health team, conveying acceptance and understanding of feelings, and utilization of social support systems

PATIENT TEACHING   Prevention must start early:

- Children must be taught to avoid unprotected sun exposure and to avoid sunburn by use of sunscreen and lip balm with SPF of 15 or higher.
- Avoid mid-day sun (10 AM to 3 PM) when UV rays are most intense.
- Avoid tanning beds and use of sun lamps.
- Wear protective clothing, hats with brims to protect ears and nose and long sleeves.

Periodic, systematic examination of skin to detect skin lesions early:

- Examine your body in a mirror from all sides, with arms raised, and lift any folds.
- Check both arms by bending elbows and looking carefully front and back, hands and palms.
- Check the backs of both legs and feet, including between each toe.
- Examine back and buttocks with a hand held mirror, looking at all surfaces including crevices.
- Examine the head and scalp with a hand-held blow dryer to move hair.
- See your dermatologist immediately for any suspicious lesion (refer to "What's wrong with my patient") that you can see or feel.

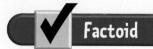

Factoid

Tiny little actinic keratoses are pre-cancerous lesions. They may be felt (rather than seen) as little, dry rough crusty places that form on sun exposed areas: face, neck, ears, back of hands, and arms and can be skin colored, pink, or tan.

Care of the local site of incision, excision, electro- or cryosurgery, or Mohs micrographic surgery and beam radiation:

- Keep incisional dressings clean and dry until advised to leave open to air.
- Be gentle and patient with wounds that heal naturally after electro- or cryosurgery, allowing tissue to slough away (no picking).
- Monitor for radiation dermatitis and avoid sun exposure. (See additional cutaneous precautions with previous radiation teaching.)

Cutting edge

While clinical trials of existing melanoma vaccines continue, the newest preclinical work by researchers in Houston, TX may prepare the way for a new immunotherapy modality. T-cells have been genetically engineered to recognize a ganglioside antigen (GD2) that is expressed on cell lines of most primary melanomas, so they can attack and disrupt the targeted melanoma cells.

After the initial staging, the treatment plan will be formulated, based on the type of cancer, the location, and extent and possible metastasis of the lesion. Table 15-7 explains various treatment modalities, indications, and implications.

Table 15-7 Treatment modalities for skin cancer

Treatment modality	Indications and implications	Complications and adverse effects
Conventional surgery: • Excisional (removal by cutting it *out*) • Incisional (cutting *into* tissue for removal of a part)	Indicated for basal cell cancer (BCC), squamous cell cancer (SCC). Some small, superficial malignant melanomas (MM) without metastasis can be excised. • Excision is the method of choice for removing small lesions where they can be cut away with margins that are safe based on the micro-stage of the primary lesion. • Incision is reserved for deep or large cancers whereby an entire full thickness of tissue is removed with closure of the incision. • Sentinel lymph nodes biopsy is indicated with deep incisional removal of MM or suspected invasive SCC. • Grafting may be necessary for incisional wound closure.	Excisional surgery is accomplished with local anesthetic. Incisional surgery carries anesthesia risk of and common complications of hemorrhage and infection. • A safe margin for a melanoma of 2 mm or less is a 1 cm radius around the tumor. • Incidence of recurrence depends on the type of lesion and the extent of growth. • May be followed with adjuvant chemotherapy. • Used in conjunction with IL-2 and investigational tumor vaccine now in clinical trials. • Effects of incisional surgery are related to the extent of surgery and metastasis to organs.

(Continued)

Table 15-7 Treatment modalities for skin cancer (*Continued*)

Treatment modality	Indications and implications	Complications and adverse effects
Cryosurgery: • Exposure of selected tissue to extreme cold (as with a probe containing liquid nitrogen) to eliminate abnormal tissue and cells • Destroys a tumor by freezing the tissue using a thermocouple apparatus and liquid nitrogen directed to the center of the lesion	Indicated for BCC and SCC • Moist tissues adhere to the cold metal of the probe and freeze. • Cells are dehydrated as their membranes burst.	A second treatment after frozen tissue thaws assures the tissue kill and afterward as refrozen tissue thaws, it becomes gelatinous. • Postprocedural swelling and edema are expected. • The dead lesion undergoes varied changes during normal healing by granulation. • Complete healing may take up to six weeks depending upon adequacy of local blood supply • Scarring occurs when the dermis is in the damage zone.
Mohs micrographic surgery (MMS): • Each layer of tissue is analyzed microscopically to ensure adequate margins of normal tissue. • Additional tissue is shaved and examined until only normal tissue remains.	The treatment of choice with superior cure rates for BCC and SCC at high risk for local recurrence. Indicated for lesions around eyes, nose, lips, and ears. The Mohs technique allows for: • Precise microscopic marginal control by using horizontal frozen sections • Maximum tissue conservation	Almost exclusively performed under local anesthesia, reducing operative risks. • Cosmetic effects are dependent upon the amount of tissue that has to be removed to obtain "clean" margins all around the lesion. • Low incidence of recurrence.
Electrosurgery: • Electrodessication • Curettage	Electrodessication is indicated for small BCC and SCC lesions (<1–2 cm). • The softer tumor is first scraped away with curettage (a spoon- or scoop-like instrument). • The base of the lesion is cauterized after curettage.	Repeating the procedure twice ensures removal of the entire lesion and cautery stops the bleeding. • Scars occur when the dermis is damaged. • Healing is usually complete in 4 weeks.
Chemotherapy: • Hydroxyurea and analogs (like drugs) • Dacarbazine • Interleukin-2 (IL-2)	Indicated for use in conjunction with surgical excision of metastatic melanoma to control the rate of growth. • Regional perfusion of chemotherapy is indicated for melanomas located in extremities, where higher concentrations of the agent can be attained while avoiding systemic and toxic effects.	None of the three FDA-approved agents for metastatic melanoma have had a significant impact on overall survival after melanoma metastasis. • Clinical trials are in progress using vaccines (immune therapy), tyrosine kinase inhibitors, and angiogenesis inhibitors.

(Continued)

Table 15-7   Treatment modalities for skin cancer (*Continued*)

Treatment modality	Indications and implications	Complications and adverse effects
Immune therapy: • Interleukin-2 (IL-2), a type of cytokine immune system signaling molecule that binds itself to receptors expressed by lymphocytes, the cells responsible for attacking foreign substances • Melanoma vaccines: Available in clinical trials only! Made from melanoma cells (proteins) vaccines help the body to recognize the cancer cell as "foreign," revving up the immune system to attack melanoma cells.	Treatment of choice for melanoma (after excision of primary tumor) or metastases to boost the immune system to prevent recurrence or to hold the tumor in check; compliments chemotherapy or radiation	Interleukin-2 combined with a melanoma vaccine has shown promising results in phase III clinical trials to double the length of survival.
Radiation: • Photon beam therapy concentrates on the focal lesion keeping effect to normal tissue low. • Carbon ion beam has increased cell killing effect. • Hypofractionated radiation using intensity-modulated radiation therapy (IMRT).	Indicated to achieve tumor control for locally advanced mucosal melanoma (head, neck, sinuses) and eye tumor (including uveal melanoma) and cutaneous melanomas after surgical excision. Whole-brain radiotherapy is indicated for brain metastases in conjunction with surgery, stereotactic radiosurgery, and chemotherapy to improve neurologic function and quality of life.	Once melanoma has spread, it does not respond well to chemotherapy or radiation. • Can cause acute toxicity and mucositis. • Can cause local erythema (redness) and blistering of the skin. • Better overall results are obtained with cutaneous lesions than with the more rare mucosal lesions. • The site must be protected from UV rays indefinitely. • Ablative dose can destroy surrounding tissue.

Source: Created by the author from Reference 86.

Once the skin cancer has been removed with progression halted or slowed, rehabilitation consists of improving cosmetic appearance (rebuilding ears, noses, lips, etc from donor tissue), releasing strictures from scarring (hands, feet, joints) as well as physical and occupational therapy with counseling and group support to help patients regain strength and confidence to return to previously enjoyed activities, work, and recreation (with appropriate sun protection). Lifelong monitoring for recurrence is recommended.

LEUKEMIA

There were an estimated 44,790 new cases of leukemia in 2009 with 21,870 deaths during this same time period.

Let's get the normal stuff straight!

Blood cells are formed in red bone marrow, the soft, fatty inner material found in the hollow of bones that supports growth of stem cells.

- A stem cell is an undifferentiated cell that can become different kinds of blood components: white blood cell to fight infection, red blood cells to carry oxygen, or platelets to aid in clotting.
- Myeloid stem cells produce erythrocytes, platelets, monocytes, and granulocytes (neutrophils, basophils, eosinophils).
- Lymphoid stem cells produce B-lymphocytes, T-lymphocytes, and natural killer cells.
- B-lymphocytes (B-cells) of lymphoid origin produce antibodies when encountering antigens in the blood.
- T-lymphocytes that originate from lymphoid stem cells in the bone marrow mature in the thymus and function to mediate cellular immune response.
- Natural killer cells (of lymphoid origin) seek out anything "not self" and launch an attack on tumors and viruses with their cytotoxic ammunition of perforin and granzyme to cause death of the foreign material.
- Leukocytes (granulocytes, lymphocytes, and monocytes) normally constitute only 1% of total blood volume.
- Neutrophils (granulocytes) comprise 50% to 70% of all leukocytes (white blood cells) and their primary job is to destroy bacteria in the blood.

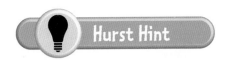

Factoid

T-lymphocytes (T-cells) get their "T" name for thymus because this is where they reside while maturing.

Hurst Hint

A neutropenic patient (not enough neutrophil granulocytes) could have a wound infection with no pus!

What is it?

Acute leukemia is a cancer of the blood forming stem cells and is classified according to the predominant cell type (lymphocytic/lymphoblastic or myelocytic/myeloblastic).

Acute lymphocytic leukemia (ALL) is primarily a childhood disease, less commonly affecting adults while acute myelogenous leukemia (AML) is chiefly a disease of middle adults. All types of leukemia are characterized by an unregulated production of leukocytes in the bone marrow with release of immature cells that don't function properly, crowding out normal cells. Either variety of leukemia can be acute or chronic depending on whether symptoms appear abruptly with rapid progression or evolve and progress slowly over months or years.

Table 15-8   Comparison of leukemia types

Type of leukemia	Characteristics	Complications/Prognosis
Acute myeloid leukemia (AML): • Primary (cause unknown) • Can stem from myelodysplastic syndrome due to abnormal development of myeloid cell lines • Secondary disease from cancer chemotherapy (see "Causes and why?")	Onset: without warning symptoms develop over weeks to months. Progression: The patient becomes very ill (infections, bleeding, severe mucositis, diarrhea) during induction therapy with chemotherapy in an attempt to eradicate leukemic cells.	Variable prognosis: younger patients fare better than older patients; those with pre-existing myelodysplastic syndrome have the worst prognosis with resistance to treatment. If secondary to alkylating agents survival is less than a year, with high incidence of septic or hemorrhagic deaths.

(Continued)

Table 15-8 Comparison of leukemia types (*Continued*)

Type of leukemia	Characteristics	Complications/Prognosis
Chronic myeloid leukemia (CML) • Arises from a mutation of the myeloid stem cell. • Blast cell production is pathologically increased.	Onset: gradual and insidious onset with few symptoms occurring in greater frequency with advancing age (55–60). Progression: Normal cells continue to be produced but the malignant cells continue to increase production of blast cells. During the transformation phase more and more lymphocytes are produced and the patient becomes increasingly symptomatic until the blast crisis of the accelerated phase becomes evident.	Prognosis: Usual life expectancy from diagnosis of CML is three–five years; however, once the disease converts to the acute (accelerated) phase it is typically followed by a terminal blast crisis. Death due to hemorrhage or sepsis commonly results within months of the acute phase. Cure is possible with ablation of malignant cells and a bone marrow transplant or peripheral blood stem cell transplant while still in the chronic phase of the disease.
Acute lymphocytic leukemia (ALL): • B-lymphocytes are affected primarily. • T-lymphocytes affected in 25% of cases. • BCR-ABL translocation occurs in 20% of cases.	Onset: Dramatically symptomatic because lymphocytes sludging in the bone marrow inhibit the development of normal myeloid cells and leukemic cells commonly infiltrate other organs and the central nervous system with meningeal involvement. Progression: When relapses occur, resuming the induction therapy chemotherapy regime can produce complete second remission.	More common in children with better overall survival (80%) compared with adult five-year survival rate of 40%. Bone marrow transplant is successful when ALL is caused by translocation of the Philadelphia chromosome.
Chronic lymphocytic leukemia (CLL): • B-lymphocyte malignancy results in identical mature cells lacking the programmed apoptosis, so they continue to be manufactured, but none die. • Most common form of leukemia.	Onset: Begins in the after 60 age group usually starting as enlarged, painful lymph nodes where immature B-cells get trapped. Progression: As the disease progresses, hepatomegaly and splenomegaly is common and treatment is initiated in late stages when anemia and thrombocytopenia develop.	Since the B-lymphocyte is a small cell, CLL doesn't have the pulmonary and cerebral complications due to vascular congestion seen in myeloid leukemias. The duration of the early phase is about 14 years and average survival is 2 years (or shorter for males) once the disease progresses to late stage. Autoimmune complications (such as hemolytic anemia and idiopathic thrombocytopenia) can occur at any stage. End stage autoimmune processes annihilate the reticuloendothelial system, red cells, and platelets.

Source: Created by the author from Reference 87.

Causes and why?

The cause of most types of leukemia is unknown; some are associated with bone marrow damage related to:

- Exposure to high levels of radiation.
- Chemotherapy (mechlorethamine, procarbazine, cyclophosphamide, chloramphenicol, and epipodophyllotoxins).
- Congenital disorders (Down's syndrome and Fanconi's syndrome).

- The human T-cell lymphotropic virus type I (HTLV-I).
- Epstein-Barr viral infection can lead to Burkitt's leukemia, an aggressive form of lymphocytic leukemia.

In most cases of chronic myeloid leukemia (CML) the cause results from translocation of two chromosomes:

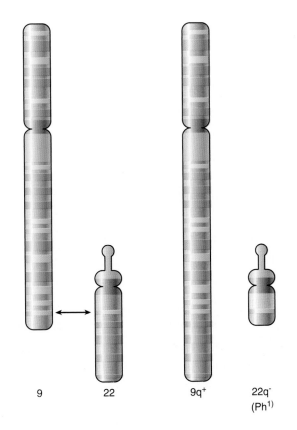

◀ Figure 15-12. Origin of the Philadelphia chromosome.

9   22   9q⁺   22q⁻ (Ph¹)

- Chromosomes number 9 and number 22 exchange places on their respective long arms.
- A large part of number 22 (see orange segment in Fig. 15-12) goes to number 9 from below the break-point cluster (BCR) (see pink dots in Fig. 15-12).
- The small segment from chromosome 9 containing a proto-oncogene of the Abelson murine leukemic virus (ABL) attaches at the break-point cluster (BCR) of chromosome 22.1

A proto-oncogene is a normal gene that codes proteins to regulate cell growth and differentiation. When the proto-oncogene translocates (as in the reciprocal exchange between chromosome 9 and chromosome 22) a hybrid protein is born, causing the normal gene to become an oncogene (a tumor inducing agent).

- A new gene code originates with fusion of these two genes (BCR and ABL).
- Unlike the normal ABL gene, the hybrid gene (BCR-ABL) has a new blueprint because it possesses tyrosine kinase activity which transforms genes.

- Once a single hematopoietic stem cell acquires the Philadelphia chromosome, its tyrosine kinase allows that cell to bypass the normal signals that control growth.
- Leukocyte production is out of control, and invariably CML develops.

Testing, testing, testing

Many times chronic leukemia is discovered accidentally when "routine" lab work detects abnormalities in the blood count (decreased normal cells and an abundance of immature "blast" cells):

- White blood cell count and differential
- Absolute neutrophil count
- Hematocrit/hemoglobin level
- Platelet count
- Bone marrow analysis (specimen obtained via bone marrow aspiration shows > 5% blasts)

Signs and symptoms and why?

Patients usually seek treatment within 3 months of onset of symptoms:

- Weakness and fatigue due to anemia causing decreased oxygen combining power
- Shortness of breath due to pulmonary capillary congestion from excessive leukocytes
- Weight loss due to increased proliferation and hypermetabolism of leukemic cells
- Easy bruising (ecchymoses, petechiae), bleeding tendencies due to thrombocytopenia
- Gingival hyperplasia and bleeding gums due to leukostasis and low platelets
- Low grade fever and night sweats
- Infection if neutrophil count falls below 500 cells/mL (diminished phagocytosis of bacteria)
- Enlarged spleen, lymph nodes, and liver due to infiltration and congestion of leukemic cells
- Abdominal pain from enlarged liver or spleen
- Bone pain due to expansion of the bone marrow secondary to proliferation of cells

What can harm my patient and why?

When leukemic cells cross the blood-brain barrier and enter the CNS, the patient may develop:

- Nerve palsies
- Headache
- Nausea and vomiting
- Seizures and coma

Following allogenic (from a donor other than the patient) peripheral blood stem cells or bone marrow transplants, the patient may develop graft-versus-host disease or possible complications from ablative therapy (chemotherapy or total body irradiation to wipe out all existing bone marrow and the malignancy) or from immunosuppressant agents given to prevent graft-versus-host disease:

- Life threatening neutropenic sepsis
- Hemorrhage when platelets fall below 10,000/mm^3
- Hemorrhagic cystitis, severe stomatitis, fluid and electrolyte imbalance from diarrhea resulting from high-dose chemotherapy or body irradiation
- Recurrent pneumonia and restrictive pulmonary conditions
- Formation of cataracts after total body irradiation
- Tumor lysis syndrome

  Acute tubular necrosis and renal failure.

- Chronic graft-versus-host disease affecting skin, GI tract, joints, and vaginal mucosa.

Interventions and why?

Provide supportive care during induction therapy (cytarabine, daunorubicin, mitoxantrone, idarubicin, etoposide):

- Administer blood and blood products (PRBCs, platelets, granulocytes) as prescribed for hemorrhage, anemia, or infection.
- Initiate bleeding precautions (see previously outlined interventions).
- Administer granulocytic growth factors (Neupogen or Leukine) for significant neutropenia to stimulate bone marrow production of leukocytes.
- Initiate protective isolation (see earlier precautions outlined for immunosuppressed patients).

  Postremission therapy (when neutrophil and platelet counts return to normal)

- Administer treatment cycles (usually lower dose) of cytarabines.
- Monitor intake and output.
- Maintain high fluid intake and administer allopurinol as prescribed to avoid urate nephropathy.
- Monitor uric acid levels.
- Notify physician if granulocyte count is below 1000/mm^3 or platelets are less than 50,000/mm^3.
- Provide diligent mouth care to help prevent stomatitis.
- Monitor for signs/symptoms of infection (fever, sore throat, fatigue).

  Following bone marrow transplant, monitor for signs or effects of graft-versus-host disease:

- Chills, fever
- Shortness of breath, dyspnea
- Tachycardia and chest pain
- Instability of blood pressure (hypotension or hypertension)

- Fluid retention, ascites, abdominal tenderness (hepatomegaly), jaundice
- Signs of CNS involvement (encephalopathy)

When the patient has an infection (bacterial, viral, fungal, protozoan):

- Obtain appropriate specimens for culture and sensitivity and notify physician of results promptly.
- Administer prescribed antibiotic therapy and monitor patient response.

PATIENT TEACHING   Patient teaching is indicated because of risk for infection and risk for bleeding previously outlined with introductory general guidelines and chemotherapy (Table 15-3).

Cutting edge

Eat sugar and die! Most treatment protocols call for the addition of a glucocorticoid (a sugar based steroid, and adding low doses of 2-deoxy-glucose (2-DG). This adds an extra punch for the big knockout! It is well known that glucocorticoids decrease glycolytic enzymes and thereby raise blood sugar, and coadministration of 2-DG inhibits glycolysis causing transient hyperglycemia. Upon cellular uptake, 2-DG is immediately changed by the enzyme hexokinase (with the addition of 6-phosphate) and has the effect on the leukemic cell of decreasing energy metabolism and increasing mitochondrial susceptibility to damage. Pow! The synergistic action of the glucocorticoid plus the 2-deoxy-glucose adds killing power, enhancing apoptosis of the malignant cells.

The patient with acute myelogenous leukemia (AML) (also called acute nonlymphocytic leukemia) needs a sufficiently aggressive induction regimen to effect complete remission because partial remission does not increase survival. When AML is related to alkylating agents it usually makes its appearance five to six years after exposure to the mutagenic agent, and the patient initially has symptoms of bone marrow failure but later develops myelodysplastic syndrome, which has a high mortality rate. The following treatment regimens are commonly used for AML:

- A two-drug regimen (daunorubicin in conjunction with cytarabine) produces a 65% response rate.
- When patients are at high risk for treatment failure, even though high dose cytarabine is controversial, it has been shown to prolong disease-free survival.
- In younger adults idarubicin may be the preferred agent over daunorubicin.
- Sometimes a third drug (thioguanine or etoposide) is added to the combination to improve response duration.
- Patients who develop myelodysplasia secondary to cytotoxic chemotherapy seem to do just as well with allogenic bone marrow transplantation without the adverse and toxic effects of induction chemotherapy.
- Low dose cytarabine for older adults may be a more acceptable option than intensive remission induction therapy and has a better survival rate than hydroxyurea.

Lymphoid blast cells are very responsive to vinca alkaloids and corticosteroids, therefore initial treatment for acute lymphoblastic leukemia (ALL) consists of a combination of vincristine, prednisone, and anthracycline. Asparaginase may or may not be included in the initial combination therapy. The goal of induction therapy is complete remission, which occurs in 80% of cases but many times duration is only approximately 15 months and when relapse occurs, prognosis is not good. If the patient is less than 55 years of age and a suitable donor is available, bone marrow transplant may provide an option for disease management.

Peripheral blood stem cell transplant from a donor is safe and cost effective. Bone marrow transplant may be autologous (from the patient), allogenic (from a family member or a matched donor (available from the national registry or cord blood registry), or syngeneic (from an identical twin). Immunosuppressant drugs (cyclosporine, tacrolimus, or sirolimus) are administered to allogenic transplant recipients to prevent graft-versus-host disease.

PRACTICE QUESTIONS

1. Which patient teaching is appropriate for secondary prevention of cancer?

    A. Perform a monthly breast self-exam beginning at age 20 to 25.

    B. Use sunscreen when engaging in outdoor activities, even on cloudy days.

    C. Have a baseline mammogram (2 views) at age 35 to 40, and yearly thereafter.

    D. Avoid first-hand or second-hand smoking and the use of tobacco in any form.

2. Which focus for patient teaching might result in a decreased incidence of bladder cancer?

    A. Stop smoking.

    B. Limit pickled meats.

    C. Reduce dietary alkalines.

    D. Increase daily fluid intake to 2500 mL.

3. Which component of the nursing care plan would be inappropriate for the patient who has a temporary sealed radiation implant in the uterus?

    A. Offer a low-residue diet.

    B. Restrict all visitors.

    C. Administer antidiarrheal agents.

    D. Maintain bedrest and log-roll for position change.

4. A sealed radioactive uterine implant is found in the patient's bed during routine Foley catheter care. Which next nursing action is priority?

   A. Place the implant in a plastic Ziploc specimen bag for removal from the room.

   B. Finish catheter care, change gloves, and call the nuclear medicine department from the patient's room phone.

   C. After completing catheter care, wrap the implant in four thicknesses of blanket material and place in the restroom with the door closed.

   D. Cover the patient and caution her not to move, and then leave the room to notify nuclear medicine that a container is needed for implant removal.

5. Which statement by a new mother following brachytherapy using an unsealed radioactive source would indicate the priority need for further discharge teaching?

   A. My parents are keeping our new baby for the next 48 hours.

   B. My husband can deliver pumped breast milk to our new baby.

   C. My husband and I will sleep in separate bedrooms for the next 72 hours.

   D. I will refrain from using the microwave and my computer for the next two days.

6. Immediately following bronchoscopy with monitored anesthesia care using propofol (Diprivan), which nursing assessment would be a cause for alarm?

   A. Loss of the gag reflex

   B. Respiratory depression

   C. Decreased mental alertness

   D. Expectoration of blood streaked sputum

7. Following mastectomy with dissection of lymph nodes, the patient complains of a "tight feeling" underneath the pressure dressing that was applied in surgery. There is a small amount of bright red blood in the bulb of the JP drain. Which next action by the nurse is priority?

   A. Notify the physician of this subjective complaint.

   B. Remove the dressing to assess the surgical incision.

   C. Obtain vital signs and repeat in 15 minutes for comparison.

   D. Reassure the patient that a pressure dressing always feels snug.

8. Which of the following measures is the most effective primary prevention of cancer in women?

   A. Referral to a smoking cessation program.

   B. HPV quadrivalent vaccination at an early age.

Hurst Hint

When answering priority questions always pick the "killer" answer! If you pick a wrong answer that does not cause any harm, you will receive another question at the same level of difficulty. The question is still counted as a "miss" but you are not penalized with CAT (computer adaptive testing).

C. High school health classes promoting sexual abstinence.

D. Routine gynecological exams and pap smear for evaluation.

9. Which statement(s) by a patient(s) in the gynecologic clinic would require further teaching by the clinic nurse?

   A. Patients B and D both require further teaching.

   B. A postmenopausal woman states that she will continue to have regular pap smear tests every two to three years.

   C. A sexually active 13-year-old desiring birth control pills states that she should have a first pap smear at age 18.

   D. A 20-year-old woman with a low-grade squamous intraepithelial lesion states that she hopes the scheduled six-month colposcopy will reveal normal tissue.

10. A patient with leukemia is receiving high dose induction therapy with cytarabine (Tarabine PFS). Several hours after the initial dose, the patient complains of both eyes "jumping" while he is trying to watch television. Which action by the nurse is priority?

    A. Notify the prescribing physician.

    B. Turn off the television and dim the lights.

    C. Ask the patient to place cupped hands over tightly closed eyes.

    D. Tell the patient that this is a common side effect of the chemotherapy.

References

1. Beers MH, ed. Diabetes. *The Merck Manual of Medical Information.* Whitestation, NJ: Merck Research Laboratories; 2003.

2. MedicineNet Search. T-cell immune response. Available at http://search.medicinenet.com/search/search_results/default.aspx?Searchwhat=1&query=T-cells&I1.x=36&I1.y=1. Accessed September 15, 2009.

3. Maggee, E. The super veggies: cruciferous vegetables. *WebMD.* Available at http://www.webmd.com/food-recipes/news/20070419/super-veggies-cruciferous-vegetables. Accessed September 11, 2009.

4. National Cancer Institute. Ovarian cancer screening using ultrasound and CA125 finds both early and late stage cancers, but also many false positives. Available at http://www.cancer.gov/newscenter/pressreleases/PLCOOvarian2005Release.

5. Bohnenkamp S, LeBaron V, Yoder LH. The medical-surgical nurse's guide to ovarian cancer: Part II. *Medsurg Nurs 16*(6): 323–331, 2007.

6. American Cancer Society. Cancer statistics. Available at http://www.cancer.org/docroot/STT/stt_0.asp. Accessed September 12, 2009.

7. American Cancer Society. Eating lots of red meat linked to colon cancer. Available at http://www.cancer.org/docroot/NWS/content/

NWS_1_1x_Eating_Lots_of_Red_Meat_Linked_to_Colon_Cancer. Accessed October 5, 2009.

8. American Cancer Society. Prevention and early detection: Environmental carcinogens. Available at http://www.cancer.org/docroot/PED/ped_1_1.asp. Accessed September 27, 2009.

9. Hurst M. A critical thinking and application NCLEX Review. Brookhaven, MS: Hurst Review Services; 2008.

10. American Cancer Society. Seven warning signs of cancer. Available at http://www.cancer.org/docroot/CRI/content/CRI_2_4_3X_What_are_the_signs_and_symptoms_of_cancer.asp. Accessed September 12, 2009.

11. American Cancer Society. Cancer facts and figures 2008. Available at http://www.cancer.org/downloads/STT/2008CAFFfinalsecured.pdf

12. La TH, Minn AY, Su Z, et al. Multimodality treatment with intensity modulated radiation therapy for esophageal cancer. *Dis Esophagus* 23(4):300–308, 2010 [Epub ahead of print]. Available at http://www.ncbi.nlm.nih.gov/pubmed/19732129?ordinalpos=33&itool=EntrezSystem2.PEntrez.Pubmed.Pubmed_ResultsPanel.Pubmed_DefaultReportPanel.Pubmed_RVDocSum. Accessed September 15, 2009.

13. National Cancer Institute. Fact sheet: Tumor staging. Available at http://www.cancer.gov/cancertopics/factsheet/Detection/staging. Accessed September 20, 2009.

14. National Cancer Institute. Fact sheet: Tumor grading. Available at http://www.cancer.gov/cancertopics/factsheet/Detection/tumor-grade. Accessed September 20, 2009.

15. Stonecypher K. Going around in circles: Is this the best practice for preparing the skin? *Crit Care Nurs Q 32*(2):94–98, 2009.

16. Kelly SS, Wheatley, D. Prevention of febrile neutropenia: Use of granulocyte colony-stimulating factors. *Br J Cancer 101*(S):S6–S10, 2009.

17. Comerford K C, Labus D, eds. *Nursing 2010 Drug Handbook.* Wolters Kluwer/Lippincott Williams & Wilkins: Philadelphia; 2010.

18. World Health Organization. WHO's pain ladder. Available at http://www.who.int/cancer/palliative/painladder/en/. Accessed September 21, 2009.

19. Rockwell S, Dorbucki IT, Kim EY, et al. Hypoxia and radiation therapy: past history, ongoing research and future promise. *Curr Mol Med 9*(4):442–458, 2009.

20. National Cancer Institute. Cancer topics: Breast cancer. Available at http://www.cancer.gov/cancertopics/types/breast. Accessed September 28, 2009.

21. Breast Cancer.org. Symptoms and diagnosis: Types of breast cancer. Available at http://www.breastcancer.org/symptoms/types/. Accessed September 28, 2009.

22. American Cancer Society. What is breast cancer in men? Available at http://www.cancer.org/docroot/CRI/content/CRI_2_4_1X_What_is_male_breast_cancer_28.asp. Accessed October 3, 2009.

23. National Cancer Institute. Breast cancer screening and testing. Available at http://www.cancer.gov/cancertopics/screening/Breast. Accessed October 8, 2009.

24. American Cancer Society. After the tests: Staging. Available at http://www.cancer.org/docroot/CRI/content/CRI_2_2_3X_After_the_tests_Staging_5.asp?sitearea. Accessed October 8, 2009.

25. Fu MR, Ridner SH, Armer J. Lymphedema post-breast cancer: Part 2. *AJN 109*(8):34–41, 2009.

26. National Cancer Institute. Metastatic cancer: Questions and answers. Available at http://www.cancer.gov/cancertopics/factsheet/Sites-Types/metastatic. Accessed October 3, 2009.

27. Fu MR, Ridner SH, Armer J. Lymphedema post-breast cancer: Part 1. *AJN, 109*(7):48–54, 2009.

28. American Cancer Society. Lymphedema: What every woman with breast cancer should know. Available at http://www.cancer.org/docroot/MIT/content/MIT_7_2x_Lymphedema_and_Breast_Cancer.asp. Accessed October 7, 2009.

29. National Cancer Institute. Managing lymphedema. Available at http://www.cancer.gov/cancertopics/pdq/supportivecare/lymphedema/Patient/page2. Accessed October 7, 2009.

30. National Lymphedema Network Medical Advisory Committee. Position statement of the National Lymphedema Network: Lymphedema risk and reduction practices. Available at http://www.lymphnet.org/pdfDocs/nlnriskreduction.pdf. Accessed October 7, 2009.

31. Boneti C, Korourian S, Diaz, Z, et al. Scientific Impact Award: Axillary node reverse mapping (ARM) to identify and protect lymphatics draining the arm during axillary lymphadenectomy. *Am J Surg 198*(4):482–487, 2009.

32. Sparano JA, Hortobagyi GN, Gralow JR, et al. Recommendations for research priorities in breast cancer by the Coalition of Cancer Cooperative Groups Scientific Leadership Council: Systemic therapy and therapeutic individualization. *Breast Cancer Res Treat 119*(3):511–527, 2010. Advance online publication. doi:10.1007/s10549-009-0433-y.

33. Martens JE, Smedts F, van Muyden R, et al. Reserve cells in human uterine cervical epithelium are derived from müllerian epithelium at midgestational age. *Int J Gynecol Pathol 26*(4):463–468, 2007.

34. Medeiros LR, Rosa DD, da Rosa MI, et al. Efficacy of human papillomavirus vaccines: A systematic quantitative review. *Int J Gynecol Cancer 19*(7):1166–1176, 2009.

35. National Cancer Institute. What you need to know about cancer of the uterus. Available at http://www.cancer.gov/cancertopics/wyntk/uterus. Accessed October 15, 2009.

36. National Cancer Institute. Cervical cancer. Available at http://www.cancer.gov/cancertopics/types/cervical/. Accessed October 27, 2009.

37. Burnett AF, Stone PJ, Duckworth LA, Roman JJ. Robotic radical trachelectomy for preservation of fertility in early cervical cancer: Case series and description of technique. *J Minim Invasive Gynecol* *16*(5):569–572, 2009.

38. National Cancer Institute. Testicular cancer: Questions and answers. Available at http://www.cancer.gov/cancertopics/factsheet/Sites-Types/testicular. Accessed October, 2, 2009.

39. MayoClinic.com. Testicular self exam. Available at http://www.mayoclinic.com/health/medical/IM02157. Accessed October 5, 2009.

40. Carkaci S, Ozkan E, Lane D, Yang WT. Scrotal sonography revisited. *J Clin Ultrasound* *38*(1):21–37, 2010 [Epub ahead of print] DOI: 10.1002/jcu.20642.

41. National Cancer Institute. Prostate cancer treatment. Available at http://www.cancer.gov/cancertopics/pdq/treatment/prostate/HealthProfessional/page2. Accessed November 13, 2009.

42. Prostate Cancer Foundation. Prostate cancer information. Available at http://www.prostatecancerfoundation.org/. Accessed October 30, 2009.

43. Lundin JI, Alexander BH, Olsen GW, Church TR. Ammonium perfluorooctanoate production and occupational mortality. *Epidemiology* *20*(6):921–928, 2009 [Epub ahead of print]. Available at http://www.ncbi.nlm.nih.gov/pubmed/19797969?ordinalpos=1&itool=EntrezSystem2.PEntrez.Pubmed.Pubmed_ResultsPanel.Pubmed_DefaultReportPanel.Pubmed_RVDocSum. Accessed October 4, 2009.

44. Guo Y, Werehere PN, Narayanan R, et al. Image registration accuracy of a 3-dimensional transrectal ultrasound guided prostate biopsy system. *J Ultrasound Med* *28*(11):1561–1568, 2009.

45. Zhang J, Hricak H, Shukla-Dave A, et al. Clinical stage T1c prostate cancer:Evaluation with endorectal MR imaging and MR spectroscopic imaging. *Radiology* *253*(2):425–434, 2009.

46. Pagana KD, Pagana TJ. *Mosby's Diagnostic and Laboratory Test Reference.* 5th ed. St Louis: Mosby; 2001.

47. Nguyen PL, Chen MH, Beard CJ, et al. Radiation with or without 6 months of androgen suppression therapy in intermediate- and high-risk clinically localized prostate cancer: A postrandomization analysis by risk group. *Int J Radiat Oncol Biol Phys* *77*(4): 1046–1052, 2009. Available at doi: 10.1016/ijrobp.2009.06.038. Accessed October 30, 2009.

48. National Cancer Institute. Low risk seen in monitoring, not treating some prostate cancers. *NCI Cancer Bulletin* *5*(4):3–4, 2008.

49. National Cancer Institute. Prostate cancer prevention: Summary of evidence. Available at http://www.cancer.gov/cancertopics/pdq/prevention/prostate/HealthProfessional/page2#Section_93. Accessed November 13, 2009.

50. Brown DA, Lindmark F, Stattin P, et al. Macrophage inhibitory cytokine 1: A new prognostic marker in prostate cancer. *Clin Cancer Res* *15*(21):6658–6654, 2009.

51. Dilger JA, Walsh MT, Warner ME, et al. Urethral injury during potassium-titanyl-phosphate laser prostatectomy complicated by transurethral resection syndrome. *Anesth Analg 107*(4):1438–1440, 2008.

52. Faraq E, Baccala AA Jr., Doutt RF, et al. Bladder perforation from photoselective vaporization of prostate resulting in rhabdomyolysis induced acute renal failure. *Minerva Anestesiol 74*(6):277–280, 2008.

53. National Cancer Institute. Fact sheet: Lung cancer. Available at http://www.cancer.gov/cancertopics/types/lung. Accessed September 24, 2009.

54. Becze E. Manage patients with non-small cell lung cancer. *ONS Connect 23*(10):20–21, 2008.

55. Tyson LB. Non-small cell lung cancer: New hope for a chronic illness. *Oncol Nurs Forum 34*(5):963–870, 2007.

56. Wagner KJ. Surgical management of non-small cell lung cancer. *Semin Oncol Nurs 24*(1):41–48, 2008.

57. National Cancer Institute. National lung screening trial. Available at http://www.cancer.gov/nlst/what-is-nlst#4. Accessed October 2, 2009.

58. Collins AS, Garner M. Caring for lung cancer patients receiving photodynamic therapy. *Crit Care Nurse 27*(2):53–60, 2007.

59. Yoder LH. An overview of lung cancer symptoms, pathophysiology and treatment. *Medsurg Nurs 15*(4):231–234, 2006.

60. deNijs EJM, Ros W, Grijpodonck MH. Nursing intervention for fatigue during treatment for cancer. *Cancer Nurs 31*(3):191–206, 2008.

61. Walker S. Updates in non-small cell lung cancer. *Clin J Oncol Nurs 12*(3):587–596, 2008.

62. National Cancer Institute. Laryngeal cancer treatment: General information. Available at http://www.cancer.gov/cancertopics/pdq/treatment/laryngeal/HealthProfessional/page2. Accessed November 14, 2009.

63. National Cancer Institute. Cancer of the larynx: Who's at risk? Available at http://www.cancer.gov/cancertopics/wyntk/larynx/page4. Accessed October 21, 2009.

64. National Cancer Institute. What you need to know about cancer of the larynx: Nutrition. Available at http://www.cancer.gov/cancertopics/wyntk/larynx/page16. Accessed October 21, 2009.

65. Van As-Brooks CJ, Fuller D. Prosthetic tracheoesophageal voice restoration following total laryngectomy. In: Ward EC, van As-Brooks CJ, eds. *Head and Neck Cancer Treatment, Rehabilitation and Outcomes.* San Diego: Pleural Publishing, Inc.; 2006.

66. Hsin LJ, Fang TJ, Chang KP, et al. Transoral endoscopic CO_2 laser microsurgery for early laryngeal cancers. *Chang Gung Med J 32*(5):517–525, 2009.

67. National Cancer Institute. Colon and rectal cancer. Available at http://www.cancer.gov/cancertopics/types/colon-and-rectal/. Accessed November 15, 2009.

68. The United Ostomy Association. Home page. Available at http://www.uoaa.org/. Accessed November 18, 2009.

69. National Cancer Institute. Spotlight: Probing the effects of circadian rhythms on cancer. *National Cancer Bulletin 5*(4):6, 2008.

70. National Cancer Institute. Bladder cancer treatment: General information. Available at http://www.cancer.gov/cancertopics/pdq/treatment/bladder/HealthProfessional/page2. Accessed: November 15, 2009.

71. American Cancer Society. Can bladder cancer be found early? Available at http://www.cancer.org/docroot/CRI/content/CRI_2_4_3X_Can_bladder_cancer_be_found_early_44.asp?rnav=cri. Accessed November 18, 2009.

72. Laudano MA, Barlow LJ, Murphy AM, et al. Long-term clinical outcomes of a phase I trial of intravesical docetaxel in the management of non-muscle-invasive bladder cancer refractory to standard intravesical therapy. *Urology 75*(1):134–137, 2009. [Epub ahead of print]. doi:10.1016/j.urology.2009.06.112

73. Lotan Y, Elias K, Svated RS, et al. Bladder cancer screening in a high risk asymptomatic population using a point of care urine based protein tumor marker. *J Urol 162*(1):52–57, 2009.

74. National Cancer Institute. Stomach (gastric) cancer. Available at http://www.cancer.gov/cancertopics/types/stomach/. Accessed November 19, 2009.

75. Hyatt BJ, Paull PE, Wassef W. Gastric oncology: An update. *Curr Opin Gastroenterol 25*(6):570–578, 2009.

76. Strong VE, Devaud N, Karpeh M. The role of laparoscopy for gastric surgery in the west. *Gastric Cancer 12*(3):127–131, 2009.

77. National Cancer Institute. Breast cancer drug helps patients with gastric cancer. *NCI Cancer Bull 6*(11):3, 2009.

78. American Cancer Society. Tanning beds may increase skin cancer risk. Available at http://www.cancer.org/docroot/NWS/content/NWS_1_1x_Tanning_Beds_May_Increase_Skin_Cancer_Risk.asp. Accessed November 20, 2009.

79. Abbasi NR, Shaw HM, Rigel DS, et al. Early diagnosis of cutaneous melanoma. *JAMA 292*(22):2771–2776, 2004.

80. Yvon E, Del Vecchio M, Savoldo B, et al. Immunotherapy of metastatic melanoma using genetically engineered GD2-specific T-cells. *Clin Cancer Res 15*(18):5852–5860, 2009.

81. Mansfield AS, Markovic SN. Novel therapies for the treatment of metastatic melanoma. *Future Oncol 5*(4):543–557, 2009.

82. National Cancer Institute. Treatment vaccines for cancer perform well in clinical trials. *NCI Cancer Bulletin 6*(11):4, 2009.

83. Walbert T, Gilbert MR. The role of chemotherapy in the treatment of patients with brain metastases from solid tumors. *Int J Clin Oncol 14*(4):299–306, 2009.

84. Register SS. Pathologic complete response of a solitary melanoma brain metastasis after local ablative radiation therapy: case report.

Med Oncol 27(4):1208, 2009 [Epub ahead of print.] Available at doi 10.1007/s12032-009-9360-3.

85. Wu AJ, Gomez J, Zhung JE, et al. Radiotherapy after surgical resection for head and neck mucosal melanoma. *American Journal of Clin Oncol.* 33(3):281–285, 2010. Available at DOI: 10.1097/COC.0b013e3181a879f5.

86. National Cancer Institute. Melanoma: Treatment options. Available at http://www.cancer.gov/cancertopics/pdq/treatment/melanoma/HealthProfessional/page5. Accessed November 25, 2009.

87. National Cancer Institute. Leukemia home page. Available at http://www.cancer.gov/cancertopics/types/leukemia. Accessed November 26, 2009.

88. Venes D, ed. *Taber's Clyclopedic Medical Dictionary.* Philadelphia: F.A. Davis Co; 2001.

89. Eberhart K, Renner K, Ritter I, et al. Low doses of 2-deoxy-glucose sensitize acute lymphoblastic leukemia cells to glucocorticoid-induced apoptosis. *Leukemia* 23(11):2167–2170, 2009. [Epub ahead of print]. Available at doi: 10.1038/leu.2009.154.

16 Alterations in Integumentary Function

OBJECTIVES

In this chapter you will review:

- The key concepts and priorities associated with nursing care of the patient having alteration in integumentary function.
- Nursing interventions to improve the quality of life when integumentary dysfunction results in change in body image secondary to disfigurement and disability.

Let's get the normal stuff straight!

The integument system is the largest system in the body. The skin comprises 15% of the total body weight and has various thicknesses and functions. Specifically the skin:

- Protects the body from germ invasion, dehydration, and injury
- Helps regulate body temperature by controlling the amount of heat loss through vasodilation, vasoconstriction, and perspiration
- Provides sensory perception, including hot, cold, pressure, and pain
- Manufactures vitamin D, which is needed for absorption of calcium
- Serves as a storage area for fat, glucose, water, and salt
- Absorbs certain materials and chemicals from the surface of the body
- Excretes water, salt, and waste products

The skin is composed of two major tissue layers: the epidermis and the dermis. There is also an underlying foundation known as the hypodermis or subcutaneous tissue, but it is not considered a true part of the skin (Fig. 16-1).

▶ Figure 16-1. Anatomy of the skin (cross-section).

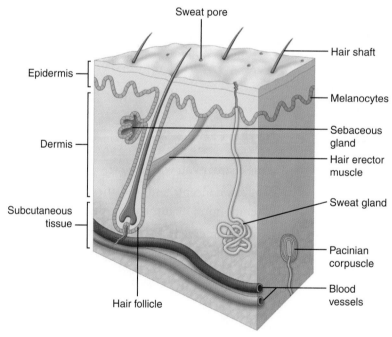

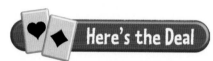

Here's the Deal

Untreated or improperly treated injuries to the skin are the most common way bacterial infections develop.

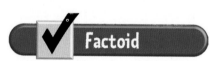

Factoid

Bacterial infections can spread when contaminated nails are used to scratch or rub healthy skin.

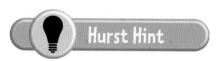

Hurst Hint

Bacteria like to settle in the warm, moist environment of the hair follicle. This is why most bacterial skin lesions originate from this site.

The skin also contains several structures:

- Sudoriferous glands (sweat)
- Sebaceous glands (oil)
- Hair
- Nails

The skin serves as the body's protective covering. Intact skin is effective in acting as a barrier to microorganisms. It also provides protection from harmful rays of the sun and protects underlying tissues from fluid loss.

Approximately one-third of the body's blood circulates through the skin, allowing the regulation of temperature. This process is obtained through vasoconstriction and vasodilation of the vessels on the skin surface. Sudoriferous glands, which produce sweat, also assist in temperature regulation by cooling the body surface through diaphoresis (sweating). The skin contains nerve endings that sense cold, heat, pressure, and pain. Skin also has the capability of absorbing certain chemicals and medications through its surface by way of hair follicles, glands, and mucus membranes.[11]

The skin's protective qualities are so crucial to the human body's survival that even a small amount of loss can compromise an adult's health.

✛ Skin infections

Infectious skin conditions can be caused by a bacteria, fungus, or virus. Table 16-1 describes the different types of infections, signs and symptoms of each infection, and the associated interventions.

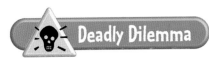

If cellulitis is not treated, gangrene can occur.

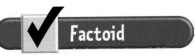

Impetigo is a highly contagious infection and can easily be transferred from one person to another. Clothing and towels of the affected person should be sterilized and frequent handwashing performed.

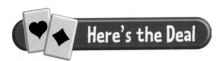

Generally speaking, Tinea loves a susceptible host (diabetics, immunosuppression) and a warm/moist environment.

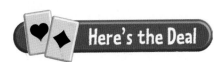

Tinea capitis is commonly seen in children.

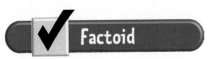

Tinea is also referred to as Ringworm because of the "ring" that forms with this infection.

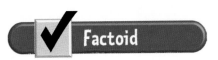

You may have heard of thrush—a *Candida* infection of the mouth. It frequently occurs in children and people taking long-term antibiotics.

Table 16-1 Skin infections

Type of infection/What is it?/Causes and why?	Testing, testing, testing	Signs and symptoms and why?	Interventions and why?
Bacterial **Define time** Cellulitis is a diffuse infection of the dermis or subcutaneous layer of the skin. Causative organisms: • Streptococcus • Staphylococcus Risk factors: • Injury or trauma causing a break in the skin • Excoriations from scratching insect bites • Ulcers from diabetes or peripheral vascular disease • Peeling or cracking of skin between the toes. Folliculitis (infection of the upper portion of the hair follicle) usually caused by Staphylococcus aureus, Pseudomonas aeruginosa Furuncles (infection occurring in the lower portion of the hair follicle); known as boils; usually caused by Staphylococcus aureus Impetigo (superficial skin infection most commonly affecting the pediatric population); usually caused by Staphylococcus aureus, Streptococcus pyogenes **Fungal** Tinea is a catchall term for fungi. It is the most common fungal infection of the skin. There are many different types of fungi. Tinea infections can be located in different parts of the body. When tinea infects the scalp it is referred to as tinea capitis; tinea cruris is a fungal infection of the groin; and tinea pedia is a fungal infection of the foot; and tinea corporis can be found anywhere on the body (back, abdomen, etc).	• Obtain history and complete physical assessment • Culture and sensitivity of wound (if necessary) Many times the diagnosis is made by clinical observation and treated accordingly **Assessment** What does the lesion look like? Where is the lesion? Scales (if present) from the lesions are scraped and placed on a slide with KOH (looking for spores or hyphae). Hyphae (threadlike structures) are indicative of a fungal infection.	Symptoms vary depending on the severity of the infection. • Pain/tenderness/heat • Local edema with an orange peel appearance • Localized fluid-filled blisters that vary in size • Fever, malaise, chills, enlarged lymph nodes **Folliculitis** *Signs and Symptoms* Skin rash of tiny white pimples at base of hair follicle **Furuncles** *Signs and Symptoms* One or more raised reddened areas with a white center; commonly called boils **Impetigo** *Signs and Symptoms* Yellow-crusted sores and/or small blisters with yellow fluid that vary in size and typically spread to other areas. Tinea is associated with insufficient hygiene, direct contact with those already infected (including inanimate objects), and frequent contact with animals. It is possible the family pet may have to be given away. **Tinea pedis** *Signs and Symptoms* Scaling and redness of soles and between toes Blistering may also occur in severe cases Itching Pain	• Daily antibacterial cleansing of skin • Avoid excessive moisture at affected areas, which decreases bacterial growth. • Prevent spread through hand hygiene. • Use standard precautions. • In the hospitalized patient, if Staphylococcus is antibiotic resistant (MRSA), strict isolation precautions are taken. • Use arm compresses BID for comfort. • Mild infections usually are treated with topical antibiotics (eg, neomycin sulfate, Polysporin, Bactroban) • Severe cellulitis requires systemic antibiotics depending on results of culture and sensitivity (C&S) **Treatment** • Antibacterial cleansing of skin daily • Avoid excessive moisture at affected areas, which decreases bacterial growth • Employ standard precautions for all bacterial infections and isolation precautions for Staphylococcus that is resistant to antibiotics • Antibiotics are given topically or systemically: neomycin sulfate (Mycifradin), gentamicin sulfate (Gentacidin), cephalexin hydrochloride (Keflex) • Warm compresses relieve folliculitis **What can harm my patient?** The greatest concern associated with bacterial skin infections is the risk of sepsis (spread of infection through the blood), which can result in organ failure and death if not treated promptly. • Antifungal creams • Hydrocortisone • Oral antifungals • Keep skin clean and dry • Avoid tight-fitting clothes and shoes **Interventions** **Tinea pedis** Topical antifungals (Miconazole [Absorbine foot powder], Nystatin (Mycostatin), Clotrimazole (Lotrimin AF).

Tinea capitis = scalp

Tinea pedis = athlete's foot

Tinea corporis = anywhere on the body

Tinea cruris = jock itch

Have to have impaired skin integrity first, and then come in contact with something that has tinea (person, animal, caps, pillow case, brush).

Dermophytes mainly live on animals, on humans, or in the soil. Most fungal infections occur on direct contact with an infected animal or person. Sometimes fungal infections can be transmitted by an inanimate object (using the towel of a person who has a fungal infection). Environmental factors may also contribute to transmission, such as athletes using showers in locker rooms, which can cause athlete's foot.

Candidiasis typically occurs during hot, humid weather and when clothing prevents moisture from leaving skin surfaces. People using antibiotics and those with compromised immune systems are at risk for developing candidiasis.

Candidiasis (yeast infection) is a fungal infection affecting mucous membranes and moist areas of the skin. *Candida* is a normal finding in the GI system and vagina, but under certain conditions an infection can occur.

Oral candidiasis (thrush) may be the first opportunistic infection seen in people with human immunodeficiency virus (HIV).

Tinea pedis

Has patient used a communal shower/swimming pool?

Clinical Observation
Tinea capitis

Patient may have come in direct contact with an infected person or object (hairbrush, pillowcase, cap)

Clinical Observation
Tinea corporis

located on nonhairy skin of the body; increased frequency in hot, humid climates

Clinical observation
Tinea cruris

Seen frequently in athletes and the obese. Associated with tight-fitting clothing; diabetes

Clinical observation
Tests

History and physical examination: Confirm diagnosis.

Culture of lesions: Microscopic examination determines specific type of fungi.

UV light: Spores and fungal infections appear blue-green under UV light.

Tinea capitis
Signs and Symptoms

One or more round/oval red scaling patches with small pustules around the edges. Any time a child has scaling at the scalp it is considered tinea capitis until proved otherwise.

Bald patches with classic black dots may develop as the fungus invades the hair, causing it to become brittle and break off at the scalp surface—temporary loss.

Severe itching.

Tinea corporis
Signs and Symptoms

- Single or multiple red patches with raised borders, scaling with a clear center
- Itching

Tinea cruris
Signs and Symptoms

- Single or multiple red patches with raised borders, scaling with a clear center
- Itching

Candidiasis
Signs and Symptoms

- Painful, itching, erythematous pustules (inflamed blisters filled with cloudy fluids)
- Vaginal candidiasis produces a white cottage cheese-like discharge

Candidiasis of the mucous membranes (thrush) produces painful white ulcers with reddened surrounding tissues

Systemic antifungals for severe cases (Griseofulvin).

Soak feet in a water and vinegar solution.

Instruct the patient:

Avoid sharing shoes and socks with others.

Dry well between the toes after bathing,

Place small pieces of cotton between the toes at night.

Keep the feet as dry as possible by

Wearing cotton socks and hosiery.

Wearing perforated shoes such as sandals.

Avoiding rubber or plastic-soled shoes.

Avoiding sneakers or other constrictive footwear.

Alternating shoes to allow for complete drying between wearing.

Interventions
Tinea capitis

Practice good hygiene, including washing hair two or three times a week with a topical antifungal preparation such as Ketoconazole (Nizoral).

Use a separate comb and brush and avoid sharing headgear with others.

All family members need to be assessed because the disease is easily transmitted.

Inside pets need to be examined also.

Administer the antifungal agent Griseofulvin.

Topical agents are not effective because the infection is within the hair shaft below the scalp surface.

If topical agents are used it is to eliminate the organisms on the hair and decrease the spread of the fungi.

Treatment is the same for tinea corporis (topical or oral antifungals).

Treatment with topical or oral antifungals.

Treatment for candidiasis includes topical and/or oral antifungals OR antifungal mouth wash for thrush.

What can harm my patient?

- Secondary bacterial infections of the skin.
- Oral candidiasis (thrush) can lead to inadequate nutritional intake. Close monitoring of children and immunocompromised individuals is needed to prevent dehydration and wasting.

(continued)

Table 16-1 Skin infections (*continued*)

Type of infection/What is it?/ Causes and why?	Testing, testing, testing	Signs and symptoms and why?	Interventions and why?
Viral Infections Viral skin infections are the result of one of several viruses that can infect the body. There are several viral infections that result in rashes and lesions of the skin. They include chickenpox, measles, and scarlet fever. This section focuses on three of the most common skin-associated viruses. **Causes and why?** Viral skin infections are a result of a virus that is spread through direct contact from an infected person to a healthy person and may reoccur after a period of dormancy in the body. Herpes simplex • Herpes simplex 1 (cold sores) • Herpes simplex 2 (genital herpes) Both types are caused by either the herpes simplex 1 or 2 virus • Herpes zoster	• Many times the diagnosis is made by clinical observation. • Skin culture and biopsy determine specific virus responsible for the infection. • Occasionally a serum antibody for herpes will be drawn. Diagnosis is usually made by clinical observation.	*Prodromal stage:* Period of time between contact with virus and skin changes • Burning and itching of mouth or genitals • Fatigue • Elevated temperature *Active stage:* • One or more small fluid-filled blisters on the mouth, face, nose, or perineal area • Rash of numerous vesicles on one side of the body following a nerve pathway (zoster) • Pain (all types)	**Herpes simplex virus** • Oral or topical antiviral drugs such as acyclovir (Zovirax) **Herpes zoster** • Analgesics for pain management • Antivirals (Acyclovir [Zovirax]) to decrease replication of virus • Corticosteroids to reduce the risk of long-term pain complications • Oral or topical antiviral drugs such as acyclovir (Zovirax) • Analgesics for pain management • Antivirals (Acyclovir, Zovirax) to decrease replication of virus • Corticosteroids to reduce the risk of long-term pain complications **What can harm my patient?** • Certain strains of HPV that cause warts can lead to the development of cervical cancer. • Secondary bacterial infections can develop at areas of lesions. • HSV can spread from mother to infant during delivery. • Herpes zoster can spread internally, causing increased morbidity. • Postherpetic neuralgia (pain lasting longer than 1 month) may occur in people with herpes zoster. • Corneal damage can occur with herpes zoster. **Treatment** **Warts**
Warts		• Common warts: rough gray, yellow, or brown skin growths • Plantar warts: hard, flat, thickened, gray or brown growths with a black center • **Genital warts:** cauliflower-textured growths on the penis, vagina, labia, or anal area	• Most common warts disappear within a few years and require no treatment unless they become painful or cause self-esteem issues. Genital warts may be treated because they tend to be more contagious than other warts. • Freezing (cryotherapy): liquid nitrogen or commercial freezing probes • Chemical removal: salicylic acid, formaldehyde, or other skin irritants to stimulate and immune reaction • Burning or cutting • Laser removal

PSORIASIS
. . . .

What is it?

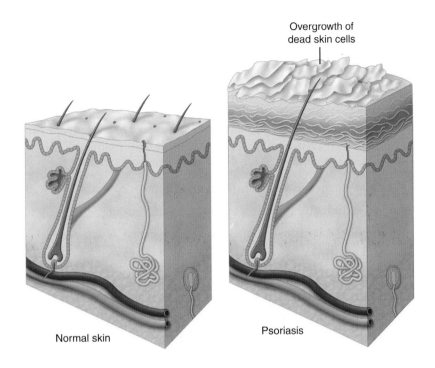

Overgrowth of
dead skin cells

◀ Figure 16-2. Psoriasis.

Normal skin

Psoriasis

Psoriasis is a common chronic inflammatory condition that is characterized by an overgrowth of skin cells (Fig. 16-2). The most commonly
occurring form is psoriasis vulgaris (plaque psoriasis) characterized by
plaques (skin overgrowth) containing silvery scales with borders that are
sharply defined.[1] Psoriasis is incurable and noncontagious, and the
course of the disorder is marked by remissions and exacerbations (flareups). The average age of onset of the disease is the late twenties.

Causes and why?

Table 16-2 displays the causes and why of psoriasis.

Table 16-2 Causes and why of psoriasis

Causes	Why?
Improper immune response of T cells (white blood cells that are used to fight foreign substances)	Immune system is stimulated by the Langerhans' cells in the skin. T lymphocytes target the keratinocytes, leading to formation of scaly areas on skin.
Genetics	Evidence shows that most cases of psoriasis have a genetic foundation.
Trauma	Traumatic injury such as sunburn, surgery, or other breaks in skin can trigger the development of psoriatic patches. This is known as Köbner's phenomenon.

Source: Created by the author from References 1, 2, and 3.

Exacerbations (flareups) of psoriasis can be brought on by:

- Hormonal changes (puberty, pregnancy)
- Streptococcal infections
- Exposure to cold weather
- Stress response
- Drugs such as beta-blockers, corticosteroids, or lithium (Eskalith)
- Endocrine disorders

Signs and symptoms and why?

Psoriasis lesions are seen predominantly in the areas of the elbows, knees, scalp, and lower back. Psoriasis can be limited to a few lesions or can involve large areas of the skin. However, for most patients the condition tends to be mild.

- Dry, red patches covered with silvery scales.
- Inflammation and irritation of the outer skin surface.
- Itching with bleeding when patches are scratched or scraped.
- Symmetric distribution.
- Face is rarely affected.
- Thick and pitted nails.

What can harm my patient and why?

Body image may be negatively affected as a result of unsightly lesions. Psychologic stress can be debilitating and severe. There is reluctance to appear in public because of others' reactions to the lesions (many mistakenly fear that lesions are contagious).

   Psoriasis is the largest risk factor for developing psoriatic arthritis. This is a chronic disease that is characterized by joint as well as skin inflammation.

Interventions and why?

- Have the patient identify factors that provoke outbreaks.
- Assess the physical, psychosocial, and occupational impact of psoriasis.
- Create a climate wherein the patient feels comfortable discussing feelings, concerns, and fears.
- Explore coping strategies used for dealing with outbreaks while attempting to maintain usual activities, and family and social interactions.
- Apply topical emollients for moisturizing.
- Apply topical corticosteroids to decrease inflammation.
- Initiate measures to reduce pruritus (itching).
- Apply prescribed topical medications after warm (not hot) bath with mild soap and scrubbing scales to maximize absorption and therapeutic value.
- Outpatient use of ultraviolet light (phototherapy) to promote healing (ie, tanning bed).

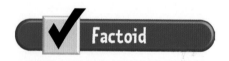

Factoid

Patients who have psoriasis of the nails are at higher risk for developing psoriatic arthritis.

Because there is no cure for psoriasis, instructions are focused on extending periods of remission and coping with the exacerbations of this chronic skin disorder.

- Use moisturizing soaps, emollients, and scalp oils to soften scales followed by gently soft brushing while bathing.
- Moisturize and lubricate affected areas to avoid fissures.
- Pat dry rather than rubbing, which is more irritating to the skin.
- Maintain a healthy lifestyle: balanced diet, regular exercise, and stress reduction.
- Notify your health care provider if you develop painful joints.
- Avoid exposure to cold to minimize wintertime exacerbations.
- Avoid prolonged sun exposure because burning can trigger outbreaks.
- Various topical treatments (ointments and creams applied to the affected area) alone or in conjunction with ultraviolet light rays is usually the first line of therapy:
  - Corticosteroids (ointments or cream) to suppress cell division
  - Vitamin A and D cream to lubricate and moisturize the skin by creating a moisture barrier
  - Coal tar preparations in the form of gels, creams, or bath soaks to suppress cell division and reduce inflammation
  - Colloidal baths (oiled oatmeal preparations) and bath salts (Dead Sea salt, Epsom salt)
  - Retinoids in gel or cream such as acitretin (Soriatane), tazarotene (Tazorac)
  - Anthralin (Anthraforte) works similarly to coal tar.
  - Tazarotene (Tazorac), a topical cream commonly used to treat acne, may be given in conjunction with steroids.
  - Calcipotriene (Dovonex) is a vitamin D derivative used to regulate cell division.
  - Salicylic acid preparations (a peeling agent) given with other ointments thin psoriasis patches.

Systemic therapy is reserved for psoriasis that responds poorly to topical agents and phototherapy:

- Immunomodulators (reserved for psoriasis resistant to topical treatments)
  - Methotrexate (Folex), cyclosporine (Sandimmune), alefacept (Amevive), efalizumab (Raptiva), or azathioprine (Imuran) to decrease cell turnover.[12]
  - Hydroxyurea is somewhat less effective than methotrexate or cyclosporine and is sometimes combined with UV treatments. Anemia and a decrease in white blood cells and platelets may occur.

What works for one patient may not work for another, and patients may become resistant to treatment that works well initially. This makes a

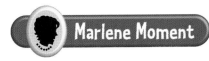
Marlene Moment

Be picky about the company you keep. Psoriasis exacerbations are more likely following psychological stress.

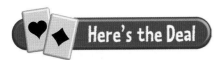
Here's the Deal

Applying topical medication on top of scales doesn't do much good! Much of the therapeutic value of the agent will be lost because it doesn't penetrate the overlapping scales! Apply occlusive dressings (moist dressing covered with outer wrap of nonpenetrating material like a plastic bag) to enhance penetration of topical medications as ordered by the physician.

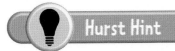
Hurst Hint

Never apply occlusive dressing over topical steroid application without a doctor's order. This is risky because in addition to enhancing tissue absorption it also enhances systemic absorption of the steroid!

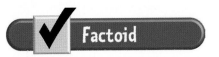
Factoid

Patients have fewer symptoms of psoriasis during summer months and more flareups during the winter season.

trial-and-error approach to treatment commonplace. Other members of the health care team are involved as needed:

- Referrals for psychological counseling and group therapy may be helpful to counteract fear of social rejection and self-isolation.
- Rheumatology referral for signs of inflammatory joint disease unrelieved by nonprescription nonsteroidal anti-inflammatory drugs (NSAIDs)

BURNS

Approximately 2 million people in the United States sustain burn injuries yearly. Burns are accidental injuries except for the type that occur through radiation therapy (cancer treatment). Most burns occur in the home setting. The patients most likely to have severe complications or death are the very young or very old. The younger the patient is, the more body surface area the burn will affect. The more body surface area affected, the greater the chance of death and complications. When an elderly person is burned, the burn tends to go deeper because of the decreased amount of subcutaneous fat.

Let's get the normal stuff straight!

The skin is the largest organ in the body, and it has a large job to perform too!

- The skin serves as a barrier to bacteria. (It is our first line of defense!)
- The skin prevents loss of body fluids.
- The three layers of the skin are the epidermis (outermost layer), the dermis (inner layer), and a layer of subcutaneous fat.
- The dermis has an abundant supply of nerves, allowing the skin to receive sensory input from the environment.
- After injury, the epidermis heals by regeneration, but deep dermal and subcutaneous tissue is replaced with scar tissue.[2]

What is it?

Burns are generally categorized into three or four types (or degrees) depending on tissue layer involvement.

They are also classified as *major* or *minor* according to the depth, surface area, and body parts involved, which helps to predict risk of complications and capacity for healing and recovery.

A burn is determined to be *minor* or *major* based on the following additional criteria:

- Any burn involving the eyes, ears, face, hands, feet, and perineum (genitals) is major.
- Burns are major in the very young and the very old because this age group is more seriously affected when complications occur.
- Superficial and partial-thickness burns are considered minor if they are <15% of the total body surface area (TBSA) burned.

- Any full-thickness burn <5% of the TBSA is considered minor unless any of the other criteria are present (very old, very young, hands, eyes, ears, feet, face, genitals).

Causes and why?

Burns can result from a variety of sources: heat, electricity, radiation, or exposure to extreme cold (frostbite).

Most burns are caused by contact with a heat source (thermal injuries):

- Fire, flames
- Steam or scalding liquids

Chemical burns are caused by caustic substances that contact the skin. Household products that can produce burns are:

- Products containing lye (drain cleaners, paint removers)
- Phenols (disinfectants and deodorizers)
- Sodium hypochlorite (in disinfectants and bleaches)
- Sulfuric acid (toilet bowl cleaners)

Electrical burns are caused when the patient is exposed to direct or alternating current that passes through the body (an electrical source or lightning).

Signs and symptoms and why?

The patient's major complaint is pain unless the majority of the burned area is full thickness, which destroys nerve endings. The patient's injury can be a combination of partial, deep partial, and full thickness burns (Table 16-3; Fig. 16-3).

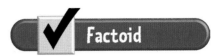
Factoid

The deepest burns cause the least pain because sensory nerves are destroyed.

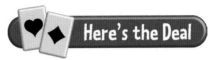
Here's the Deal

Burns can also be classified as *iatrogenic* (from a prescribed treatment or diagnostic procedure) such as radiation used in cancer treatment or application of heat (defective heating pads, improperly insulated hot packs).

Table 16-3   Assessment and evaluation of burn wounds

Type of burn	Signs and symptoms	Why
First-degree: superficial partial thickness	Red, dry skin; blanches with pressure; minimal or no edema; possible blisters; tingling; hyperesthesia (supersensitivity); pain is soothed by cooling	Damage to epidermis, possibly a portion of dermis
Second-degree: deep partial-thickness	Redness; pain; weeping surface; hyperesthesia; sensitive to cold air; broken epidermis; thick blisters with edema	Damage to epidermis, upper dermis, portion of deeper dermis, nerve involvement
Third-degree: full-thickness	Pain free; shock; hematuria (blood in urine); entrance and exit wounds (electrical burn); broken skin with fat exposed; edema; dry; pale white or cherry red, leathery, or charred	Damage to epidermis, entire dermis, subcutaneous tissue (sometimes); nerve endings destroyed; destruction of lymph and blood vessels
Fourth-degree: deep full-thickness	Pain free; exposed muscle, bone, and tendons	Damage extends beyond skin and affects the muscle, bone, and internal tissues

Source: Hurst M. *Hurst Reviews: Hurst Pathophysiology* New York: McGraw-Hill; 2008.

▶ Figure 16-3. Classification of burn wounds.

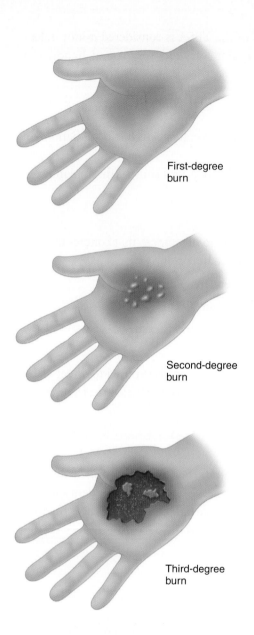

First-degree burn

Second-degree burn

Third-degree burn

Physiologic Changes Occurring after a Major Burn

The symptoms listed in Table 16-3 are the "basics" of what you may see with a burn. Depending on the severity of the burn, other things could be occurring in the body that would bring about additional signs and symptoms. Let's look at some of these now.

- The injury (the burn itself) has damaged the vessels so that fluid begins to leak out → vascular volume decreases → hypotension/shock/ decreased renal perfusion.
- Any time vascular volume leaks out of the body (whether into the tissue or out of the body completely), cardiac output will begin to decrease and BP will drop further.
- The sympathetic nervous system kicks in (a response to the burn shock), causing the heart rate to increase; peripheral vasoconstriction occurs (vessels clamping down on less fluid), which makes it even harder for the heart to pump blood out against the increased pressure (further decreasing cardiac output).

- The majority is fluid leakage out of the vascular space, which occurs during the first 24 to 36 hours. After this time the vessels begin to heal and the fluid begins to return to the vascular space. If the heart and kidneys are working properly, diuresis will begin and will last for up to 2 weeks.
- The patient could possibly be anemic because of red blood cell (RBC) destruction (burns destroy RBCs). The HCT could be up as the blood stream is concentrated because of plasma leakage. (The patient may need a blood transfusion.)
- Platelets may be decreased because of burn injury, which puts the patient at risk for bleeding.
- Hyponatremia: Leaky (highly permeable) vessels cause plasma fluid to leak out of the vascular space → sodium is lost. Hyponatremia is common during the first week after the burn (acute phase) as fluid begins to shift back into the vascular space, causing dilution (which makes serum Na decrease).
- Immediately after the burn injury, hyperkalemia will be present. (As cells are destroyed and rupture, K^+ is released into the blood stream.)
- Severe burns suppress the immune system greatly.
- Hypothermia occurs initially resulting from skin loss because skin holds in body heat. During the healing phases hyperthermia may occur even when there is no infection.
- Hypermetabolism of the body occurs after it has stabilized. All of the body systems are hyperfunctional. This is caused by a surge in catecholamines, cortisol, and glucagon. This hypermetabolism causes muscles to breakdown, depleted stores of glycogen, and decreased protein production. This hypermetabolic state is why the patient must have increased calories and nutrition throughout recovery.

Testing, testing, testing

When inhalation injury is suspected, additional tests are performed:

- Monitor laboratory indicators of nutritional status: prealbumin, total protein, or albumin.
- The most sensitive indicator of overall nutritional status is prealbumin.
- The prealbumin test measures a protein that reflects current nutritional status and is monitored closely, because prealbumin changes more quickly than albumin or total protein, making it more useful for detecting changes in short-term nutritional status.
- Serum carboxyhemoglobin levels (COHb) detects carbon monoxide poisoning.
- Fiberoptic bronchoscopy can actually visualize damage to the mucosal surfaces and structures of the airways.
- Xenon 133 (^{133}Xe) ventilation perfusion scans provide a noninvasive study of physiologic lung function.[4]
- Pulmonary function studies are a group of tests that measure lung function, including forced vital capacity (FCV) and forced expiratory volume (FVE-1). (Refer to Chapter 4 for an explanation of these tests.)

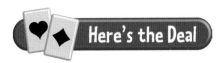

Severely burned patients may have an increase in their metabolic rate by as much as 200%! This will decrease over time, but the patient will continue to have an increased metabolism for up to one year.

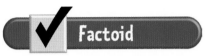

Arterial blood gases (ABGs) reveal metabolic acidosis, because when sodium leaves the leaky (permeable) vascular space with the plasma fluid, bicarbonate accompanies the sodium, leaving the patient with a base-bicarbonate deficit.

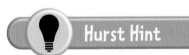

Concentration makes numbers go UP! In fluid volume deficit the vascular space is concentrated, so the hematocrit goes UP!

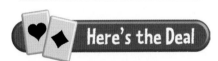

Under normal circumstances of fluid volume deficit (FVD) when the vascular volume is depleted (concentrated), the sodium is elevated along with the hematocrit, but what is different after a major burn? Increased capillary permeability, enabling the sodium to leave with the water! Therefore the patient will have an FVD (shock) but it will be accompanied by *hyponatremia*.

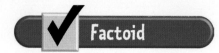

Factoid

Inhalation injury increases the mortality rate of burns.[5]

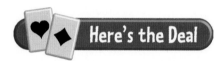

Here's the Deal

A burned patient may have several wounds with varying degrees of burn depth. The area of the wound closest to the burn source (flame, chemical) will be the most severely affected (Table 16-4).

As long as the kidneys are still working (ie, are able to produce, concentrate, and dilute urine), the urinalysis will reveal:

- High specific gravity associated with intravascular dehydration (FVD) during the first 24 hours, when fluid is leaving the vascular space, and with the fluid shift when vessels recover a degree of permeability, fluid moves back into the vascular space and specific gravity decreases as urine becomes more dilute.

- With severe damage to muscles (full thickness burns, electrical burns), destruction of skeletal muscle cells causes release of free myoglobins in circulation, which are filtered out by the kidneys. Urinary myoglobin levels get very high with sudden and severe muscle damage.

- In the presence of acute tubular necrosis (owing to hypovolemia and/or sludging of the kidneys with cellular debris), a large number of granular casts will be present in the urine.

Following any form of electrical injury, the patient will have tests to determine injury to the heart and other internal organs:

- Heart injury: Serial cardiac biomarkers (CK-MB, LDH, and troponin) are drawn to identify myocardial injury. Stat 12 EKG is standard and may be repeated if any set of biomarkers is elevated.

- Kidney injury: BUN and creatinine (to identify renal damage because electricity travels to vascular areas).

- Liver injury: SGOT (now called aspartate transaminase [AST]) and SGPT (now called alanine transaminase [ALT]). Note that this organ is also very vascular.

Table 16-4 Respiratory injuries

Burns of the upper torso with inhalation of sooty debris, heat, and smoke.	Burns are visible about the face or neck: • Singed nasal hair • Hoarseness, raspy voice • Sooty or blood-streaked sputum • Dyspnea (difficulty breathing), tachypnea (fast breathing) • Decreased oxygen saturation • Patchy discoloration and/or blistering of oropharyngeal membranes	• Burns occurring within an enclosed area predispose to upper airway injury. • Thermal injury causes vessels about the face and neck to be highly permeable, causing edema that can close off air passageways. • Air passageways can become occluded with edema within the pharynx, larynx, or trachea. • Injury to the type 2 (surfactant-producing) cells of the alveoli can cause lung water to pour into the alveoli, halting diffusion of oxygen.
Impending acute renal failure, which can lead to acute tubular necrosis; greatest risk is during the plasma to interstitial fluid shift when vascular fluid leaks out into the tissues, leaving the vascular compartment dehydrated.	Hypovolemia, fluid volume deficit culminate in shock and acute renal failure: • Urinary output <30 mL/h • Hematuria • Hemoglobinuria • High level of myoglobins present in urine • Granular casts present in the urine	• As blood pressure falls secondary to FVD, renal perfusion diminishes, causing urine output to drop. • Sludge released by damaged, hemolyzed cells can plug renal tubules. • Decreasing urinary output means one of two things: either the kidneys are trying to help the problem of FVD by conserving fluid, or they are not being perfused and therefore are unable to produce urine.

Source: Created by the author from References 2 and 6.

What can harm my patient and why?

After a major burn, harm can occur because of the pathophysiological changes that accompany a major burn (Table 16-5).

- Inhalation injuries
- Acute respiratory distress syndrome
- Respiratory failure
- Hyperkalemia, hypokalemia (depending on stage of recovery)
- Bleeding (caused by thrombocytopenia)
- Anemia (caused by RBC destruction)
- Decreased cardiac output (caused by decreased vascular volume)
- Shock (loss of volume)
- Hyponatremia
- Acute tubular necrosis and/or renal failure
- Compartment syndrome (swelling of tissues decreasing perfusion to an area)

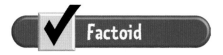

Shock kills kidneys!

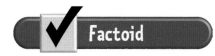

Increased capillary permeability causes blood vessels to become leaky!

Table 16-5 What can harm my burned patient and why?

Burn injury: pathophysiology	Rationale: the whys	What can harm my patient?
Plasma seeps from the vascular space into the tissues (interstitial space)	Because of increased capillary permeability of vessel walls secondary to damage from the burn injury.	During the first 24 hours after a burn is when the majority of vascular fluid is lost into the interstitial space leading to: • Fluid volume deficit • Hypotension • Shock • Edema into the local burn wound about the head and neck, or if heat has been inhaled can obstruct air passageways
Tachycardia	Secondary to FVD • The heart increases in effort to circulate the decreased remaining volume.	Increased heart rate increases the demand for extra oxygen, and elderly patients or those having comorbidities can decompensate.
Decreased cardiac output	Secondary to FVD • Less volume means less pressure! • If there's not much volume in the vascular space, the cardiac output decreases.	Decreased tissue perfusion as a result of hypotension.
Decreased urinary output: oliguria or anuria	• Can result from fluid volume deficit, causing the kidneys to reabsorb water for conservation of fluid. • Can be caused by decreased renal perfusion secondary to decreased cardiac output.	• Acute renal failure can occur after only 20 minutes of low or no perfusion. • Acute tubular necrosis causes permanent kidney damage.

(Continued)

Table 16-5 What can harm my burned patient and why? *(continued)*

Burn injury: pathophysiology	Rationale: the whys	What can harm my patient?
Increased secretion of epinephrine and norepinephrine (fight or flight hormone signs and symptom stress hormones)	• Initially the blood pressure drops owing to generalized vasodilation secondary to the thermal injury. • Secretion of epinephrine and norepinephrine is a compensatory response activated by hypotension and decreased cardiac output. • These catecholamines cause vasoconstriction to raise the blood pressure and shunt blood to vital organs (heart, brain, lungs, and kidneys).	If there is inadequate blood volume to perfuse all four of the vital organs (heart, brain, lungs, and kidneys), the kidneys will be "voted off the island" first, and the available blood supply will be diverted to the heart, brain, and lungs.
Increased secretion of ADH and aldosterone	• Aldosterone causes the patient to retain sodium and water, thereby replacing blood volume. • ADH causes the patient to retain water to increase blood volume.	ADH and aldosterone are wonderful for building up the blood volume, which is much needed (especially during the first 24 hours when the patient is "shocky"), but when fluid begins to shift back into the vascular space the patient will be at risk for fluid volume excess.
Airway injury owing to heat inhalation and inhaled carbon monoxide	• Being burned in an enclosed space will result in more airway injury. • Normally, oxygen should bind with hemoglobin. • Carbon monoxide can run much faster than oxygen; therefore, it gets to the hemoglobin first and binds. • Oxygen cannot bind once carbon monoxide is in place (bound) because there is no place for it.	Carbon monoxide poisoning results in hypoxia, hypoxemia, and possible death.

Source: Created by the author from Reference 6.

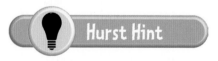

Less volume means less pressure.

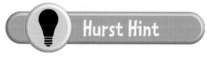

Hypotension equals hypoperfusion.

Complications of electrical burns:

• Blood within the vessels is electrocoagulated (congealed), stopping blood flow and can shut down circulation to an entire limb.

• Everywhere there is a blood vessel, a nerve runs right alongside, and nerves sustain similar damage.

Refer to Table 16-6 for complications of electrical burns due to poor circulation and nerve damage and massive tissue destruction (similar to a huge crushing injury) associated with full thickness burns.

Table 16-6 Complications of Electrical Burns

Ventricular fibrillation and sudden death	Muscle necrosis, and "mummification" of hands and feet, leading to limb loss
Other cardiac arrhythmias (conduction blocks, PVCs from myocardial irritability)	Hemolysis and renal failure as tubules plug up with cellular debris, free hemoglobins, and myoglobins
Seizures/coma and various kinds of mental changes	Anemia owing to hemolysis because the burn causes blood cells to break open
Eye disorders: cataracts and retinal detachment	Paresis/paralysis and any other kind of neurologic defect known. (This complication may be immediate or delayed.)

Source: Created by the author from Reference 6.

Additional later harm can occur as the burn wounds are evolving:

- Infection owing to microbial contamination can complicate burn wounds and lead to sepsis and/or death.
- Dry hard eschar that forms from dead tissue in circumferential burns can cut off blood supply to a limb, leading to necrosis and amputation.
- Eschar on the thorax can limit respiratory excursion to impair breathing.
- Contractures may develop because scar tissue shrinks (contracts) as it heals and can restrict movement of joints.

Interventions and why?

Adequate fluid resuscitation is essential during the early postburn period to treat burn shock and ensure renal perfusion.

- Various fluid resuscitation formulas are used as guides to determine the volume and type of fluid needed.
- The maximum daily fluid volume is generally set at 10,000 mL for the most severe burn.
- Hypertonic saline may be required during the initial postburn shock phase when sodium and water leave the vascular space.
- Blood transfusions and blood products (serum albumin) may be required based on bleed loss of blood and plasma proteins.
- Serial determinations of hematocrit, serum electrolytes, osmolality, calcium, glucose, and albumin can help direct appropriate fluid replacement.
- Persistent metabolic acidosis on arterial blood gases may indicate ongoing hypoperfusion from hypovolemia.

Invasive hemodynamic monitoring with central venous catheters, arterial lines, and Swan-Ganz catheters may be required with inhalation injury, but because of the additional risks for sepsis, thrombophlebitis, and endocarditis, the risks and benefits are carefully weighed. Noninvasive is the rule unless the patient's condition mandates such procedures.

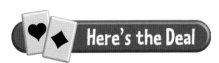

A certain amount of blood pressure to is necessary to perfuse vital organs. Any time the systolic blood pressure drops to 90 mm Hg or below, inadequate organ perfusion can occur, and that is very dangerous.

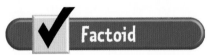

Carbon monoxide poisoning is the most common airway injury.

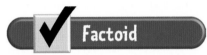

Respiratory involvement greatly increases the postburn mortality rate.[7]

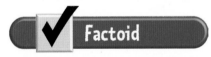

Albumin is necessary for creating the capillary osmotic pressure required to hold fluid in the vascular compartment. Albumin can help to correct a fluid volume deficit by pulling fluid out of the extracellular space and into the vascular space.

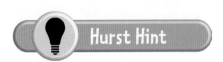

Albumin can pull too much fluid into the vascular space too quickly and cause fluid volume excess, heart failure in susceptible individuals (the very old, the very young, heart patients, and renal patients), and pulmonary edema.

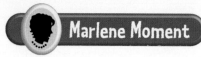

Marlene Moment

I know some humans that act like pigs. Does that mean that their donated skin would be considered a heterograft? Haven't you known a few such individuals that should be freeze-dried?

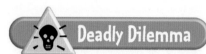

Deadly Dilemma

Clues that should make you suspect airway injury: singed eyelashes and facial hair, reddened face, singed nasal hair—soot smears over the face and coughing up dark, sooty sputum. Patchy discoloration of the nasal and oral mucosal surfaces can occur as a result of breathing heat and smoke.

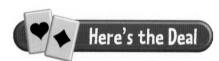

Here's the Deal

Carbon monoxide takes up the only available seat (binds) on the hemoglobin, making it impossible for oxygen to bind for transportation to the cells. Administering 100% oxygen will decrease the half-life of CO to 45 minutes versus 2.5 hours on room air.

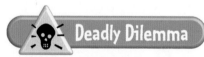

Deadly Dilemma

Cherry red skin and an O_2 sat of 95% will make you think the patient is doing great, but they are hypoxic. The pulse oximeter is reading the CO as O_2 and the cherry red skin is a hallmark of CO poisoning.

- Successful management of the postburn hypermetabolic hinges upon:
  - Adequate nutritional support
  - Warming the external environment
  - Preventing burn sepsis by achieving early wound closure

Patients with high voltage electrical burns and crush injuries have an increased risk of renal tubule obstruction from myoglobinuria and hemoglobinuria, and aggressive fluid resuscitation may not be enough in the presence of acute kidney injury:

- Diuretics may be prescribed (Lasix or mannitol).
- Ultrafiltration: continuous venovenous hemofiltration (CVVH) until evidence of renal recovery is seen (0.5 mL/kg/urine volume for 24 hours).
- Aggressive treatment of shock with protocols using vasopressin, dobutamine, and norepinephrine.[3]

Mechanical debridement uses instrumentation to separate eschar from viable tissue is followed by hemostatic agents and pressure dressings to staunch bleeding. Surgical debridement involves excision with removal of nonviable and necrotic tissue, reducing the risk of sepsis and hastening wound healing.

- Biologic dressings (homografts/allografts or heterografts/xenografts) are used for small burns with clean wound beds to provide temporary wound coverage to reduce pain and fluid loss through evaporation and burn exudates, provide a barrier to entry of bacteria, and promote healing.

Define time

Autografts = me! My own skin from a donor site on my body. These can be whole sheets of skin, meshed (to stretch and cover a larger surface area), or postage stamp size.

Homografts = not me, but like me: from fresh or frozen human sources (cadaver skin, tissue banks, processed amniotic membranes).

Heterografts = not me, not even like me: from pigs, rabbits, lizards! These are fresh, frozen, or freeze dried.

- Biosynthetic and synthetic dressings are used for large areas requiring wound coverage until the wound bed is clean, granulating, and ready to receive an autograft.
- Autografts provide permanent wound coverage.

Physical therapy is indicated for all patients recovering from serious burn injuries, and is useful in conjunction with other treatments to hasten recovery and prevent complications, especially contractures.

Moderate to major burns:

- Nursing care begins with a rapid perusal of the A-B-Cs: airway, breathing, and circulation.
- With burns to the face, head, or neck or if the burn occurred in an enclosed space, think airway first!

- Prepare to assist with prophylactic endotracheal intubation to protect the airway before edema into the burn wound can close off the airway.
- ABGs: monitor for metabolic acidosis.
- Serum carboxyhemoglobin levels.
- For hypoxemia secondary to carbon monoxide poisoning: give 100% oxygen!

Use large gauge venous access devices for placement in nonburned areas to gain immediate IV access:

- A minimum of two reliable sites is indicated for fluid volume replacement.
- Insert a Foley catheter and measure the immediate return and hourly urine output.
- Determine the time that the burn injury occurred (not the time of arrival in the emergency department) because half of the total 24-hour fluid resuscitation must be delivered within the first 8 hours (Parkland formula).

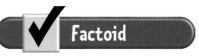

Factoid

It is important to remember that all fluid replacement formulas are estimates and must be titrated based on the patient's physical response.

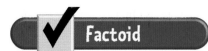

Factoid

The single best indicator of fluid replacement in this situation is urine output.

Parkland Formula

(4 ml of LR) × (body weight in kg) × (% of TBSA burned) = total fluid requirements for the first 24 hours after burn

first 8 hours = ½ of total volume

second 8 hours = ¼ of total volume

third 8 hours = ¼ of total volume

- Assess the percentage of body surface burned by using the "rule of 9s" (Fig. 16-4).

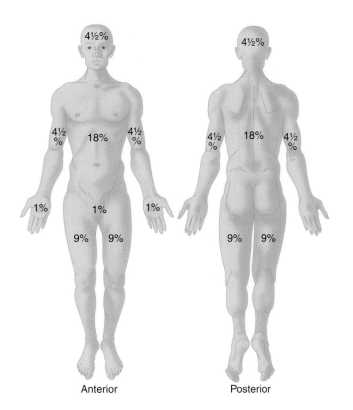

◀ Figure 16-4. Anterior and posterior views: the rule of 9s.

Anterior   Posterior

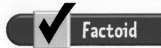

Factoid

Blood pressure readings can be obtained using an arterial line for continuous blood pressure monitoring if using a blood pressure cuff would cause further harm to the patient's injuries.

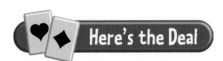

Here's the Deal

There are two reasons that analgesia for the patient with a major burn must be given by the IV route:

- The burned patient needs immediate relief, and IV analgesia works fast!
- Absorption of IM analgesia requires good muscle perfusion, and the burned patient does not meet these criteria!

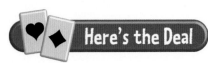

Here's the Deal

When the burn wound extends into blood vessels and muscle tissue, free hemoglobins and myoglobins are released into circulation and can plug the renal tubules. Pigments seen in the urine give evidence of these substances being filtered through the kidneys and the doctor will want to hurry up and flush out the kidneys.

Fluid resuscitation with isotonic fluids is given to restore circulating volume and raise the blood pressure to improve renal perfusion.

- Weigh the patient, converting pounds to kilograms.
- Place the patient NPO.
- Monitor bowel sounds frequently. Paralytic ileus may develop.
- Monitor hourly urinary output to evaluate efficacy of fluid resuscitation and renal perfusion.
- Monitor urine-specific gravity and serum hematocrit to evaluate vascular space hydration status.
- Monitor continuous blood pressure readings to evaluate fluid volume status and organ perfusion.

My patient needs analgesia as soon as possible after the initial A-B-C priority needs have been satisfied and other injuries have been ruled out:

- Administer prescribed morphine IVP starting with the lowest dose in the prescribed range (usually titrated slowly until relief is obtained).

Albumin may be prescribed after 24 hours to increase vascular volume and increase renal perfusion.

- Administer IV slowly and monitor patient response because increased fluid volume increases the workload on the heart.
- Monitor CVP hourly being alert to sudden increases as well as trends.
- Monitor for signs of fluid volume excess: increasing blood pressure, CVP, distended neck veins, basilar rales.
- Monitor emesis for evidence of coffee ground appearance because the patient is at high risk for developing a Curling's ulcer.
- Administer prescribed GI-protective medications such as Mylanta, Protonix, and Pepcid.
- Observe urinary output for color changes (red, brown, black) and notify the doctor immediately.

General components of the nursing care plan for any burn patient should include burn wound care:

- Burn would must be cleansed initially and daily with a mild antibacterial agent and sterile saline or water.
- Cleansing of the wound and gentle debridement of eschar, using scissors and forceps, can be accomplished using hydrotherapy, shower, shower cart, bathtub, or at the bedside.

Regardless of the method, chilling must be avoided because this adds unnecessary metabolic stress:

- The room temperature should be 80°F to 85°F.
- The water temperature should be 100°F.
- Limit wound cleaning to 20 to 30 minutes.

General components of the nursing care plan for any burned patient should include:

- Meticulous daily hygiene for nonburned skin and hair as well as oral care.

- Premedication prior to daily hydrotherapy, which will clean and gently debride nonviable loose skin from the wound bed.
- Application of prescribed topical antibacterial agents (Table 16-7) and sterile dressings.

Table 16-7 Topical agents for wound management

Topical agent	Side effects/ adverse effects	Nursing implications
Silvadene (silver sulfadiazine): • Acts on the cell membrane and cell wall • Has bactericidal action on many gram-positive and gram-negative bacteria	• May cause leukopenia but this usually resolves • May cause sulfa crystals in the urine • Hypersensitivity reaction can occur if allergic to sulfa. • Can cause erythema multiforme	• Check allergy to sulfa. • Pat dry and apply cream after daily wound cleansing. • Apply thin layer (1/16 in). • Reapply if it rubs off. • Monitor WBCs. • Inspect skin and discontinue if rash occurs. • Monitor for burning, pain, or pruritus and report promptly. • Monitor for hepatic or renal dysfunction.
Sulfamylon (mafenide acetate): • Effective against many gram-positive and gram-negative organisms and some strains of anaerobes. • Active even in the presence of pus and produces marked reduction of bacterial growth in avascular tissue, diffusing rapidly through eschar • Agent of choice for electrical burns because of ability to penetrate eschar	• Hypersensitivity reaction possible, but cross-sensitivity to other sulfonamides not established • Intense stinging, burning pain up to 20 minutes after application • Acid–base imbalance	• Premedicate before application. • Apply to clean debrided skin with a sterile gloved hand. • Keep burn covered with cream, and apply more if it rubs off any area. • Be alert to signs of metabolic acidosis, especially with extensive burns.
Silver nitrate 0.5% (aqueous solution): • Has bacteriostatic and fungicidal action • Does NOT penetrate eschar • Solution is hypotonic and acts as a wick for sodium and potassium	Electrolyte imbalance • Stains everything (dressings, bed linen, clothing) black. • Burning and skin irritation. • Absorbed nitrate can cause hyponatremia. • Toxic effect: methemoglobinemia (inactivated hemoglobin).	• Dressings must be kept wet: remoisten every two hours. • Cover with gauze or blankets to reduce vaporization. • Monitor electrolytes (Na^+ and K^+).
Betadine (povidone-iodine)	• Stings. • Stains. • Allergic reactions. • Acid–base problems.	• Question about allergy to iodine. • Avoid using near the eyes: can cause ocular burn. • Avoid use with occlusive dressings.

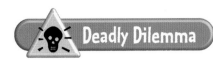

Deadly Dilemma

- The patient receiving cleansing in a hydrotherapy tub is at risk for cross-contamination of wounds from one area of the body to the other, loss of electrolytes from open would areas, and chilling.
- Enzymatic agents may be applied to the burn wound for a more rapid debridement of eschar.
- Application of topical anti-infectives and either bulky dressings or a warm environment and a bed cradle to keep linens from touching the skin. A variety of techniques are used for wound cleaning depending upon whether the patient is ambulatory or nonambulatory and the extent of the burn.
- Hydrotherapy tanks.
- Showers and shower chairs.
- Washing on a stretcher with a spray nozzle.

(Continued)

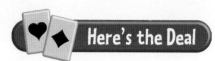

Topical medications must be alternated because the bacteria can build up a tolerance or resistance to the drug.

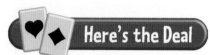

All burns are contaminated wounds! People "stop-drop-and roll" to put out flames, and guess where tetanus lives? In the soil! Tetanus toxoid is given to produce active immunity, which means that two to four weeks after the injection of a weak antigenic substance, the body will produce antibodies against the tetanus bacillus. But the burned patient cannot wait two to four weeks! He or she needs immediate protection, which is why immune serum globulin is administered—to supply the patient with needed antibodies for passive immunity and immediate protection!

Never administer tetanus toxoid (or any other vaccine) to anybody who is immune suppressed (eg, HIV-positive patients, patients taking chemotherapy, or elderly patients with poor nutrition), because rather than making antibodies against the tetanus bacillus, they could develop tetanus!

Table 16-7 Topical agents for wound management (*continued*)

Topical agent	Side effects/adverse effects	Nursing implications
Acticoat (metallic silver): • Consists of two layers of silver-coated high-density polyethylene mesh enclosing a single layer of nylon/polyester non-woven fabric. • Exhibits pronounced anti-bacterial activity against a wide range of gram-positive and gram-negative bacteria including strains resistant to many types of antibiotics. It is also effective against clinically important strains of yeasts and fungi. • Can be left in place for 3 days without changing the dressing. Acticoat 7 is changed weekly (good for 7 days).	• Hypersensitivity reaction may occur. • Stinging occurs in some partial thickness burns.	• Darker blue surface must be in direct contact with the skin. • Moisten dressing with sterile water (NOT saline). • Cover with a secondary dressing. • Do not use concurrently with oil based products or topical antimicrobials. • Change dressing more frequently for heavily exudating wounds. • If adherence occurs soak the dressing off to avoid trauma to underlying tissue.[6]
Topical enzymatic drugs for debridement of burn wounds: • Travase • Collagenase	• May cause scarring because of its digestive action. • Supports growth of organisms by creating a warm, moist environment.	• Wear gloves. • Discontinue and remove from skin in the event of bleeding or pain. • Use concomitantly with topical anti-infectives to prevent sepsis. • Do not use on face, if pregnant, over large nerves, or near any area opened to a body cavity.

Source: Created by the author from Reference 8.

Broad-spectrum antibiotics are used initially because all burn wounds are contaminated. These drugs will be discontinued as soon as C&S reports are returned.

• Protect wounds undergoing surgical intervention (debridement, grafting) from trauma and microbial contamination.

• Monitor biologic grafts (temporary wound coverage) for signs of infection or rejection.

• Monitor the burn wounds for any evidence of infection: redness, breakdown, or suppuration (formation of pus).

• Maintain strict asepsis and handwashing to prevent cross-contamination.

• Implement protective or reverse isolation.

• Administer tetanus prophylaxis and/or immune serum globulin as indicated.

Ensure adequacy of nutrition to support hypermetabolic state and wound healing:

- Monitor and record intake: three high-calorie, high-protein meals with ample vitamin C and three high-calorie snacks.
- Calculate and record daily calorie count to aid in evaluating adequacy of nutritional intake.
- Administer nutritional supplements as prescribed.
- Administer nasogastric or G-tube feedings if indicated, checking gastric residuals prior to each feeding and auscultating bowel sounds.
- Administer prescribed total parenteral nutrition (TPN) and lipids according to established protocols.
- Weigh patient daily and record, evaluating trends and correlating with urinary ketones.

The nurse is constantly on the alert for complications of burn wounds:

- Monitor serum electrolytes, being alert to the development of hyperkalemia and hyponatremia.
- Monitor ABGs, being alert to the development of metabolic acidosis and hypoxia.
- Monitor Sao₂ and differentiate restlessness from a pain response.

Because tight dressings, edema, or eschar can compromise circulation, the nurse must:

- Monitor pulses, skin color, skin temperature, and capillary refill.
- Be especially alert to circumferential burns (those that encircle a limb).
- Notify the doctor immediately for any indicators of impaired circulation and prepare to assist with escharotomy or fasciotomy to relieve the pressure and restore circulation.

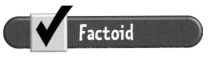

Overfeeding is to be avoided because the resultant increased metabolism increases oxygen consumption and production of carbon dioxide, all of which add to the existing metabolic stress imposed on the body by burn trauma.

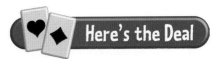

If the burned patient has ketonuria, obviously he or she is burning body fats for energy, and the doctor must be notified to re-evaluate the level of nutritional support and caloric needs.

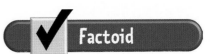

Restlessness and tachycardia are early signs of hypoxia.

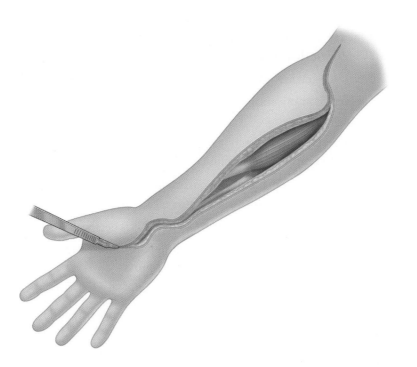

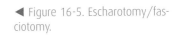

◄ Figure 16-5. Escharotomy/fasciotomy.

Escharotomy is an incision into the eschar to create a slit to relieve constriction of blood vessels. Fasciotomy is a deeper incision that relieves a pressure in a compartment to relieve pressure on blood vessels and nerves (Fig. 16-5).

▶ Figure 16-6. Mesh autograft.

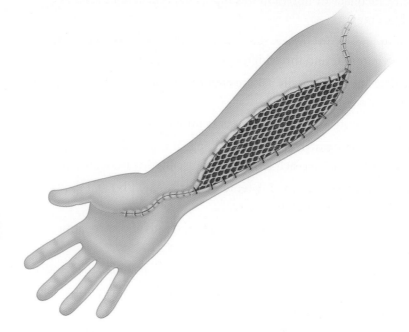

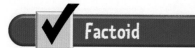

A bluish or cool graft indicates poor circulation and a risk for loss of the graft (Fig. 16-6).

PATIENT TEACHING   Prevention is the best medicine!

- Photosensitive medications increase risk for burns! Limit exposure, and wear protective clothing and sunscreen for prevention.
- Install smoke detectors, check them weekly, and change batteries every six months.
- Have chimneys and fireplaces inspected and cleaned yearly.
- Never leave burning candles unattended.
- Set the temperature of the hot water heater to "low-medium" if there are elderly or diabetic persons in the home.
- Never use electrical appliances or cords in or near water.

To prevent complications from a burn wound (infection or impaired circulation):

- If the burn is on a leg, keep it raised or propped up for the first 24 hours to help reduce swelling.
- Go to the nearest emergency department for swelling, numbness, or tingling below a burn on your arm or leg.
- Keep the bandage clean and dry. Change it if it gets wet.
- Immediately report any fever, increasing pain, and redness around the burn, or bad-smelling drainage from the burn.

Care of an autograft (recipient site/donor site):

- Donor site (partial thickness) heals in 7 to 14 days. Be gentle with tender new skin.

- No smoking, and don't be around smokers. Nicotine is a powerful vasoconstrictor, and you need good blood flow into the graft.

- Don't lie on the recipient graft site or have any pressure on the site.

- Don't wear a watch or carry a purse over the graft site.

- Notify your doctor immediately if the graft becomes blue or cool.

  Care of healing burned skin:

- Protect burned skin from the sun. Wear wide-brimmed hats and use sunscreen.

- Use fragrance-free lubricating creams and mild soaps.

- Avoid any further trauma to healing skin. Don't scratch, and leave blisters intact.

Cutting edge

Newly emerging drug-resistant pathogens are forcing burn care providers to find alternate drugs that are effective. At the Galveston, TX Shriners Burn Hospital an old drug (Colistin) is making a reappearance in the battle against burn infections. First isolated in Japan in 1949, Colistin (also called polymyxin E) has re-emerged as a highly effective antibiotic against multiresistant *Pseudomonas* and *Acinetobacter* burn infections. Vancomycin and clindamycin remain the drugs of choice for methicillin-resistant *Staphylococcus aureus* (MRSA) infection.[9,10]

At another renowned burn center (Ft. Sam Houston, TX), the continuous venovenous hemofiltration (CVVH) technique (a form of hemofiltration) has shown a promise of extrarenal effects in critically ill burned patients: reversal of shock and improvement of acute respiratory distress syndrome (ARDS) with the additional benefit of immunomodulatory effects and patients being weaned off vasopressors by 48 hours.

PRACTICE QUESTIONS

1. Which recommendation is most appropriate to a massage therapist with chronic dermatitis on both hands?

   A. Wear gloves to avoid contact with lotions and oils used for massage.

   B. Use soybean oil and add the fragrance effect from a candle or simmer pot.

   C. A patch test should be performed to determine the source of this obvious allergy.

   D. Consider a career change to cosmetology because this would give the hands a rest yet satisfy service-oriented inclinations.

2. When the patient has psoriasis, which of the following self-reported practices would require further teaching?

   A. Soaking a warm bath to scrub scales with a soft brush and mild soap.

   B. Skin is carefully examined for changes between phototherapy treatments.

C. Occlusive dressings over topical medications are never left in place longer than eight hours.

D. Dry shaving over thick scaling lesions with a safety razor before application of prescribed topical agents.

3. Which question is most important to ask an adolescent girl with severe acne vulgaris before administering the prescribed initial Accutane tablet?

A. Are you sexually active?

B. Are you allergic to any antibiotics?

C. Have you ever taken this acne drug previously?

D. Have you been eating chocolate in the last 24 hours?

4. The patient with an acute outbreak of dermatitis herpetiformis has tiny pruritic blisters over elbows, knees, buttocks, and the nape of his neck. From the list of patient problems upon admission, to which need will the nurse direct immediate attention?

A. Intense pruritus

B. Gluten-free diet and snacks

C. Evidence of anemia

B. Bowel assessment for celiac disease

5. The patient has sustained burns to the upper torso, face, and neck as a result of a steam injury when a pressure cooker exploded. Which priority nursing intervention is of the most immediate concern?

A. Administer prescribed morphine.

B. Make preparations for endotracheal intubation.

C. Prepare to administer prescribed isotonic IV fluid resuscitation.

D. Have the bag-mask device readily available to support respirations.

6. Which short-term goal is the most appropriate for a depressed burn patient facing long-term rehabilitation? The patient will:

A. Demonstrate increased participation in unit activities.

B. Make realistic plans for coping with physical disability.

C. Assign meaning to the life events contributing to current depression.

D. Communicate with other patients on the unit about common problems rather than talking about his depression.

7. Your patient was tightening the coupling on a rusty steam pipe when the pipe split, spewing a large stream of hot steam over his body. All of the following burn wounds are painful; blanch and refill promptly with fingertip pressure.

● Red patches on the front of his left arm and hand

● Blisters across one-half of his left chest and abdomen

- Blisters over the anterior thigh to the knee
- Posteriorly the entire trunk has equal areas of red patches and blisters

Use the anterior/posterior burn map (Fig. 16-4) for calculating TBSA and choose the most accurate assessment. Select all that apply.

A. TBSA 36%

B. TBSA 41.5%

C. TBSA 32.5%

D. TBSA 45%

E. Superficial partial thickness 13.5%

F. Superficial partial thickness 18%

G. Deep partial thickness 22.5%

H. Superficial partial thickness 23.5%

I. Minor burn

J. Major burn

8. Following escharotomy of a circumferential burn to the arm, which provides the best means for evaluating the effectiveness of this procedure?

A. Absence of pain in the extremity

B. Prompt capillary refill after blanching

C. Absence of bleeding at the site of the incision

D. Ability of the patient to wiggle his or her fingers

9. Upon removing the bulky dressing, the nurse notes that a greenish pigmented slime is covering the burn wound over the chest and arm. Which next nursing action is most appropriate?

A. Collect a specimen of the burn exudate in a sterile tube.

B. Apply the prescribed topical agent and re-dress the wound.

C. Have the patient lather up with antibacterial soap in a warm shower.

D. Question the patient about recent ingestion of green leafy vegetables.

10. An autograft becomes accidentally dislodged from the wound bed as a dressing is being removed. Which next action is priority?

A. Call for bedside assistance.

B. Call the doctor from the bedside.

C. Halt any additional unwrapping and rewrap the site.

D. Apply sterile saline moistened gauze to the wound bed and graft.

References

1. National Psoriasis Foundation. Home page. Available at http://psoriasis.org/netcommunity/home. Accessed November 7, 2009.

2. Porth CM. *Pathophysiology: Concepts of Altered Health States.* 7th ed. Philadelphia: Lippincott Williams & Wilkins; 2007.

3. Chung KK, Lundy J, Matson JR, et al. Continuous venovenous hemo-filtration in severely burned patients with acute kidney injury: A cohort study. *Crit Care* 13:R62, 2009.

4. Simon BA. Regional ventilation and lung mechanics using X-ray CT. *Acad Radiol* 12(11):1413–1422, 2005.

5. Metzger JC, Eastman AL, Pepe PE. Year in review 2008: Critical care-trauma. *Crit Care* 13(5):226, 2009.

6. SMLT Datacard. Acticoat dressing. Available at http://www.dressings.org/Dressings/acticoat.html. Accessed September 26, 2009.

7. Mustonen K-M, Vuola J. Acute renal failure in intensive care burn patients (ARF in burn patients). *J Burn Care Res* 29(1):227–237, 2008.

8. Hurst M. *A Critical Thinking and Application NCLEX Review.* Brookhaven, MS: Hurst Review Services; 2008.

9. Hachem RY, Chemaly RF, Ahmar CA, et al. Colistin is effective in treatment of infections caused by multidrug-resistant *Pseudomonas aeruginosa* in cancer patients. *Antimicrob Agents Chemother* 51(6):1905–1911, 2007.

10. Branski LK, Al-Mousawi A, Rivero H, et al. Emerging infections in burns. *SurgInfect* 2009.

11. Williams JD, Tate BJ. Occupational allergic contact dermatitis from olive oil. *Contact Dermatitis* 55(4):251–252, 2006.

12. Comerford KC, Labus D, eds. *Nursing 2010 Drug Handbook.* Philadelphia: Lippincott Williams & Wilkins; 2010.

APPENDIX A

✚ Formulas for fluid volume replacement in burns

There are various formulas as guides for fluid volume replacement in burn patients. The physician is responsible for calculating the IV fluid needed during the first 24 hours, and the amount of colloids (usually serum albumin) after 24 hours. The nurse is responsible for monitoring the patient response to fluid replacement therapy, which determines the efficacy of IV fluid replacement.

• All formulas use the patients total body surface area burned (TBSA) and weight in kilograms.

• All IV solutions are balanced solutions of electrolytes (isotonic) such as Lactated Ringer's and normal (0.9%) saline.

• Colloids are added after the first 24 hours when the injured vessel walls have regained a degree of permeability (not leaking so badly), and serum albumin is the solution most commonly used.

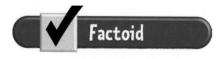

Factoid

Serum albumin (a colloid) is necessary for creating the osmotic pressure that holds vascular fluid inside the vascular compartment (so it doesn't leak out).

✚ Brooke Army formula

- Electrolyte solution (Lactated Ringer's): 1.5 mL × kg body weight × TBSA burned
- Glucose (D5%W): 2000 mL for insensible loss
- Colloids (serum albumin): 0.5 mL × kg body weight × percent TBSA
- Day 1: Give one-half of the total volume in the first 8 hours, and give the remaining one-half over the next 16 hours.
- Day 2: Give one-half of the total colloids plus one-half of the daily calculated electrolyte solution, and all of the replacement for insensible loss (D5%W).
- When partial- and full-thickness burns (second and third degree) are in excess of 50% TBSA, the fluid requirements will be based on 50% TBSA.

✚ Consensus formula

- Lactated Ringer's solution (or other isotonic saline solution): 2 to 4 mL × kg weight × TBSA burned
- Give one-half of the total in the first 8 hours.
- Give the remaining one-half total volume over the next 16 hours.

✚ Evans formula

- Colloids: 1 mL × kg body weight × percent TBSA burned
- Electrolytes (normal saline): 1 mL × kg body weight × TBSA burned
- Glucose (D5%W): 2000 mL for insensible loss
- Day 1: give one-half of the total in the first 8 hours, and the remaining one-half over the next 16 hours.
- Day 2: Give one-half of the colloids and one-half of the electrolyte solution plus all of the insensible loss replacement.
- The maximum fluid volume is 10,000 mL per 24-hour period.
- When partial and full thickness burns (second and third degree) are in excess of 50% TBSA, the fluid requirements will be based on 50% TBSA.

✚ Parkland/Baxter formula

- Lactated Ringer's solution: 4 mL × kg body weight × total body surface burned (TBSA).
- Day 1: Give one-half of the total in the first 8 hours; give the other one-half over the next 16 hours.
- Day 2: The flow rate varies according to the patient response (heart rate, blood pressure, and hourly urine output). Colloids (serum albumin) are added after 24 hours.

ANSWERS AND EXPLANATIONS FOR THE PRACTICE QUESTIONS

Chapter 1

1. Correct Answer: C. Things can happen on a busy medical-surgical unit. Patients can suddenly become more acutely ill, and the nurse manager must be available to troubleshoot and to assist if emergency situations occur on the unit.

Answer A: is not cost effective, but this remains a viable option for staffing in an emergency situation.

Answer B: is also a viable option; however, caution in selecting patient assignments is required if the nurse is unfamiliar with medical-surgical patients.

Answer D: does not help with the existing patient load, but will reduce the additional consumption of time and manpower associated with patient admissions.

2. Correct Answer: C. Although all other nursing actions (A, B, D) may be indicated to prevent future similar action by this physician, this is the only option that will help *this* patient by allowing surgery to proceed, providing real and immediate help for the identified patient problem, which is not being fully informed of risks, benefits, and options before authorizing surgery.

3. Correct Answer: B. This important hint could mean that the patient carries the genetic defect that when combined with certain inhaled anesthetics and the muscle relaxant succinylcholine produces the potentially deadly malignant hyperthermia (MH).

Answer A: could mean that she also carries the breast cancer gene, which is can be cured with early detection and excision, and can be treated with chemotherapy and radiation IF the patient lives through surgery and is NOT one of the 10% of patients who DIE from malignant hyperthermia.

Answer C: Knowing that the patient is susceptible to nausea and vomiting can enable the nurse to plan proactive means to prevent this postoperative complaint IF the patient survives surgery.

Answer D: Knowing about the latex allergy that could cause anaphylaxis is good, as it enables the surgical team to make sure that the patient is not exposed to any latex.

NOT knowing about the potential for malignant hyperpyrexia could lead to lack of preparedness for dealing with the deadly MH.

4. **Correct answer: A.** Hemorrhage will always be the priority over pain, infection, or psychosocial concerns. This is the KILLER answer!

Answer B: If the patient hemorrhages, he or she will not live long enough for the nurse to re-evaluate the effectiveness of the analgesia.

Answer C: If the patient hemorrhages, he or she will not live long enough for the fever to spike from an infection (about 3 days).

Answer D: Maslow's hierarchy of needs states that physiologic needs (02) are more essential that psychosocial needs such as body image.

5. **Correct Answer: B.** Loss of fluids from anywhere can cause shock, especially in the elderly! Monitoring the systolic blood pressure and cardiac output (central perfusion to vital organs and peripheral perfusion) in addition to watching for early signs of shock (restlessness and tachycardia) are priority because shock is a killer!

Answer A: *Clostridium difficile* (*C. diff*) may be the infecting organism; this is common with bowel surgery, and anti-infective rather than antidiarrheal agents are effective.

Answer C: Dumb answer! People strain with constipation, not diarrhea! Well, maybe the patient could strain his rectal sphincter, trying to "hold it!"

Answer D: The purpose of protective isolation is to keep the immunosuppressed patient from getting a hospital acquired infection because of cross-contamination. This patient needs isolation of fecally contaminated articles to avoid infecting others.

6. **Correct Answer: B.** Hemorrhage can be a killer complication after amputation because major arteries have been interrupted, and a tourniquet at the bedside can be lifesaving. Did you think that this was a sociocultural question? No, it was a hemorrhage question!

Answer A: Visualize this: As the patient is dying from hemorrhage, the nurse reads aloud "As I walk through the valley of the shadow of death, I will fear no evil." No! A Bible would be a socioculturally appropriate article to have available, but Maslow's hierarchy deems physical needs more basic, and priority over higher level needs such as spiritual needs. Spiritual needs won't kill you, but hemorrhage will!

Answer C: Again, according to Maslow's hierarchy, oxygen is a more basic need than elimination. Don't read anything into the question! I didn't say the patient was a cardiac who might die on a bedpan from straining at stool!

Answer D: An article to measure blood pressure would be indicated when hemorrhage is suspected and one must monitor for early shock (restlessness and tachycardia), but without a tourniquet to stop the flow of blood, the blood pressure cuff will only enable you to watch the cardiac output fall as early shock progresses to late shock, from which there is no coming back. Killer! If tachycardia and restlessness are present, you can put on the tourniquet and then call for someone to bring a blood pressure machine.

7. Correct Answer: C. The patient was in a dorsal lithotomy position for vaginal surgery and is predisposed to venostasis from surgical positioning. A deep vein thrombosis (DVT) can be a killer complication if the clot becomes an embolus and travels to the lung causing a pulmonary embolus (PE). This is the nurse's major concern!

Answer A: Numbness and tingling could be another serious complication secondary to surgical positioning in stirrups, because this could indicate nerve injury, which could lead to disability. Calf pain is still the priority assessment, because this can lead to sudden death caused by PE! Physical rehab may be indicated for nerve injury, but burial may be indicated for a sudden massive PE! No question about the major concern now, is there?

Answer B: Because the bladder is a pelvic organ, this subjective complaint should cause the nurse to palpate the bladder for distention. Inability to void may be a transient problem, easily remedied with "in-and-out" catheterization (a nursing concern, but not a killer complication like a possible DVT).

Answer D: Nausea is a frequent uncomfortable side effect of codeine, and the nurse will notify the physician for a different analgesic order, and notify the pharmacy of a drug reaction, but again, not a killer answer! Nobody ever died from nausea.

8. Correct Answer: B. Serum creatinine is a test to evaluate glomerular function, and when elevated (normal = 0.5–1.5 mg/dL) above 2.5 mg/dL is an indicator of renal impairment. The creatinine is especially relevant in diabetic patients because they tend to have renal disease secondary to vascular damage. When the kidneys cannot effectively excrete X-ray dye, acute renal failure can result.

Answer A: Blood urea nitrogen (BUN) is a good test for renal function, but serum creatinine is a more sensitive and specific indicator of renal disease than BUN and is not influenced by diet or fluid intake. A slight BUN elevation (normal = 5–25 mg/dL) is expected in the elderly patient, but could also result from hypovolemia secondary to NPO status.(P.S. Did you pick up on the word "most"? This is a qualifier in the question that forces you to pick creatinine instead of BUN.)

Answer C: A slightly elevated urine specific gravity (>1.026) can be seen with dehydration and is not a cause for concern.

Answer D: Blood sugar in upper limits of normal is expected of a diabetic patient, and may be helpful in avoiding hypoglycemia caused by missing breakfast and possibly lunch because of NPO status. This is not a cause for concern!

9. Correct answer: C. Serum albumin. Albumin is a protein that is a good indicator of nutritional status because protein is the basic building block for muscle tissue. If protein is adequate, all other nutrients are also adequate. If protein (albumin) is lacking, fluid will leak out from the vascular space into the tissues or will "third space" into body cavities. Albumin is necessary for maintaining the osmotic pressure that keeps fluid in the vascular space.

Answer A: Glucose level has no relationship with edema. Hyperglycemia would cause particle-induced diuresis (PID) and fluid loss rather than edema.

Answer B: Sodium is the only electrolyte that even cares about water and could cause fluid retention. You would not want to send a patient to surgery with hyponatremia or hypernatremia because of blood pressure or cardiac issues, but sodium has nothing to do with nutritional status (readiness) related to postoperative wound healing.

Answer D: Magnesium is an electrolyte that is important in most metabolic processes, but is mainly important in cardiac patients. Low levels increase cardiac irritability, causing arrhythmias, and high levels delay neuromuscular conduction to widen the PR interval and the QRS. Even though magnesium deficiency does occur in malnutrition, it does not indicate a positive nitrogen balance and "good" nutrition for wound healing. All symptoms associated with magnesium are neuromuscular.

10. Correct answer: D. The RN must monitor and interpret the blood pressure reading in order to regulate the nitroglycerin drip, and the flow rate may or may not change with each reading based on nursing judgment of the primary nurse. Maintenance of blood pressure within a specific range cannot be compromised by possibly invalid readings or time delay when the UAP or licensed personnel is looking for the primary nurse for purpose of reporting each of the frequent reading. The primary nurse must also be at the bedside in this circumstance to evaluate the adequacy of the patient's cardiac output.

Answer A: This task is within the scope of practice and level of competency, but the responsibility and authority of this patient belongs to the primary nurse who should retain care of this patient. Reporting back and forth with the frequent blood pressure reads would be a waste of precious RN time, and may place the patient in jeopardy while waiting for titration of the medication after reporting from one RN to another. The primary nurse has to be at the bedside anyway to titrate, so titrating in conjunction with blood pressure monitoring is actually conserving a valuable resource.

Answers B and C: Incorrect. This is not within the scope of practice because of the circumstance and level of nursing judgment required.

Chapter 2

1. Correct Answer: A. Because the patient is already sitting straight up, the most immediate thing the nurse can do while remaining at the bedside (awaiting a second nurse to bring the morphine) is to dangle the patient's legs over the side of the bed, hanging them dependent to trap venous blood in the periphery, away from the heart, immediately reducing preload. This action will reduce any further backflow into the lungs. Rule: Never leave an unstable patient!

Answer B: It is always appropriate to assess prior to selecting an implementation answer, but you've already assessed labored respirations, verified by the patient. Also, the posterior auscultation can be accomplished while the patient is dangling legs over the bedside.

Answer C: A nurse should be able to apply oxygen per mask without calling for respiratory therapy. Putting your work off on somebody else will always be wrong!

Answer D: Morphine is an excellent choice to relax smooth muscles of the bronchus, to vasodilate and trap venous blood in the periphery, promoting ease of breathing, but it takes time to get the drug from the medicine room, signout the drug, and administer, not to mention having to leave the patient to do so!

Hurst Rule

Never leave an unstable patient: This is always wrong!

---

2. **Correct Answer: C.** Rule: Always assume the worst! Many diuretics may cause the patient to excrete calcium (which acts like a sedative). A twitchy eyelid is a muscle spasm that may forewarn of tetany. Latent tetany can be verified with a positive Trousseau's or Chvostek's sign, in which event the doctor must be notified. A tracheostomy set had better be at the bedside with an amp of calcium gluconate and a 60-mL syringe taped to the top of the tray.

Answer A: Halting the IVP medication is appropriate, but hypotension does not make an eyelid twitch! Better worry about hypocalcemia rather than hypotension!

Answer B: Rapid IVP Lasix will drop the blood pressure by relaxing the smooth muscle around the blood vessels (tunica media), and a twitching eyelid does not represent a relaxed muscle, rather a rigid tight (not sedated) muscle as evidence of latent tetany.

Answer D: Nothing is wrong with obtaining a nursing history of previous twitchy eyelids, but would a previous happening 10 years ago be significant now? And do you want to finish administering the dose of Lasix, because this may be the culprit that has lowered the serum calcium? I don't think so...not without notifying the doctor and checking electrolytes first!

3. **Correct Answers: A and D.** Hypotension <90 mm Hg is not sufficient for adequate renal perfusion. Dyspnea and air hunger are late signs of shock usually accompanied by cyanosis, which indicates that the lungs are not receiving adequate perfusion, so perfusion to the kidneys has already been compromised, because the kidneys are the first of the four vital organs to be eliminated.

Answer B: Sustained tachycardia >140 reduces the cardiac output, and any significant decrease in CO can reduce renal perfusion, and if coupled with other signs of shock could lead to acute renal failure, but this is not a definite indicator.

Answer C: Cold clammy skin is caused by systemic vasoconstriction to raise blood pressure and shunt blood to vital organs (namely, the kidney...so this is a good sign—actually intended to restore renal perfusion—when something bad is happening!).

4. Correct Answer: B. Do not question this order! The patient with hyponatremia has too much water and not enough sodium. The patient having neurologic changes needs hypertonic saline 3% or 5%. The patient does not need any more water!

Answer A: D5W **(A)** is isotonic initially, but when metabolized creates free water (becoming hypotonic) to further dilute the existing sodium, making the sodium level plunge even lower. NS with KCL

Answer C: **(C)** is a killer answer, because the patient with hyponatremia is already dilute and NS (isotonic=equal amounts of sodium and water) stays in the vascular space but does nothing to correct the imbalance, but potassium actually makes the hyponatremia worse! Because sodium and potassium have an inverse relationship, the added potassium will only drive the existing sodium lower!

If NS 0.5% were given (slightly more than ½ NS=hypotonic), this solution cannot supply enough saline to correct such a severe imbalance (neurologic changes), hypotonic solutions LEAVE the vascular space: they go OUT of the vascular space to hydrate the cells that already have too much water on board. The problem is NOT hydration. This patient has too much water, and not enough sodium!
Better question these incorrect answers **A, C, and D.** See rationales above!

5. Correct Answer: A. Feeding tube patients tend to get dehydrated, especially patients on bed rest, because bed rest induces diuresis! If the patient is already having neurologic signs, a grand mal seizure may be next! Better take seizure precautions while awaiting the serum sodium results.

Answer B: When hypernatremia is present, the brain cells shrink because when the body is dehydrated, water is drawn from the cells into the vascular space.

Answer C: Until serum sodium is corrected, the patient will be unable to process information regarding time, place, and person, but more importantly, safety issues always take priority over psychosocial issues (remember Maslow?).

Answer D: While you're taking vital signs, your patient is having a seizure! Safety first!

6. Correct Answer: C. The patient's problem is hypermagnesemia. You'd better count the respirations! Magnesium acts like a sedative: The bowel prep (a magnesium containing cathartic) cannot be excreted if the patient is in the oliguric phase. All the clues point to neuromuscular problems, and because the diaphragm is a big important muscle, you better check respirations! With hypermagnesemia, the patient

may develop hypotension caused by vasodilation secondary to hypermagnesemia, but respirations are still the priority assessment because the nurse has to remember the A-B-Cs! Breathing (respirations) always comes before circulation (blood pressure).

7. **Correct Answer: C.** Chvostek's sign is an early indicator of neuromuscular irritability associated with hypocalcemia, and as the trigeminal nerve (crossing the cheekbone) is tapped, that side of the face and eye will go into spasm. The most serious concern is impending tetany and laryngospasm, which will close off the airway.

    Answers A, B, and D: Vital signs are late indicators of a problem. Forget counting the respiratory rate if the patient isn't breathing because of laryngospasm, which has blocked the airway. As soon as latent tetany (as evidenced by a positive Chvostek's and Trousseau's signs) is detected, the patient will be given IV calcium to prevent airway obstruction. When does NCLEX© want you to intervene? Early or late? Early, of course, before the patient gets into trouble!

8. **Correct Answer: D.** What electrolyte are you worried about? Potassium!! You had better be worrying about a fatal arrhythmia! Let's put the patient on a heart monitor please! Heart is priority!

    Answers A and B: Blood pressure and weight point to fluid retention and FVE, which increases workload on the heart and can lead to heart failure. If you are worried about heart failure, the priority is to auscultate the lungs!

    Answer C: The patient must be scheduled for dialysis as soon as possible; however, the patient must be alive to obtain hemodialysis. Better put him or her on a heart monitor while you attempt to contact the hemolysis center.

    Answer: E: Maslow's hierarchy mandates that physiologic needs take priority over psychosocial needs, and the patient is in the emergency department where physiologic needs (namely an arrhythmia) are being taken care of.

9. **Correct Answer: D.** Ordinarily, you think that a loop diuretic would be helpful because serum potassium is lowered by diuresis, but all you need to know is that fluid is leaving the vascular space immediately after a burn owing to capillary permeability. If the vascular space is dry, Lasix would be contraindicated, because what little fluid remains in the vascular space would be excreted, leaving the patient in FVD (shock).

    Insulin and glucose (**A**) is good because this drives the potassium back into the cells. Calcium gluconate is good (**B**) because it decreases arrhythmias secondary to cardiotoxic effects of hyperkalemia. Albuterol (**C**) pushes potassium into the cells for short periods (2–4 hours) usually used for patients on hemodialysis to buy some time while dialysis is in progress if arrhythmias are problematic.

10. Correct Answer: A.

Hurst Rule

If the patient begins having new or different symptoms after onset of a medication, always stop the infusion and call the doctor. You can always re-start the medication after collaboration with somebody who knows more than you! The burning is caused by irritation of the vessel lining, and the doctor may prescribe a slower flow rate, or increase the dilution of the potassium.

Answer B: Draining the vein will not stop the irritating effect of the potassium. More is coming behind it because the infusion is still in progress.

Answer C: Even though a warm compress will promote vasodilation, the irritating chemical is still in contact with the venous wall.

Answer D: Even though this is a true statement, the patient is symptomatic, and this answer does nothing to correct the problem, which is venous irritation accompanied by a local inflammatory reaction.

Chapter 3

1. Correct Answer: B. Your patient has metabolic alkalosis. If she is vomiting, vomiting, vomiting … then she is losing acid, acid, acid! Which means she is alkaline on the inside, and the problem is not her breathing (therefore you can just forget about answers A and C, which go with a respiratory problem). If the lungs were trying to compensate for the metabolic alkalosis, the PCO_2 would be up (not down) because she would be trying to conserve some acid by holding on to her carbon dioxide.

Answer D: This is just plain wrong. If you vomit, you lose acid … so why would she want to excrete her base? That's a dumb answer. (Sorry!)

2. Correct Answer: D. Your patient has hyperphosphatemia, which is the exact same thing as hypocalcemia, which is why she should be on her side (dysphagia = risk for aspiration). The mental changes are caused by metabolic acidosis. The incidence of hyperphosphatemic acidosis and other severe electrolyte imbalance induced by the traditional phosphate salts is well documented.

Answer A: If the doctor accidentally perforated her bowel, she won't be sore or have a tender abdomen immediately.

Ditto for Answer B: What's the belly got to do with the problem her brain is having? (How's your brain? I don't know. Let me check your belly!)

Answer C: This tells me you think she is overdosed on 5 mg of Valium. Get real!

3. Correct Answer: A. We've depressed her CNS with the narcotic, and her breathing center will be depressed too! Because she's got on the abdominal binder, I don't assume that she is taking any nice deep breaths, so she is retaining CO_2 and may already be in early respiratory acidosis. You'd better wake her up and make her blow off some CO_2 (acid).

Answer B: If you chose this answer, you need to run on back to the nurse's station and pick up one of those laminated RIP signs. Be sure to put it on the door, so nobody else will wake her up either. You're a KILLER! You're not going to get a license in the mail.

Answer C: Duh … oxygen is not her problem. Her problem is CO_2. If you wait on her to get hypoxic too … well, you're a KILLER! She will be blue and bradycardiac to go with the low O_2 saturation now that she's hypoxemic.

Answer D: When she fails the LOC and orientation test, she may already be brain dead from the respiratory acidosis that you could have remedied early on … with the incentive spirometer. The NCLEX lady wants you to intervene early, not LATE!

4. **Correct Answer: C.** This patient has all the symptoms of occult metabolic acidosis owing to subclinical hypoperfusion. A serum lactate will identify anaerobic metabolism by-products (lactic acid), which may warrant ABGs to confirm the diagnosis.

Answer A: This choice lists only one GI symptom, which could be drug related; all others are characteristic of low perfusion/oxygen lack acidosis.

Answer B: This is unfounded because no symptoms of infection are displayed. Usually the patient has to spike a fever or have purulent drainage to warrant collaboration with infection control.

Answer D: This is dangerous because increasing activity level will increase oxygen demand and worsen the patient symptoms, increasing acidic by-products of anaerobic metabolism.

5. **Correct Answer: A.** In acidosis, hydrogen leaves the vascular space and is pushed into cells, exchanging places with potassium, which leaves the cells, going into the blood stream, so the patient becomes hyperkalemic.

Answer B: Calcium is associated with acidosis, but levels go UP, rather than down.

Answers C and D: Magnesium and phosphorus levels are not significantly affected in acidosis.

6. **Correct Answer: B.** A central nervous depressant depresses respirations and leads to increased levels of CO_2 and because the patient has obstructive lung disease and already has high levels of CO_2, respiratory acidosis can occur.

Answer A: Blood pressure readings are considered "significant" if a 20-mm Hg change in systolic measurement occurs; 10 mm Hg can represent a normal fluctuation and is not significant.

Answer C: Low level oxygen does not affect the hypoxemic drive of the chronic lung patient; warm, pink, moist skin may result from fever.

Answer D: Tenting represents decreased skin turgor, which could signify dehydration (which also could result from fever), but tenting on hands is common. Forehead and sternum tenting more accurately represent hydration.

7. **Correct Answer: A.** In metabolic acidosis the pH is low, but the P_{CO_2} is also low because the patient in DKA has Kussmaul respirations in an effort to blow off more acid (CO_2).

Answer B: This is respiratory alkalosis, pure and simple. The pH is high (not low), but the base is normal, because kidneys are so slow to compensate. However, the CO_2 is low, because the patient is blowing it off.

Answer C: Maw-Maw keeps forgetting that she already took the prescribed aspirin dose and now she has respiratory alkalosis because recent salicylate poisoning is a respiratory stimulant in the early phase. The late phase after aspirin overdose causes high ion gap acidosis. See answer B for hyperventilation.

Answer D: This is metabolic alkalosis! Gastric acid is lost to suction and vomiting, leaving the body in an alkaline state.

8. **Correct Answer: A.** Metabolic acidosis because high concentrations of hydrogen ions keeps calcium from binding to plasma proteins (hypercalcemia), and an attempt to lower serum levels of hydrogen by movement into the cell causes potassium to move out (hyperkalemia)!

Answer B: Alkalosis cannot be correct because of the above rationales (see A).

Answer C: Acidosis is correct (see preceding rationales), but there is no evidence of dietary respiratory depression noted that could cause CO_2 to be retained.

Answer D: Alkalosis is incorrect (see rationale A), and there is no evidence of a respiratory problem associated with a restrictive diet (unless you hyperventilated when you saw the "Death by Chocolate" dessert on the menu).

9. **Correct Answer: B.** Brain trauma (especially in the medulla) and ICP can decrease the respiratory rate and depth. Retaining CO_2 leads to respiratory acidosis.

Answers A and C: This is a lung problem because the respiratory center in the brain is depressed, so "metabolic" makes both these answers incorrect.

Answer D: Respiratory alkalosis would result from too rapid respirations (blowing off CO_2), not too slow or shallow.

10. **Correct Answer: B.** Mechanical ventilation is required for patients who cannot breathe effectively without help, so compensation for respiratory insufficiency/acidosis is underway, because several days have passed and the "slow-poke" kidneys have finally kicked in to begin excreting excess hydrogen.

Answer A: The patient had respiratory insufficiency and acidosis or he or she would not have been placed on the ventilator in the first place.

Answer C: Ventilator support gets more oxygen to the tissues to halt further anaerobic metabolism and buildup of lactic acid.

Answer D: Acidic urine is good because bacteria don't like an acid environment, but we're supposed to be evaluating the patient's acid–base imbalance and response to the ventilator! Oxygenation is priority over infection, unless of course the patient is in septic shock, because *then* you have metabolic acidosis caused by cellular hypoperfusion.

Chapter 4

1. **Correct Answers: A, B, C, and E.** All are components of metabolic syndrome.

   Answer D: High levels of high-density lipoproteins (HDLs) are cardioprotective! They act like a detergent in blood vessels, keeping them clean and free of the foam cells, the fatty streaks, and eventually the atheromatous plaques of CAD (physiologic integrity).

2. **Correct Answer: A.** Grapefruit juice increases the bioavailability of calcium channel blockers, thereby raising blood levels excessively, which could precipitate a dangerous drop in blood pressure and decrease cardiac output.

   Answer B: Resting is a good thing for someone with angina, but what has rest got to do with taking a calcium channel blocker? This drug should improve a person's work performance!

   Answer C: The patient doesn't need more blood flow to the heart muscle during sleep, better coronary blood flow is needed during the waking hours when a person is up and about performing activities of daily living!

   Answer D: While the patient is attaining therapeutic blood levels of amlodipine, chest pain may still occur with activity, a warning signal that the heart muscle is not receiving adequate oxygenation. Nitroglycerin must be taken SL to restore the balance of oxygen rapidly, and will continue to be used for prompt relief of any acute attack of angina (pharmacologic and parenteral therapies).

3. **Correct Answer: B.** Further teaching is needed! B-complex vitamins (B_3, niacin included) taken with Lipitor may lead to development of a serious muscle disorder (rhabdomyolysis), which can cause renal failure.

   Answers A, C, and D: All are indicated as a part of self-care while taking antianginal medications. The heart rate should be monitored.

   Answer A: Beta-adrenergic blockers/calcium channel blockers decrease heart rate.

   Answer C: Removal of the transdermal Nitro patch for 8 to 12 hours daily is necessary to prevent the development of a tolerance to the medication.

Answer D: Orthostatic hypotension is a valid concern with drugs that reduce the cardiac output (pharmacologic and parenteral therapies).

4. **Correct Answer: C.** Sex can be resumed when the patient can walk around the block or climb a flight of stairs without chest pain.

   Answer A: Staying indoors is good when a heat advisory is issued, but this patient needs air conditioning. Fans only blow hot air. If the patient does not have an air conditioner, transportation into a day center or air-conditioned mall is advised.

   Answer B: The patient with angina should not be outside in the snow doing any heavy work, no matter how light the shovel is!

   Answer D: Large, heavy meals are contraindicated, as they cause a huge shift of blood flow to the GI tract for digestion, and may compromise coronary blood flow (physiologic integrity).

5. **Correct Answer: A.** Levitra. This is the killer answer! Nitroglycerin is contraindicated if Viagra, Cialis, or Levitra have been taken in the past 24 hours because of resultant profound hypotension and drop in cardiac output.

   Answers B, C, and D: These are all compatible with nitroglycerin infusion: Lovenox (anticoagulant), Integrilin (GP IIb-IIIa inhibitor), and Atromid-S (anti-lipidemic) (pharmacologic and parenteral therapies).

6. **Correct Answer: A.** Morphine first!! In addition to relieving the pain and anxiety, morphine causes vasodilation, which will reduce preload, reducing the workload on the heart, as blood is pooled out in the periphery, away from the heart.

   Answers B, C, and D: Each have a role in limiting the size of the infarction.

   Answer B: Oxygen, yes, according to the AHA ACLS protocols. Oxygen is a drug! It keeps the ischemic myocardial cells from dying and becoming more necrotic.

   Answer C: Nitroglycerin opens up coronary vessels to improve blood flow, again, keeping ischemic cells alive.

   Answer D: Aspirin has antiplatelet properties that keep the existing clot in the coronary artery from getting any larger.

7. **Correct Answer: A.** Applying cold may buy some time while preparations for surgery are underway. Cold reduces oxygen requirements of the tissue, and can delay tissue necrosis. Notifying the doctor can be accomplished while directing a coworker to apply the ice (or vice versa).

   Answer B: This will make arterial insufficiency even worse! You elevate vein problems, but you "hang art."

   Answer C: Pain never killed anybody, and is not the immediate priority. Life and limb will always come first!

   Answer D: This is delaying treatment. Why is the leg cold? Because there is no blood flow owing to an arterial thrombus! Maybe if we can warm it up some, vasodilate the artery perhaps, the thrombus can break loose and take out the lungs too! Now the patient can have a pulmonary embolus to go with his dead leg. Killer!

8. **Correct Answer: C.** The function of the left ventricle is to keep blood moving forward. As long as the lungs are clear, the failing ventricle is at least adequate. In shock, the damaged heart can hardly perfuse itself, let alone the other vital organs. The urine output will be diminished and the skin will be cold and clammy from diaphoresis caused by vasoconstriction, which raises the blood pressure and shunts blood to vital organs.

   Answers A, B, and D: These are excellent indicators of cardiac output, but the nurse cannot know if the low blood pressure is adequate for keeping blood moving forward without auscultation. Auscultation is the priority, because by the time the patient feels short of breath and dyspneic, the lungs are already filling with fluid.

9. **Correct Answer: A.** Always assess first before selecting an intervention answer.

   Answer B: This does not match symptoms of left heart failure! JVD signals right heart failure. Shortness of breath implies left failure. Remember, L = lungs!

   Answers C and D: These are both indicated after assessing for moist rales.

   Answer C: Morphine is the drug of choice for pulmonary edema because it relieves the restlessness, anxiety, and agitation that accompany difficult breathing, while it also vasodilates to reduce preload and afterload.

   Answer D: Lasix is a rapid-acting diuretic, which also vasodilates but does nothing to relieve associated agitation.

10. **Correct Answer: A.** The patient with valvular dysfunction may not notice any problems until he or she becomes short of breath, usually with exertion.

    Answer B: Pale, ashen skin color usually accompanies cardiogenic shock, a very late sign.

    Answer C: Substernal chest pain is a sign of acute coronary syndrome.

    Answer D: Cyanosis is a late sign of hypoxia.

Chapter 5

1. **Correct Answer: B.** The patient in Addisonian crisis has a deficit of aldosterone and is at risk for hypovolemia because sodium and water losses result in decreased circulatory volume.

   Answer A: The acute MI patient is prone to develop *cardiogenic* shock.

   Answer C: The patient who had a central line inserted may have had the right atrium nicked, causing iatrogenic cardiac tamponade (circulatory shock, but obstructive type).

Answer D: The young man with the PE is at risk for obstruction to outflow from the heart (also obstructive type).

2. **Correct Answer: D.** The hypotension accompanying acute MI is unrelated to a deficit of circulating volume. Replacing plasma volume is not indicated and will be harmful in that the increased preload would place more workload onto an already failing heart.

Answer B: Vasopressor agents are used cautiously to raise systolic blood pressure while carefully monitoring the effect of increased afterload.

Answers A and C: Both are indicated as standard treatment modalities to restore and maintain perfusion to the myocardium to improve contractility.

3. **Correct Answer: B.** Septic shock is a form of distributive shock, triggered by systemic inflammatory mediators that cause the person to be hypotensive because of vasodilation, which gives rise to warm flushed skin.

Answers A, C, and D: The classic presentation of cold and clammy skin owing to vasoconstriction, which is the sympathetic response, is found in burn, hemorrhagic, and cardiogenic shock.

4. **Correct Answer: B.** When the vascular space is unusually large (because of vasodilation), administering a fluid bolus will add volume to improve cardiac output and raise the blood pressure to better perfuse the placenta and save the unborn baby from certain hypoxemia.

Answer A: This would further compromise fetal oxygenation by reducing chest expansion of the woman with pressure of a gravid (35-lb) uterus on the maternal diaphragm, and forcing blood flow away from the uterus by gravity. Lowering the head of the bed could also have a very dangerous effect by allowing the spinal anesthetic to migrate farther up the spinal canal and paralyze the woman's diaphragm.

Answer C: This would also aggravate the problem by trapping maternal venous blood, keeping it out in the periphery and away from central circulation. Both legs can be *raised* to drain blood into central circulation for the effect of a physiologic fluid bolus.

Answer D: This is ineffective for an obstetric emergency, which requires 100% oxygen by tight-fitting face mask to salvage a fetus in distress.

5. **Correct Answer: C.** There is no substitute for prompt administration of epinephrine, which relaxes bronchospasm and opens up the airway. Without epinephrine, the patient is dead and none of the other interventions will bring him or her back.

6. **Correct Answer: C.** Generalized vasodilation produces hypotension, leading to poor tissue perfusion. You better go for the vasopressors or the patient won't live long enough for the culture to grow!

Answer A: If you picked culture as a first intervention … your patient is dead, but at least you know what bug killed him! However, we do obtain cultures before starting antibiotic therapy.

Answer B: This may be indicated, because shock activates a systemic inflammatory response, but if you don't get the blood pressure up first, the patient is dead.

Answer D: It is always important to keep family members informed of changes in patient status (when they are on the accepted list and have a "code" word to receive information), but Maslow's hierarchy places unmet physiologic lower-level needs before higher-level psychosocial needs.

7. Correct Answer: C. Iatrogenic cardiac tamponade should be suspected because a common site of bleeding is the right atrium after insertion of a central line. Oxygen is indicated when cardiac output is decreasing because of cardiac compression.

    Answer A: This is indicated after the immediate intervention of applying oxygen. (Rule: If there is something you can do first to help reduce a complication, do it!)

    Answers B and D: Trapping blood in the periphery or increasing blood flow to the brain does nothing to improve cardiac output or tissue oxygenation.

8. Correct Answer: A. Administer oxygen.

    Answer B: This is delaying treatment. Damp clothing never killed anybody!

    Answer C: This can further depresses the central nervous system that is already depressed because of lack of oxygen.

    Answer D: This is a bit premature for EARLY shock, which, if treated promptly and aggressively, may be reversed to restore effective circulation.

9. Correct Answer: C. Epinephrine and antihistamines are the only options to relieve a bronchospasm in anaphylactic shock.

    Answers A and B: Providing oxygen will be ineffective when the airway is obstructed. (The ET tube cannot be introduced if the airway is in a spasm.)

    Answer D: This does not solve an airway problem.

10. Correct Answer: A. A hallmark sign of a congenital hiatal hernia. Abdominal organs sucked upward into the thoracic cavity result in the concave appearance of the abdomen.

    Answer B: Acrocyanosis is normal in the newborn.

    Answer C: Systolic blood pressure will be low rather than high because the cardiac output falls when the heart is being compressed by encroaching abdominal organs.

Answer D: High-pitched crowing is associated with bronchospasm. Ventilatory efforts will be shallow because of lack of room for lung expansion.

Chapter 6

1. **Correct Answer: A.** A leukotriene receptor antagonists (eg, Singular) or alternates such as cromolyn, nedocromil, or an inhaled short-acting beta$_2$-agonist are recommended by the NHLBI-3 as pre-exercise strategies to avoid EIB.

   Answers B, C, and D: (B) The asthmatic patient who has EIB must warm-up before ALL exercise, not just exercise in a cold environment. A cold environment will additionally require a covering over the mouth to avoid the environmental trigger of cold air entering the airways. (C) LABAs are not used for premedication before exercise, because they can mask poorly controlled asthma. (D) Inhaled corticosteroids are appropriate for immunotherapy against allergens, and allergens are not implicated in exercise-induced asthma.

2. **Correct Answer: B.** Here's the strategy: You only have one chance to tell the NCLEX-lady what is the most important thing to do! This patient has had a pulmonary embolus, so if you don't do anything else, you'd better apply 100% oxygen! Otherwise, the patient may not live to be a candidate for clot busting!

   Answer A: The patient is anxious because he or she cannot breathe!

   Answer C: We don't clot bust dead people! We're in the business of keeping living people alive. Clot busting is important, but what comes first? A-B-C!

   Answer D: The upright position is fine, but the extra time and effort to position the patient forward with arms up would be interpreted as delaying treatment by the NCLEX® people.

3. **Correct Answer: A.** These foods reduce the risk of developing COPD, and help to prevent decline in lung function for those who have obstructive lung disease.

   Answers B, C, and D: Meats actually increase the production of CO_2, and does the patient with COPD need any more RBCs? No! They already have polycythemia because of chronic hypoxemia. You're a killer: Viscous blood can lead to a stroke or a PE! And we certainly don't want to dehydrate them by withholding their water!

4. **Correct Answer: D.** If she is *planning* surgery, this means she hasn't had it yet, and the birth control pill plus smoking is asking for a thrombus, which could become an embolus.

   Answer A: This patient is up and walking the halls and ready to go home after uncomplicated minor surgery.

   Answer B: Older patients have a lesser amount of total body water, but fluid resuscitation is in progress, so dehydration is not a problem.

Answer C: This patient does not require prolonged bed rest, and there is no indicator of dehydration, which would make the blood more viscous and prone to clotting.

Answer E: We would like for the patient to walk, but as long as the SCDs are in place, venous return to the heart is as good as walking, because the rhythmic squeezing of the sleeves over the lower leg simulates the "muscle pump" to return venous blood to the heart, avoiding venostasis. Also, there is no evidence of venostasis or dehydration.

5. **Correct Answer: C.** You had better be trying to get as much oxygen into what little lung the patient is able to perfuse with blood. The "triple s" chest pain means pulmonary embolus! And if your postoperative patient became suddenly acutely breathless, the PE is a big one!

   Answer A: Not bad, if this is all that I have. However, I'd rather have more oxygen, please.

   Answer: B: Again, not enough oxygen for the acutely breathless patient with a PE.

   Answer D: I'm glad you know that with a PE there is pulmonary hypertension because circulation through the lung is obstructed, but this is why the patient may require mechanical ventilation with PEEP. Low pressure hasn't got a prayer of going where it needs to go. It will take higher pressure to get oxygen into this lung.

6. **Correct Answer: C.** The patient with COPD has chronically high levels of CO_2, which is acidic. Fruits and vegetables produce alkali, which will help neutralize excess acid, and they also have a protective effect on the lungs.

   Answers A and B: These choices are loaded with calories and protein, but too much at one serving! COPD people tire and achieve satiety quickly, so small frequent meals are better.

   Answer D: This choice is nutrient dense (except for non-nutrient coffee) and is a good second choice because the bacon is actually a fat rather than a meat source, and fat supplies need calories. No fruits or vegetables (alkaline) are contained herein and too many carbohydrates can increase production of carbon dioxide.

7. **Correct Answer: D.** Pressure from the buildup of fluid or air on the injured side pushes everything to the opposite side. As the heart shifts to compress the unaffected lung, the trachea will also be pulled toward the unaffected side.

   Answer A: Distant or muffled heart sounds is a sign of cardiac tamponade.

   Answer B: Blood in the airways occurs with pulmonary contusion, which most probably accompanies the trauma that caused the broken ribs.

   Answer C: Breath sounds will be absent on the AFFECTED side, the side that is collapsed and not moving air. Only very late (when the patient is in respiratory failure) the severely compressed unaffected lung can no longer move air, but by that time the patient has already shocked from low perfusion because the great vessels are compressed and there is virtually no cardiac output.

8. **Correct Answer: D.** Your patient is experiencing respiratory failure, which is defined by PaO_2 <60 mm Hg and $PaCO_2$ >50 mm Hg. He or she will require immediate help to breathe, and this help comes in the form of immediate intubation with mechanical ventilation.

Answer A: You will actually need to lower the head of the bed so that endotracheal intubation can be quickly accomplished. While the patient was struggling to breathe, the head of the bed should have been raised, but it's time now to let the ventilator take over the work of breathing.

Answer B: Forty percent oxygen is not enough to save vital organs. While you are sprinkling a thimble full of water on a raging fire (Get the picture?), your patient is having a fatal arrhythmia from low perfusion to the heart muscle.

Answer C: If this intervention had been accomplished earlier, at the first sign of restlessness and tachycardia, the patient might not be experiencing the present respiratory failure. This option is too little, too late.

9. **Correct Answer: B.** Most adult patients with cystic fibrosis report having thought about end of life care, but few actually have made plans. It's time to talk. Actually, it's past time to talk, but better late than never!

Answer A: How do you know your patient is ready to die?

Hurst Rule

Always assess before you select an intervention answer! You will never go wrong with this strategy!

Answer C: How do you know your patient is ready to die? (See above Hurst rule.)

Answer D: This is a true fact, but do you want to give false hope to somebody who may be dying? Better find out what the patient wants first. (Refer to Hurst rule above).

10. **Correct Answer: A.** Prone! Several intervals of prone positioning to accomplish 18 hours out of each 24 hours in the prone position will shift lung tissue forward to clear airways, decrease atelectasis, reduce lung inflammation, and enhance oxygenation and perfusion. Aeration improves because the heart no longer compresses the left lateral posterior lung. This position is alternated with kinetic therapy and rotational therapy to recruit collapsed airways. Positioning must begin early in the course of ARDS.

Answers B, C, and D: A supine position promotes perfusion of the dependent posterior surface of the lungs only and the heart compresses the posterior left lateral lung surface. This is the worst position for the ARDS patient. A semi-Fowler's position places the lower lobes dependent, and the Trendelenburg position shifts the abdominal organs upward to compress the diaphragm. Not good!

Chapter 7

1. Correct Answer: A. Amitriptyline is the only abortive medication listed that is effective for migraine headaches.

   Answers B, C, and D: These are all prophylactic medications used for headaches.

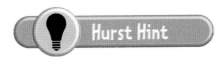

2. Correct Answer: A. Do not disturb the patient after abortive medication has been given! The patient needs to sleep it off without any disturbances.

   Answer B: Do not awaken the patient. Record that the patient appears to be sleeping. Sleep is what the patient needs! If you awaken this patient, he or she may not be able to return to sleep.

   Answer C: The patient does not need to eat! The patient needs to sleep off the headache! The patient can eat later, when he or she feels more like eating (after the headache is gone).

   Answer D: This intervention should have been accomplished BEFORE the abortive medication was administered.

3. Correct Answer: C. A falling GCS score equates decreasing arousal, and ability to process information and respond, which is always bad.

   Answer A: This reflects a wonderful papillary reaction and indicates good cerebral perfusion pressure (CPP).

   Answer B: This symptom is characteristic of a tension headache and is unrelated to what should be your primary concern—increasing intracranial pressure that is compressing neural tissue.

   Answer D: A drop in systolic blood pressure of 10 mm Hg is not significant unless the blood pressure is already <90 systolic; otherwise, 20 mm Hg is considered significant. I wonder what kind of analgesia somebody gave to a head-injured patient? I hope it wasn't anything that would depress respirations or an aspirin-containing compound that would increase the bleeding.

4. Correct Answer: A. This *first* action provides some immediate relief to drop the pressure while you are **(B)** looking for bladder or bowel distention, which is a common precipitating cause of autonomic dysreflexia. If the trigger cannot be found quickly **(D)**, Apresoline will be administered. The physician will be notified **(C)** after the nurse intervenes quickly with appropriate nursing measures (in this order) to relieve the patient's symptoms.

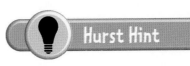

5. Correct Answer: C. Patients who have HNP can walk, stand, or lie down, but sitting aggravates the pain because increased lumbar pressure is generated. The patient should be advised to lie down in good alignment for reassessment in 15 to 30 minutes.

   Answers A, B, and D: These answers are not necessarily correct based on the available data provided.

6. Correct Answer: B. Warm compresses give immediate relief (reported by patients at 2 minutes and 5 minutes), and can result in increased compliance with therapy. Warm compresses vasodilate, which promotes more rapid absorption from the local tissues into the blood.

Answers A and D: A subcutaneous needle (24–25 gauge) is implied because the injection is SQ, but even a 22-gauge needle would cause pain because the medication is irritating, so moving down from a 22- to a 24-gauge needle or the push and pause method would not be helpful.

Answer C: This would not be helpful for the immediate local reaction because the medication will take 20 to 30 minutes to get into systemic circulation. However, NSAIDs are VERY helpful in reducing the flu-like symptoms that accompany these injections.

7. Correct Answer: A. Most patients (two-thirds of cases) experiencing GBS report infection within two weeks of symptom onset.

Answer B: Multiple sclerosis and Parkinson's disease are linked to family history, but heredity and genetics are not implicated in the development of GBS.

Answer C: Poorly controlled diabetes predisposes the patient to cranial nerve and peripheral neuropathies, but is unrelated to the development of GBS.

Answer D: Enlargement of the thymus gland (or tumor in the gland) is seen in up to 80% of patients who develop myasthenia gravis, but is not implicated in the development of GBS.

8. Correct Answer: B. Large international randomized trials have proved the effectiveness of (**A**) plasmapheresis and (**B**) IVIG, but steroids have been deemed ineffective.

Answer D: Plasmapheresis and IVIG ARE effective, making "None" incorrect.

9. Correct Answer: B. Elavil (a tricyclic antidepressant combined with selegiline) will cause hypertensive crisis and possibly death.

Answer A: Colace is a stool softener, needed by the patient with Parkinson's disease because of the tendency toward constipation. Colace does not interact with any antiparkinson medications.

Answer C: Benadryl (antihistamine and anticholinergic) should not be given with tricyclic medications (Elavil) either. However, it is not contraindicated with levodopa or selegiline.

Answer D: Ibuprofen (an NSAID) increases the risk for gastric ulceration and bleeding if taken with the Alzheimer medications, which are all irritating and should be taken with food, but the anti-Parkinson medications do not create a high risk for bleeding, so there is no contraindication for concurrent use of NSAIDs.

10. Correct Answer: C. Lighting should be increased before dusk, and food to digest will increase metabolic energy expenditure, enhancing sleep.

Answer A: Ativan given to the elderly will actually increase restlessness, and have the opposite effect.

Answer B: Turning on the TV will provide more undue stimuli, and closing the door will encourage the patient to open it.

Answer D: A family member may be needed later if efforts to get the patient quiet and ready for bedtime are unsuccessful (notice the qualifier "initial"). This is the next best answer, but it is still incorrect! Sorry.

Chapter 8

1. **Correct Answer: B.** Costovertebral tenderness means that the lower UTI has become an upper UTI and the patient has a kidney infection rather than a bladder or prostate infection. Test-taking strategy: Always assess first before intervening!

    Answer A: Cranberry juice is great for acidifying the urine to prevent UTIs, but the problem is not in the urine (the filtrate) now; the problem is within the glomerulus.

    Answer C: Obtaining a clean catch is an intervention that was performed when the UTI was diagnosed. The doctor will prescribe further in-depth testing of the upper urinary tract.

    Answer D: The problem is recurrent urinary tract infection, so the next logical step is that possibly the lower urinary tract pathogen has ascended to the kidney.

2. **Correct Answer: B.** Crystals may form in the urine when fluoroquinolones are given; therefore, the patient must stay well hydrated to prevent formation of stones. There are no clues in the question to let you know that this patient has a urinary tract infection that originated in the prostate gland, but if you know that fluoroquinolones have a high concentration in the bladder, you always force fluids to promote excretion and flush out the bladder.

    Answer A: Fluoroquinolones cause gastric upset and but should be taken on an empty stomach to enhance absorption.

    Answer C: Fluoroquinolones do not cause color changes in the urine. Pyridium (a urinary antiseptic) turns the urine red, and nitrofurantoin (Bactrim, Septra) stain the urine brown.

    Answer D: Going blind just sounds like a bad complication of something, but when you select an answer, it should always be relevant to the subject. In this case visual changes are not associated with fluoroquinolones.

3. **Correct Answer: B.** A dead kidney cannot filter the blood to produce urine. Necrosis means dead. Nephrons are no longer functional. The person's life has been saved by aggressive treatment to restore circulating volume and blood pressure, which saved the heart, brain, and lungs, but the kidneys are gone! Acute renal failure can occur after only 20 minutes of low or no perfusion.

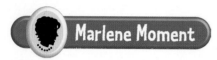

Marlene Moment

That only worked for Jesus!

Answer A: The patient cannot be dehydrated if there is normal circulating volume and blood pressure!

Answer C: If unrelieved, pre-renal failure can progress to intrarenal failure because blood flow and oxygen are what keep the kidney alive and functional, but it cannot progress to postrenal failure (ie, caused by a big prostate), which obstructs outflow of the urine from the kidney.

Answer D: Three days is the time that it takes the kidney to correct an acid–base imbalance (as opposed to three hours for the lungs), but if the kidneys are dead, they will not be resurrected in three days.

4. **Correct Answer: A.** The urine can be black or red or brown after a major burn because the burn wound causes cells to lyse (rupture), and we expect this because free hemoglobulins and myoglobulins are released in the blood when RBCs rupture or the burn damages muscle tissue. However, sludging can occur in the tubules, plugging them up; therefore, the doctor must be notified immediately so you can get an order to hurry up and start flushing out the kidneys, thereby preventing acute renal failure, which could progress to acute tubular necrosis and death.

Answer B: The MI patient will experience a drop in blood pressure with nitroglycerin because it dilates veins and arteries, but the blood pressure comes back up or the nurse would still be with the patient. The rule is to NEVER leave the unstable patient, and the MI patient is unstable as long as he or she is hypotensive. Nothing in the question said that the MI patient was unrelieved of pain or hypotensive.

Hurst Rule

Don't read anything into the question! Don't be imagining symptoms that are not there!

Answer C: Saturating a V-pad in one hour is okay for a newly delivered patient, but saturating MORE than one is a red flag for hemorrhage! So if I check her and the uterus is firm, I will not call the doctor, because I expect lochia rubra to saturate one pad per hour.

Answer D: The thyroidectomy patient is at high risk for bleeding, but if I check and find the dressing dry with no pooling to the back, I am not worried (baseline vitals for comparison not showing a 20 mm Hg drop) because a systolic pressure of 100 is adequate to perfuse vital organs.

5. **Correct Answer: D.** When the specific gravity is fixed after a fluid bolus, this tells you that the kidney is nonfunctional. It is no longer able to concentrate and dilute according to the body's needs. This only occurs in bilateral renal failure.

Answer A: A systolic blood pressure of 90 should be able to minimally perfuse kidneys to keep them alive, but stable only means that the blood pressure is not bouncing around. The kidneys could already be dead, yet the blood pressure is 120/80 (perfect).

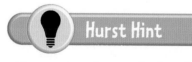

Hurst Hint

Always select the most basic and fundamental concept relevant to the priory need (which in this case is bacteriologic safety).

Answer B: Stable just means not bouncing around. They could be stable but sky high!

6. Correct Answer: A. If the patient cannot learn handwashing you can forget all the rest. Otherwise I would be doing my site care with dirty hands, and what have I accomplished? Duh, peritonitis!

   Answer B: Site care is important, but handwashing (medical asepsis) is more fundamental than anything else.

   Answer C: There are no dietary restrictions (ie, normal sodium or potassium intake) because the dialysis is continuous, and with each drain these substances plus toxins are being removed. Protein may be restricted if the patient has a high BUN.

   Answer D: The peritoneal dialysis patient can play golf, work, shop, work in the home or yard as desired, as well as a number of other activities. Swimming in a lake would not be a good idea, nor would any activity in which a fall might occur because of clumsiness (roller blading) secondary to a change in the center of gravity caused by the 2000 to 2500 mL of dialysate in the abdomen at all times.

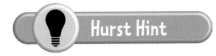

Hurst Hint

Always select the most concrete, definite answer that would not be affected by other variables.

7. Correct Answer: D. Cloudy effluent is the most concrete indicator of peritonitis, which is a killer complication of peritoneal dialysis. Abdominal pain is another indicator, but standing alone, this complaint could be linked to anything from a transient stomach virus or an ulcer.

   Answer A: Abdominal pain could be related to menstrual cramps and who knows what else? See above rationale.

   Answer B: Low-grade fever could be related to a mild URI or another common variable. Also, the fever associated with peritonitis is different. Expect a spike!

   Answer C: Constipation is a common complaint of patients who undergo peritoneal dialysis because the constant fluid in the abdominal cavity leads to decreased peristalsis and the stretched out abdominal musculature reduces bearing efforts owing to decreased muscle tone. But when we are looking for PRIORITY concerns, ask yourself, "Can constipation kill my patient?" I don't think so!

8. Correct Answer: B. If the stone is blocking urine outflow, the urinary output will decrease. This is the priority because hydronephrosis can kill a kidney from the back pressure. Straining urine will provide evidence that the stone has (or has not) been passed.

   Answer A: Pain never killed anybody. Poor Paw-Paw … what did he die of? A kidney stone? If you believe that, I have a bridge I want to sell you in Brooklyn!

   Answer C: The hematuria produced by a renal calculi is not the hemorrhage variety! Kidney stones are not little smooth stones; they have sharp spinous processes and claw their way down the ureters (producing renal colic). The calculi scratch the ureters, and these scratches are responsible for blood in the urine. Can you hemorrhage from a scratch? I don't think so! And nobody ever died from hemorrhage of the ureteral artery either! (There is NOT a ureteral artery. I just made that up!) Nobody is going to die (or even become anemic) from the blood lost in the urine because of a kidney stone!

Answer D: It is possible to develop a kidney infection that is related to an infected stone, but infection is not the immediate threat. The most immediate threat (killer answer) is the risk for hydronephrosis because of blockage of urinary outflow. Losing a kidney is a greater threat than an infection, which can be treated with antibiotics.

9. **Correct Answer: D.** The sediment that you are seeing is what remains of the stone that has been busted up (and passed via the Foley catheter) by sound waves (extracorporeal shock wave lithotripsy). This answer provides visible PROOF that the renal calculi has been busted up and passed!

   Answer A: Renal colic occurs because of spasm of smooth muscle when the stone is moving! The renal calculi could still be present, but not moving (lodged) and the pain has subsided.

   Answer B: The blood could be free of RBCs because the stone is lodged and is no longer moving and clawing its way down the ureter.

   Answer C: If the urinary output has doubled, it is possible that the one remaining kidney has taken over the work of the dead (nonfunctional) kidney and the stone is still in place, causing hydronephrosis.

10. **Correct Answer: A.** Ultrafiltration only pulls water and is used in conjunction with hemodialysis and peritoneal dialysis when the vascular space is still too dilute, as evidenced by the hyponatremia and the added "water" weight.

    Answer B: CRRT is used for the hemodialysis patient who cannot tolerate regular (more aggressive hemodialysis). Only 80 mL of blood is in the filter at any time during dialysis, and because filtration is continuous (over 24 hours instead of 3–4 hours) this is a more "gentle" pull that is used when the patient has an unstable cardiovascular status.

    Answer C: If hemodialysis (the regular kind) is performed again, more water and more electrolytes will be pulled off. The serum sodium is low because the blood is still too dilute. The patient cannot tolerate the additional loss of sodium with the water!

    Answer D: The patient receiving hemodialysis does NOT have a peritoneal catheter in place! This answer is totally inappropriate! The patient has functional access device and puncturing into the peritoneum is an added invasive procedure that carries risk of injury and infection.

Chapter 9

1. **Correct Answer: C.** The right side position is helpful for gastric emptying, but lying down is incorrect because recumbency allows acid reflux into the esophagus. This patient must sit up after meals!

Answers A, B, and D: These are all indicated patient teachings and would not require further teaching. (**A**) Portion control means smaller meal size and less pressure in the stomach. Less pressure means less gastric reflux. (**B**) Pizza, spaghetti, and ravioli all contain acidic tomatoes, onions and garlic (not a good GERD diet). (**D**) The PPI should be in circulation by the time food is introduced for maximum effect.

2. **Correct Answer: A.** Anytime the patient with a hiatal hernia consumes a large meal and overdistends the portion of stomach that has herniated upward into the chest cavity, the increased pressure will cause heartburn and severe pain.

Answer B: A fatty meal will relax the lower esophageal sphincter and allow more reflux causing heartburn, but research has documented that painful symptoms with hiatal are not related to what the person eats but rather how much the person eats. It is the stretching and distention of the stomach that creates hiatal hernia pain that sends patients to the emergency department.

Answer C: Alcohol increases gastric acidity and produces more GERD, but is unrelated to the pain of hiatal hernia caused by entrapment of the stomach in the thoracic cavity.

Answer D: Physical activity after a meal will divert blood flow from the gastric circulation to the skeletal muscles, which have greater need for oxygenated blood flow. This will produce muscle cramps (not chest pain) and is unrelated to the hiatal hernia.

3. **Correct Answer: C.** NSAIDs break down the gastric mucosal barrier that protects the stomach from being digested by gastric acid. When blood in the GI tract is digested, a black tarry stool results. Anemia from constant blood loss reduces hemoglobin and thereby reduces oxygen combining capacity (oxyhemoglobin) for transport of oxygen to cells. Expect fainting if your brain isn't getting enough oxygen! In this real case, a hemoglobin of 5.0 from a chronic bleed actually caused the fall, but the elderly woman thought her vitamins were making her stools black.

Answer A: Who cares what she was doing? She could have been doing anything! She was actually standing at the sink washing dishes. Not relevant! She has a chronic bleed from an NSAID ulcer!

Answer B: Inner ear problems can cause a person to be dizzy, but so can a million other things. The hint is "NSAIDs." If this wasn't important, it would not have been in the question.

Answer D: Get out your clipboard and get ready to write down every single medication! You may need extra paper because polypharmacy is an issue with geriatric patients. Yes, she could have also been taking an anticoagulant, but if the NCLEX® lady thought you needed more data, it would have been included in the question.

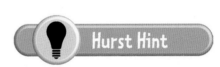
Hurst Hint

Only answer what is asked, using the data provided! You will get into trouble by trying to invent more problems!

4. **Correct Answer: A.** Iatrogenic transmission through contaminated endoscopes has been documented in the United States and is particularly problematic in developing countries where resources for full disinfection procedures are lacking.

> **Define Time**
>
> Iatrogenic means that the infection is hospital acquired.

Answer B: Reverse isolation is used when the patient is at risk for developing an infection (large burns, immunosuppressed patients, etc) so persons entering the room must avoid introducing organisms.

Answer C: *H. pylori* is transmitted by the fecal-oral and oral-oral route. There is no evidence to indicate blood borne infection.

Answer D: *H. pylori* is not an airborne infection! But let's try it! Maybe a mask will help keep dirty fingers out of your mouth!! I don't think so! Let's try handwashing, which is the first line of defense!

5. **Correct Answer: B.** The pancreas lies in the upper abdomen posterior to the stomach directly underneath the tenderness, and pancreatitis is a complication of ERCP affecting one in six patients who undergo this procedure. This patient must be evaluated by the physician prior to being discharged because acute pancreatitis could rapidly become fatal.

Answer A: Sounds right because we are talking about gallstones, which may be plugging up the common bile duct and blocking bile from the liver and gallbladder into the intestine. It is bile pigment that gives stool the characteristic brown color. Without bile the stools are pale (clay colored) and grayish. If the stone has just been removed, don't expect brown stool in the distal descending colon yet! It will take another meal or two for normal colored stools to make their way into the rectum. You know what you eat doesn't come out immediately unless you've got "short gut" syndrome or something!

Answer C: Transient vertigo is related to orthostatic hypotension. Because vital signs are normal, a three-step blood pressure may be indicated. The patient may possibly be dehydrated from being NPO, or maybe this is a side effect of one of her medications, but it is unrelated to the ERCP. The questions said: a complication of *this* procedure.

6. **Correct Answer: A.** Obviously the dysfunctional pancreas is unable to supply adequate enzymes for digestion of fats if the stool (which is probably greasy also) floats! Pancreatic enzyme supplements will be prescribed, urine will be checked for ketones, and the blood sugar will be monitored because the pancreas may be failing in both the endocrine function and the exocrine function.

Answer B: He is probably dreaming that he is in a room with all of his favorite brands of liquor, but they are all just out of his reach! Just kidding! Frightening dreams are very distressing and disturbing to the psyche, and should be addressed. But remember Maslow: which is

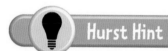
Hurst Hint

Don't just say, "Well I know that means *something*, and I should not let her go until I tell the doctor." Only answer what is asked: stay focused if you want to get more questions right than wrong!

priority? A physical need or a psychosocial need? Starvation or sleep deprivation? Case closed.

Answer C: If the blood pressure is normal (120/80) and the pulse pressure (40) increased by 20%, the current blood pressure is now 120/72. I'm not worried….are you? Here's the deal, I would be worried if this patient had a head injury because a widening pulse pressure means he's getting worse: intracranial pressure is increasing. Were you afraid that maybe he got drunk and fell on his head? Sorry, answer is still wrong!

Answer D: I know what you're thinking! Shame on you! He is not drinking again, he hasn't missed an AA meeting (I know because he sat by me)! Alcoholics have those spidery dilated blood vessels on their noses even when they are not drinking, and I told you he was up all night having bad dreams! Your eyes would be blood shot too! Shame on you!

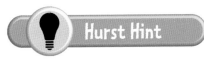

Don't make up stuff that is not there: answer only what the NCLEX® lady asks you, using only the data that you were given! This guy is so malnourished that his pancreas will probably never get well!

7. **Correct Answer: D.** New CAPD patients can quickly develop bad habits and experienced CAPD patients can start taking shortcuts that lead to contamination of the catheter or the dialysate during exchanges. The best way to stop these breaks in techniques is to schedule regular reviews for everybody to closely watch what they are doing and fix the problem *before* they develop an infection.

Answer A: "Yearly" in December is too late for those 11 patients who developed peritonitis because of poor technique in January through November! Reviews to prevent peritonitis have to be ongoing on a regular basis because new patients can develop bad habits after training and "old" patients get complacent after being infection free for two to three years.

Answer B: Teaching handwashing one time will not accomplish the goal! How do you know they are actually doing what you taught them to do? Don't you have to monitor their technique for opening the dialysate and connecting and disconnecting the port also? Handwashing will always be the most important way of stopping the chain of infection, and it seemed like the correct answer…but one word made it wrong: before! You *do* need to make sure somebody is "teachable" before peritoneal dialysis is even considered, but this question is dealing with patients who are *already* performing dialysis exchanges into their peritoneum four times each day. Don't you think it would be helpful to reinforce the technique on an ongoing basis for somebody who already has the catheter in their abdomen? Yes, most definitely!

Answer C: Never consult the doctor for a problem that the nurse is supposed to know how to handle! That answer will always be wrong! Also, because this patient is doing four exchanges per day, 365 days a year for the rest of their life, I guess they just have to be on prophylactic antibiotics for the rest of their life. It only takes one mistake, one short cut to save time, one contamination to develop peritonitis!

Don't pick an answer that says to call the doctor if there is anything that the nurse can do to help the problem in any way. Only call the doctor if there is absolutely nothing a nurse can do to prevent a complication or safeguard the patient!

8. **Correct Answer: A.** The most common and most dangerous symptom of IBD is frequent watery diarrheal stools, which can lead to the

priority nursing diagnosis of FVD. You had better be monitoring the patient's fluid status!

Answer B: Antidiarrheal agents only work in mild cases, and if the IBD is mild, the patient is obviously not losing much fluid. Antidiarrheal agents do not work with severe IBD. You had better be worried about FVD!

Answer C: These assessments help you to evaluate whether the treatment (steroids, hydration, antibiotics, immune modifiers, biologic treatments) have been effective. This is not an evaluation question! The NCLEX® lady needs to know whether or not to trust you! Yes, she would like for you to be able to recognize symptoms of IBD, but she wants to know if YOU know the most important thing to do for this patient! Be alert to signs of FVD, because that is the priority!

Answer D: Pain never killed anybody! The patient may think he or she is dying, and pain will always be their priority, but you are the nurse, and you better be the most concerned about FVD because a big time FVD is called shock!

Hurst Hint

Evaluation questions usually ask something like this: "If the treatment plan has been effective, the nurse will note...blah, blah, blah." If you know all of your signs and symptoms, you can expect to get all your assessment and evaluation questions right!

Hurst Hint

Always pick the "killer" answer! And remember: pain never killed anybody!

Hurst Hint

Don't read anything more into the question than what is asked. If details are not specified, assume they are talking about the conventional way of kissing.

9. **Correct Answer: B.** Hepatitis A is transmitted by the fecal-oral route and handwashing is most important, especially before preparing food (that could be contaminated with the HAV virus)!

Answer A: The baby is not contaminated—it is the Mama who has Hepatitis A! The baby cannot contract hepatitis A from having a diaper change. The organism lives in feces, and it is MAMA's feces that is contaminated!

Answer C: Hepatitis A is not transmitted by body fluids such as saliva, so kissing does not support a fecal-oral mode of transmission (but maybe it depends on which end you are kissing!).

Answer D: The patient with hepatitis A is no longer communicable by the time that jaundice appears. The pre-ictal period (before onset of jaundice) is when the HAV is most highly communicable. Fecal-oral contamination would have to occur during sexual activity for transmission to occur because blood and body fluids are not a mode of transmission of the hepatitis A virus.

10. **Correct Answer: A.** You better get a doctor on the way stat while you are trying to find the Sengstaken Blakemore tube that you should have already had in readiness because you knew your patient had cirrhosis. The doctor is the only one who can insert this tube to apply tamponade to the esophageal varix and stop the bleeding.

Answer B: Oxygen sounds good and it is always indicated with hemorrhage and with patients who are anemic, but you're a killer! Look at your assessment data again. A tight fitting mask will drown him in his own blood when that mask fills up with blood and he aspirates it into his lung. A nasal cannula would be safer, but this would still not be the priority answer.

Answer C: You never leave an unstable patient! (That is the iron-clad rule!) But if you pick this answer, you are telling the NCLEX® lady: "I'll just hold this basin and keep catching blood until it stops and you are dead!" You can't do that!

Answer D: Yes, let's put a tourniquet around his neck! You are NOT going to get a license in the mail picking answers like this!

Chapter 10

1. **Correct Answer: C.** Alcohol contains calories and four beers exceed the "moderation" recommended by the ADA. Alcohol is toxic to nerves, so there is greater incidence of pain, burning, tingling, and numbness. Alcohol is also caloric, which raises blood sugar. Hyperglycemia (sugar) destroys blood vessels and the retina is a wall of tiny vessels at the back of the eye.

Answer A: Diabetics are supposed to develop routines, and running is great to include in a daily routine because it helps to lower blood sugar, improve circulation, and maintain weight control.

Answer B: You should be worried about hypoglycemia if the diabetic is unable to eat and has taken oral hypoglycemic medication. *Occasionally* and *transient* are the key words! It doesn't happen often and it goes away relatively quickly, so the patient would be able to eat when nausea subsides.

Answer D: Again, the key is occasional. Blood sugar goes up when diabetic patients forget to take oral medications, but this does not mean that they go for long periods without medication.

2. **Correct Answer: B.** Pain with palpation is not neuropathy. Typical burning, aching, numbness, and paresthesias are continuous. Many times infected ulcers are masked by thick, hard calluses that have a mushy necrosis underneath. A relevant lab would be the white count report, as well as heart rate and temperature. All of these point to infection, which must be addressed quickly before development of gas gangrene or necrotizing fasciitis.

Answer A: Assumes this is chronic neuropathy and the patient could be septic and the limb could become unsalvageable before the doctor realizes that there is a need for surgical intervention.

Answer C: This intervention assumes that the patient has developed a possible DVT. Patients don't get DVTs in their toe! And there was no mention of local erythema and heat or redness,

Answer D: Medicating the patient will mask the symptoms, and as long as you don't palpate the toe, the warning symptom of pain will go unnoticed until the onset of gas gangrene.

Answer E: This intervention would be appropriate for arterial insufficiency, to get more blood flow into the tissues. This patient has peripheral neuritis and pain to touch warns of additional pathology underneath the callous. Better alert the doctor to the priority issue!

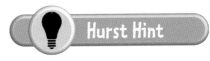

Hurst Hint

If there is nothing that the nurse can do to stop the problem or prevent a complication, you have to get some help for your patient by calling the doctor. Priority means that you have to pick the ONE thing that will help this hemorrhaging patient the most. This strategy will help you weed out all those other things!

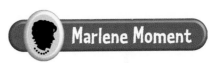

Marlene Moment

Routines are good for the diabetic patient, but the routine practice of drinking four beers a day is not recommended. One drink is all women can have per day, and guys can have two drinks. And NO, having a sex change operation does NOT mean that now you can have three drinks a day!

3. Correct Answer: B. Increasing the caloric value of the bedtime snack will offset the early morning (2–3 AM) drop in blood glucose.

Answer A: The patient is experiencing a drop in blood sugar between the hours of 2 and 3 AM, and a snack at this time would be needed, unless of course you had planned in advance for this occurrence and provided a heavier bedtime snack! Is it better to let the patient "bottom out" and then give food, or would it be better to prevent the drop in blood sugar?

Answer C: By early morning the patient will be rebounding with hyperglycemia when you awaken him or her at 5 AM to eat, thereby raising blood glucose even higher! Not good!

Answer D: Administering the intermediate-acting insulin later in the evening is the treatment of choice when the patient is experiencing the Dawn phenomenon, wherein the blood glucose starts rising around 3 AM. This intervention would worsen the drop in blood glucose associated with the Somogyi effect.

4. Correct Answer: C. The Type 2 diabetic who has normal liver function will convert excessive amounts of glycogen to glucose at night, which raises blood glucose. A bedtime snack could increase glucose levels even more. Hold the bedtime snack.

Answer A: It's okay to call the doctor to report that the bedtime snack is not necessary because the patient isn't taking NPH insulin, but you had better hold the bedtime snack as a next action. If you call the doctor, and he or she says don't give the bedtime snack, you would really hate to have to drop an NG tube to retrieve the bedtime feeding!

Hurst Rule

If there is anything that the nurse can do to help the patient or prevent a predictable complication, do that first before calling the doctor!.

Answer B: This intervention sends the message, "Hey, I don't really believe my reading is correct, and this will be interpreted as delaying treatment." Besides that, in real life nursing, the lab is only consulted for repeat blood glucose when levels are >200 mg/dL or <70 mg/dL.

Answer D: Yes, let's give you some more calories so your night time blood glucose will go even higher, causing microvascular injury. Remember: Sugar destroys blood glucose just like fat!

5. Correct Answer: C. Diabetes is under control and no medications are being given that would cause the blood sugar to drop during the night.

Answers A and D: Both of these patients have Type 1 (insulin-dependent) diabetes, one of which has no warning symptoms of hypoglycemia.

Answer B: The bedtime glucose of 140 mg/dL will be even higher in the morning because glycogen will be converted to glucose during the night, which will raise the serum glucose.

6. **Correct Answer: D.** Applying external heat is incorrect and should not be included in the plan of care for a patient with hypothyroidism no matter how careful you are. Heat will cause vasodilation and drop the blood pressure. Slow warming with extra clothing, layered coverlets, and closing air conditioning vents are all appropriate means of maintaining body heat.

    Answer A: The patient with hypothyroidism does not have the energy for self-care, and it is highly probable that hygiene (oral as well as body hygiene) has been neglected, so meticulous hygiene is appropriate for inclusion in the plan of care.

    Answer B: Patients with hypothyroidism have coronary artery disease because altered metabolism of fats, and cholesterol/triglyceride levels are usually elevated. They don't need any more animal fat, so this restriction is appropriate for the patient with hypothyroidism!

    Answer C: Because of slowed cognition, using simple concrete terms will enhance comprehension when giving instructions to the hypothyroid patient, who may have decreased ability to process information.

7. **Correct Answer: A.** Always remember A-B-C if it is relevant, and it is with hyperparathyroidism. (Too much PTH means too much calcium, which acts like a sedative.) Flaccid muscle tone and hypoventilation requires that the most immediate priority is airway and breathing.

    Answer B: Circulation is important, this priority comes *after* attention has been directed toward airway and breathing. What good would come of circulating *deoxygenated* blood, and how long can the heart muscle last without oxygen? Always remember A-B-C when prioritizing in emergency situations.

    Answer C: Critical symptoms are treated first! Getting the serum calcium levels down is priority over diagnostics. If the patient isn't breathing, you don't send him or her down for an imaging study!

    Answer D: Surgery is indicated "when medically feasible." Patient who are not breathing and in a code situation because of an arrhythmia or shocky from polyuria are not good candidates for surgery!

8. **Correct Answer: A.** You had better be worried about this urine output! The amount and color is abnormal for someone who has been NPO for surgery. The patient may be developing diabetes insipidus (DI) and you are not going to let her go home! You will call the doctor and collaborate to keep her at the hospital for further observation! If you think, "Wow, what good kidneys you have" and let the patient go home, she could "D" = diuresis until she is "D" = dead! If the problem is DI the doctor will prescribe ADH replacement:

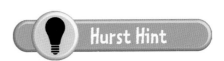

Hurst Hint

Circle the "D" in DI and remember: the "D" stands for diuresis!

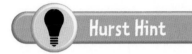

Greater than 20 mm Hg constitutes a significant change in systolic blood pressure. A 10% increase means that instead of a heart rate of 80, the heart rate is increased to 88! You're not worried about this minor fluctuation!

DDAVP (desmopressin acetate) or vasopressin (Petersen) and she will be fine when her ADH secretion goes back to normal.

Answer B: Pain never killed anybody. She hasn't had brain surgery, so you don't need to worry about ICP. A mild headache is not a cause for alarm.

Answer C: Small amounts of bright red blood are normal and expected after sinus surgery. If the dressings were saturated (rather than soiled), I might be worried!

Answer D: A 10 mm Hg decrease is not significant: 120/80 versus 110/80 is not a cause for alarm and can be attributed to normal pre-operative anxiety.

9. **Correct Answer: D.** Any commercially prepared food can be consumed as long as the food does not contain vanilla or caffeine (CNS stimulant that would speed up the heart by increasing sympathetic and catecholamine production.)

Answer A: Sweets such as vanilla Coke®, chocolate pie, and fudge brownies contain both caffeine and vanilla, which would alter the VMA test. Most cakes and pastries contain vanilla, so patients are advised to avoid desserts prior to the test. Other specific foods to avoid are citrus fruits and bananas.

Answer B: The test requires a 24-hour urine specimen, which is assessed for the presence of catecholamines (epinephrine and norepinephrine). The patient must always discard the first voiding (starting with an empty bladder) and keep the last voided specimen within the 24-hour time frame.

Answer C: During the urine collection the patient must rest in a cool, quiet, nonstimulating environment so that stress hormones (epinephrine and norepinephrine) are not excreted in the urine. Exercise causes a burst of catecholamines, as does smoking, which would cause a false-positive result, because the urine would be full of stress hormones from the adrenal medulla.

10. **Correct Answer: D.** Metyrapone blocks the enzyme needed to produce cortisol, so circulating levels of cortisol will drop, producing negative feedback, which would cause the pituitary to produce ACTH. If the adrenal insufficiency is caused by autoimmune destruction of the adrenal glands (primary hypocortisolism), the little existing cortisol production will be blocked and the patient will rapidly develop hypotension, shock, hyponatremia, and hyperkalemia, leading to cardiovascular collapse or a fatal arrhythmia, whichever comes first. DON'T let them give your patient this drug if it is even remotely possible that your patient could have primary Addison's disease. Their diseased glands won't be able to produce more cortisol once the metyrapone knocks out what little existing hormone the gland has been able to produce.

Answers A, B, and C: The assessment clues point to adrenal cortical insufficiency: Addison's disease. Symptoms of bronzing skin, weakness, hypotension, and weight loss are classic. Not enough of the mineralocorticoid aldosterone causes this patient to lose sodium and water (hypotension and weight loss) and retain potassium; therefore, serum electrolytes are appropriate and needed to establish a diagnosis. Insufficient glucocorticoids will cause a decrease in blood glucose; therefore, fasting blood glucose is also indicated for this patient, and should not be questioned.

Answer E: Cosyntropin is a drug that mimics ACTH and is given to stimulate the production of cortisol. If this stimulation test is performed and the cortisol level does NOT increase, it means that the adrenal glands are incapable of responding, and verifies the diagnosis of primary adrenal insufficiency (Addison's disease). Based on the "clues" given, this test is appropriate as a diagnostic aid for this patient.

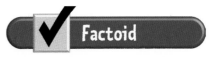

If the cosyntropin stimulation test is prescribed for a patient suspected of Cushing's syndrome, the result would be a huge increase in cortisol production if the patient has adrenal hyperplasia! The overactive gland gets a little taste of stimulation and goes crazy!

Chapter 11

1. Correct Answer: B. The first and foremost intervention following chemical exposure to the eye will always be to flush, flush, flush! This dilutes and removes the chemical to decrease damage to the delicate tissue of the eye.

    Answer A: This is delaying treatment! Flush first and then call 911!

    Answer C: This is delaying treatment! Flush first and remove the contact lens after a few minutes of flushing (comes out easier), and then resume flushing.

    Answer D: Blinking will distribute the chemical throughout the eye, increasing the chemical damage.

2. Correct Answer: A. Obviously the retina has suffered damage because the patient has lost his or her central vision (cones in the macula) being able to only see peripherally (a "rod" function). This assessment should be reported to the ophthalmic surgeon immediately!

    Answer B: Papillary edema (papilledema = a "choked" disc) produces swelling of the blind spot in the optic disc, which has no photoreceptor cells, so the brain uses the mechanism of "filling in" to compensate for light focused on the disc area. This is a sign of significantly increased intracranial pressure, which is dangerous because swelling can compress the optic nerve causing permanent blindness.[1]

    Answer C: This may or may not be true. If the macula is gone, central vision is gone!

    Answer D: Surgical repair involved suctioning out the vitreous that leaked out behind and laser or cryotherapy to seal the hole that was in the posterior retina. *Successful* surgical repair means that there is not a hole in the retina, so vitreous cannot be leaking out.

3. Correct Answer: B. The patient has sustained blunt trauma to the head and is exhibiting signs of retinal detachment. You had better call the doctor stat because there is nothing else that the nurse can do to prevent a complication or remedy this problem.

Answer A: Yes, let's darken the room so he or she can see the flashing lights better! No! This will do nothing to help a detached retina and will be interpreted by the NCLEX® lady as delaying treatment.

Answer C: A detached retina neither causes pain nor causes any alteration in the vital signs. Flashing lights are an early sign, and the speed of reattachment of the retina may influence the prognosis if intervention can be accomplished before full detachment.

Answer D: This is just a nice little thing to do, but it does not help the problem. Again, this answer is wrong because it delays treatment.

4. **Correct Answer: B.** This is a safety issue because of decreased visual acuity, especially in terms of night vision. Many elderly patients awaken to void at least once during the night, and the potential for falls is increased.

Answer A: Cycloplegic drops are prescribed to paralyze the ciliary muscle (responsible for accommodation), which keeps the pupil from dilating or constricting! Why would that be indicated the night *before* surgery to remove the lens? It wouldn't. Gong! That's a dumb answer!

Answer C: Sounds really good, doesn't it? Bed low, rails up … what can be wrong with that? Nothing, it's just not the best answer! If your patient needs to void, he or she will crawl over the side rails and will probably not fall until he or she trips over something in the dim light. Visual acuity is the problem, not muscle weakness or physical debilitation! It will be impaired vision that causes the fall, so pick an answer that will help the stated problem!

Answer D: Nothing is wrong with this answer. Preop anxiety is always a possibility because of fear of the unknown, but physical needs will always take priority over psychosocial needs (Maslow's hierarchy), and safety is the priority. Sorry.

5. **Correct Answer: A.** Redness with visible blood vessels in the ordinarily white sclera can mean infection or other acute disorders of the eye! Cataract surgery will be canceled for an infected eye or for acute angle-closure glaucoma (which is a medical emergency), and the doctor must be notified so that an evaluation can take place immediately.

Answer B: Glaucoma (with controlled IOP) is not a contraindication for cataract surgery; however, postop steroid medications may be re-evaluated and NSAID drops used instead to reduce inflammation.

Answer C: Don't call the doctor for this patient complaint! Cycloplegic drops normally cause a transient stinging sensation.

Answer D: Preoperative anxiety can account for this insignificant rise in systolic blood pressure. No need to worry about a blood pressure fluctuation unless it is 20 mm Hg (or greater) elevation above baseline.

6. **Correct Answer: C.** African Americans are three times more likely to develop primary open-angle glaucoma than Caucasians, and they do so at a younger age (beginning at age 40 rather than the Caucasian risk age >60 years). Additional risk factors for this patient, who requires earlier and

more frequent exams and measurement of intraocular pressure, are hypertension and diabetes, which produce peripheral vascular spasm.

Answer A: Risk for glaucoma is increased when a first-degree relative (mother, father, sister, brother) has the disease. Her gender, her age, and her family history are not high-risk factors for primary open-angle glaucoma.

Answer B: Hispanics are at greater risk for glaucoma than Caucasians, but like Caucasians, the risk increases after age 60. Her headaches do need to be diagnosed, and possibly she has a refractive error, needing visual field testing

Answer D: Ethnic risks for glaucoma are found in Hispanics, African Americans (primary open-angle glaucoma), and persons from East Asia (Japanese, Chinese from Hong Kong and Singapore) and Eskimos (Inuit descent) Close work causing eye strain may be associated with progression of myopia (which is a risk factor for glaucoma); however, having myopia is not stated and therefore should not be assumed.

7. Correct Answer: A. If retinal detachment is suspected, shouldn't the emergency physician consult with an ophthalmologist? Yes, most definitely, and the eye specialist would never dilate an injured eye on a person with a congenitally narrow anterior chamber (East Asian) for fear of precipitating yet another medical emergency—acute closed-angle glaucoma—which will rapidly shoot up the intraocular pressure, causing damage to the optic nerve.

Answer B: Even if the patient didn't have all the other musculoskeletal injuries from the MVA, the cornea alone is screaming with pain! Morphine causes pinpoint pupils, which would be a good thing if the damaged cornea has any swelling that could also close off the angle. Dilating the pupil would be terrible for this patient, but constricting the pupil would be an added benefit that accompanies analgesia.

Answer C: Fluorescein dye is needed prior to inspecting the cornea because the yellow stain will more clearly define any scratches on the cornea. A tiny scratch could be missed upon direct visualization without the dye.

Answer D: Proparacaine is a topical local anesthetic to relieve pain so the patient can open her eye. Corneal abrasions are severely painful and it is helpful to numb the pain so the lid can be opened enough to examine the cornea.

8. Correct Answer: C. The nurse should check the temperature of the water because a cold solution in the ear will produce these symptoms.

Answer A: The position of the bed has nothing to do with the patient symptoms.

Answer B: The intactness of the eardrum should have been checked BEFORE initiating any irrigation. If you had applied too much pressure and caused a rupture of the membrane, the patient would experience pain, not nausea and nystagmus.

Answer D: Do not call the doctor. There is nothing wrong with the patient. Your water is too cold, and this is the "normal" response that cold water will elicit.

9. **Correct Answer: B.** The stapes that was "fixed" could no longer transmit sound waves to the inner ear, so the foot of the stapes was replaced with a prosthesis, which corrects the conductive hearing loss in the affected ear.

   Answer A: You can only hear out of both ears equally, if all conditions are equal. The unaffected ear canal could be occluded with impacted cerumen for all we know!

   The surgery only helps the affected ear to transmit sound waves through the middle ear to reach the oval window.

   Answer C: Tinnitus is not a reason for having a stapedectomy. This is a sensorineural symptom indicating damage within the hair cells of the cochlea.

   Answer D: Whirling vertigo is a symptom of Ménière's disease, which is NOT the problem when a stapedectomy is performed.

10. **Correct Answer: A.** This surgical procedure provides an avenue for shunting fluid away to reduce the endolymphatic fluid, which will hopefully reduce attacks.

    Answers B and C: Both of these options destroy the inner ear (one chemically, the other surgically), and these options are always a *last* resort because they result in permanent deafness.

    Answer D: A ventilation tube goes into the middle ear to equalize pressure therein with (outside) atmospheric pressure when the eustachian tube is not doing its job of equalizing pressure.

Chapter 12

1. **Correct Answer: C.** Delayed compartment syndrome following a contusion (bleeding within the muscle) plus the constricting effect of the brace may be compromising blood flow to the nerves and tissue. Upon inspection, the affected leg may appear to be bulging outward, noticeably larger than the unaffected thigh. Release pressure first, and then call the doctor to report your concern. Were you afraid that you couldn't remove a brace? Braces are for support, not like a cast that you cannot remove for bathing. But consider this, if this same patient were in a cast and the toes sticking out were blue and numb, would you bivalve the cast to release the pressure? Remove the cast? The correct answer is to do whatever you have to do to restore blood flow if you suspect that tissue circulation is compromised!

   Answer A: Not only does this answer delay treatment, but it is unsafe as well because elevating the leg would drain more blood downward toward the affected thigh muscle, one compartment of which is already overstretched and ischemic.

Answer B: Call the doctor is not an unsafe answer since you are getting help for the patient, therefore you will not be dropped to a lower level question on NCLEX®, but you are delaying treatment because the brace was not removed first.

Answer D: This is an unsafe answer! Giving analgesia and waiting 30 minutes to reassess provides the opportunity for another half hour of ischemic damage to the leg. If the analgesia provides enough relief enough for the patient to tolerate the pain, treatment for the ischemic condition could be even further delayed.

Always pick an answer that helps the patient's problem before calling the doctor. Everything else delays treatment.

A strategy for answering test questions is to read the question and then before even looking at the possible answers, ask yourself, "What's wrong with my patient?"

2. **Correct Answer: A.** Pain in this patient situation is the priority! Using the Hurst hint that "pain never killed anybody" would be inappropriate under these circumstances. When the nurse is monitoring for a complication of orthopedic surgery, compartment syndrome should be the first thing that pops into your mind! Compartment syndrome can lead to an amputation or death if not detected and treated.

Answer B: External fixation means that a rod has been placed through the skin into the bone to hold it in place temporarily. Low-grade fever would be expected and normal because the first line of defense (the skin) has been breached. The nurse should monitor the temperature, but infection is not the priority when the patient is at risk for compartment syndrome.

Answer C: You do not have to worry about alignment because the bone has been "fixated" externally. A rod with screws is holding the bone in the normal anatomical position.

Answer D: Equal warmth of the extremities is an important nursing assessment because this tells the nurse that blood flow going into the extremity is equal compared with the unaffected extremity. This is the *second* best answer. Poikilothermia (body temperature the same as that of the environment) is the sixth "P" of the traditional 5 Ps that comprise the neurovascular check: pulse, pallor, pain, paresthesia, paralysis, and capillary refill ("PRESS") the nail bed to see if it refills promptly (<2 seconds). By the time a limb becomes cold, the tissues have long since been ischemic. This is a very *late* sign. Don't ever wait for the limb to get cold. Intervene as soon as the patient's nerve endings start to tingle. If you wait for blood flow to totally shut down (warm blood is what makes the skin warm), the limb probably won't be salvaged.

The SEVEN "Ps" in the neurovascular check are: pain, pulse, paresthesia, pallor, paralysis, poikilothermia, and PRESS nail beds to check capillary refill.

3. **Correct Answer: C.** The web between the big toe and the next toe is the specific area innervated by the deep peroneal nerve. Take an applicator and prick the wooden end into the web and see if the patient feels the sensation.

Ask the patient to look away so he or she does not see what you're doing. We want to know if the patient feels the sensation between his or her toes and is not just interpreting a visual cue.

Hurst Rule

Always assess before you implement!

Answer A: There is nothing wrong with elevating the foot, but we aren't finished with the assessment yet!

Hurst Rule

Least invasive first! This rule will never fail you. Trust me.

Answer B: Petaling a cast is nice, but not priority at this time when there may be compression of the peroneal nerve even in the presence of adequate blood flow.

Answer D: The data given (a warm foot—which is probably pink too—and palpable pulses) are enough to determine that circulation is at least adequate. The nail bed blanch will give further validation, and is a part of the neurovascular check, but because we only have assurance of motor movement (not sensation) and the location of the fracture, it is a priority to determine that the peroneal nerve is not being compressed!

4. **Correct Answer: C.** If the patient has a paralytic ileus, bowel sounds will be absent and the doctor needs this information as soon as possible (asap).

Answer A: This is not a bad option, because the patient may actually have an impaction that can be manually removed (gently, please) with a lubricated gloved finger. This is not the correct answer because it is an invasive procedure (your gloved finger is going as far as you can reach into the patient's anus).

Answer B: You're a killer! This answer will get you a lower level next question. If the patient didn't already have abdominal compartment syndrome, he or she does now! Way to go! Normal abdominal pressure is 0 to 5 mm Hg, and with straining and bearing down, expect the pressure to rise even more. Abdominal perfusion pressure of 12 mm Hg or more defines intra-abdominal hypertension.

5. **Correct Answer: B.** This is a classic fat embolus! Long bones (femur) and pelvis fracture are at high risk for fat embolism within the first 36 hours postinjury. The patient needs oxygen, so pick an answer that will help the patient!

Answer A: I know what you're thinking! Always assess before picking an intervention answer. Your patient gave you all the assessment you need to know that he or she needs oxygen. Obtaining the other data to further confirm hypoxia (absent breath sounds and tachycardia) will delay treatment. The doctor will want to be notified so a stat VQ scan can determine the extent of hypoperfusion.

Answer C: Were you thinking the patient had compartment syndrome? Did you think having more room in the thorax would improve oxygenation if the lungs are blocked by a plug of fat (yellow marrow)? Think again.

Answer D: Turning the patient to the opposite side from the site of chest pain means that the airless occluded lung is upright and the patient is lying on the only lung that can ventilate and perfuse oxygen. The patient can only deep breathe as far as the cast over the thorax will allow, which is not a good choice.

6. **Correct Answer: E.** Keeping the toes dry and cool will slow metabolism and improve viability to support successful reattachment of the severed toes.

   Answer A: The toes need to be transported to the hospital, but unless kept cool for transport, surgical reattachment may not be an option upon arrival.

   Answer B: The toes should be kept clean and dry, not submerged in water.

   Answer C: Depending upon the thickness of the shoe, uniformity of external ice may not penetrate the distal tip of the shoe, or may be too cold for proximal toes where they have been amputated from the foot. Bacteria in the shoe may also invade the toes at the amputation site.

   Answer D: Maybe the toes can be saved! They should be kept cool and dry (see option E) and transported to the hospital. The vascular surgeon will make the determination to offer the toes to the family for burial or authorize disposal with surgical waste if the patient or family decline a burial option.

7. **Correct Answer: A.** The duration of pain (acute or chronic) makes the greatest difference in the treatment protocol. Acute pain will be managed with NSAIDs to reduce the inflammatory response, but with chronic back pain (>3 months duration) the inflammatory response has subsided and NSAIDs are no longer indicated.

   Answer B: Both acute and chronic pain are localized in the lower back and may radiate if nerves are involved.

   Answer C: If the patient could get relief, he or she would probably not be at the doctor's office or emergency department in the first place.

   Answer D: This is important and with both acute and chronic low back pain the intensity could vary from moderate to severe, but the choice of medications is dependent upon whether the low back pain is acute or chronic (inflammation versus no inflammation).

8. **Correct Answer: C.** This is the best answer considering that three rather than four nurses are required, and sliding rather than physically lifting are safer options for nurses. One nurse is required to hold the bar whereupon are the 5 lb of weights, so that when they say "go" or "on the count of three" the nurse removes the 5 lb of inertia by lifting up while beginning to pull the patient upward.

   Answer A: You never discontinue weights without a doctor's order, not even for a few minutes. What will happen? Without the traction applied to overcome muscle spasm at the site of the injury, the huge thigh muscle goes into a tense spasm and causes bone ends to move, cutting through muscle tissue, nerves, and blood vessels. Could this

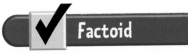
Factoid

When you and your friends are out of gas, and you are pushing a car off the road, you all push together on the count of three. Once the car is moving (inertia overcome), a single person can push the car with ease. This is the same physics principle (work and inertia).

added trauma lead to compartment syndrome and possible loss of a limb? Yes. So, don't do it!

Answer B: If you are dragging the patient (95 lb) and the weights (5 lb) up in bed, the force exerted by the nurses must overcome the inertia of the weights, which would apply additional pressure on the fractured hip. This is a seriously BAD answer that will get you a lower level of difficulty on your next computer adaptive testing (CAT) item. The doctor ordered 5 lb for a reason. Don't drag the patient up and let his or her broken hip bring the weights up!

Answer D: This is not good utilization of staff! Also, it will be difficult to find two other nurses to help you on a busy med-surg unit. If the patient is physically lifted, his or her body weight will not be included in the friction pull, but when the four nurses begin to pull, they have to pull harder to overcome inertia of the dead hanging weights. While the four are pulling in the opposite direction, before having overcome inertia, added traction (force) is applied to the injured hip, which could cause bones to move. More energy is exerted by the four nurses who physically lift the upper and lower torso of the patient so that no body part touches the bed on the way up. Lifting rather than sliding also places the health care worker at greater risk for back injury.

9. **Correct Answer: B.** Nuclear medicine does this test. The highly vascular bone tissue takes up the nuclide and reveals the characteristically enlarged Pagetic lesions and possibly deformed bones. This test lets the doctor confirm the diagnosis without a shadow of doubt and also give information about the extensiveness of the disease process.

   Answer A: Why should the woman be subjected to unnecessary radiation from an X-ray of her pelvis when the doctor already has a more valuable US image? (Dumb answer.)

   Answers C and D: Both these urinary tests are infrequently used because they are less specific for Paget's disease.

10. **Correct Answer: B and C.** A very rare but very serious adverse effect can occur with Reclast—osteonecrosis of the jaw—in which dissolution (disintegration) of the gums can expose the necrotic bone of the jaw. All patients should have a routine oral exam before treatment with Reclast, especially those with poor oral hygiene, cancer patients taking chemotherapy or any patient taking corticosteroids.

    Answer A: Within three days of infusion, zoledronic acid may cause fever, chills, muscle aches, aching bones and joints, and/or headache similar to flulike syndrome. These mild to moderate symptoms are self-limiting and resolve spontaneously within four days. Nurses should forewarn patients that this reaction may occur (so patients won't think they are sick) and recommend acetaminophen or an appropriate OTC nonsteroidal anti-inflammatory agent.

    Answer B: The patient taking Reclast needs more than simply dietary calcium! The patient must understand the need to take daily calcium

1500 mg in divided doses and vitamin D (800 IU/day) supplements for two to four months. Diet alone will not be sufficient to prevent serious hypocalcemia.

Answer D: The patient must have a creatinine clearance >35 mL/min that is confirmed PRIOR to the IV administration of this agent. The patient must drink enough fluids prior to receiving the drug to ensure that he or she is adequately hydrated. The recommended follow-up lab is repeat ALP.

Chapter 13

1. **Correct Answer: C.** Microorganism → Portal of exit → Mode of transmission → Portal of entry → Host.
   Microorganisms colonize in the infected body and leave the body via a *portal of exit* such as coughing or sneezing. The microorganisms are then transferred via a *mode of transmission* such as person to person contact, entering the susceptible host through a *portal of entry* such as the respiratory tract. A *host* is a person that is susceptible to infection for reasons such as young or advanced age or immunodeficiency.

2. **Correct Answers: A, B, and D.** A urinary tract infection is characterized by fever of 100.4°F or greater, urgency, frequency, dysuria (painful urination), and suprapubic tenderness (pain over the bladder area). Hypotension is not a symptom of urinary tract infection, but may indicate sepsis related to harmful microorganisms in the blood.

3. **Correct Answer: C.** Community-acquired infections are acquired at home or in the community. A patient may have symptoms of infection upon admission or be asymptomatic; developing symptoms within 24 to 48 hours after admission. The time frame suggests that the patient was exposed to a pathogen and already incubating the disease **prior to admission.** Hospital-acquired infections generally occur 48 to 72 hours after admission with no evidence of incubation on admission. *Endemic* is a term that means the usual or expected level of disease seen within a geographic area. An epidemic is disease above the expected or usual level.

4. **Correct Answers: A, B, C, and D.** The nurse's hands should be washed before and after work, after using the toilet, nose blowing, or covering a cough or sneeze, before eating, drinking, or handling food, when visibly soiled, before and after every patient contact, between care of different sites on the patient, before all dressing changes, after contact with blood and body fluids, after contact with objects near the patient, and before putting on or after taking off personal protective equipment. Don't forget to take care of your hands!

5. **Correct Answer: C.** Depending on the specific organization's policy, most IVs should be restarted every 72 hours. Others have increased

the time to 96 hours. However, restarting an IV every 96 hours is not acceptable on the NCLEX®-RN exam.

6. **Correct Answers: A, C, and D.** Methicillin-resistant *Staphylococcus aureus* (MRSA) is spread by either direct contact or contact with contaminated items. Nurses caring for patients with MRSA should wear gloves and a gown, dedicate equipment (eg, stethoscopes, blood pressure cuffs, and thermometers) to the patient's exclusive use, and wash hands immediately after removing contaminated personal protective equipment. Care should be taken not to touch the face, door handles, door frames, or ink pens when wearing gloves. Because MRSA is spread through contact, wearing a mask is not required.

7. **Correct Answer: D.** The 50-year-old man who is HIV positive is the best choice. The question does not state that this patient has AIDS, but only that he is HIV positive. HIV is spread through direct contact with infected blood and body fluids. The new patient is placed at no additional risk by being assigned to a room with an HIV-positive patient. Remember, when caring for patients, nurses utilize standard precautions under the premise that all patients may be HIV positive.

Answer A: The 20-year-old woman with a broken femur is not the best option because most facilities do not make co-ed room assignments.

Answer B: The 42-year-old man with MRSA is not a suitable roommate. This patient should be under contact isolation. Because of the risk of infection, no other patient would be assigned to his room.

Answer C: The 25-year-old man with pneumonia is also not a good choice because an infection is probably causing his pneumonia. Recall that patients with chronic illnesses, such as diabetes, are at an increased risk for infection. Assigning an at-risk patient to a room where there is a suspected or known infection is never a good idea.

8. **Correct Answers: A, C, and D.** Tetanus, diphtheria, and pertussis are vaccine-preventable diseases. All children receive the vaccine through the DPT vaccination that covers diphtheria, pertussis (whooping cough), and tetanus.

Answer B: Tuberculosis is acquired by inhaling the organism *Mycobacterium tuberculosis,* via the airborne route such as coughing, sneezing, or speaking. There is no vaccine to prevent individuals from becoming infected with tuberculosis.

9. **Correct Answers: B and D.** The nurse should suspect that the patient may have been exposed to both hepatitis B and HIV. Hepatitis B may be caused by exposure to infected blood and body fluids, transfusion of blood and blood products, and hemodialysis. Symptoms of hepatitis B include fatigue; fever; nausea and vomiting; abdominal pain; anorexia; and clay-colored stools. Although not as easily spread as hepatitis B, HIV is transmitted via infected blood and body fluids as well. Early signs of

HIV infection also include fatigue, fever, and GI disturbances. Because the patient recently received a homemade tattoo, it is possible that contaminated needles were used placing the patient at risk for both hepatitis B and HIV. Even though there may be other illnesses that cause these symptoms, both hepatitis B and HIV infections are possible and should be ruled out when evaluating the patient. Hepatitis A is generally acquired through contaminated food. Hepatitis C is also spread via blood and body fluids; however, 80% of all cases are asymptomatic.

10. **Correct Answer: B.** Gonorrhea is a sexually transmitted infection also known as the "clap" or "drips." It is caused by the bacterium *Neisseria gonorrhea* and is easy to transmit. Ejaculation does not have to occur to spread this disease. Men can be asymptomatic or have painful urination and white, yellow, or green discharge from the penis. The bacterium may also spread to the anus causing rectal itching. Syphilis is characterized by a firm, round, small, painless sore that appears at the spot where syphilis entered the body. Trichomoniasis is more common in women and can only be transmitted to men by infected women. Men are usually asymptomatic. Pediculosis is caused by the pubic or crab louse, which causes intense itching and may be visualized on the pubic hair.

Chapter 14

1. **Correct Answer: A.** Patients typically report feeling fatigued.

   Answer B: Patients are usually prescribed medications during exacerbations and over the long-term.

   Answer C: Patients can expect periods of remissions and exacerbations, few symptoms to critical symptoms.

   Answer D: Patients should be told that sun exposure and UVL exposure will worsen skin symptoms.

2. **Correct Answer: A.** Many body systems are involved including skin manifestations, joint changes, respiratory and renal systems.

   Answer B: Many body systems are affected, thus the term systemic.

   Answer C: Neurologic symptoms may include psychotic symptoms, seizures, headaches, and others. Other systems are also involved with SLE.

   Answer D: The skin is affected and the patient may exhibit with rashes, scaring lesions, and hair loss.

3. **Correct Answer: C.** The erythrocyte sedimentation rate, called sed rate is useful in monitoring the course of the disease. Generally, the higher the sed rate, the more severe the illness.

   Answer A: Decreased red blood cells indicates anemia, which may have many causes. That value alone would not indicate the severity of RA.

   Answer B: Many patients who have RA have a positive titer; however, not all positive titers indicate the presence of RA.

Answer D: The C-reactive protein test may be used to assess for presence of inflammation. It may also be used in tandem with other lab tests, such as those listed in the answer options.

4. **Correct Answer: D.** Inflammation affects the synovial membrane, and granulation tissue erodes the cartilage and eventually affects the bone as well.

   Answer A: Osteoarthritis may be associated with aging.

   Answer B: RA is very debilitating and deformity results.

   Answer C: Women are more commonly affected by RA.

5. **Correct Answer: B.** Patients with fibromyalgesia may experience fatigue, chest pain, pelvic pain, and abdominal pain.

   Answer A: Pain occurs in many sites.

   Answer C: Patients may experience intermittent pain. It may worsen with increased activity or stress.

   Answer D: Pain is typically described as a burning pain.

6. **Correct Answer: C.** Symptoms may be episodic; however, symptoms may be aggravated by increased activity, increased stress, and some patients report increased pain with changing weather conditions.

   Answer A: Typically, the onset of symptoms is in middle age.

   Answer B: Fibromyalgia occurs most often in women.

   Answer D: The symptoms are not unique to this illness alone; therefore, diagnosis is difficult.

7. **Correct Answer: B.** The butterfly rash is a classic manifestation of skin involvement with SLE.

   Answer A: Lesions may appear on areas of the body exposed to the sun.

   Answer C: Lesions may occur, as well as rashes, may occur on areas of the body that are exposed to the sun.

   Answer D: The rash is typically dry and scaly. Itching may or may not be present.

8. **Correct Answer: C.** The disease may be treated aggressively until remission occurs; however, patients may receive steroid therapy for long periods or for a short duration.

   Answer A: The patient may be treated with high doses for brief periods or low doses over time.

   Answer B: The approach may differ with patients and the disease process.

   Answer D: Therapy may be decreased over time.

9. **Correct Answer: B.** Exercise is important; however, overactivity may increase pain.

Answer A: There are no dietary recommendations for treatment of fibromyalgia.

Answer C: Pain control usually requires prescription medications, including NSAIDS, antidepressants, and medications for nerve pain.

Answer D: Moderate and low-impact aerobic and stretching exercises are recommended.

10. **Correct Answer: A.** The discoid lesions produce scarring.

Answer B: Scarring results from the discoid lesions.

Answer C: The lesions are disc shaped, and may be described as coin-like.

Answer D: Alopecia is common.

Chapter 15

1. **Correct Answer: C.** This screening test for breast cancer is a form of secondary prevention because it does not prevent breast cancer; rather it is a means for early identification that can detect cancer at an early stage when the prognosis for cure more likely.

Answer A: The monthly BSE should begin regardless of the age.

Answer B: Use of sunscreen is recommended as a means of *primary* prevention of cancer.

Answer D: Tobacco is the biggest preventable cause of cancer, making this means for *primary* (not secondary) prevention very important.

2. **Correct Answer: A.** Smoking is the leading cause of bladder cancer.

Answer B: Pickled and smoked meats increase risk for stomach cancer (not bladder).

Answer C: Alkalines increase risk for kidney stones (calcium) rather than cancer.

Answer D: Fluid intake keeps toxins flushed out, but the nicotine in the blood remains as a constant irritant to bladder mucosa.

3. **Correct Answer: B.** All visitors are not restricted! Only restrict children and pregnant women who because of rapidly growing cells will be more susceptible to the effects of radiation. All other visitors are restricted to a 30 minute daily visit.

Answer A: Low residue diet is indicated because dietary fiber will distend the bowel and push out the implant.

Answer C: Many times antidiarrheal agents such as Lomotil (diphenoxylate) will be prescribed to prevent a bowel movement that would cause the implant to be expelled.

Answer D: Bedrest is indicated because being upright or out of bed would favor dislodgement of the implant due to gravitational force. Log rolling prevents hip action when turning in bed which could also displace the implant.

4. **Correct Answer: D.** Distance yourself from the implant as quickly as possible and get somebody from nuclear medicine to come to the room stat for removal of radioactive material. Do not allow anyone else (visitors or other healthcare providers) to enter the room until the implant has been safely removed. You are responsible for protecting yourself and others from radiation exposure!

Answer A: The implant must be placed in a lead lined container as soon as possible. You wouldn't remove the implant from the room and irradiate yourself and everybody else in the hall on the way to nuclear medicine for disposal of the implant.

Answer B: You limit your exposure to radioactivity by getting away from the implant as soon as possible.

Answer C: The nuclear medicine department will come with tongs and a lead-lined container to remove the implant from the room. Don't touch the implant.

5. **Correct Answer: B.** Body fluids (breast milk) will contain radioactivity and may not be given to the new baby, so obviously further discharge teaching is needed since the priority is to protect the baby.

Answer A: No further teaching is needed because the woman knows that she should not be around babies for 48 hours. She should also stay away from pregnant women. Any radioactivity from an unsealed source can be transferred to the fetus because rapidly dividing cells are most radiosensitive.

Answer C: The radioactivity is gone (decayed) in 48 hours, making this answer incorrect, but protecting another adult from skin contact is not the priority. Children under the age of 16 and pregnant women are most susceptible to radioactivity. Sleeping in the bed is allowed but there should be no intercourse (because of body fluid precautions) for 48 hours.

Answer D: These activities are not indicated.

6. **Correct Answer: B.** Please be alarmed if your patient's respirations are depressed! Hypoventilation causes metabolic acidosis relatively quickly! "Depressed" means a rate less than 12. This is never normal, not even after general anesthesia!

Answer A: We *expect* loss of gag reflex after this procedure and keep the patient NPO until the gag reflex returns.

Answer C: Again, this is expected following sedation. Patients are instructed not to operate machinery, drive, or engage in hazardous activities that require alertness and good coordination until the effects of the drug are known.

Answer D: A streak is just a tiny amount of blood in the sputum which is a common occurrence following bronchoscopy. This is not hemorrhage. The NCLEX lady thinks that as soon as you see the word "blood" you are going to be scared and grab this answer! Don't get distracted by questions like these.

7. **Correct Answer: A.** When the NCLEX question says "priority" you better pick the one answer that you promise you will do if you don't do anything else! And before you pick any answer (really, before you even look at the possible choices) what should you ask? What's wrong with my patient? If you are assuming the worst (like you are supposed to do with every NCLEX test item), you will fear that a hematoma is developing at the surgical site. Call the doctor stat!

Answer B: You cannot remove a surgical dressing. If you remove the pressure that is applied for compression to reduce bleeding, what could happen? Bleeding!

Answer C: Obtaining vital signs (or anything other than calling the doctor) is delaying treatment. If the patient is bleeding into the tissues, there is nothing that a nurse can do to stop the bleeding.

Answer D: Always assume the worst, and you will not be guilty of overlooking something that could turn out to be a big problem! In reality, you would "decompress the bulb of the JP drain." That is something the nurse can do if you suspect that the suction has been lost. If there is something that the nurse can do to help the problem, you always want to do that before you call the doctor, but if there is nothing the nurse can do to help the patient, you must always call the doctor. In our test question above, this was not an option. Your best answer was to call the doctor.

8. **Correct Answer: B.** 70% of all cancers of the cervix are caused by the human papillomavirus of which there is a vaccine for four of the subtypes that cause 70% of all cervical cancers: HPV 6, 11, 16, and 18, all of which are covered by the quadrivalent vaccine.

Answer A: Smoking cessation is great as a means for primary prevention of lung cancer and cancer of the bladder (both of which are cancers that MEN as well as women develop). The question is relating to WOMEN so you have to ask yourself, "What kind of cancers do women get?" Gynecological cancers! Smoking is not known to cause cancer of the cervix!

Answer C: Education is always good, but how do you know that the person will comply with abstinence? Patient compliance makes this answer less effective than the vaccine that will prevent HPV infection if she chooses to have sex anyway and contracts the virus.

Answer D: An exam and a pap smear cannot prevent a viral infection or cancer because screening tests are not primary prevention. This is an example of *secondary* prevention: detection after the infection or cervical cancer from the HPV has occurred.

9. **Correct Answer: C.** Pap smear testing should begin no longer than 3 years after first becoming sexually active. This girl's first pap smear should be scheduled by age 16 at the latest.

Answer A: (which actually includes **B and D**): These patients do not require further teaching because a postmenopausal woman should still continue to have regular pap smears at least until age 70, at which time she may discuss discontinuing this screening test if the last three pap smears (over the last 10 years) have been normal and she has few or no risk factors. The majority of low-grade squamous intraepithelial lesions very commonly return to normal over months to several years in young women.[34] It is the high-grade squamous intraepithelial lesions that commonly become malignant. Colposcopy uses a light source and magnification to visualize tissues of the cervix, vagina, and vulva as a follow-up to low-grade intraepithelial lesions in young women. Using high-powered magnification, many distinctive characteristics (such as vascular patterns of malignant and nonmalignant lesions) can be clearly identified, and if questionable, tissue can be obtained during this exam for a biopsy, which would provide a definite diagnosis.

10. **Correct Answer: A.** The first sign of neurotoxicity that may occur with high dose cytarabine is nystagmus, which precedes ataxia and cerebellar dysfunction. The physician must be notified of this early sign of toxicity.

Answer B: This is a nice thing to do, but you are looking for the *priority*! If you picked this answer, you are telling the NCLEX® lady that you don't know the signs of neurotoxicity. The Hurst rule is to always worry if your patient develops a new symptom after receiving a new drug. This answer is delaying treatment for toxicity.

Answer C: Covering up his eye won't stop the nystagmus or the neurotoxicity, which may progress to cerebellar syndrome. Call the doctor.

Answer D: This is not a common side effect! Nystagmus is a serious adverse effect that should be reported to the doctor immediately.

Chapter 16

1. **Correct Answer: B.** Many people are allergic to tree oils and products containing fragrance. A recommendation to change the carrier oil removes the element of skin contact with fragrance (aroma in the room rather than in the oil or lotion) and therefore may remove the source of irritation. These are common sense things that nurses teach patients with dermatitis to do!

Answer A: The dermatitis should clear up very quickly, because nobody wants a gloved massage! As soon as business begins to slack off, his or her hands will begin to show a terrific improvement, making this answer bad for business. This answer can also be bad for already irritated hands that are in contact with latex or plastic gloves (with or without the added allergen of the powder) continuously during a busy workday.

Answer C: It is not within the scope of nursing to prescribe and diagnose, which makes this answer incorrect. Even if a patch test were indicated, initial steps use the process of elimination to find a possible cause rather than a painful, inconvenient, and expensive test.

Answer D: Again, this is not within the scope of nursing. You are not a career guidance counselor, and again, aren't we jumping the gun just a little bit? First things first: See if a particular allergen is the offending agent and stop using that product when doing massages.

2. **Correct Answer: D.** Further teaching is needed! Shaving (even with a safety razor) can be dangerous because razor pressure exerted to remove the patches of dead and living skin can traumatize the beefy red base of the lesion, causing bleeding and creating a portal for entry of microorganisms for resultant skin infection. Debridement is necessary prior to topical applications to promote optimal absorption and therapeutic effects of prescribed lotions, creams, or ointments, and this can be safely accomplished in the bath (see option B) with a soft brush and some soap.

   Answer A: Warm baths are good (no further teaching needed) for hydrating the skin to enhance removal of the layers of dead skin with gentle scrubbing motions. Note that too-frequent washing is discouraged because dry skin worsens psoriasis.

   Answer B: Ultraviolet light therapy treatments are usually scheduled two to three times weekly, but an interim period of 48 hours is needed because it could take this long for a burn to become apparent. Watching for changes is good because a subsequent treatment may need to be delayed.

   Answer C: Plastic wraps or vinyl body suits cannot be worn for more than eight hours because of the risk for development of folliculitis, so it is a good practice (no further teaching needed) to remove occlusive dressings in a timely manner.

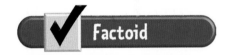

UV irradiation to already burned skin would not be good!

3. **Correct Answer: A.** Most important means "What is the ONE question you had better ask if you don't ask anything else?" This could be a sexually active (and maybe pregnant) 17 year old! Taking isotretinoin (Accutane) requires a pregnancy test two weeks before initiating therapy, and reliable birth control must begin one month before beginning treatment and must continue for one month after discontinuing the drug. Obviously the drug is highly teratogenic and will result in severe birth anomalies.

   Answer B: Accutane is not an antibiotic. Did you think it was? And there is no cross-sensitivity to antibiotics either! Accutane is a highly toxic metabolite of retinol (vitamin A), which reduces sebum production and shrinks the size and number of sebaceous glands.

   Answer C: It would be nice to know if she has taken the drug before, but why am I asking now? To see if she had any toxic effects, or if she knew about its teratogenic effects? We don't really need to be beating around the bush on this important issue, do we?

   Answer D: What has chocolate got to do with anything? Nothing, not even if she ate a whole box of chocolates. Were you thinking hyperglycemia or something? ACCU-tane sounds a little like ACU-check? Don't do any wild guessing on NCLEX®. It will get you in trouble!

4. Correct Answer: A. The itching is very intense with this autoimmune disease, and scratching is to be avoided to prevent ruptured vesicles and skin excoriations that will be a portal of entry for microorganisms. The patient needs prompt interventions to relieve pruritus, and it is also a safety issue.

Answer B: The patient only develops this type of dermatitis in the context of gluten sensitivity, but who can eat when they are clawing themselves to death? What if the choice were, "Teach the patient about the need for a lifelong gluten-free diet?" Hey, who can be receptive to teaching when they are itching to death?

Answer C: You're thinking that if the patient has celiac disease, he will automatically have anemia also because typically this bowel disease results in malabsorption of folate and iron. Well you can check his conjunctiva to see if it is pale and ask him if he is tired, and he will say emphatically, "YES! I'm tired of itching!" Besides, patients don't even know that they have gluten sensitivity because the bowel disease is typically subclinical.

Answer D: Ask him about his bowel pattern, diarrhea, bloating, and steatorrhea (bulky, fatty stools) because you will need this for the admission history, but the history can be obtained later, after you have some Benadryl on board, and have gotten an order for some ice packs or cooling gel for the intensely pruritic skin lesions.

5. Correct Answer: B. Airway is always the priority when applicable! Don't just pick airway if it doesn't apply, but it is correct here because of capillary permeability in the local area around the neck. Edema can very rapidly close off the airway and intubation must be accomplished quickly while a tube can still be inserted.

Answer A: The patient definitely needs analgesia, and administration of morphine will not only ease the pain, but will enhance intubation, but when you are picking *priority* answers, you have one chance to tell the NCLEX® lady that this is what you will do, if you don't do anything else! You better make sure she can breathe.

Answer C: This is another critical answer because fluid will be lost from the vascular space quickly after a major burn owing to increased capillary permeability from the thermal injury to the vessel walls. So now you have to pick between two killer answers: airway (for breathing) and circulation. Which comes first? Duh … you know it's airway if you have to pick!

Answer D: Bag breathing is fine as long as the airway is patent. You will not have a patent airway with this patient. If his or her neck is swollen tight, you can't manually pump the air into the lungs … an endotracheal tube will be required. You're a killer if you picked this answer!

6. Correct Answer: A. Depressed people like to be alone, so an appropriate goal that can be realistically accomplished in a short time span is to get him or her out of the room and involved in unit activities,

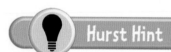

Hurst Hint

Pain never killed anybody (but a collapsed airway will do it every time!).

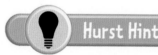

Hurst Hint

Did you have to know anything about burns or burn rehabilitation to answer this question? No you did not! This is not a burn question. This is a depression question! One of the first things you have to figure out with each NCLEX question is, "What are they asking me?"

which will generate more psychic energy while providing opportunities to experience accomplishment, which will increase self-esteem.

Answer B: Coping with physical disability is the goal of long-term rehabilitation, and the patient is not there yet. However, we do want this to happen as a result of successful rehabilitation.

Answer C: Oooh ... this is heavy! This long-term goal may take years of psychotherapy!

Answer D: It will always be wrong to want the depressed patient to stop talking about his thoughts and feelings, even if they are all focused on depression. It is therapeutic to get depressed feelings out rather than turning the focus inward.

7. Correct Answer: A. The total TBSA is 36%.

- One-half of the left arm 9% = 4.5%
- One-half of the left chest 18% = 9%
- One-half of the anterior leg 9% = 4.5%
- Entire posterior trunk = 18%
- Total BSA = 36%

Answer E: Superficial partial thickness (first-degree burns) are shallow, only affecting the top layer of the epithelium and are red and tender .

- One-half of left arm 9% = 4.5%
- One-half of posterior trunk 18% = 9%
- Total superficial partial thickness = 13.5%

Answer G: Formation of blisters occur when the deeper dermis is affected as well as the epidermis. Blanching with capillary refill tells you that the capillaries are alive and well, and pain tells you that the nerve endings are intact and functional.

- One-half of chest and abdomen (one-half of the anterior trunk) 18% = 9% blisters
- One-half of anterior leg 9% = 4.5%
- One-half of posterior trunk 18% = 9%
- Total deep partial thickness burn = 22.5%

Answer I: This a major burn for two reasons. First, a hand is involved, which means that the risk for disability is increased because if the fingers develop contractures, the patient will lose fine motor ability and opposition of thumb to fingers. The second reason (even if you can't remember the numbers) is the extent of the burn: 36% is more than a third of the body. This is a huge burn! A major burn!

Answers E, G, I: All others are incorrect for the reasons explained above. Don't you hate alternate items? Everybody does! Here is the good news: If you take 100 questions on the NCLEX®, you might get two alternate items that actually count.

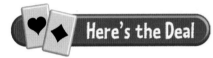
Here's the Deal

Many alternate items are currently being field tested. That means that these items are experimental (or pilot) test questions that do not count for you or against you. They are tagged to be placed in a separate folder for the NCLEX® people to evaluate them according to how graduate nurses across the country are answering them, to see if there are problems with the questions or the answers. Many of the alternate items in the "select all that apply" category are difficult to write because all the correct responses have to apply all the time, and that means that every single variable has to be considered. So if you get 15 alternate items, remember that most of them are still experimental items!

8. Correct Answer: B. An escharotomy is performed only when circulation is compromised by restrictive eschar. The objective of creating an

opening through the eschar is to relieve the pressure and restore circulation. If nail beds blanch and refill promptly, blood is flowing into the limb.

Answer A: There is no pain with a third-degree (full-thickness) burn because nerve endings have been destroyed. Pain is ordinarily an indicator of ischemia to a limb because lactic acid builds up when the muscles undergo anaerobic metabolism, but in this instance absence of pain is not an indicator of circulation to a limb.

Answer C: No bleeding means no blood flow. We are looking for an indicator that blood is flowing into a limb. We expect some oozing blood from viable tissue if the incision is deep enough to relieve the pressure.

Answer D: I know what you are thinking: dead fingers can't wiggle! And you are correct; however, *dying* fingers can still move if the muscles and tendons are working. Movement (motor) is a neurologic check, and the right answer involves a circulatory (vascular) check!

9. **Correct Answer: A.** The doctor may want a culture of the burn exudates to determine the organism that has infected the burn wound, although if the greenish pigment points toward *Pseudomonas*, a C&S is still indicated because many pathogens are becoming resistant to antimicrobials.

Answer B: Don't ever put ointment on top of infectious material! The wound bed should be clean before any topical agent is applied.

Answer C: We are looking for the NEXT nursing action. We would not want to wash away the green slime before getting a sample of it for wound culture.

Answer D: Turnip greens will not leak out through a burn wound. Don't be silly!

10. **Correct Answer: D.** The "next" action means that you may be doing more than one of the things listed and you are supposed to decide what to do FIRST.

The priority here is that the autograft must be salvaged! It has to be protected between layers of sterile normal saline until the doctor can replace and/or realign the graft onto the wound bed. The integrity of the graft and the wound bed is damaged if drying occurs. Help the patient first, and then call the doctor.

Answer A: What kind of assistance are you calling for? You are supposed to know what to do. If supplies were needed, calling for assistance would be indicated because you cannot leave the patient to go get what you need. (He or she might be touching the graft or lifting it up to see what has happened.) Assume you have the supplies that you need if you are given the option to apply moist saline gauze.

Answer B: Calling the doctor is not the best answer because there is something that the nurse can do to save the graft; however, this answer will (eventually) get some help for the patient so your next question

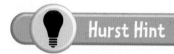

Hurst Hint

If there is something that the nurse can do to help the patient or prevent a predictable or potential problem, you always do that first and then call the doctor.

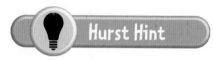

Hurst Hint

Never leave an unstable patient.

on the NCLEX® computer adaptive test (CAT) will be at the same level of difficulty.

Answer C: Rewrapping the dressing material over the dislodged graft will cause the graft to stick in a wrong position, so that when it is lifted, damage may occur to the graft and to fragile capillaries in the wound bed underneath. Besides this, if you lay the graft back down, you just became a plastic surgeon, and I don't think this is within your scope of practice!

INDEX